Advances in Pain Research and Therapy
Volume 7

RECENT ADVANCES IN THE MANAGEMENT OF PAIN

Advances in Pain Research and Therapy
Volume 7

Recent Advances in the Management of Pain

Editors

Costantino Benedetti, M.D.
Department of Anesthesiology
Multidisciplinary Pain Center
University of Washington
Seattle, Washington

C. Richard Chapman, Ph.D.
Department of Anesthesiology
Multidisciplinary Pain Center
University of Washington
Seattle, Washington

Guido Moricca, M.D.
National Cancer Institute
Regina Elena
Rome, Italy

Raven Press ■ New York

Raven Press, 1140 Avenue of the Americas, New York, New York 10036

Made in the United States of America

Library of Congress Cataloging in Publication Data
Main entry under title:

Recent advances in the management of pain.

(Advances in pain research and therapy; v. 7)
"Originated with the International Symposium on Recent Advances in the Management of Pain held in Palermo, Italy, to honor Dr. John J. Bonica"—Pref.
Includes bibliographies and index.
1. Pain—Treatment—Congresses. 2. Bonica, John J. (John Joseph), 1917–   . I. Benedetti, Costantino. II. Chapman, C. Richard. III. Moricca, Guido. IV. Bonica, John J. (John Joseph), 1971–
V. International Symposium on Recent Advances in the Management of Pain (1981: Palermo, Sicily) VI. Series.
[DNLM: 1. Pain—therapy—congresses. W1 AD706 v. 7 / WL 704 R295 1981]
RB127.R4 1984   616'.0472   84-15111
ISBN 0-88167-021-9

The material contained in this volume was submitted as previously unpublished material, except in the instances in which credit has been given to the source from which some of the illustrative material was derived.

Great care has been taken to maintain the accuracy of the information contained in the volume. However, Raven Press cannot be held responsible for errors or for any consequences arising from the use of the information contained herein.

Dedication

The authors and editors dedicate this volume to honor Professor John Joseph Bonica, whose lifetime commitment to the conquest of human pain and suffering has made this field a major area of inquiry in medical science, and who has spearheaded the dissemination of medical knowledge about painful states and their therapies. Dr. Bonica is Chairman Emeritus and Professor of the Department of Anesthesiology, and founder and Director Emeritus of the Multidisciplinary Pain Center of the University of Washington, Seattle, Washington.

Giovanni Giuseppe Bonica was born in Filicudi, Italy, in 1917 and came to the United States in 1928. He graduated from New York University in 1938 and in 1942 he received his M.D. Degree from Marquette University where he was an honor student. Dr. Bonica completed his internship and residency in anesthesiology at St. Vincent's Hospital in New York City, and in 1944 he was appointed Chief of Anesthesia and Operating Section of Madigan (Army) General Hospital, Fort Lewis, Washington. There he developed and managed a pain therapy service and, as a result of these experiences, Dr. Bonica initiated and practiced the far reaching concept of the multidisciplinary approach to pain research, diagnosis, and therapy. After his military service, he became Director of Anesthesia of Tacoma General and Pierce County Hospitals, Tacoma, Washington, where he put the multidisciplinary pain clinic concept into practice in a civilian private hospital.

In 1960, Dr. Bonica was appointed Chairman of the Department of Anesthesiology of the University of Washington, and a year later he established its Multidisciplinary Pain Clinic. For over two decades he worked to develop full cooperation and collaboration between clinicians and basic scientists concerned with pain. In 1980, the cooperative group he had formed was formally designated the University of Washington Multidisciplinary Pain Center. In 1973, he sponsored and organized the First International Symposium on Pain, during which the International Association for the Study of Pain was founded and the mechanisms for publishing the interdisciplinary journal *Pain* were set in motion.

Professor Bonica has published several hundred scientific articles, six comprehensive books including *Management of Pain, Clinical Applications of Diagnostic and Therapeutic Blocks,* and the 2-volume work, *Principles and Practice of Obstetric Analgesia and Anesthesia.* He has edited and has been a major contributor to many monographs including two on regional anesthesia and three on obstetric anesthesia and seven volumes on *Pain Research and Therapy* (1974–1980). Professor Bonica has been a Visiting Professor in medical centers in the United States and abroad. He has been President of the American Society of Anesthesiologists (ASA), the Association of University Anesthetists, the Association for Research in Nervous and Mental Disease, the World Federation of Societies of Anesthesiologists, and the International Association for the Study of Pain, and also Chairman of the Board of the American Pain Society.

Professor Bonica has received many awards and honors, including Alpha Omega Alpha from Marquette University, a Doctor of Medical Science (DMSc) degree from the University of Siena, Doctor of Science (DSc) degree from the Medical College of Wisconsin, Honorary Fellowship of the Faculty of Anaesthetists of the Royal College of Surgeons of England, and the Award for Distinguished Achievement of Modern Medicine. Dr. Bonica is also an honorary member of the Association of Anaesthetists of Great Britain and Ireland and many other anesthesia and medical societies. In 1973, he was knighted Grand Officer of the Order of Merit of Italy, the highest honor awarded to foreign nationals by the President of Italy. In 1978, the Eastern Pain Association established a lectureship in his honor and a year later the University of Washington established a Visiting Professorship. More recently, a lectureship to honor Dr. Bonica was established by the International Association for the Study of Pain and the Australasian Pain Society. These and many other honors attest to the fact that Dr. Bonica has done more for the field of pain research and therapy than anyone else.

On a personal level, the editors wish to acknowledge that John J. Bonica has been a compelling and inspiring force in each of our professional lives, and we are profoundly indebted to him. Those who have had the fortune to have him as a friend, as well as a teacher and colleague, know that he fulfills the strictest definition of such a relationship. Professor Bonica has been, and continues to be, a dramatic example of what dedication can achieve in life. It has been a privilege to work with this great man and share his goals.

Preface

This volume originated with the International Symposium on Recent Advances in the Management of Pain held in Palermo, Italy, sponsored by the Italian Association for the Study of Pain and the Italian League on Pain Control, to honor Dr. John J. Bonica. In addition to critically selecting a number of papers presented at the symposium, the editors invited a number of Dr. Bonica's friends who have expertise in specific areas to contribute to the volume.

The chapters in this volume present selected, state-of-the-art information dealing with the areas of research and clinical application of knowledge in the field of acute and chronic pain. The volume is divided into three major parts: basic considerations, therapeutic modalities, and a discussion on separate pain syndromes.

In preparing this volume, the editors have addressed both the clinician and the researcher. The clinician who treats patients suffering with acute or chronic pain will find the basic considerations stimulating and helpful for appreciation of the intricate mechanisms involved in pain perception. The sections on therapeutic modalities and individual pain syndromes should be useful guidelines in the treatment of patients with particular types of pain. For the researcher we hope this volume will stimulate further inquiry and investigation since large voids are still present in our current knowledge about pain. Advances in pain therapy can be accomplished only with increased understanding of the basic substrate of nociception: its generation, transmission, and final translation to perception at the cortical level.

In the section on basic considerations, the introductory chapter deals with the concept of pain in the Western world, followed by recent advances in the field of pain research and up-to-date concepts of the neural and biochemical mechanisms of pain and analgesia. Chapters on methods of measuring clinical pain, the peculiarity of pain in elderly patients, correlations of pain and depression, and the legal and social implications of chronic pain are also discussed in this section. In the section on therapeutic modalities, different interventions for pain are described including pharmacologic agents, psychologic techniques, regional anesthesia, neurosurgical ablative procedures, and other modalities. A number of pain problems frequently encountered in medical practice are described in the last section of this volume, and their management is discussed. There is a chapter on postoperative pain management, two chapters on headache, several chapters on pain of neurologic origin, musculoskeletal pain, visceral and vascular pain, and a section on cancer pain.

This volume will serve as a source book and guide for health care professionals concerned with understanding pain at the scientific level and the care of patients in pain at the clinical level. It is intended to promote the dissemination of new information and the generation of new ideas. Its theme serves to emphasize the responsibility of scientists and clinicians alike to continually work toward improving the care of patients in pain.

The Editors

Contents

Pain and Pain Syndromes

Postoperative Pain

Headache

Pain of Neurologic Origin

Musculoskeletal Pain

Visceral and Vascular Pain

Cancer Pain

Contributors

Steen Anderson
Clinical Pain Service
University of Washington
Seattle, Washington 98195

Gualtiero Bellucci
Chair of Anesthesiology
Policlinico
53100 Siena, Italy

Costantino Benedetti
Department of Anesthesiology, RN-10
University of Washington
Seattle, Washington 98195

John J. Bonica
Department of Anesthesiology, RN-10
University of Washington
Seattle, Washington 98195

Steven F. Brena
Emory University Pain Control
  Center
1441 Clifton Road N.E.
Atlanta, Georgia 30322

Stephen Butler
University of Washington School of
  Medicine
Seattle, Washington 98195

F. Cangi
Institute of Internal Medicine and
  Clinical Pharmacology
University of Florence
Via G. B. Morgagni 85
50134 Florence, Italy

Harold Carron
Department of Anesthesiology
University of Virginia Medical Center
Charlottesville, Virginia 22908

C. Richard Chapman
Multidisciplinary Pain Center
Department of Anesthesiology, RN-10
University of Washington
Seattle, Washington 98195

Stanley L. Chapman
Emory University Pain Control
  Center
1441 Clifton Road N.E.
Atlanta, Georgia 30322

C. Conti
Institute of Clinical Medicine V
University of Rome
Policlinico Umberto I
Rome, Italy

G. Cruccu
Institute of Clinical Neurology V
University of Rome
Policlinico Umberto I
Rome, Italy

N. Deshpande
Imperial Cancer Research Fund
Lincoln's Inn Fields
London WC2A 3PX, England

Robert P. Elde
Department of Anatomy
University of Minnesota
Minneapolis, Minnesota 55455

A. Fabbri
Institute of Clinical Medicine V
University of Rome
Policlinico Umberto I
Rome, Italy

M. Fanciullacci
Institute of Internal Medicine and
  Clinical Pharmacology
University of Florence
Via G. B. Morgagni 85
50134 Florence, Italy

Emilio Favale
University of Genoa
Neurological Clinic IIa
Via A. De Toni, 5
16132 Genoa, Italy

M. Felici
Hospital of St. Giuseppe
Marino, Rome, Italy

Theresa Ferrer-Brechner
Department of Anesthesiology
Oncology Pain Management
Jonsson Comprehensive Cancer
  Center
University of California
Los Angeles, California 90024

F. Fraioli
Institute of Clinical Medicine V
University of Rome
Policlinico Umberto I
Rome, Italy

Giancarlo Gianasi
Service of Anesthesia and Intensive
  Therapy
Section of Analgesia
Bellaria Hospital
Via Altura, 3
Bologna, Italy

L. Gnessi
Institute of Clinical Medicine V
University of Rome
Policlinico Umberto I
Rome, Italy

Vay L. W. Go
Department of Gastroenterology
Mayo Clinic
Rochester, Minnesota 55905

Dieter Gross
Niederraeder Landstrasse 58
D-6000 Frankfurt
  am Main 71, Federal Republic
  of Germany

Lawrence M. Halpern
Department of Pharmacology, SJ-30
University of Washington
Seattle, Washington 98195

S. W. Harkins
Department of Gerontology
Medical College of Virginia
Virginia Commonwealth University
Box 228, MCV Station
Richmond, Virginia 23298

Gail J. Harty
Departments of Neurosurgery and
  Pharmacology
Mayo Clinic
Rochester, Minnesota 55905

James R. Howe
Departments of Neurosurgery and
  Pharmacology
Mayo Clinic
Rochester, Minnesota 55905

M. Inghilleri
Institute of Clinical Neurology V
University of Rome
Policlinico Umberto I
Rome, Italy

S. Ischia
Institute of Anesthesiology and
  Intensive Care
University of Padova of Verona
Verona Annex
37134 Verona, Italy

Louis Jacobson
University of Washington
Department of Anesthesiology, RN-10
Seattle, Washington 98195

Joseph Kwentus
Department of Psychiatry
Medical College of Virginia
Virginia Commonwealth University
Box 228, MCV Station
Richmond, Virginia 23298

Massimo Leandri
University of Genoa
Neurological Clinic IIa
Via A. De Toni, 5
16132 Genoa, Italy

Allan B. Levin
Department of Neurosurgery
University of Wisconsin Clinical
  Science Center
600 Highland Avenue
Madison, Wisconsin 53792

James W. Lewis
Department of Psychology
University of California
Los Angeles, California 90024

John C. Liebeskind
Department of Psychology
University of California
Los Angeles, California 90024

Ulf Lindblom
Department of Neurology
Karolinska Hospital
Box 60500
S-104 01 Stockholm, Sweden

A. Luzzani
Institute of Anesthesiology and
  Intensive Care
University of Padova of Verona
Verona Annex
37134 Verona, Italy

Jose L. Madrid
Department of Anesthesiology and
  Pain Clinic
City Hospital "1ˢᵗ October"
Madrid, Spain

G. F. Maffezzoli
Institute of Anesthesiology and
  Intensive Care
University of Padova of Verona
Verona Annex
37134 Verona, Italy

M. Manfredi
Institute of Clinical Neurology V
University of Rome
Policlinico Umberto I
Rome, Italy

Marco Maresca
Pain Center
Institute of Clinical Medicine and
  Therapy
University of Florence
Via G. B. Morgagni 85
50134 Florence, Italy

G. Mazzetti
Department of Orthopedics
Regional Hospital
36100 Vicenza, Italy

Paul E. Micevych
Department of Neurosurgery
Mayo Clinic
Rochester, Minnesota 55905

Daniel C. Moore
Department of Anesthesiology
University of Washington
Seattle, Washington 98195

C. Moretti
Institute of Clinical Medicine V
University of Rome
Policlinico Umberto I
Rome, Italy

Terence M. Murphy
Clinical Pain Service
University of Washington
Seattle, Washington 98195

Giovanni Nattero
Headache Center
Institute of Internal Medicine
Turin University
Via Genova, 3
10126 Turin, Italy

Giuseppe Nuzzaci
Department of Cardiovascular
  Diseases
Institute of Clinical Medicine
University of Florence
Via G. B. Morgagni 85
50134 Florence, Italy

L. Pacini
Institute of Anesthesiology and
  Intensive Care
University of Padova of Verona
Verona Annex
37134 Verona, Italy

Carlo Alberto Pagni
2nd Chair of Neurosurgery and Aldo
  Pasetti
Center for Pain Research and
  Therapy
University of Turin
10126 Turin, Italy

Vittorio Pasqualucci
Second Department of
  Anesthesiology and Pain Therapy
Ospedale Policlinico
06100 Perugia, Italy

U. Pietrini
Institute of Internal Medicine and
  Clinical Pharmacology
University of Florence
Via G. B. Morgagni 85
50134 Florence, Italy

Donald D. Price
Department of Anesthesiology
Medical College of Virginia
Virginia Commonwealth University
Box 228, MCV Station
Richmond, Virginia 23298

Paolo Procacci
Pain Center
Institute of Clinical Medicine and
  Therapy
University of Florence
Via G. B. Morgagni 85
50134 Florence, Italy

Lincoln L. Ramirez
Department of Neurosurgery
University of Wisconsin Clinical
  Science Center
600 Highland Avenue
Madison, Wisconsin 53792

R. Rizzi
Department of Anesthesiology
Intensive Care and Pain Relief
Regional Hospital
I-36100 Vicenza, Italy

Joan M. Romano
Pain Center
Department of Psychiatry and
  Behavioral Sciences, RP-10
University of Washington
Seattle, Washington 98195

F. Sicuteri
Institute of Internal Medicine and
  Clinical Pharmacology
University of Florence
Via G. B. Morgagni 85
50134 Florence, Italy

Anders E. Sola
Department of Anesthesiology and
  Pain Service
University of Washington Medical
  School
120 Northgate Plaza, Rm 340
Seattle, Washington 98125

Richard A. Sternbach
Scripps Clinic and Research
  Foundation
La Jolla, California 92037

Karen L. Syrjala
Multidisciplinary Pain Center
Department of Anesthesiology, RN-10
University of Washington
Seattle, Washington 98195

Gregory W. Terman
Department of Psychology
University of California
Los Angeles, California 90024

Judith A. Turner
Pain Center
Department of Psychiatry and
  Behavioral Science, RP-10
Department of Rehabilitation
  Medicine
University of Washington
Seattle, Washington 98195

V. Ventafridda
Division of Pain Therapy
National Cancer Institute
Via Venezian, 1
20133 Milan, Italy

M. Visentin
Department of Anesthesiology
Intensive Care and Pain Relief
Regional Hospital
36100 Vicenza, Italy

P. D. Wall
Department of Anatomy
Cerebral Functions Group
University College London
Gower Street
London WC1E 6BT, England

Tony L. Yaksh
Department of Neurosurgery
Mayo Clinic
Rochester, Minnesota 55905

Massimo Zoppi
Department of Rheumatology
Institute of Clinical Medicine
University of Florence
Via G. B. Morgagni 85
50134 Florence, Italy

RECENT ADVANCES IN THE MANAGEMENT OF PAIN

*Advances in Pain Research
and Therapy, Vol. 7,*
edited by C. Benedetti et al.
Raven Press, New York © 1984.

Pain Concept in Western Civilization: A Historical Review

Paolo Procacci and Marco Maresca

*Pain Center, Institute of Medical Clinic and Therapy,
University of Florence, 50134 Florence, Italy*

Bonica (11–13) and Keele (36), among others (19,52), have emphasized that pain has been a major concern of humankind since its beginning and the subject of ubiquitous efforts to understand and control it. It is likely that pain relief was the primary reason for the advent of the Shaman, healer, and later the physician; even today it remains one of the most important raison d'être of all health professionals. Both rational and superstitious means have been used from prehistoric time to the present. In this chapter, we will discuss the concept of pain in the Mediterranean region, and subsequently among Western civilizations. The concept of pain in Eastern civilization is not considered because, in our opinion, it is necessary to have knowledge of Eastern languages (53).

PRIMITIVE CIVILIZATIONS

Prehistoric people had no difficulty in understanding pain associated with injury, but they were mystified by pain caused by disease. Such pain was linked with an intrusion into the human body of magic fluids, objects, or demons. It was believed that arrows, swords, and spears were objects that allowed the magic fluid or demon to enter the body, and produce spontaneous pain (11,13,16,36,52). To treat the pain, the Shaman or sorcerer made small wounds in the patient to allow the bad fluid, or spirit, to escape. Among some prehistoric tribes, the Shaman sucked the spirit directly from the wound, taking it into himself, and neutralizing it with magic power—a therapy that still survives in some countries.

The concept of intrusion of the body as a cause of pain remained, with some variation, in the two great Mediterranean civilizations, the ancient Egyptians, and the Assyro-Babylonians (13,16,36). We can read in the Ebers (23) and Berlin papyri (58) that the routes of departure of the intruding demons could be vomit, urine, the sneeze of the nose, or the sweat of the limbs. It was in these civilizations that the question arose of where the center of sensation (the *sensorium commune*) was localized. According to the Egyptians, a widely distributed network of vessels called "metu" carried the breath of life and sensations to the heart (36). This was the beginning of the concept that the heart was the center of the *sensorium commune*, an idea that lasted more than two thousand years. This concept is also common in the Indo-European languages where we find such expressions as "hard heart," "a man without heart," and "my heart says to me."

In the Assyro-Babylonian and Hebraic civilizations there was a typical evolution from the concept of demons to the concept of sin, with the typical relationship of sin-punishment (10,16,35). This relationship, pain-sin-punishment is particularly important because it was largely adopted in the Christian ethic and is the fundamental significance of the word "pain" in English, derived from the Latin word *poena* meaning punishment.

ANCIENT GREECE

The ancient Greeks were intensely interested in the nature of sensory data, and the sense organs of the body found a prominent place in their physiologic speculations (11,16,36). Pythagoras (566–497 B.C.), the first great Greek thinker who traveled widely to Egypt, Babylon, and India, and finally settled in Croton in Southern Italy, apparently stimulated his disciple Alcmaeon to carry out intensive studies of the senses (26). Alcmaeon, without apparent precedent, produced the idea that the brain, not the heart, was the center for sensation and reason. Anaxagoras (500–428 B.C.) (2) held the view that all sensation, indeed all life, contained its element of pain, the perception of which was located in the brain. Despite the support of Anaxagoras and also of Democritus and others, Alcmaeon's view did not gain widespread acceptance due, in part, to the opposition of Empedocles and, above all, Aristotle. According to Empedocles (24), the capacity for all sensations, especially pain and pleasure, was located in the heart's blood.

It is not easy to interpret the thought of Hippocrates (34) because the *Corpus Hippocraticum* was written by different authors at different times (47). The main importance was the theory of the four humours: blood, phlegm, yellow bile, and black bile. Pain was felt when one of these humours was in defect or excess (*dyscrasia*). The brain was considered a gland, the center of thought and perhaps of sensations.

For the history of the concept of pain, the theories on sensations of Plato and Aristotle are important because they remained a fundamental part of the teaching in medical school during the Renaissance and, in part, until the present time. Plato's concepts on sensations were mostly exposed in *Timaeus* (50). According to Plato, the heart and liver were the center for appreciation of all sensations. The function of the brain in sensory processes was not clearly described: this organ was considered mainly active in elaborating the concepts derived from the sensations. The relationship between pain and pleasure was considered. Plato observed that pleasure often derived from pain relief. In the dialogue *Phaedo* (49), this concept is exposed by Socrates: when the chain has been taken off of his leg, Socrates observes that the disappearance of pain induced pleasure; Plato therefore deduced that pain and pleasure, although opposite sensations, are linked together, as originating from the same head (49).

Plato's concepts on sensations were further developed by Aristotle (384–322 B.C.), mainly in *De Anima* (3) and in *Ethica Nicomachea* (4). Aristotle distinguished five senses: vision, hearing, taste, smell, and touch. According to Aristotle, the brain had no direct function in the sensory processes; the *sensorium commune*, center of sensory perception, was located in the heart, according to the concepts of the Egyptians and of other ancient civilizations. The heart was considered by Aristotle as the most important organ of the body, i.e., as the center of all the fundamental life functions and as the location of the soul. For Aristotle, the function of the brain was to produce cool secretions that cooled the hot air and blood arising from the heart. Pain sensations were considered a result of an increased sensitivity of every sensation, especially touch. This concept was stressed in *De Anima* (3), where Aristotle said that "sensations are pleasant when their sensible extremes such as acid and sweet are brought into their proper ratio, whilst in excess they are painful and destructive." Aristotle's work had a great influence on science in the Middle Ages, during the Renaissance, and until recent times.

Soon after Aristotle's death, his direct successor, Theophrastus (372–287 B.C.), cast serious doubt about his master's views. Stratton, who succeeded Theophrastus, propounded the view that the center of sensation, including pain, was in the brain (13,36). Later, Herophilus (335–280 B.C.) and Erasistratus (310–250 B.C.) of Alexandria provided anatomic evidence that the brain was part of the nervous system and nerves attached to the neuraxis were of two kinds: those for movement and those for feeling (13,36).

ANCIENT ROME

Among the Roman writers, it is important to note that Celsus (17) considered pain in relation to the phenomenon of inflammation. Pain was mentioned as one of the typical symptoms of inflammation (along with redness, swelling, and heat) in the famous definition of Celsus, which remains one of the best examples of an accurate observation of natural phenomena. Although Celsus recognized the concept of Herophilus and Erasistratus regarding pain, particularly that of internal disease, he failed to mention the concept about the brain, the spinal cord, and motor and sensory nerves. For nearly four centuries, the work of the Egyptians was lost to the Roman World, until rescued by Galen (130–201 A.D.) (27,36).

Galen, who had studied in Greece and Alexandria, settled in Rome and became court physician to Marcus Aurelius. He carried out extensive studies on sensory physiology and reestablished the importance of the central and peripheral nervous system (27). He clearly established the anatomy of the cranial and spinal nerves and the sympathetic trunks. On the basis of experiments of nerve and discrete section of the spinal cord on newborn pigs, Galen elaborated a complex theory of sensation. He classified nerves as "soft," concerned with sensory functions, as "hard," concerned with motor function, and a third type related to the lowest form of sensibility, i.e., pain sensation. Soft nerves contained invisible tubular cavities in which a "psychic pneuma" flowed and which, according to Galen, served different senses: every organ had a nerve supply suited to its physiologic function. The largest nerves subserved the special senses. The center of sensibility was the brain, which was softer than any nerve and received all kinds of sensations. Despite Galen's great contribution on the function of the nervous system in sensation, the Aristotelian concept of the five senses and of pain as a "passion of the soul" felt in the heart, prevailed for 23 centuries.

After Galen, it is important to consider the writers of the third and fourth centuries because they often summarized ideas expressed by ancient authors whose works are lost. Two of these writers, Nemesius and Caelius Aurelianus, are noteworthy for their concept of pain. Nemesius (36) first considered the cerebral ventricles as the center for sensory perception; this concept was accepted by many authors during the Middle Ages and the Renaissance. Caelius Aurelianus (15) used for the first time the term *passio cardiaca propria* for pain of the heart. This is an important point because it was not until the latter part of the eighteenth century that Heberden called pain in the heart *angina pectoris* and *dolor pectoris* (32).

THE MIDDLE AGES

In the Middle Ages, during the Renaissance, and up to the time of Heberden, it is not easy to trace the concept of pain because many words were used: *dolor*, *spasmus*, and *angor* or *angina*. Heberden in the Commentarii (33) told that an old British physician said to him that angina pectoris was well known as a typical attack of chest pain, but with another name. Unfortunately, Heberden did not give that name.

In the Middle Ages the philosophy of Aristotle dominated, but the concept of the sensory heart was not accepted by all scientists. During this period the center of medicine shifted to Arabia where Avicenna (980–1038 A.D.) (5) quantified all available knowledge and distinguished five "external" senses and five "internal" senses. He located the internal senses in the cerebral ventricles. Avicenna was especially interested in pain and described the etiology and mechanism of 15 different types of pain due to different kinds of humoral changes.

In Europe during the Middle Ages the shift of the center of sensory perception from the heart to the brain began with the work of Albertus Magnus (1), who located the *sensorium commune* in the anterior cerebral ventricle.

According to the *Anathomia* of Mondino (43), which remained as a fundamental text for over 200 years in many medical schools, the brain was not
only the site of sensations, but also had the power to cool the heart. It is
apparent that in this book Mondino presents an overlapping of Aristotelian
and Galenic thought.

THE RENAISSANCE

The Renaissance fostered a great scientific spirit to encourage many remarkable advances in chemistry, physics, physiology, and anatomy, but
especially the anatomy of the nervous system. During this period, Plato's
and Aristotle's works were studied with particular interest in the Greek
originals and not in Arabian translations. Comments were made especially
by Marsilio Ficino, Pico della Mirandola, and the other members of the
famous *Academia Platonica* founded in Florence by Lorenzo the Magnifi-
cent. A great scientist and artist of the Renaissance, Leonardo da Vinci,
represented the relationship of pain and pleasure in a famous drawing (39).
Leonardo's concept was very similar to the one exposed by Plato in *Phaedo*:
pleasure and pain were represented as a man with two faces to indicate that
they were strictly linked together. Leonardo's concepts on sensory processes were clearly illustrated in Windsor manuscripts on anatomy (38).
According to Leonardo, nerves had a tubular structure and pain sensibility
was strictly related to touch sensibility. The *sensorium commune* was located in the third ventricle of the brain and he considered the spinal cord
as a conductor that transmitted sensations to the brain.

During the sixteenth century, other scientists, including Vesalius (54) and
Varolius (36), followed Leonardo's concept on the anatomy and physiology
of sensations. In their works the brain was considered the center of sensation; the nerves were generally considered as tubular structures. Despite
the evidence presented on the role of the brain in sensation up to that time,
the Aristotelian concept still prevailed. Thus William Harvey, who in 1628
discovered circulation, still believed that the heart was the site where pain
was felt (36).

In contrast, Descartes (1596–1650 A.D.), Harvey's contemporary, adhered
to Galenic physiology and considered the brain the seat of sensation and
motor function. In his book, *L'Homme* (Man), published in 1664 (14 years
after his death), Descartes described the results of his extensive anatomic
studies, including sensory physiology (22). He considered nerves as tubes
in which there was a sort of marrow composed of fine threads that started
from the proper substance of the brain and ended in the skin or other tissues.
Sensory stimuli were transmitted to the brain by means of these threads.
The sensations became conscious in the pineal gland where the *res cogitans*
and the *res extensa* were connected. The nervous pathways of heat and pain,
from the periphery to the pineal gland, were depicted by Descartes in a

famous figure of a boy with his foot near a fire which stimulated the skin of the foot and thus pulled on "delicate threads" in the nerves that were connected to the pineal gland in the brain.

We must remember, however, that up to the eighteenth century the main textbooks of medicine contained the works of Hippocrates and Aristotle. Consequently, the idea of the heart as the *sensorium commune* remained parallel to the theory that considered the brain the center of sensory perception. Erasmus Darwin (20), grandfather of Charles Darwin, followed the Aristotelian idea regarding pain as a phase of unpleasantness and said that pain resulted "whenever the sensorial motions are stronger than usual. . . . A great excess of light . . . of pressure or distention . . . of heat . . . of cold produces pain." He thus anticipated the intensive pain theory that was introduced several decades later.

THE NINETEENTH CENTURY

The scientific study of sensation in general, and pain in particular, in the modern sense began in the first half of the nineteenth century when physiology emerged as an experimental science. This era was initiated in part by the publications of Bell in 1811–1827 (6,7) and later those of Magendie (41), who demonstrated with animal experiments that the function of the dorsal roots of spinal nerves is sensory and that of the ventral roots is motor. The impetus to the scientific study of pain was further enhanced by the writings of Weber and of Müller. In contrast to the older concepts, Weber (56) distinguished between touch and pain by classifying touch as a sense of the skin and pain as *Gemeingefühl*, an expression denoting common sensitivity possessed by skin and the internal organs. In 1826, Müller (44) proposed his "Doctrine of Specific Nerve Energies," which was later amplified (45). This doctrine stated that the brain received information on external objects and body structures only by way of sensory nerves and the sensory nerves for each of the five senses carried a particular form of specific energy for each sensation. Müller's concept then was that of a straight-through system from the sensory organ to the brain center responsible for the sensation. He considered pain as due to the excitation of specific sensory receptors and nervous paths as did Galen over 1600 years before. Müller's ideas were widely accepted because of their simplicity. During the ensuing half century, anatomic, physiologic, and histologic studies were done that eventually prompted the formulation of two physiologic theories of pain: the specificity theory and the intensive theory.

The *specificity (or sensory) theory* stated that pain was a specific sensation with its own sensory apparatus independent of touch and other senses. This theory was formulated by Schiff (51) in 1858 following his analgesic experiments in animals. Noting the effects of various incisions in the spinal cord, he found pain and touch were independent. Section of the gray matter of the spinal cord eliminated pain but not touch, and a cut through the white matter caused loss of touch but pain was unaffected. The results of these vivisections were promptly corroborated by clinical evidence as a number of clinicians reported pathologic cases of disease or injured spinal cords with similar sensory defects (for references, see 13). The theory was reaffirmed by evidence examined during the ensuing decade by others, including Blix (9) and Goldscheider (28), who discovered separate spots for warmth, cold, and touch in the skin. A decade later von Frey (55) extended these studies to map out pain and touch spots. He also did histologic examinations of the skin, intending to identify specific end organs responsible for each sensation.

Definite relationships between morphology and function were proposed: (a) Meissner's corpuscles and Merkel's disks and basket endings were considered the specific receptors of touch; (b) Krause's end bulbs were considered the receptors of cold; (c) Ruffini's corpuscles were considered specific for warmth; and (d) free nerve endings were assumed to be the pain receptors. On the basis of his findings and imaginative deductions, von Frey expanded Muller's concept of the sense of touch to four major cutaneous modalities: touch, warmth, cold, and pain. Von Frey's theory, which dealt only with receptors, prompted others to believe that pain was subserved by specific fibers from the receptors to the spinal cord and specific pathways in the neuraxis (13).

The *intensive theory*, suggested by Weber and others in Germany, was explicitly formulated by Erb (25) in 1874, who maintained that every sensory stimulus was capable of producing pain if it reached sufficient intensity. This theory received subsequent support from others, including Blix and Goldscheider. His studies in 1884 lead Blix (9) to believe that pain was a specific sensation, but afterwards he discarded this view (10). Goldscheider also shifted views: at first he did not believe that pain was specific, but by 1885, just as Blix was shifting in the other direction, Goldscheider (29) concluded that the evidence favored specificity. He held this view until 1891, when he shifted once more because of the results obtained by Naunyn (46) 2 years earlier, which led the latter to conclude that pain was the result of summation. In 1894 Goldscheider (30) developed the theory that stimulus intensity and central summation were the critical determinants of pain.

By the end of the nineteenth century there existed three conflicting concepts on the nature of pain. The specificity theory and the intensive theory, which were in opposition to each other, were embraced by physiologists and a few psychologists. These two theories opposed the traditional Aristotelian concept that pain was an affective quality, which at the time was supported by most philosophers and psychologists.

PRESENT CENTURY

During the present century, research on pain has continued and the published data acquired were used to support either the specificity theory, the

intensive theory, or a modification of these. The intense controversy between von Frey and Goldscheider continued until the late 1920s and each
rallied supporters (13). Experiments in peripheral nerves were carried out
to show there was a one-to-one relation between receptive type, fiber size,
and quality of experience. Other animal experiences suggested the anterolateral quadrant of the spinal cord was critically important for pain sensation,
a concept reinforced by Spiller's observation of analgesia with pathologic
lesions of this part of the cord (11) and early results of anterolateral cordotomy by Spiller and Martin (11) and many others subsequently. All of
these tended to support the specificity theory.

Weddell and his co-workers (37,57) of the Anatomical School of Oxford
University, on the basis of experimental studies, strongly criticized the concept of receptive specificity. After a careful sensory examination of a given
skin area, a biopsy was performed and a histologic examination of the excised skin carried out. The results did not confirm the strict relationships
that had been proposed between morphology and function of sensory receptors. Moreover, some nervous endings were found that had an intermediate aspect between the known forms of receptors. Some receptors were
identified that had the same function but a different aspect in hairy skin and
in glabrous skin (57). Analysis of their data prompted Lele et al. (37) to
propose the "pattern theory" as an alternative to the theory of receptor
specificity. According to this theory, there are no specific cutaneous receptors for the different sensory modalities, but different stimuli provoke the
excitation of nonspecific receptors according to different spatio-temporal
patterns of activation. The different spatio-temporal patterns induce the
onset of various sensations in the central nervous system.

The theory proposed by Weddell and his co-workers was accepted by
many (31), especially neurologists and neurosurgeons who found it suitable
to interpret complex clinical conditions such as postherpetic neuralgia, causalgia, and central pain. In these conditions, it is difficult to explain the pain
mechanisms based on the specificity of receptors and nervous pathways;
pain can be better explained as resulting from a modification of spatio-temporal patterns of excitation. On the other hand, Weddell's theory was not
accepted by many neurophysiologists who proved the existence of some
receptors and nervous fibers with a high specificity for some types of stimuli
(35,60). Other experimental studies suggested a relative specificity ("double
specificity") of some receptors and the concept of modulation of end organs,
which seems to mediate the two opposing theories (21,40).

CURRENT STATUS

The question is still open and being debated. At the periphery in the skin
there are high threshold end organs that can be considered nociceptors (8,14).
It is important to point out, however, that no receptors with similar char-

acteristics have been identified in the viscera (18,42). In our opinion, we accept the concept that in some parts of the body there are receptors that are selectively or mainly excited by noxious stimuli. Regarding the polymodal receptors, it must be noted that these receptors probably cannot give rise to the quality of pain (e.g., pricking, burning). This is clear in some pathologic conditions where only C fibers can be activated and the pain does not have a well-defined quality, but is diffuse and unpleasant.

We can say that neither the electrophysiologic approach nor the biochemical research solved the problem of "physical" pain. Electrophysiologic studies have demonstrated that many paths and centers are excited during pain sensation, but the relative importance of definite paths and centers is still a question of debate. On the other hand, the extensive experimental studies on neurotransmitters, neuromodulators, and opioid peptides have not yet defined their role in pain (48,59). It is highly probable that many substances (e.g., acetylcholine, noradrenaline, 5-hydroxytryptamine, peptides) are involved in the integration of pain.

In conclusion, our knowledge has greatly increased in recent years, but the main problems are still a matter of debate as they were in Aristotle's and Galen's works. As has been repeatedly emphasized by Bonica (13), to settle these issues and many other aspects of pain, more research needs to be done, not only on experimental animals, but on humans with pathologic pain (12,13).

REFERENCES

1. Alberti Magni opera omnia, curavit Institutum Alberti Magni Coloniense, Bernhardo Geyer praeside. Monasterii Westfalorum, in aedibus Aschendorff, 1951.
2. Anaxagorae Clazomenii fragmenta quae supersunt, omnia, collecta commentarioque illustrata ab Eduardo Schaubach. Lipsiae, sumptibus Hartmanni, 1827.
3. Aristotelis de anima libri tres. Ad interpretum Graecorum auctoritatem et codicum fidem recognovit commentariis illustravit Frider. Adolph. Trendelenburg. Berolini, sumptibus W. Weberi, 1877.
4. Aristotelis Ethica Nichomachea. Edidit et commentario continuo instruxit G. Ramsauer. Lipsiae, in aedibus B. G. Teubneri, 1878.
5. Avicenna (Ibn Sina) (1562): Liber canonis. Venetiis, apud Juntas.
6. Bell, C. (1811): *Idea of a New Anatomy of the Brain Submitted for the Observations of his Friends*. Strahan and Preston, London.
7. Bell, J., and Bell, C. (1827): *The Anatomy and Physiology of the Human Body, 5th Am. ed.* Collins, New York.
8. Bessou, P., and Perl, E. R. (1969): Response of cutaneous sensory units with unmyelinated fibers to noxious stimuli. *J. Neurophysiol.*, 32:1025–1043.
9. Blix, M. (1884): Experimentelle Beitrag zur Losung der Frage uber die specifische Energie der Hautnerven. *Z. Biol.*, 20:141.
10. Blix, M. (1885): Experimentelle Beitrag zur Losung der Frage uber die specifische Energie der Hautnerven. *Z. Biol.*, 21:160.
11. Bonica, J. J. (1953): *Management of Pain*. Lea & Febiger, Philadelphia.
12. Bonica, J. J. (1977): Introduction. In: *Facial Pain, 2nd ed.*, edited by C. C. Alling. Lea & Febiger, Philadelphia.
13. Bonica, J. J. (1979): Introduction. In: *Pain*, edited by J. J. Bonica, pp. 1–17; 381–387. Raven Press, New York.

14. Burgess, P. R., and Perl, E. R. (1967): Myelinated afferent fibres responding specifically to noxious stimulation of the skin. *J. Physiol. (Lond.)*, 190:541–562.
15. Caelius Aurelianus (1722): *De morbis acutis*. Ed. Wetsteniana, Amsterdam.
16. Castiglioni, A. (1947): *A History of Medicine*. Knopf, New York.
17. Celsus, Aulus Cornelius (1891): De medicina libri octo. Ad fidem optimorum librorum denuo recensuit, adnotatione critica indicibusque instruxit C. Daremberg. Lipsiae, in aedibus B. G. Teubneri.
18. Cervero, F. (1980): Deep and visceral pain. In: *Pain and Society*, edited by H. W. Kosterlitz and L. Y. Terenius, pp. 263–281. Verlag Chemie, Weinheim.
19. Dallenbach, K. M. (1939): Pain: History and present status. *Am. J. Psychol.*, 52:331–347.
20. Darwin, E. (1794): *Zoonomia, or the Laws of Organic Life*. J. Johnson, London, Sec. 14, pp. 76–90.
21. Davis, H. (1961): Some principles of sensory receptor action. *Physiol. Rev.*, 41:391–416.
22. Descartes, R. (1664): *L'homme*. Angot, Paris.
23. Ebers, Papyros. (1875): *Das hermetische Buch uber die Arzneimittel der alten Aegypter von Georg Ebers*. Engelmann, Leipzig.
24. Empedoclis agrigentini fragmenta disposuit recensuit adnotavit Henricus Stein. Bonnae, apud Adolphum Marcum, 1852.
25. Erb, W. H. (1874): Krankheiten der peripherischen cerebrospinalen Nerven. (Quoted from G. W. A. Luckey, Some recent studies of pain.) *Am. J. Psychol.*, 7:109.
26. Freeman, K. (1948): *Ancilla to the Pre-Socratic Philosophers*. Blackwell, Oxford.
27. Galeni opera (1597): Venetiis, apud Juntas, 1597.
28. Goldscheider, A. (1884): Die spezifische Energie der Gefuhlsnerven der Haut. *Monatsschr. Prakt. Dermatol.*, 3:282.
29. Goldscheider, A. (1885): Neue Tatsachen uber die Hautsinnesnerven. *Arch. Anat. Physiol.*, (Physiol. Abth. Suppl. Bd.) 1–110 (Gesammelte Abhandlungen 1, 1989, 197).
30. Goldscheider, A. (1894): *Ueber den Schmerz in Physiologischer und Klinischer Hinsicht*. Hirschwald, Berlin.
31. Gooddy, W. (1957): On the nature of pain. *Brain*, 80:118–131.
32. Heberden, W. (1772): Some account of a disorder of the breast. *Med. Trans. R. Coll. Physic* [*Lond.*], 2:59.
33. Heberden, W. (1802): *Commentaries on the History and Cure of Disease*. Wells and Lilly, Boston.
34. Hippocratis medicorum omnium facile principis opera omnia quae extant. Chouet, Geneva, 1657.
35. Iggo, A. (1965): The peripheral mechanisms of cutaneous sensation. In: *Studies in Physiology*, edited by D. R. Curtis and A. K. McIntyre, pp. 92–100. Springer, Berlin.
36. Keele, K. D. (1957): *Anatomies of Pain*. Blackwell, Oxford.
37. Lele, P. P., Weddell, G., and Williams, C. (1954): The relationship between heat transfer, skin temperature and cutaneous sensibility. *J. Physiol. (Lond.)*, 126:206–234.
38. Leonardo da Vinci: Corpus of the anatomical studies in the collection of Her Majesty the Queen at Windsor Castle. By K. D. Keele and C. Pedretti. Johnson Reprint Company, H. B. Jovanovich, London, 1978–1980.
39. Leonardo da Vinci (1981): *Il codice di Leonardo da Vinci nella biblioteca del principe Trivulzio in Milano* (Trascritto ed annotato da Luca Beltrami.) Fratelli Dumolard, Milano.
40. Livingston, R. B. (1959): Central control of receptors and sensory transmission systems. In: *Handbook of Physiology: Neurophysiology, Vol. 1*, edited by J. Field, H. W. Magoun, and V. E. Hall. American Physiological Society, Washington.
41. Magendie, F. (1822): Experiences sur les fonctions des racines des nerfs rachidiens. *J. Physiol. Exp.* 2:276–279.
42. Malliani, A. (1982): Cardiovascular sympathetic afferent fibers. *Rev. Physiol. Biochem. Pharmacol.*, 94:11–74.
43. Mondino de' Liucci (1538): Anathomia. Venetiis, in officina D. Bernardini.
44. Müller, J. (1826): *Zur vergleichenden Physiologie des Gesichtssinnes des Menschen und der Thiere nebst einem Versuch uber die Bewegungen der Augen und uber den Menschlichen Blick*, pp. 32, 462. Cnobloch, Leipzig.
45. Müller, J. (1840): *Handbuch der Physiologie des Menschen fur Vorlesungen*. Hollscher, Koblenz.
46. Naunyn, B. (1889): Ueber Die Auslosung von Schmerzempfindung durch Summation sich zeitlich folgender sensibler Erregungen. *Arch. Exp. Pathol. Pharm.* 25:272–305.

47. Pascucci, G. (1948): *Storia Della Letteratura Greca*. Sansoni, Firenze.
48. Pepeu, G., and Marconcini Pepeu, I. (1982): La terapia farmacologica del dolore. In: *Fisiopatologia e terapia medica del dolore*, edited by U. Teodori, M. Maresca, C. A. Pagni, G. Pepeu, P. Procacci, and M. Zoppi, pp. 63–80. Pozzi, Roma.
49. Plato (1885): *Phaedo* (Edited with introduction and notes by W. D. Geddes.) Macmillan, London.
50. Plato (1888): *Timaeus*. (Edited with introduction and notes by R. D. Archer-Hind.) Macmillan, London.
51. Schiff, M. (1848): *Lehrbuch der Physiologie, Muskel, und Nervenphysiologie*, pp. 1, 228. Lahr, Schavenburg.
52. Tainter, M. L. (1948): Pain. *Ann. NY Acad. Sci.* 51:3.
53. Tu, W. (1980): A religiophilosophical perspective on pain. In: *Pain and Society*, edited by H. W. Kosterlitz and L. Y. Terenius. Verlag Chemie, Weinheim.
54. Vesalius, A. (1543): *De humani corporis fabrica*. Oporinus, Basileae.
55. Von Frey, M. (1894): Beitrage zur Physiologie des Schmerzsinnes. *Ber Verhandl konig Suchs Ges Wiss Leipzig*, 46:185–196, 288–296.
56. Weber, E. H. (1846): Der Tastsinn und das Gemeingefuhl. In: *Handworterbuch der Physiologie, Vol. 3*, edited by R. Wagner, pp. 481–588. Vieweg, Braunschweig.
57. Weddell, G., and Miller, S. (1962): Cutaneous sensibility. *Annu. Rev. Physiol.*, 24:199–222.
58. Wreszinski, W. (1909): *Der grosse medizinische Papyrus des Berliner Museums*. Hinrichs, Leipzig.
59. Zimmerman, M. (1979): Peripheral and central nervous mechanisms of nociception, pain and pain therapy: Facts and hypotheses. In: *Advances in Pain Research and Therapy, Vol. 3*, edited by J. J. Bonica, J. C. Liebeskind, and D. G. Albe-Fessard, pp. 3–32. Raven Press, New York.
60. Zotterman, Y. (1962): Nerve fibres mediating pain: A brief review with a discussion on the specificity of cutaneous afferent nerve fibres. In: *The Assessment of Pain in Man and Animals*, edited by C. A. Keele and R. Smith, pp. 60–73. Livingstone, Edinburgh.

*Advances in Pain Research
and Therapy, Vol. 7,*
edited by C. Benedetti et al.
Raven Press, New York © 1984.

Neurophysiology of Acute and Chronic Pain

P. D. Wall

*Department of Anatomy, Cerebral Functions Group, University College London,
London WC1E 6BT, England*

Every clinician and every patient in pain knows that pain does not remain static. It evolves from the moment of injury, if that can be defined, or from the time when the patient becomes aware of the pain. Even in those lucky circumstances after acute injury where pain steadily dies down, there is a sequence of changes in the nature and location of the pain. Some changes of pain can be explained by the obvious change of the location or extent of the damage. No one is surprised that the process of childbirth includes a shifting sequence of pains as different structures become involved. Similarly carcinoma, with spreading metastases and evoked secondary changes such as bone erosion, would be expected to change in its signs and symptoms. Even arthritis, which spreads to involve more and more tissue, is reasonably likely to demonstrate a pathologic history as it moves from early to late stages.

Similarly it is not surprising that the patient's attitude changes as the condition progresses. A sudden onset of pain is naturally associated with alarm and an emergency action to avoid the unpleasant circumstances. This emergency period is likely to move into a period of tension and anxiety where the patient wonders if the right thing is being done. It is a period when the patient will assess the future consequences of how long this state will last and how it will affect the patient's life and relations with others. If pain persists, periods of desperation, irritation, worry, and depression are likely. The disappointment of failure to recover and of failure of treatment contribute to what has come to be called the chronic pain state.

In this chapter are presented summaries of recent advances in our knowledge of the changes in local tissues, peripheral nerves, and spinal cord that follow injury; new data derived from animal and human behavioral studies; the role temporal, spatial, and cognitive factors play in influencing pain perception; and some of the most important changes and factors involved in the transition from acute pain to chronic pain.

SEQUENTIAL CHANGES OF PAIN SENSITIVITY AFTER INJURY

The obvious organic change in the location of abnormal tissue and the reasonable change of attitude of the patient to a disease and its pain are real enough, but they should not submerge the equally obvious fact that sequences of change other than these are also in progress. The first of these is the nature of the peripheral inflammatory process, which extends far beyond the immediate region of damage even when the region shows no signs of infection. There are clear signs that changes occur in the nerves supplying the damaged area and that these spread centrally to involve the central nervous system. These changes are also equally obvious to the thinking clinician and patient.

The long-range spread of the effect of a simple fracture is not to be explained by the local reparative inflammatory processes that surround the fracture. The entire limb becomes tender with hyperalgesia and allodynia (the production of pain by normally innocuous stimuli). The reflexes evoked from areas far distant from the injury change. These secondary changes have the obvious function of splinting the limb by long-range neural loops and increase the chances of healing. Beyond these relatively mechanical but complex widespread neurologic changes, the whole organism changes.

A wounded man or animal exhibits a syndrome of whole body changes (19). Overall activity is reduced, appetite changes, the sleep pattern is disturbed and prolonged, attention shifts, concentration drops, and sociability changes. These global changes are not to be dismissed as expressions of the individual psychology. They are observed and felt to some degree over a wide range of psychologic types. One is tempted to suggest that they are part of a general syndrome of reaction to injury because very similar changes are seen in a number of species of wild and domesticated animals who express their particular sickness by a general change in their way of acting. Each species has its recognizable peculiarities but at the same time shows changes that are common to all wounded animals and humans. We should be aware of these widespread consequences of even highly localized injury, and we should seek to understand their mechanisms.

Classical Studies of Pain Concentrated on the Consequences of Abrupt Stimuli

Scientists have quite rightly concentrated initially on the circumstances associated with the immediate time epoch after injury. This was a necessary tactical first step. They first worked on the nature of normal tissue and the nerve impulses that flowed from it. They then introduced single definable step changes in the state of the tissue. Such stimuli generate a rapidly rising and falling barrage of nerve impulses from the periphery, which penetrate the nervous system.

This maneuver of an abrupt stimulus that generates a clearly recognizable message well distinguished from the background has certain inherent dangers. It has the great scientific advantage that the times of onset and cessation of the stimulus and the generated message can be defined accurately. It might not matter that such stimuli do not occur in nature if this type of artificial event could be considered a cartoon that incorporates crucial factors of naturally occurring injurious events. Unfortunately this is not so.

The nervous system has evolved to handle certain types of events. If it is presented with unnatural concatenations of events, it may demonstrate unnatural responses. These are most easily demonstrated by examining the consequences of electrical stimulation of nerves, a stimulus much favored by basic scientists. First, one must accept that the stimulus will bring into action a mixture of nerve fibers that would never be simultaneously active in any known situation that occurs in nature. The problem here is that the major lesson taught us by such masters as Sherrington is forgotten.

Afferent nerve fibers evoke both excitations and inhibitions in the central nervous system. The proper functioning of an integrated nervous system depends on its ability to weave these conflicting influences into meaningful patterns. To present the nervous system with an abnormal temporal and spatial input of conflicting afferents means that inevitably it will generate an abnormal response. These abnormal responses have their scientific use in revealing the existence of minimal linkages between cells.

One of the particular problems of these test stimuli is the temporal aspect in which the postsynaptic element detects a very rapidly rising excitatory front so that there is a precipitous fall of membrane potential. Such excitatory postsynaptic potentials can easily be so large that they not only reach the firing threshold of the cell but reach far beyond it to deliver a grossly supramaximal stimulus. Such a stimulus will produce such marked depolarization that it is quite impossible for the most powerful available inhibitory mechanisms to prevent the firing of the cell. Such test stimuli are therefore only suited to reveal maximal abrupt excitatory mechanisms and are quite unsuitable for detecting the lurking presence of inhibitory control mechanisms.

Do "Natural" Stimuli Solve Problems Unanswered by Electrical Stimuli?

If the scientist decides to move away from these obvious inherent dangers of single brief electrical stimuli and turns to stimuli such as pressure or temperature that may well occur in nature, the problems of generating artificial responses do not disappear. The nineteenth-century tradition of challenging a system with a minimal isolated perturbation persists for good reason. In the time dimension, the obsession with being able to define the instant of the stimulus persists so that brief short-lasting stimuli retain a fascination for scientists. The problem does not disappear even when the most sophisticated stimuli are used, such as brief laser flashes applied to the skin.

Exaggerating this interest in defining stimulus onset is the appearance of equipment designed to extract signal from noise. The most obvious of these is the signal averager, which necessarily has to be timed from some event, usually the stimulus. Only rarely have such machines been used in a more subtle manner, in which a response is identified as the trigger signal followed by averaging in the time epoch before the response.

Many of the rapidly rising natural stimuli still suffer from the same temporal problem as that of electrical stimuli in that they produce such a rapidly rising supramaximal stimulus that tonic or phasic inhibitory mechanisms are overwhelmed. The remarkable book by Beecher (1) reviews the huge number of test stimuli that have been used in attempts to provide useful experimental pain models. The problem with such tests is that they fail to imitate the obvious characteristics of clinical pain, including response to narcotics.

As soon as the experimental scientist begins to face this problem by administering a less intense stimulus over a more prolonged time, a series of changing phenomena are encountered. These include adaptation, accommodation, habituation, sensitization, desensitization, and learning. Obviously the scientist would prefer to delay involvement with these processes until the nature of the primary event has been solved. The implication of this aim is that there is indeed a primary event detected by the nervous system, which is then followed by a series of secondary events that tend to counteract or exaggerate the primary event. It will be seen immediately that this may be based on a false assumption.

While there is no doubt that the arrival of a stimulus will trigger reactions that will affect the reception of subsequent stimuli, there is the basic assumption that the simplest situation for study is to present a set of nerve cells that are "tabula rasa" with a sudden change. That assumption might be valid for some idealized tissue culture situation in which the interaction between two isolated cells was being investigated. In fact, any real nervous system is set in a particular mode for stimulus reception.

The simplest of nerve cells are contacted by the dominant afferents at only a minority of their synapses, for example, in lamina 4 of the spinal cord where cells are dominated by afferent inputs from low-threshold cutaneous mechanosensitive afferents (18). The other contacts originate from many nearby and distant sources. These sources set the receptivity of the cell by a selective mixture of detailed and different excitatory and inhibitory mechanisms. It may appear that such cells are specialized to receive impulses from a strictly delineated area of skin, the receptive field. True as this conclusion may be, it neglects the huge number of other endings on the cell that determine the receptivity of the cell to its dominating input.

In a remarkable series of reports (3), just this type of cell is examined in the fifth nerve nucleus of the awake behaving monkey. It is shown at first that the firing pattern of the cells reflects in a most lawful fashion the temperature of the face skin within the receptive field. In fact, this particular relationship differs very little between the awake animal and the same animal and cell in the generally anesthetized state.

Up to this point one may be encouraged to think of these cells as relatively mechanical reporters of the state of the skin as signaled by the afferent nerve fibers. This would seem a highly satisfactory conclusion for those who postulate an early stage of sensory systems that collect and encode information from a restricted specific group of afferents. However, it appears that even these first central cells radically change their state, depending on the behavioral set of the animal. The monkey is presented with a warning light that he is about to be given a sensory task that he must discriminate. When the stimulus occurs, he must decide if it is the type of stimulus to which he should respond for reward. Then he may respond by pushing a button to deliver his reward. Some of these cells respond at all three phases of the task.

This impressive experiment removes these cells from any simple relay role and shows them to be playing a subtle role in the overall behavioral sequence in the learned series of events between warning and alerting through discrimination to selective relevant response. Given that this is the nature of our first central receiving cells, it is not surprising that we learn little of the actual state, let alone the potentialities of our sensory systems, by presenting them with abrupt and arbitrary stimuli.

LESSONS LEARNED FROM ANIMAL BEHAVIOR STUDIES

We are most fortunate to be able to benefit from the prolonged and detailed studies of Vierck et al. (17). They have studied their own reactions and those of primates to brief stimuli from which they can escape. Their first conclusion is that any normal human or animal will turn off a stimulus before it becomes painful rather than after waiting for it to become painful. This apparently obvious conclusion has escaped many who have designed animal tests. Many such tests, such as the hot plate test, the tail flick test, and the titration test where the animal chooses to turn off a rising stimulus, are all threshold measurements for some predictive type of behavior that is likely to be far below the pain threshold.

Instead of relying on such single-measure tests of threshold with a doubtful meaning in relation to pain, Vierck et al. (17) have observed in detail many aspects of their own behavior and that of monkeys in escaping from painful shocks. In this way they have defined a number of measures that have been used by others, which they find fail to measure the intensity of the stimulus or the evoked pain that they sense. These include the number of escape responses in which any normal animal or human will just as reliably interrupt a small pain as well as a big one. Similarly the latency of response is the same for small or large pains in their tests. The most reliable immediate measure was the strength or force used to pull the lever to stop the pain. In between the tests they measured the amount of behavioral disturbance.

When they had accurate measures for animals that matched their own human responses, they proceeded to the most meaningful and obvious test to see if this measure of pain related to the human experience that morphine is an analgesic. Vierck et al. (17), like Beecher (1), were well aware that abrupt tests failed to demonstrate such analgesia, and therefore there was something wrong with the tests. Despite this, animal tests are used routinely to assess narcotic potency. The experiments use as typical systemic doses of morphine 5 to 10 mg/kg in rats or mice, 3 to 6 mg/kg in rabbits, and 1 to 12 mg/kg in monkeys. The use of these gigantic doses traditionally has been justified by the untested assumption that nonhuman species are resistant to narcotics.

It will now be seen that there are two interrelated matters of doubt: first, the relation of the tested behavioral response to pain, and second, the possibility that the morphine was affecting the perception of pain or some other ability. Vierck et al. (17) found, in fact, that 0.5 mg/kg systemic morphine produced a large decrease of the animals' ability to detect touch.

This raised the suspicion that much smaller doses than those needed to disrupt so-called pain behavior were greatly disturbing the animals' ability to respond to minimal stimuli that are not grossly disturbed in a human under narcotic analgesia. They proceeded to test monkeys' ability to play a game in which they got a food reward on hearing a tone and pulling a lever. A dose of 1 mg/kg systemic morphine was sufficient to produce a huge disorganization of this performance.

In other words, the doses of morphine that have been used in animals to demonstrate analgesia are many times higher than those that produce severe behavioral disturbances of neuronal functions unrelated to pain. The failure of these animal tests to measure analgesia as experienced by humans does not mean that they are useless; it may be that these other pharmacologic actions of morphine give a useful index of relative potency of morphine to other narcotics.

Like Beecher (1), Vierck et al. (17) turned to seek some index of pain that showed the expected and required response to narcotics. In both solutions, it is interesting that the prolonged action of stimuli was chosen after the failure to find meaningful changes in responses to abrupt stimuli unless gigantic doses were used. For Beecher, the answer was provided by the subacute effort tourniquet test. Blood flow to the arm is occluded, a fixed series of finger grips against a measured load is carried out, and the time to onset of severe pain is measured. The test and the pain are ended by release of the blood pressure cuff. Doses such as 0.1 mg/kg of morphine prolong the period before this type of pain becomes intolerable.

Vierck et al. (17) turned to another phenomenon: "second pain." In a number of situations, a sudden stimulus such as dipping a finger in hot water results in a rapid pain followed some seconds later by a second pain with a different quality from the first. With the acceptance of the existence of two types of afferent fibers, the relatively rapidly conducting A delta fibers and the slow unmyelinated C fibers, it was natural to propose that these two pains are caused by the arrival of two temporally separated volleys in afferent fibers. There are strong reasons to doubt this simple interpretation (15).

Whatever the explanation, the phenomenon is real enough and is abolished preferentially in humans by a systemic dose of 0.15 mg/kg morphine.

Trials of Pain Tolerance Give Variable Results

Our sensory systems have evolved to extract a meaning from events and to express that meaning in terms of relevant response. It is therefore not surprising that our nervous systems have severe problems in making meaningful responses to meaningless stimuli. A painful stimulus that does not signify injury is a paradox. Yet that is exactly what we have to interpret as trained experimental subjects in a trial of pain tolerance. For example, we have to say to ourselves, "I know that this stimulus will not injure me, but I guess that if it increased it would be dangerous." No wonder that we each, as individuals, give different answers to that guess in pain tolerance tests. No wonder that experimenters are puzzled that their subjects keep reaching a tolerance level that the experimenter does not feel as pain. It is not surprising then that different laboratories with carefully trained subjects give very different answers for pain tolerance in identical tests (16).

We have seen that the response of first central cells varies depending on the general circumstances of the animal. This is a specific example of the gate control mechanism (13) in which the response of a first central cell depends on three factors: (a) the activity of afferent fibers activated by the stimulus, (b) the afferent barrage generated by other nearby fibers, and (c) the activity of intrinsic mechanisms within the central nervous system, particularly the descending influences from the brain to the spinal cord. It is not surprising, and is, in fact, a crucial test of the existence of such a gate control mechanism, that the whole organism also reflects the existence of selection of relevance, which begins at the first central synapse and continues presumably at all subsequent relay and analysis stations.

We see this in action in two careful psychophysical studies carried out by Gracely and Wolskee (6) and McGrath et al. (10) in which they measured the response of humans to tooth stimulation. The response of their subjects varied fundamentally depending on whether the subject was concentrating on the intensity of the stimulus or on its painfulness. Intensity is a neutral quality that does not imply imperative action, whereas the painful aspects of an identical stimulus refer to qualities that imply a threat to the integrity of the organism and require imperative action. With this type of analysis, which dissects different factors from the same stimulus, we begin to see why there has been such a chaotic and unsatisfactory history of pain testing in humans and animals. The problems are well reviewed in *The Textbook of Pain* (25).

Very rapidly rising stimuli, whether electrical, mechanical, or thermal, will tend to overwhelm normal analysis mechanisms and to set off nondifferentiable artificial sensations mixed with alerting startle responses. More slowly rising stimuli not only evoke counterreactions within peripheral nerves and the central nervous system but are channeled and interpreted in quite different ways, including a cognitive analysis of different aspects of the same stimulus. The subject under hypnotic analgesia is capable of giving conflicting reports on the temperature and on the painfulness of ice water covering a hand (7). The trained subject has been directed to report on some particular aspect of the stimulus. The untrained patient will report on a personal choice of aspects (28).

Training is not the monopoly of psychologists and psychiatrists. The fisherman working on the deck of a trawler in the Arctic in conditions far beyond most people's pain tolerance is an extreme example of training. He is in no sense insensitive, as he can tell you the water and air temperature with great accuracy. He believes as a result of his background that these conditions are not tissue-threatening. In the long run he may be wrong, but his tradition and his mates and his income assure him that to continue in these dreadful conditions is good. Subject such a man to painful stimuli other than cold water, and he will join the general population and will not show a generally elevated pain tolerance threshold.

Spatial, Temporal, and Cognitive Aspects Determine Pain

The temporal aspects of stimulation and the problems they raise for testing pain mechanisms have been stressed. Spatial aspects also play a crucial role. If a sharp pencil is gradually pressed into the fingertip, a conical pit will form extending over several millimeters before there is a sensation of pain. Once sensed, the pain will appear to be exactly localized at the tip of the pencil, and there is no sensation associated with the very large area of skin that is obviously grossly distorted far beyond the threshold for sensation. This is an illustration of the power of inhibition that may operate on our senses to concentrate the apparent stimulus to a much smaller area than is actually involved.

It is possible to trick these inhibitory mechanisms by applying stimuli to very restricted areas. A fine filament touched to particular points on the lips or nose evokes massive responses with prolonged sensory aftereffects (15). An identical mechanical distortion of skin applied over a larger area produces minimal innocuous sensations. The extension of stimuli to distant areas involves more and more extensive inhibitory mechanisms (8). Although these inherent inhibitory processes represent an important part of pain mechanisms and influence responses to applied test stimuli, their failure to operate produce severe pathologic variants of normal pain with hyperalgesia, summation, and radiation.

TRANSITION FROM ACUTE TO CHRONIC PAIN

The simplest way to explain chronic pain would be to propose that it represents a tonic continuation of the process of acute pain. In part, this may be true. Many tonic biologic processes such as striped muscle contractions are explained largely by proposing a steady repetition of the processes of phasic action. However, it is clear that certain new factors emerge as time passes after injury and after nerve impulses have begun to bombard the central nervous system.

Soft Tissue and Nerve Ends

A series of breakdowns, migrations, and differentiations of cells represents the inflammatory and scar tissue formation changes. The nerve fibers themselves play a part in these inflammatory changes (9). Some of the tissue changes are mediated by way of the axon reflex in the unmyelinated C fibers. There are three separate but interrelated changes. First, blood vessels dilate to produce the heat and flare; they leak independently to produce the swelling and wheal; and third, there are three separate changes in the response of the nervous system to stimuli. First, there can be a sensitization of endings that have been stimulated in the original injury (2). Second, endings at some distance that were not involved in the original stimulus become more sensitive (5). Third, there are indirect secondary changes within the central nervous system that increase the excitability of cells so that afferent signals from normal tissue by way of normal afferents trigger abnormal central responses, secondary hyperalgesia.

We do not know the fundamental mechanism of any of these slowly developing changes, but there is a strong suspicion that the C fibers are involved in all of them. Since C fibers contain peptides such as substance P, cholecystokinin, vasoactive intestinal peptide, and somatostatin, there are those who propose that these peptides play a role in inducing the slow secondary challenges that follow many minutes after injury.

Nerve Fibers

Even trivial and superficial injuries will smash nerve fibers and will be followed by sprouting and repair. More extensive injuries will involve larger and larger nerves, and the prognosis for complete recovery drops. Although attention naturally is directed to the point where the nerve is cut across, it has been shown that 12 locations should be considered in the vicinity of the central and peripheral extension of the neuron that is damaged (20).

Peripheral to the injury, Wallerian degeneration will progress and surround cells, end stations will react, and neighboring intact nerves will sprout to move into the territory vacated by the degenerating terminals. At the instant of injury, an injury discharge is emitted from the cut end, but this dies down within seconds (27). The ends rapidly seal over and sprouts begin to probe out into damaged tissue.

The subsequent course depends critically on the tissue encountered by these outgrowing sprouts. In the extreme case of a simple crush, there is complete Wallerian degeneration in the periphery, but the basement membrane remains intact and guides the sprouts and the Schwann cells into apposition. This is followed by a steady progress of the sprout toward its original peripheral destination. Such sprouts are rapidly surrounded by a "normal" environment for a nerve fiber. In contrast, if the nerve has been physically disrupted, the space into which the sprout has grown will be invaded by fibroblasts, other nerve sprouts, debris, blood vessels, and so on. As we shall see, the presence of nerve sprouts in this foreign environment triggers a number of central reactions, many of which do not occur after crush injuries.

Multiple sprouts grow out from the severed axon and probe out, seeking a suitable environment. Some curve back into the parent nerve, utilizing the presence of Schwann cells covering the proximal axon. After 1 to 2 weeks, the total number of sprouts per axon decreases, but even when the axon's sprouts fail to find a suitable medium for growth, they remain as an immature sprout and form a neuroma.

As the sprouts grow out, they develop three properties that they do not share with the mature membrane of their parent axon (24). They become spontaneously active, which rises in intensity for 2 weeks and then sinks to zero if the sprout extends successfully to the periphery, but not if it remains trapped in the neuroma. The outgrowing sprouts develop a marked mechanical sensitivity, which explains the Tinel sign. Last, they become extremely sensitive to sympathetic amines with an alpha sensitivity, which explains one aspect of the sympathetic dystrophies.

Effects Central to the Injury

After peripheral nerve injury, a cascade of changes sweeps centrally over the proximal part of the cut nerve. Conduction velocity decreases. There are chemical changes in the dorsal root ganglia associated with chromatolysis. The dorsal root ganglion cells also undergo physiologic changes in their membrane properties in the same three ways as occur in the peripheral sprouts. This means that a damaged nerve fiber is producing two abnormal sources of nerve impulses to bombard the spinal cord, one from the cut end of the axon and the other from the dorsal root ganglion cell. With these changes there is an alteration of metabolism of dorsal root ganglion cells that is apparent in the small cells, which decrease their synthesis of peptides so that there is eventually a decrease of peptide content of unmyelinated fiber terminals in the spinal cord.

Slow Effects in Spinal Cord Produced by Nerve Impulses

Peripheral nerve injury produces an immediate afferent barrage that is handled by the fast-reacting mechanisms of the gate control system, which transmit the impulses to the brain and to the reflex circuits. However, the arrival of this injury barrage produces some readjustments of central excitabilities, which depend on a different mechanism from those handling the normal rapid synaptic excitations and inhibitions. These changes, which appear in tens of minutes after the injury, are to be correlated with the secondary hyperalgesia and involve much wider areas of input than those involved in the original injury. For example, the area from which a flexion reflex in a particular muscle can be evoked spreads and the threshold is decreased.

A particular group of cells in the most dorsal lamina of dorsal horn that take part in these changes has been identified (11). The receptive fields of these cells normally have an ameboid quality in which they sometimes are excited from one area of skin and sometimes from another (4). If skin is damaged near the area of skin that normally excites a particular cell, the receptive field of the cell moves after a latent period of some 10 min and incorporates the area of damage.

This magnetic effect of the injury involves a change of the effective input to the cell, a connectivity control. It is dependent on prolonged and slow reaction to the barrage of nerve impulses in unmyelinated fibers. It does not occur if the C fibers' central synaptic excitation has been inactivated by capsaicin (21). If the area of damage is anesthetized after the shift of connectivity has occurred, the receptive field remains in the abnormal location for tens of minutes before slowly drifting back to its original location. These experiments show that the spinal cord possesses a slowly acting mechanism that is capable of focusing reaction onto certain active inputs.

Slow Effects in Spinal Cord Produced by Transport Mechanisms

If the sciatic nerve of the rat is cut across, a series of physiologic changes begin within the spinal cord after 3 to 4 days. These include a reduction of dorsal root potentials, which are associated with presynaptic inhibition, and a reduction of postsynaptic inhibitions. The immediate effect of nerve section is the loss of drive to those cells whose receptive fields are in the area supplied by the cut nerve.

As the inhibitions disappear, many cells that have lost their normal input begin to respond to nearby intact nerves. This type of connectivity control is dependent on C fibers because it is not necessary to cut the entire nerve. The change of connectivity is produced by poisoning the C fibers with capsaicin (22). The effect is not caused by an absence of nerve impulses, since the connections do not change if nerve impulses are chronically blocked with tetrodotoxin (26).

The final proof that these changes are caused by the transport of substances from the periphery is shown by the fact that they are prevented if a transport blocker such as colchicine is placed central to the nerve section

(M. Devor, *personal communication*). Reasons are given elsewhere to suggest that these slow changes of connection represent an unmasking of existing connections rather than the sprouting of new fibers (25).

SUMMARY AND CONCLUSIONS

I have described here in some detail a sequence of slow changes in tissue, in peripheral nerve, and in the spinal cord. There is no reason to stop at that point, since it is inevitable that such changes will have a direct effect on the reaction of more central structures. However, it is equally possible that the sequence of changes that reach to the spinal cord might also trigger slow secondary changes in more rostral structures. McMahon and Wall (12) found that, unlike spinal cord change, peripheral nerve injury does not change the organization of dorsal column nuclei. However, there are signs of changes of organization in the mapping of cerebral cortex (14,23), but we do not yet know if these are entirely attributable to changes at the first central synapses or if deeper structures also change.

What is apparent is that the signs and symptoms of the patient show a sequence of changes after tissue damage. Pain, tenderness, hyperpathia, guarding, abnormal reflexes, and changed motor patterns spread far beyond the region of the original injury. Each of these changes must have its physiologic basis, and not all can be attributed to changes in the immediate area of damage.

These secondary changes are as much a source of the patient's suffering as the primary cause and are therefore an important therapeutic target. We can now see that their prevention may be possible as we understand their mechanisms. Early treatment may be needed, and it may be necessary to consider blocking not only nerve impulses but also transport mechanisms. The changes undoubtedly contribute to the problems of the patient with chronic pain, and we need most urgently to understand how much of the patient's state is the consequence of these automatic adjustments of a nervous system trying to counteract injury and how much of the state is produced by high-level cognitive reactions to misery.

REFERENCES

1. Beecher, H. K. (1959): *Measurement of Subjective Responses.* Oxford University Press, New York.
2. Campbell, J. N., and Meyer, R. A. (1983): Sensitization of unmyelinated nociceptive afferents in monkey varies with skin type. *J. Neurophysiol.*, 49:98–110.
3. Dubner, R., Hoffman, D. S., and Hayes, R. L. (1981): Neuronal activity in medullary dorsal horn of awake monkeys trained in a thermal discrimination task. III. Task-related responses and their functional role. *J. Neurophysiol.*, 46:444–446.
4. Dubuisson, D., Fitzgerald, M., and Wall, P. D. (1979): Ameboid receptive fields of cells in laminae 1, 2 and 3. *Brain Res.*, 177:376–378.
5. Fitzgerald, M. (1979): The spread of sensitization of polymodal nociceptors in the rabbit from nearby injury and by antidromic nerve stimulation. *J. Physiol.*, 297:207–216.

6. Gracely, R. H., and Wolskee, P. J. (1983): Semantic functional measurement of pain: Integrating perception and language. *Pain*, 15:389–398.
7. Hilgard, E. R., and Hilgard, J. R. (1975): *Hypnosis in the Relief of Pain*. William Kaufmann, Inc., Los Altos, Calif.
8. Le Bars, D., Dickenson, A. H., and Besson, J. M. (1979): Diffuse noxious inhibitory controls DNIC. Effects on dorsal horn convergent neurones in the rat. *Pain*, 6:283–304.
9. Lewis, T. (1942): *Pain*. Macmillan, London.
10. McGrath, P. A., Gracely, R. H., Dubner, R., and Heft, M. W. (1983): Non-pain and pain sensations evoked by tooth pulp stimulation. *Pain*, 15:377–388.
11. McMahon, S. B., and Wall, P. D. (1983): A system of rat spinal cord lamina I cells projecting through the contralateral dorso-lateral funiculus. *J. Comp. Neurol.*, 214:217–223.
12. McMahon, S. B., and Wall, P. D. (1983): Plasticity in the nucleus gracilis of the rat. *Exp. Neurol.*, 80:195–207.
13. Melzack, R., and Wall, P. D. (1965): Pain mechanisms: A new theory. *Science*, 150:971–979.
14. Merzenick, M. M., and Kaas, J. H. (1982): Reorganization of mammalian somatosensory cortex following peripheral nerve injury. *Trends Neurosci.*, 5:434–436.
15. Sinclair, D. (1981): *Mechanisms of Cutaneous Sensation*. Oxford University Press, Oxford.
16. Sternbach, R. A., and Turskey, B. (1964): On the psychophysical power function in electric shock. *Psychosom. Sci.*, 1:217–218.
17. Vierck, C. J., Cooper, B. Y., Franzen, O., Ritz, L. A., and Greenspan, J. D. (1983): Behavioural analysis of CNS pathways and transmitter systems involved in conduction and inhibition of pain sensations and reactions in primates. *Prog. Psychobiol. Physiol. Psych.*, 10:113–165.
18. Wall, P. D. (1967): The laminar organization of dorsal horn and effects of descending impulses. *J. Physiol.*, 188:403–423.
19. Wall, P. D. (1979): On the relation of injury to pain. The John J. Bonica Lecture. *Pain*, 6:253–264.
20. Wall, P. D., and Devor, M. (1982): Consequences of peripheral nerve damage in the spinal cord and in neighbouring intact peripheral nerves. In: *Abnormal Impulse Generators in Nerve and Muscle*, edited by J. Ochoa, pp. 267–283. Oxford University Press, Oxford.
21. Wall, P. D., and Fitzgerald, M. (1981): Effects of capsaicin applied locally to adult peripheral nerve. I. Physiology of peripheral nerve and spinal cord. *Pain*, 11:363–377.
22. Wall, P. D., Fitzgerald, M., and S. J. Gibson (1981): The response of rat spinal cord cells to unmyelinated afferents after peripheral nerve section and after changes in substance P levels. *Neuroscience*, 6:2205–2215.
23. Wall, P. D., Fitzgerald, M., Nussbaumer, J. C., Van der Loss, H., and Devor, M. (1982): Somatotopic maps are disorganised in adult rodents treated with capsaicin as neonates. *Nature*, 295:691–693.
24. Wall, P. D., and Gutnick, M. (1974): Ongoing activity in peripheral nerves: II. The physiology and pharmacology of impulses originating in a neuroma. *Exp. Neurol.*, 43:580–593.
25. Wall, P. D., and Melzack, R. (Eds.) (1984): *The Textbook of Pain*. Churchill-Livingstone, Edinburgh.
26. Wall, P. D., Mills, R., Fitzgerald, M., and Gibson, S. J. (1982): Chronic blockade of sciatic nerve transmission by tetrodotoxin does not produce central changes in the dorsal horn of the spinal cord of the rat. *Neurosci. Lett.*, 30:315–320.
27. Wall, P. D., Waxman, S., and Basbaum, A. I. (1974): Ongoing activity in peripheral nerve: III. Injury discharge. *Exp. Neurol.*, 45:576–589.
28. Zborowski, M. (1969): *People in Pain*. Jossy-Bass, San Francisco.

*Advances in Pain Research
and Therapy, Vol. 7,*
edited by C. Benedetti et al.
Raven Press, New York © 1984.

Spinal Neurotransmitter Systems Associated with Activity in the Rostrad Transmission System by Pain-Evoking Stimuli

*Tony L. Yaksh, *Paul E. Micevych, **Robert P. Elde, and
†Vay L. W. Go

*Departments of *Neurosurgery and †Gastroenterology, Mayo Clinic, Rochester,
Minnesota 55905; and **Department of Anatomy, University of Minnesota,
Minneapolis, Minnesota 55455*

Tissue damaging stimuli of a somatic or visceral origin often will evoke behavior aimed at terminating the stimulus (i.e., escape) or a verbal report of pain. Although the characteristics of the response are organized at the supraspinal level, the initiation of the response subsequent to such a peripheral stimulus must pass through the first-order synapse in the dorsal horn of the spinal cord and be carried forward to higher centers. It is to certain aspects of this spinal segmental link in the rostrad transmission system that we will direct our attention in this discussion.

Examination of electrical activity in single primary afferents reveals that certain populations of fibers are driven preferentially by thermal, mechanical, and chemical stimuli that will evoke escape behavior in the unanesthetized animal. Measurement of the conduction velocity of such afferent fibers indicates that they belong to the category of unmyelinated and lightly myelinated fibers (33). Single-unit recording in the dorsal horn of the spinal cord of the unanesthetized, spinally transected mammal reveals that there are populations of second-order neurons that fire with increasing rapidity as a function of the activation of small, myelinated and unmyelinated primary afferents (27). The significant correlation between the discharge characteristics of these wide dynamic-range dorsal horn cells with human psychophysics suggests that such activity evoked by small afferent input could be a neural substrate for the sensory input associated with the "pain report" (26). These comments do not prove that there is a "pain pathway," but they do indicate that there are certain neural substrates, the activity of which correlates with the appearance of pain behavior. As will be discussed below, the "meaning" of the activity in any given neuron may depend on factors other than the source of its excitatory drive.

Studies on the mechanisms governing activity in these spinal units indicate that, aside from the excitatory drive coming from primary afferents, there is a variable modulation of their evoked discharge by several modulatory substrates. As described in the Chapter by T. L. Yaksh, J. R. Howe, and G. J. Harty, *this volume*, studies on the pharmacologic characteristics of the spinal cord have indicated the existence of spinopetal monoaminergic and segmental enkephalinergic systems, the activation of whose receptors in the dorsal horn results in a powerful inhibition in the processing by the spinal cord of nociceptive information.

Thus the nature of the sensory message generated in this rostrad transmission system (RTS) is dependent not only on the characteristics of the afferent input, but on the nature and magnitude of the modulatory control that is exerted at the level of the synaptic link between the primary afferent and second-order neuron in the dorsal horn. In the subsequent discussion we will examine some aspects of the pharmacology of the suspected excitatory-modulatory transmitter links in this spinal part of the RTS.

PHARMACOLOGY OF SMALL PRIMARY AFFERENTS

The electrophysiologic and behavioral data noted above clearly suggest that activity in certain populations of small myelinated and unmyelinated primary afferents is sufficient to produce pain reports. A candidate transmitter for the first-order synaptic link of the afferent fiber responsive to high-threshold somatic and visceral stimuli therefore should be found in small primary afferents, and it should have predictable physiologic consequences when applied in the system where its receptors (i.e., the afferent terminals) are found.

Prior to 1975, the only reasonable candidates appeared to be one or more of the excitatory amino acids such as glutamate or aspartate. Since that time, however, it has become apparent that certain so-called gut peptides may in fact possess some of the appropriate characteristics required for a transmitter in this first-order link for pathways serving the transmission of information through small fibers. This evidence exists to suggest that substance P (sP), vasoactive intestinal polypeptide (VIP), and cholecystokinin (CCK) are contained in primary afferents (15). Particular emphasis has been placed on the 11 amino acid peptide, sP. The characteristics of this peptide, insofar as they describe it as a candidate for primary afferent transmitter, will be the subject of this part of the discussion.

SPINAL DISTRIBUTION OF SUBSTANCE P

Substance P has been shown by radioimmunoassay and immunohistochemical techniques to be contained in high concentrations in the spinal cord, primarily in the dorsal horn (2,8,10,16). Figures 1 and 2 present the

TABLE 1. *Levels of substance P of the rhizotomized and hemisected cat lumbar spinal cord, expressed as percent of the nonlesioned side*

	N	Dorsal horn	Ventral horn	Dorsal root ganglion
Dorsal rhizotomy[a]	4	44[b]	96	278[b]
Ventral rhizotomy	4	78[b]	91	122
Hemisection	4	67[b]	71[b]	102

[a] Animals were sacrificed 10–16 days following lesions.
[b] $p < 0.05$.
From T. L. Yaksh and V. L. W. Go (*unpublished data*).

immunohistofluorescence associated with sP in the dorsal horn of the control cat and rat spinal cord. As can be seen, the densities of these terminals and fibers is primarily distributed in the substantia gelatinosa of the dorsal horn. In both species immunoreactive fibers/terminals are seen in laminae I and II, with only scattered fibers in lamina III (Fig. 2). When animals are treated with colchicine to enhance cell body staining, sP immunoreactive cell bodies are localized in laminae III, IV, and V of the dorsal horn and the most dorsal areas of the ventral horn. Further, sP immunoreactive fibers/terminals are observed in lamina X around the central canal and throughout the ventral horn in moderate to low concentrations.

To investigate the neuronal systems with which this agent is associated, various approaches have been used to manipulate the levels of this material (16). Changes in the level of sP activity after various spinal lesion experiments have permitted several laboratories, including our own, to establish that sP may be associated with several discrete systems. Table 1 presents the effect on sP levels in cat lumbar spinal cord of dorsal and ventral lumbar rhizotomies and C2 cord hemisection. Several interesting observations may be made on these results obtained in the cat. First, dorsal rhizotomies produced a significant reduction in the levels of sP in the dorsal horn. Such treatments failed to have any significant effect on the levels of sP in the ventral horn. Such lesions also increased the levels of sP in the dorsal root ganglion, presumably reflecting a block of sP transport from the ganglion. This effect on dorsal horn sP after dorsal root section shown with radioimmunoassay is corroborated by the immunohistochemistry. Figure 1 shows the effect of a rhizotomy on the levels of sP immunoreactivity in the dorsal horn after 7 days. A significant reduction can be seen in the levels of sP-associated fluorescence as compared to the contralateral side. Second, ventral rhizotomies produced a small but measurable decrease in the levels of sP in the ipsilateral dorsal horn. Third, hemisection at the cervical level produces about a 30% reduction in the levels of sP in the dorsal and ventral horns.

These data suggest that sP in the dorsal horn depends on input arising from primary afferents arriving through the dorsal root ganglia. The effects

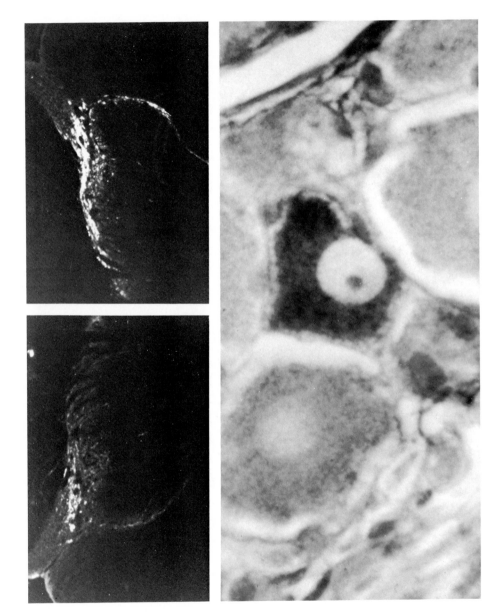

of ventral rhizotomy on dorsal horn levels is consistent with the observation that small unmyelinated primary afferents may enter the spinal cord through the ventral roots (5,6) and provides evidence for the first time that some of these afferents may be associated with a specific peptide. The hemisection experiments indicate that some sP terminals in the spinal cord may be associated with certain descending pathways that originate rostral to the spinal lesion.

Perhaps the most conclusive evidence that sP is contained in small afferents is the fact that immunohistochemistry has clearly shown sP immunoreactivity localized in the type B cells of Anders (16). These ganglion cells are generally thought to give rise to small myelinated and unmyelinated fibers. Figure 1 (bottom) presents a photomicrograph of a number of ganglion cells. As can be seen, sP immunoreactivity is located only in one of several small cells and in none of the large cells.

In short, the immunohistochemical and radioimmunoassay experiments carried out with surgical manipulation of the spinal cord strongly suggest that sP in the cord may be located in at least two pools, one associated with small primary afferent terminals and a second associated with descending pathways, presumably serotonergic in character.

Manipulation of Release

If sP serves as a neurotransmitter, then it should be contained in a releasable pool, and the physiologic stimulus for its release should be consistent with the properties of the neural system with which the peptide is thought to be associated. Experiments carried out in brain tissue have revealed that sP is contained in synaptosomal fractions and vesicles (10,25). *In vitro* experiments have demonstrated that sP is contained in a mobile fraction that is releasable by local depolarization (8,20). To examine whether sP is released *in vivo*, a spinal superfusion procedure, as described in Fig. 3, has been used. In these experiments, carried out in the cat and the rat, potassium in excess releases sP. This release is antagonized by the addition of cobalt, suggesting the possible significance of a calcium excitation-secretion coupling link.

FIG. 1. Photomicrographs of the left (**upper left**) and right (**upper right**) dorsal horn of the cat spinal cord 7 days after a left dorsal rhizotomy. All sections were incubated with anti-sP serum. The immunofluorescent pattern of staining with anti-sP in a normal cat spinal cord (**left**) is present in laminae I and II of the dorsal horn, with occasional fibers penetrating deeper into the gray matter. Note the diminished immunofluorescence staining (**right**) after a dorsal rhizotomy. Note that the immunoreactivity appears to be reduced across the entire substantia gelatinosa and marginal zone. The photomicrograph of dorsal root ganglion (**bottom**) was processed according to the PAP technique and shows sP-immunoreactivity within a small type B cell of the dorsal root ganglion. It is the central processes of these cells that inactivate the dorsal horn of the spinal cord and are interrupted by a dorsal rhizotomy.

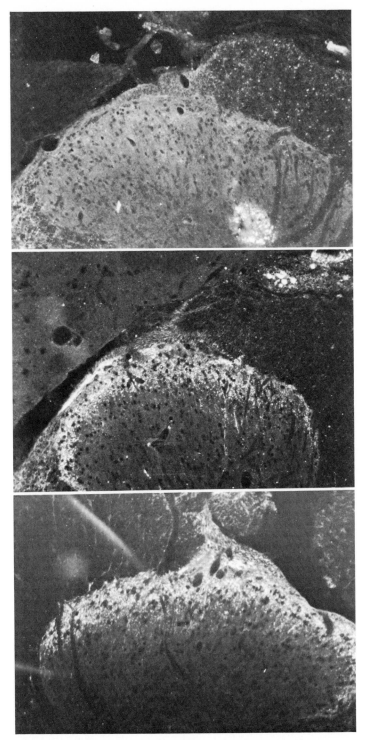

FIG. 2. Photomicrograph showing the effects in the rat on sP immunofluorescence in dorsal horn of intrathecal capsaicin (30 μg: **top**), 5,6-dihydroxytryptamine (20 μg: **middle**), or vehicle (**bottom**) injected in a volume of 15 μl, 7 days before sacrifice.

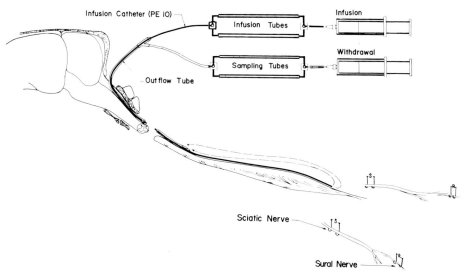

FIG. 3. Schematic representation of a system used to superfuse the cat spinal cord. Artificial cerebrospinal fluid is infused at the level of the sacral cord at the rate of 100 or 200 μl/min and collected by withdrawal syringe through an outer concentric cannula at the level of the thoracic cord. Sequential samples are taken without interrupting perfusion outflow rate or pressure by directing the perfusion pathway through parallel glass sampling tubes kept in ice.

To determine whether the activation of somatic input would increase the release of sP from spinal cord, cats were prepared with spinal superfusion systems, and the sciatic nerves were stimulated bilaterally. Figure 4 presents the results of experiments in which it is shown that low intensity stimulation of the sciatic nerve had no effect on the levels of sP from spinal cord. In contrast, high intensity stimulation resulted in a fourfold increase in the resting levels of this peptide. Importantly, the addition of morphine (5×10^{-4} M) to the intrathecal perfusate resulted in a significant attenuation of the effects of such stimulation on sP levels in spinal superfusate (40). As the release could be obtained in spinal transected animals, the sP contained in the descending apparently monoamine pathways contributed only a small amount in comparison to the material deriving from afferent input.

Physiologic Correlates of Changes in Spinal Substance P Levels

If sP plays a role in the synaptic transmission of small primary afferents, its local application should mimic the effects produced when such afferent systems are activated.

The iontophoretic application of sP has been shown to produce a delayed and long-lasting depolarization of dorsal horn neurons that have been functionally identified as spinal nociceptive neurons (14,42).

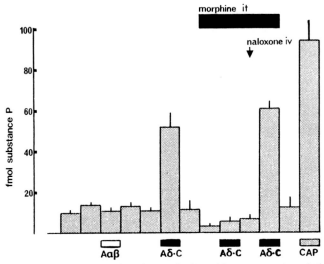

FIG. 4. Release of sP from superfused cat spinal cord in response to sciatic nerve stimulation and capsaicin (CAP). Cats were anesthetized with chloralose-urethane (100 mg/kg) and prepared with a tracheal tube and jugular and carotid catheters. Perfusion, therefore, was localized to the upper sacral and lumbar spinal cord. The sciatic nerve was stimulated with rectangular pulses (3–4 V, 0.05 msec, 50 Hz for activation of Aα and Aβ fibers and 40–50 V, 0.05 msec, 50 Hz for recruitment of Aδ and C fibers). Superfusate in all experiments consisted of NaCl, 151.1 mM; KCl, 2.6 mM; MgSO$_4$, 0.9 mM; CaCl$_2$, 1.3 mM; NaHCO$_3$, 21.0 mM; K$_2$HPO$_4$, 2.5 mM; gassed with 95% O$_2$ and 5% CO$_2$ before perfusion. Perfusion samples (3 ml) were collected into glacial acetic acid (final concentration of 2 N) and immediately frozen and lyophilized. Samples were reconstituted in 1.0-ml assay buffer, neutralized; aliquots of each fraction were used to determine the content of sP in perfusion samples by radioimmunoassay with a sensitivity of 1.5 femtomole per assay tube samples produced parallel dilution curves. Each value is the mean ± SEM from four separate experiments (40).

Increasing the levels of sP activity by the intrathecal injection of this peptide results in behavioral signs of irritation and agitation (9,18).

Capsaicin, a homovanillic acid derivative, will deplete sP in the spinal dorsal horn (21,37) and release sP from the spinal cord *in vitro* (13,30) and *in vivo* (40). In recent experiments, it has been demonstrated that the acute intrathecal administration of capsaicin in adult cats and rats will produce a significant reduction in the levels of sP in the spinal cord (1,37), particularly in the dorsal horn. Figure 4 presents the effects of such treatments on the immunohistofluorescence of sP in the dorsal horn. As compared to the section obtained from the control animals (Fig. 1), capsaicin resulted in an almost complete depletion of sP in the substantia gelatinosa. Importantly, such treatments with capsaicin have no effect on levels of monoamines in the spinal cord (T. L. Yaksh and G. M. Tyce, *unpublished observations*).

The effect of capsaicin on sP in the dorsal horn strongly suggests that it may act to alter the distribution of the peptide in a limited population of spinal cord terminals, mainly those in primary afferents. Figure 4 also indicates that intrathecal 5,6-DHT has no effect on the levels of sP in the dorsal horn (although levels of sP in the ventral horn are significantly reduced). The intrathecal administration of capsaicin has been used to examine the effects of depleting the afferent stores of sP on the nociceptive threshold. In adult animals treated acutely with intrathecal capsaicin, prolonged elevation in the nociceptive threshold as measured by thermal (hot plate and tail flick) and chemical stimuli (37) was obtained. The elevated nociceptive thresholds were correlated closely with the degree of sP depletion measured after sacrifice. These results are consistent with the early findings of Jancśo et al. (19), where systemic capsaicin was observed to induce a functionally selective inactivation of peripheral afferents (18). Pretreatment of the animal with 5,6-DHT also resulted in a significant reduction in sP levels, but this reduction in sP levels was accompanied by a reduction in the nociceptive threshold (37), presumably associated with the loss of a descending 5-HT modulatory system (see Chapter by T. L. Yaksh, J. R. Howe, and G. J. Harty, *this volume*) with which some stores of spinal sP are thought to be located (4,17). These results showing an effect in the rat on nociceptive behavior are consistent with results showing an effect of capsaicin on small primary afferents.

Postulated Role for Substance P in the Spinal Cord

Whether sP is a conventional neurotransmitter or represents something conceptually different has yet to be determined. One alternative is suggested by the work of Steinacker (28). He has proposed that this peptide may act to modulate the calcium-dependent phase of K^+ conductance that has been reported (3). If this calcium-mediated change in K^+ conductance does contribute to the characteristics of the repetitive discharge properties of the cell, then sP could serve to bias the output of neural systems activated by the more phasic actions of other transmitters. In this sense, sP, or similar compounds, may serve as the long-term regulators of rhythmic neural activity. It is significant that sP-containing vesicles are often observed in dorsal horn terminals along with smaller vesicles that do not contain sP. One might thus speculate that neural activity resulting in the release of the alternate transmitter would also evoke the release of sP. The presence or absence of this peptide would then serve to modify the ultimate characteristics of the discharge pattern of the postsynaptic cell.

An important physiologic phenomenon that may be associated with such a suggestion is the so-called wind-up response. Originally reported by Mendell and Wall (22), this effect is the facilitation of the discharge evoked in lamina V neurons by repetitive afferent stimulation. The effect is characterized by increasingly higher rates of discharge after the delivery of several peripheral stimuli at intervals of up to several seconds. Mendell and Wall had demonstrated that the effect is uniquely produced by the activation of the smaller peripheral afferents (C). Thus, in view of the proposed influence of sP on processes regulating repetitive discharge, it may be that the observed wind-up produced by small fiber activation is a consequence of the concurrent release and action of sP on the postsynaptic membrane of the lamina V cell or some connected interneuron.

The delay in onset of the effects of ionotophoretically applied sP, the presence of several different types of vesicles in the same terminals, and the probable association of sP with smaller afferents (the activity of which is required for wind-up) are suggestive data that may reflect a true modulatory role of sP released during dorsal horn activity. Such data, reviewed above, while suggesting a close correlation between sP and nociceptive transmission, are not entirely conclusive. The fact that intrathecally applied sP does not produce outright behavioral signs of intense pain, as does intrathecal capsaicin, which depolarizes small afferents, suggests that its presence alone does not constitute the total content of an Aδ/C fiber synapse. Moreover, as with all studies of neurotransmitters and physiologic systems, the sP changes produced by the several manipulations may be only ancillary to the effects of these manipulations on other systems that are associated with nociceptive transmission.

PHARMACOLOGY OF MODULATORY SUBSTRATES

As noted earlier, it is clear that the concept of the pain pathway is not one that may be defined simply in terms of the elements that promote the rostrad movement of sensory information. As discussed in detail in the Chapter by T. L. Yaksh, J. R. Howe, and G. J. Harty, *this volume*, there are modulatory substrates that control rostrad processing of information. Classically, GABA and glycine have been proposed to serve as inhibitory transmitters governing dorsal horn neuron activity by a pre- and postsynaptic action, respectively (12). More recently, we have become aware that increasing monoamine or opiate tone in the spinal cord by means of intrathecal or iontophoretic administration results in an elevation of nociceptive threshold and a reduction of the discharge of nociceptive neurons via mechanisms that are clearly related to the activation of specific receptor systems. The presence of endogenous circuits (i.e., descending monoamine pathways and intrinsic enkephalin-containing cell bodies) suggests that, under certain physiologically defined conditions, the activation of these same endogenous receptor systems would give rise to the activation of these same receptors with the attendent functional consequence (i.e., a modulation of the processing of nociceptive information at the level of the dorsal horn). An essential question is what "naturally" activates these intrinsic pathways.

In a series of experiments, we have used the classic idea that if an agent is a neurotransmitter for a particular neuronal system, increasing activity in that neuronal system will generate increased extracellular levels of that putative transmitter. Using this as a paradigm, we have sought to investigate

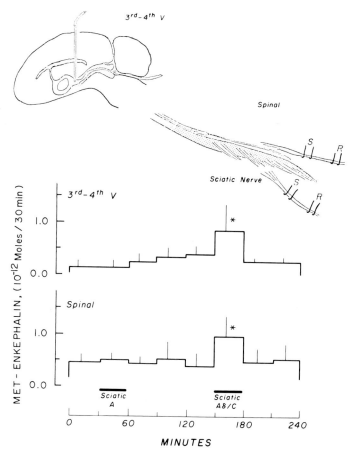

FIG. 5. Methionine-enkephalin-like immunoreactivity levels (met-enkephalin: pм/30 min; mean ± SE; $N = 5$) in ventricular (*top*) and spinal (*bottom*) perfusates. During the interval (*black bar*), stimulation of the sciatic nerves (50 Hz, 1/2 sec, 0.5 msec), as indicated in the top schematic, was carried out. During sample 2, stimulation intensity was low, and evoked a fast conducting compound-action potential at the distal recording electrodes on the sural nerve. During sample 6 (*black bar*), the sciatic nerve was stimulated at a high intensity to evoke an Aβ/Aδ/C fiber compound-action potential. *, $p < 0.05$. Other details of the perfusion are as described in Fig. 4 (36).

the release of serotonin and noradrenaline from the spinal cord, and me-thionine-enkephalin-like immunoreactivity (MELI) from the spinal cord and from the mesencephalic aqueduct—two places where increasing levels of opiate receptor activity are known to produce increases in the pain threshold in a variety of species (41). Using a spinal perfusion procedure, as described basically in Fig. 3, we sought to determine what effects somatic input (sciatic nerve stimulation) would have on the resting levels of these three materials. Figure 5 presents the effects of such stimulation on the release of MELI from the third-aqueductal perfusate and the spinal cord. As can be seen, at low-intensity stimulation of the sciatic nerve associated with Aβ active input, there was no discernible effect on the resting levels of MELI in either brain or cord superfusate. In contrast, increasing the stimulus intensity to include smaller, higher threshold fibers resulted in a highly significant elevation in MELI activity from both brain and cord.

In other experiments, we sought to determine if the release depended on an intact neuraxis. Cold block of the cervical cord attenuated MELI release into the mesencephalic aqueduct, but had no effect on spinal release. This suggested that the spinal enkephalin circuitry is segmentally organized. Further evidence for such segmental organization derived from experiments where stimulation of the infraorbital branch of the trigeminal nerve was observed to have no effect on the levels of enkephalin released from the lumbar spinal cord. In contrast, such stimulation did in fact increase levels of MELI into the mesencephalic aqueductal perfusate. Similar studies carried out with measurements of serotonin and noradrenaline revealed that, as with the release of MELI from the spinal cord, high- but not low-intensity stimulation of the sciatic nerve proved to be the effective stimulus (32). However, in contrast to the release of MELI from the spinal cord, spinal cord block at the cervical level completely antagonized the sciatic nerve-evoked release of these monoamines from the spinal cord.

This suggests that the increased levels of 5-HT and noradrenaline in the lumbar spinal superfusates, secondary to sciatic nerve stimulation, depended on an ascending supraspinal loop. Moreover, unlike MELI release, the release of 5-HT and noradrenaline from the spinal cord could be driven not only by segmental input (sciatic nerve stimulation) but by stimulation of a distal input (i.e., the infraorbital branch of the trigeminal nerve). These two observations suggest that the 5-HT/noradrenaline system is activated in a diffuse fashion by nonsomatotopically organized input. The release of enkephalin from the spinal cord is clearly related to a segmental organization. On the other hand, the release of MELI from the mesencephalic aqueduct is related to a system that receives activation from all somatic input.

FUNCTIONAL SIGNIFICANCE OF REFLEX-ACTIVATED MODULATORY SUBSTRATES

It is interesting to conjecture the significance of the reflex activation of a somatotopically and nonsomatotopically organized modulatory substrate. Under the conditions of a segmentally limited input, one would hypothesize that 5-HT and noradrenaline systems are activated throughout the spinal sensory axis, whereas the MELI system in the spinal cord is only activated in the vicinity of the segmental input. In recent experiments, Wang et al. (35) have demonstrated that the pharmacologic interaction between intrathecally administered α-adrenergic and opiate agonists in the cord is synergistic, that is, that inactive doses of α-adrenergic agonists in conjunction with inactive doses of opiates result in a highly significant analgesia. This synergistic interaction, we believe, is a consequence of the fact that the activation of opiate receptors alters the gain of the rostrad transmission system. Thus it has been shown that morphine will reduce the slope of the cell's response–skin temperature response curve (31).

The interaction between systems that alter gain would be multiplicative and not additive. These data, therefore, suggest that the conjoint activation of a local monoaminergic and opiate synaptic system in the spinal cord would result in a modulatory effect far greater than that which would be achieved if either of the systems were activated alone. Thus, under the conditions of a somatic input, as defined by the activation of a population of afferent fibers having high electrical thresholds, there is the cojoint activation of three modulatory circuits: one segmentally organized and two organized in a non-segmental fashion. The physiologic effects obtained when these receptors are activated in a pharmacologically defined fashion clearly suggests that such input serves to modulate the rostrad transmission of nociceptive information.

It should be noted that simply because the intrathecal administration of these agents produces "analgesia," this does not necessarily imply the natural function of these intrinsic modulatory systems. We suggest that these systems may serve three functions.

1. They reduce the gain of the RTS. The reason for this may have nothing to do with analgesia, but may result from the need to govern the amount of information that is traveling forward in the transmission system. Given that the spinal cord has a limited channel capacity, such a selection system would appear necessary.

2. These modulatory substrates may serve to select the stimulus modality to which a given cell responds. It has been known since the days of Sherrington that in the cerebrate versus the decerebrate spinal animal, there is a bias in the emphasis on proprioceptor versus cutaneous reflex activity. Similarly, in the dorsal horn of the spinal cord, it is known that a wide majority of the sensory neurons are wide dynamic range in character, responding to Aβ, Aδ, and C fiber activation. It is known that stimulation of corticospinal fibers inhibit the Aβ-evoked discharge, leaving the Aδ/C fiber activity intact (7). In contrast, stimulation at many brainstem sites has no effect on the Aβ-evoked discharge in a given cell but completely antagonizes the response to Aδ/C-fiber stimulation (11). In brief, such specificity would result in the creation of modality-specific sensory neurons in the dorsal horn of the spinal cord. It is interesting that much electrophysiology has been carried out on the cerebrate or decerebrate spinal animal, both of which would have a spinal cord whose characteristics are totally unlike those that occurred in the unanesthetized animal.

3. The descending pathways that we have examined have been studied mainly with relevance to the question of nociceptive transmission. It is quite clear, however, that such modulation also has great relevance to autonomic

and motor outflow. Descending pathways are known to terminate in the vicinity of motor horn cells and in the mediolateral columns, and sympathetic outflow has been shown to be sensitive to changes in such descending systems. It is quite likely that, under certain conditions, the activation of high intensity somatic input produces autonomic reflex activity, which is under a driven modulation by these descending pathways (39).

In summary, one cannot discuss the substrate for pain transmission simply as a function of the pathway through which information gains access to the higher perceptual centers. The question of pain is truly one that is described in simplest terms as a function of the outcome of a reflex activation of modulatory systems that alter the content of the sensory message at the first synapse.

ACKNOWLEDGMENTS

We would like to thank Ms. Gail Harty for her assistance in carrying out many of the spinal superfusion experiments, Mrs. Marg Mourning for her expert histologic work, and Ms. Ann Rockafellow for editorial assistance. Work reported in this chapter was supported by grants NS 14629 and NS 16541.

REFERENCES

1. Abay, E. O., and Yaksh, T. L. (1980): Effects of intrathecal capsaicin on thermal, mechanical and chemical nociceptive response in the cat. *Pharmacologist*, 22:204.
2. Barber, R. P., Vaughn, J. E., Slemmon, J. R., Salvaterra, P. M., Roberts, E., and Leeman, S. E. (1979): The origin, distribution and synaptic relationships of substance P axons in rat spinal cord. *J. Comp. Neurol.*, 184:331–352.
3. Barrett, E. F., and Barrett, J. N. (1976): Separation of two voltage-sensitive potassium currents and demonstration of a tetrodotoxin-resistant calcium current in frog motoneurones. *J. Physiol.*, 255:737–774.
4. Chan-Palay, V., Jonsson, G., and Palay, S. L. (1978): Serotonin and substance P coexist in neurons of the rat's central nervous system. *Proc. Natl. Acad. Sci. USA*, 75:1582–1586.
5. Coggeshall, R. E., Coulter, J. D., and Willis, W. D. (1974): Unmyelinated axons in the ventral roots of the cat lumbosacral enlargement. *J. Comp. Neurol.*, 153:39–58.
6. Coggeshall, R. E., and Ito, H. (1977): Sensory fibres in ventral roots L7 and S1 in the cat. *J. Physiol.*, 267:215–235.
7. Coulter, J. D., Foreman, R. D., Beall, J. E., and Willis, W. D. (1976): Cerebral cortical modulation of primate spinothalamic neurons. In: *Advances in Pain Research and Therapy, Vol. 1*, edited by J. J. Bonica and D. Albe-Fessard, pp. 271–277. Raven Press, New York.
8. Cuello, A. C., Emson, P., del Fiacco, M., Gale, J., Iversen, L. L., Jessell, T. M., Kanazawa, I., Paxinos, G., and Quik, M. (1977): Distribution and release of substance P in the central nervous system. In: *Centrally Acting Peptides*, edited by J. Hughes. Macmillan, London.
9. Dobry, P. J. K., Piercey, M. F., and Schroeder, L. A. (1980): Pharmacological characterization of reciprocal hindlimb scratching induced by intracranial substance P. *Neuroscience (Abst.)*, 6:621.
10. Duffy, M. J., Mulhall, D., and Powell, D. (1975): Subcellular distribution of substance P in bovine hypothalamus and substantia nigra. *J. Neurochem.*, 25:305–307.
11. Fields, H. L., and Basbaum, A. I. (1978): Brainstem control of spinal pain transmission neurons. *Annu. Rev. Physiol.*, 40:193–221.

12. Game, C. J. A., and Lodge, D. (1975): The pharmacology of the inhibition of dorsal horn neurones by impulses in myelinated cutaneous afferents in the cat. *Exp. Brain Res.*, 23:75–84.

13. Gamse, R., Molnar, A., and Lembeck, F. (1979): Substance P release from spinal cord slices by capsaicin. *Life Sci.*, 25:625–636.

14. Henry, J. L. (1976): Effects of substance P on functionally identified units in cat spinal cord. *Brain Res.*, 114:439–451.

15. Hökfelt, T., Johansson, O., Ljungdahl, Å., Lundberg, J. M., and Schultzberg, M. (1980): Peptidergic neurons. *Nature*, 284:515–521.

16. Hökfelt, T., Kellerth, J.-O., Nilsson, G., and Pernow, B. (1975): Experimental immuno-histochemical studies on the localization and distribution of substance P in cat primary sensory neurons. *Brain Res.*, 100:235–252.

17. Hökfelt, T., Ljungdahl, Å., Steinbusch, H., Verhofstad, A., Nilsson, G., Brodin, E., Pernow, B., and Goldstein, M. (1978): Immunohistochemical evidence of substance P-like immunoreactivity in some 5-hydroxytryptamine-containing neurons in the rat central nervous system. *Neuroscience*, 3:517–538.

18. Hylden, J. L. K., and Wilcox, G. L. (1981): Intrathecal substance P elicits a caudally directed biting and scratching behavior in mice. *Brain Res.*, 217:212–215.

19. Jancsó, G., Kiraly, E., and Jancso-Gabor, A. (1977): Pharmacologically induced selective degeneration of chemosensitive primary sensory neurons. *Nature*, 270:741–743.

20. Jessell, T. M., and Iversen, L. L. (1977): Opiate analgesics inhibit substance P release from rat trigeminal nucleus. *Nature*, 268:549–551.

21. Jessell, T. M., Iversen, L. L., and Cuello, A. C. (1978): Capsaicin induced depletion of substance P from primary sensory neurones. *Brain Res.*, 152:183–188.

22. Mendell, L. M., and Wall, P. D. (1965): Response of single dorsal horn cells to peripheral cutaneous unmyelinated fibres. *Nature*, 206:97–99.

23. Nagy, J. I., Vincent, S. R., Staines, W. A., Fibiger, H. C., Reisine, T. O., and Yamamura, H. J. (1980): Neurotoxic action of capsaicin on spinal substance P neurons. *Brain Res.*, 186:435–444.

24. Otsuka, M., and Konishi, S. (1976): Release of substance P-like immunoreactivity from isolated spinal cord of newborn rats. *Nature*, 264:83–84.

25. Pickel, V. M., Reis, D. J., and Leeman, S. E. (1977): Ultrastructural localization of substance P in neurones of rat spinal cord. *Brain Res.*, 122:534–540.

26. Price, D. D., and Browe, A. C. (1975): Spinal cord coding of graded non-noxious and noxious temperature increases. *Exp. Neurol.*, 48:201–221.

27. Price, D. D., and Dubner, R. (1977): Neurons that subserve the sensory-discriminative aspects of pain. *Pain*, 3:307–338.

28. Steinacker, A. (1977): Calcium-dependent presynaptic action of substance P at the frog neuromuscular junction. *Nature*, 267:268–270.

29. Szolcsanyi, J. (1977): A pharmacological approach to elucidation of the role of different nerve fibres and receptor endings in mediation of pain. *J. Physiol. (Paris)*, 73:251–259.

30. Theriault, E., Otsuka, M., and Jessell, T. M. (1979): Capsaicin-evoked release of substance P from primary sensory neurons. *Brain Res.*, 170:209–213.

31. Toyooka, H., Kitahata, L. M., Dohi, S., Ohtani, M., Hanaoka, K., and Taub, A. (1978): Effect of morphine on the rexed lamina VII spinal neuronal response to graded radiant heat stimulation. *Exp. Neurol.*, 62:146–158.

32. Tyce, G. M., and Yaksh, T. L. (1981): Monoamine release from cat spinal cord by somatic stimuli: an intrinsic modulatory system. *J. Physiol. (Lond.)*, 314:513–529.

33. Vallbo, Å. B., Hagbarth, K.-E., Torebjörk, H. E., and Wallin, B. G. (1979): Somatosensory, proprioceptive, and sympathetic activity in human peripheral nerves. *Physiol. Rev.*, 59:919–957.

34. Wall, P. D. (1967): The laminar organization of dorsal horn and effects of descending impulses. *J. Physiol. (Lond.)*, 188:403–423.

35. Wang, J.-Y., Yasuoka, S., and Yaksh, T. L. (1980): Studies on the analgetic effect of intrathecal ST-91 (2-[2,6-diethyl-phenylamino]-2-imidazoline): Antagonism, tolerance and interaction with morphine. *Pharmacologist (Abst.)*, 22:302.

36. Yaksh, T. L., and Elde, R. P. (1981): Factors governing the release of methionine enkephalin-like immunoreactivity from the mesencephalon and spinal cord of the cat *in vivo*. *J. Neurophysiol.*, 46:1056–1075.

37. Yaksh, T. L., Farb, D., Leeman, S., and Jessell, T. (1979): Intrathecal capsaicin depletes substance P in the rat spinal cord and produces prolonged thermal analgesia. *Science,* 206:481–483.
38. Yaksh, T. L., and Hammond, D. L. (1982): Peripheral and central substrates involved in the rostrad transmission of nociceptive information. *Pain,* 13:1–85.
39. Yaksh, T. L., Hammond, D. L., and Tyce, G. M. (1981): Functional aspects of bulbospinal monoaminergic projections: Role in modulating processing of somatosensory information. *Fed. Proc.,* 40:2786–2794.
40. Yaksh, T. L., Jessell, T. M., Gamse, R., Mudge, A. W., and Leeman, S. E. (1980): Intrathecal morphine inhibits substance P release from mammalian spinal cord *in vivo. Nature,* 286:155–156.
41. Yaksh, T. L., and Rudy, T. A. (1978): Narcotic analgesics: CNS sites and mechanisms of action as revealed by intracerebral injection techniques. *Pain,* 4:299–359.
42. Zieglgansberger, W., and Tulloch, I. F. (1979): Effect of substance P on neurones in the dorsal horn of the spinal cord of the cat. *Brain Res.,* 166:273–282.

*Advances in Pain Research
and Therapy, Vol. 7,*
edited by C. Benedetti et al.
Raven Press, New York © 1984.

Endogenous Pain Inhibitory Substrates and Mechanisms

Gregory W. Terman, James W. Lewis, and
John C. Liebeskind

*Department of Psychology, University of California, Los Angeles,
California 90024*

The last decade and a half of pain research has provided much evidence for the existence of intrinsic pain suppressive systems operating by activation of descending controls from brainstem to spinal cord. We will briefly review the literature supporting this hypothesis and summarize work investigating the activation and function of such endogenous pain inhibitory systems.

ACTIVATION OF ANALGESIA SYSTEMS BY ELECTRICAL STIMULATION AND OPIATE ADMINISTRATION

The first concrete evidence for the existence of endogenous pain inhibitory systems came from reports that electrical stimulation of the medial brainstem caused potent analgesia (56,69). This finding has since been replicated and extended numerous times in the rat (e.g., 53), cat (e.g., 49), monkey (e.g., 25), and in humans (e.g., 30,70). Stimulation-produced analgesia (SPA) has, for example, been found capable of completely inhibiting behavioral responses to numerous noxious somatic and visceral stimuli, including electric shocks applied to the tooth pulp (63) and limbs (56), heating of the skin (53), subcutaneous injections of formalin (58), intraperitoneal injections of hypertonic saline (22), and acute distension of the appendix (R. L. Nahin, *in preparation*). Mayer et al. (56) found that this reduction in pain responsiveness was regularly associated with neither motor dysfunction nor diminished sensory capacity in other than the nociceptive modality. In a particularly clear demonstration of this point, Oliveras et al. (63) showed that whereas the jaw opening reflex to noxious tooth pulp stimulation was suppressed by brain stimulation, a similar jaw opening response to innocuous tooth tap was not affected. The specificity of SPA in blocking responses to noxious stimuli also has been observed electrophysiologically in recordings from brain and spinal neurons (60,61).

43

This analgetic specificity was reminiscent of the relatively specific pain-suppressing effects of opiate drugs and suggested that SPA might share sites and/or mechanisms of action with opiate analgesia (56). This hypothesis was supported by reports that the same periaqueductal region that yields profound SPA also is exquisitely sensitive to morphine (34,73). Mapping studies have since shown that many brain sites support both SPA and morphine analgesia (54,92). In addition to sharing common sites of action, stimulation-produced and opiate analgesia have been associated in a number of other ways. For example, it has been shown that repeated brainstem stimulation manifests analgetic tolerance (52). Also, animals made tolerant to morphine showed reduced SPA, or cross-tolerance, again suggesting that SPA and opiate analgesia are mediated by a common receptor.

Lesions of the dorsolateral funiculus (DLF) of the spinal cord block both SPA and morphine analgesia, attesting to the critical importance of this descending path connecting the medial brainstem to the spinal dorsal horn (7). Opioid peptides and their receptors are well situated in the nervous system to function in a natural pain inhibitory system (37,76,78). They are found, among other places, in those brain regions where SPA and opiate microinjections appear to work best. They also are found in the DLF (60a,75) and spinal dorsal horn (18,29,75). Injections of small amounts of opioid peptides into many of these areas can cause significant increases in pain thresholds (8,84). Direct measures of endogenous opioids indicate that these substances are released by analgesic brain stimulation in humans (4,31).

Probably the most salient finding associating the mechanisms of stimulation-produced and opiate analgesic action was the demonstration that the opiate-antagonist drug, naloxone, significantly reduced SPA in the rat (2,3). This observation suggested that SPA and opiate drugs share a common receptor site, presumably the opiate receptor (3). Although some authors were unable to replicate this finding (e.g., 65,93), others were successful (e.g., 30,62).

Recent work from our laboratory seems to resolve these discrepancies. We find that, whereas SPA can be elicited equally well from dorsal and ventral parts of the rat's periaqueductal gray matter, only SPA from ventral stimulation sites in the dorsal raphe and subjacent tegmentum is antagonized by naloxone (14). Moreover, even very low doses of the drug (5 μg via the intraperitoneal route) significantly reduce SPA from these naloxone-sensitive placements, suggesting antagonistic action at a high-affinity receptor site. This localization of adjacent naloxone-sensitive and naloxone-insensitive SPA regions in the rat midbrain may explain both the failure of some investigators to obtain naloxone-reducible SPA and the curious observation that even SPA that is naloxone-sensitive is only partially reduced by the drug. That anatomically distinct opioid and nonopioid mechanisms of SPA exist was further supported by recent findings (68), indicating that bulbar raphe lesions disrupt only naloxone-sensitive SPA. It seems, then, that not one but multiple intrinsic analgesia systems exist, some opioid-mediated and some not. In the rest of this chapter, we will discuss other lines of evidence supporting this hypothesis.

STRESS MAY BE A NATURAL ACTIVATOR FOR PAIN INHIBITORY SYSTEMS

Even if one accepts the existence of one or more intrinsic analgesia systems within the brain and spinal cord, the important question still remains: Under what circumstances are such systems adaptively activated? Because noxious stimuli provide important warning signals that often lead to adaptive behaviors, an endogenous analgesia substrate should not be easily activated. On the other hand, it was reasoned (48) that, under conditions of dire emergency, the perception of pain might disrupt effective coping behavior, giving pain suppression the greater survival value.

The analgesic effect of various stressors lends credence to the view that stress is a natural or physiologic trigger for activating intrinsic pain-suppressive mechanisms. Akil et al. (1) and Hayes et al. (27) were the first to demonstrate that stress caused potent analgesia in the rat. Their findings were different, however, in that the analgesia studied by Akil et al. (1) was blocked by naloxone, whereas that studied by Hayes et al. (27,28) was not. Subsequent studies by these and other investigators (e.g., 5,6,10,15) did little to resolve this matter, and the use of diverse stressors and parameters of stress administration further complicated the issue and made comparisons among these studies difficult.

Our recent work has helped to clarify these discrepant findings. Using a single, constant-intensity stressor—inescapable footshock—we found that by varying only its temporal parameters, two equipotent forms of analgesia could be produced differing in their anatomic and neurochemical bases. Thus, for example, analgesia produced by brief (3 min), continuous footshock (2.5 mA, 60 Hz) was found to be resistant to naloxone, whereas analgesia produced by prolonged (20 min), intermittent (1 sec on every 5 sec) footshock of the same intensity was significantly attenuated by this drug (16). Thus stress certainly appears to activate intrinsic analgesia systems of the brain. Whether opioid or nonopioid systems are called into play depends, at least in part, on temporal characteristics of the stressor.

Subsequent work confirmed the existence of separate opioid and nonopioid stress analgesia systems by applying criteria other than naloxone antagonism. It was found that, with repeated exposure to footshock, tolerance developed to only the naloxone-sensitive (opioid) form of stress analgesia (44). Similarly, rats made tolerant to morphine demonstrated cross-tolerance to the opioid, but not nonopioid, stress analgesia. Repeated exposure to either footshock procedure failed to affect the animal's analgesic response to the other (82). This complete lack of cross-tolerance between the two stress paradigms points to the specificity of the tolerance phenomenon and further confirms the discrete nature of opioid and nonopioid stress analgesia systems.

Work by other investigators also supports the existence of separate opioid and nonopioid systems underlying stress analgesia and shows that such systems can be activated differentially as a function of which body region is shocked (88) and how many shocks are applied (26).

NEUROCHEMISTRY AND NEUROANATOMY OF STRESS ANALGESIA

Having determined the existence of both opioid and nonopioid forms of stress analgesia, we sought to characterize more fully their neurohumoral and neuroanatomic bases. Because the pituitary–adrenal axis has long been recognized for its role in adaptive responses to stress, and because pain suppression can be viewed as just such an adaptive response, the participation of this hormonal system in stress analgesia was studied. Because stress causes the release of beta-endorphin from the pituitary (71), we began by examining the effect of hypophysectomy on opioid and nonopioid stress analgesia. We found hypophysectomy attenuated only the naloxone-sensitive form (43). Still, it is well known that removal of the pituitary can compromise the function of both the adrenal medulla and cortex (66). Thus the effect of hypophysectomy on naloxone-sensitive stress analgesia might be due principally to a reduction in adrenal function. Indeed, as the adrenal medulla is known to contain enkephalin-like peptides and to secrete them in response to sympathetic activation (e.g., 77,85,94), we were particularly interested in its role in stress analgesia.

We next showed (47) that adrenalectomy, adrenal demedullation, and adrenal medullary denervation (celiac ganglionectomy) all cause profound blockade of opioid, but not nonopioid, stress analgesia. Because demedullation and ganglionectomy had as great an effect as removal of the entire adrenal gland, because the three adrenal surgeries had a greater effect on stress analgesia than did hypophysectomy, and because all of these procedures affected only that form of stress analgesia sensitive to naloxone, we concluded that these effects resulted from a reduction in enkephalin-like peptides of the adrenal medulla (47). In support of this view, we also found that the peripherally acting ganglionic blocking agent, hexamethonium, which reduces adrenal enkephalin secretion *in vitro* (86), attenuated opioid stress analgesia (47).

Biochemical evidence for a role of adrenal enkephalins in this type of stress analgesia also was gathered. The opioid, but not nonopioid, stress analgesia depleted opiate-like material in the adrenal medulla (46). Finally, we found that a dose of reserpine that increases the adrenal content of enkephalins and its stimulation-induced release (46,86) significantly augmented opioid stress analgesia while actually diminishing stress analgesia of the nonopioid form (47,79). Although these experiments give evidence for a peripheral source of opioids involved in opioid stress analgesia, the locus of the opiate receptor mediating this analgesia has yet to be determined. These findings in no way preclude the possibility that opioids of central origin also play an important part in stress analgesia. In fact, several groups have been able to observe changes in central opioid activity correlated with opioid stress analgesia (41,51,72).

We went on to investigate the role of neurohumors other than opioids in the mechanisms of stress analgesia. We recently reported that administration of the muscarinic cholinergic antagonist, scopolamine, but not centrally in- active methylscopolamine, reduces naloxone-sensitive but not naloxone-in- sensitive stress analgesia (40). This observation parallels anatomic evidence for the presence of muscarinic receptors in parts of the midbrain and spinal cord involved in pain modulation (87). We and others also have shown that oxotremorine, a potent muscarinic agonist, causes analgesia sensitive to opiate-antagonist blockade (32,40). Perhaps the binding of acetylcholine to certain central muscarinic receptors stimulates the release of opioid peptides involved in stress analgesia.

Although the foregoing studies have helped to define several important mediators of opioid stress analgesia, they have not similarly elucidated the neurochemistry of stress analgesia of the nonopioid sort. Because nonopioid stress analgesia manifests neither tolerance nor cross-tolerance to morphine, and therefore activating this sytem should not cause many of the undesirable effects of opiate analgesia, better characterization of the nonopioid analgesia substrate might have important clinical significance.

Recently, a role for the biogenic amine, histamine, in nonopioid stress analgesia has been suggested. We have reported that whereas nonopioid stress analgesia is unaffected by numerous drugs, including serotonin, do- pamine, and norepinephrine depletors, and receptor antagonists, and agon- ists, it is significantly reduced by the H_1 histamine receptor antagonist, di- phenhydramine (80). This effect appears to be receptor-specific in that the H_2 histamine receptor antagonist, cimetidine, did not have this effect (G. W. Terman, Y. Shavit, J. W. Lewis, J. T. Cannon, and J. C. Liebeskind, *in preparation*). The histidine decarboxylase inhibitor, alpha-fluoromethyl- histidine, disrupts histamine synthesis (36) and thus depletes this putative neurotransmitter (21). This drug significantly reduces nonopioid stress an- algesia (81). Its effect appears to be due to depletion of neuronal histamine because it is these stores that initially are affected by alpha-fluoromethyl- histidine (21) and because depletion of nonneural histamine stores by the mast cell degranulator, compound 48/80, had no effect on stress analgesia whatsoever. That neuronal histamine might be a mediator of nonopioid stress analgesia is an intriguing hypothesis requiring further investigation. Studies indicating that antihistamines potentiate morphine analgesia (12) and that histamine exerts an analgesic action on its own (23) give further impetus for this line of research.

Attempts to characterize the neuroanatomic substrates of opioid and non-opioid stress analgesia also have begun. Because of the importance of descending bulbospinal pathways, particularly the DLF, in morphine analgesia and SPA (19), the role of the DLF in opioid and nonopioid stress analgesia was investigated. Both forms of stress analgesia were reduced significantly by lesions of the DLF, although the opioid form appeared to be most affected (45). Similar findings were reported by Watkins et al. (89), studying their forms of opioid and nonopioid footshock-induced analgesia. These studies suggest the importance of descending influences in both opioid and nonopioid stress analgesia, similar to that seen in SPA and morphine analgesia.

The nucleus raphe magnus (NRM), whose neurons contribute importantly to the DLF, also plays a role in stress analgesia. Lesions of this nucleus reduce nonopioid, but not opioid, stress analgesia (13). Although additional studies are required to delineate more precisely which cell groups within the NRM are responsible for this effect, these findings nonetheless emphasize once again the separateness of the substrates mediating the analgesias activated by brief, continuous and prolonged, intermittent exposure to the same footshock stressor.

DEMONSTRATION OF TWO DISCRETE FORMS OF OPIOID-MEDIATED STRESS ANALGESIA

Our most recent studies (83; G. W. Terman et al., *in preparation*) are showing that even the analgesia produced by exposure to brief, continuous footshock is not a unitary phenomenon. We find that 2.5 mA of continuous footshock applied for 1 to 2 min elicits an analgesic effect greatly attenuated by pretreatment with either naloxone or the long-lasting opiate antagonist, naltrexone. By contrast, exposure to 4 to 5 min of the same footshock produces an equipotent analgesia insensitive to these drugs. Three minutes of continuous footshock at 2.5 mA, parameters previously seen to elicit nonopioid stress analgesia according to several criteria (39,44), seem, on reinspection, to yield stress analgesia that is neither purely opioid nor purely nonopioid in nature. In subsequent studies, we have used 1 and 4 min of continuous footshock as the shortest-duration stress parameters capable of producing significant and equipotent opioid and nonopioid analgesia, respectively.

Analgesia caused by 1 min of continuous footshock stress has been found to satisfy several additional criteria for opioid mediation. For example, although even high doses of an opiate antagonist had no effect on the analgesia elicited by 4 min of continuous footshock, as little as 0.1 mg/kg of naloxone significantly reduced analgesia from 1 min of footshock stress (83). Moreover, like the opioid-mediated analgesia produced by 20 min of intermittent footshock, analgesia produced by 1 min of continuous footshock was found to tolerate with repeated administration (14 days) and to show cross-tolerance with morphine. The analgesia elicited by 4 min of footshock, which was not blocked by an opiate antagonist, manifested neither tolerance nor cross-tolerance with morphine.

Cross-tolerance experiments between stressors also have been carried out. Animals given 14 daily sessions of the 4-min footshock (nonopioid paradigm) showed normal analgesia when administered either of the opioid stress analgesia paradigms (1 min continuous or 20 min intermittent). Animals receiving either of the opioid analgesia paradigms for 14 days showed cross-tolerance to the other opioid stress analgesia procedure, although analgesic responsivenss to the nonopioid form of stress remained unaffected.

Opioid stress analgesia, then, can be provoked by two paradigms of footshock stress differing only in their temporal parameters. Our most recent studies show that the neurohumoral mechanisms underlying these two opioid stress analgesias are quite different (G. W. Terman et al., *in preparation*). We first observed that the opioid and nonopioid forms of stress analgesia deriving from continuous footshock were unaffected by even a surgical level of pentobarbital anesthesia (55 mg/kg). No differences between awake and anesthetized animals were seen in either baseline or poststress tail-flick latencies. On the other hand, anesthesia completely eliminated the analgesic effect of 20 min of intermittent footshock stress (35), signaling a distinct difference between the two opioid stress analgesias. In other experiments, we have shown that hypophysectomy and adrenalectomy disrupt the 20-min intermittent, but not the 1-min continuous, form of opioid stress analgesia (G. W. Terman et al., *in preparation*). Similarly, we find that scopolamine reduces the analgesic effect of the 20-min, but not the 1-min, footshock stress.

We have demonstrated, then, that at least three different forms of stress analgesia can be produced by varying the temporal parameters of a single stressor, inescapable footshock. Two of these forms can be reduced by opiate antagonists, show tolerance with repetition and cross-tolerance both with morphine and each other, and therefore are considered opioid-mediated. A third form of stress analgesia demonstrating none of these characteristics is designated nonopioid. The two opioid-mediated stress analgesias differ in that only one is blocked by anesthesia, hypophysectomy, adrenalectomy, and a central muscarinic cholinergic antagonist. Both hormonally and nonhormonally mediated forms of opioid stress analgesia have been reported by others. For example, MacLennan et al. (50) have shown that their form of opioid stress analgesia relies on the adrenal cortex, whereas that studied by Watkins et al. (90) and Watkins and Mayer (91) is independent of the pituitary–adrenal axis. The fact that the former is caused by relatively long-duration intermittent stress and the latter by short-duration continuous stress suggests an obvious parallel to our results.

PROPERTIES OF STRESS THAT DIFFERENTIALLY PRODUCE DISCRETE FORMS OF STRESS ANALGESIA

Experiments investigating the underlying pharmacology and anatomy of these three discrete forms of stress analgesia are continuing in our laboratory. We are particularly interested in studying the role of histamine and the DLF in the opioid and nonopioid forms of continuous footshock-induced analgesia. Equally important, however, may be the question of what specific properties of footshock activate these different analgesia systems. As previously noted, evidence exists that activation of opioid and nonopioid stress analgesia mechanisms depends on the anatomic location of stress administration (88), the number of stressful episodes administered (26), and the temporal parameters of the stressor (39). In further parametric evaluation of stress analgesia from continuous footshock, we now find (83a) that, holding the duration of footshock constant at 3 min, the opioid or nonopioid nature of the analgesic effect is determined by the level of current administered. Lower currents (1.5 and 2.0 mA) were found to produce naltrexone-sensitive analgesia; higher currents (3.0 and 3.5 mA) produced analgesia insensitive to naltrexone treatment. The 2.5 mA-intensity value used in most of our previous work (e.g., 44) seems to provide neither a purely opioid nor purely nonopioid analgesia, much as 3 min of footshock at 2.5 mA seems in between more purely opioid (1–2 min) and nonopioid (4–5 min) temporal parameters.

In summary, we see that small increments in either intensity or duration of continuous footshock cause a complete shift from opioid to nonopioid mediation. It is intriguing that merely adding 1 mA or 2 min to the footshock yielding clearly opioid analgesia provokes a type of analgesia totally unaffected by an opiate antagonist, by footshock repetition, or by prior exposure to morphine. It must be noted, however, that variations in intensity and duration are not the sole determinants of the opioid or nonopioid nature of footshock stress analgesia. For example, by using the same total amount of footshock as that causing nonopioid analgesia (2.5 mA for 4 min), but applying it intermittently (on 1 sec of every 5 sec) for 20 min rather than continuously, an opioid form of analgesia is elicited.

SUMMARY AND CONCLUSIONS

Reports that electrical stimulation of the brainstem produced potent analgesia first suggested the existence of opioid and nonopioid pain-inhibitory systems within the central nervous system (14,56). Subsequent investigations of stress analgesia began in an attempt to find the natural activation of these intrinsic analgesia substrates. It is noteworthy, therefore, that experiments on stress analgesia are now beginning to interdigitate closely with and complement the parent series of SPA investigations. Opioid and non-opioid substrates of SPA appear to coexist in close proximity to one another in ventral and dorsal areas of the rat's periaqueductal gray matter, respectively (14). We now find that repeated exposure to either the 1- or 20-min form of opioid stress analgesia causes a significant attenuation in SPA (cross-tolerance) for the opioid (ventral), but not nonopioid (dorsal), SPA placements (64). The same exposure to nonopioid stress analgesia has no such effect. These findings support the view that opioid forms of stress analgesia and SPA share a common underlying mechanism of action.

Studies of footshock stress analgesia have proven useful as a precise, reliable, and controllable probe for elucidating anatomic substrates, neurochemical mechanisms, and environmental activators of endogenous pain-inhibitory systems within the brain and spinal cord. We have seen, for example, that even small variations in footshock parameters can shift dramatically the neurochemical and neuroanatomic foundations of stress analgesia. Clearly, we still know very little about how pain-suppressing systems are activated. Some evidence has emerged that opioid peptides are released tonically (9,33), at least during certain hours of the day (20). Still, it is widely held that such tonic release is at best minimal, and that opioids active in pain suppression are released principally in a phasic manner, triggered by specific internal or external events (42,74).

Stress analgesia studies may prove heuristic in suggesting conditions under which stress activates opioid or nonopioid substrates of pain inhibition. Although inescapable footshock merely models the stressors animals might normally encounter in nature, studies suggesting that more natural stressors such as sexual arousal (17), fighting (59), and food deprivation (11,57) also can activate opioid and nonopioid analgesic mechanisms suggest the validity of this model. Moreover, stress analgesia studies may ultimately have clinical relevance as well. Although production of analgesia by exposure to stressors probably is not itself clinically applicable, investigation of the stimuli sufficient for activating endogenous pain-suppressing systems may lead to a better understanding of reportedly opioid-mediated therapeutic techniques such as acupuncture and placebo analgesia (e.g., 38,55,67) and nonopioid phenomena such as hypnotic analgesia (24,55). Obviously, the ability to activate selectively and noninvasively the intrinsic analgesia systems of the body would have important clinical implications for the control of pain.

ACKNOWLEDGMENTS

Our work is supported by NIH grant NSO7628 and a gift from the Brotman Foundation. We are grateful to Merck, Sharp and Dohme for the gift of alpha-fluoromethylhistadine and Endo Laboratories for the gift of naloxone and naltrexone. We thank Ms. Sabrina Hulsey for her help in preparing this manuscript.

REFERENCES

1. Akil, H., Madden, J., Patrick, R. L., and Barchas, J. D. (1976): Stress-induced increase in endogenous opiate peptides: Concurrent analgesia and its partial reversal by naloxone. In: *Opiates and Endogenous Opioid Peptides*, edited by H. W. Kosterlitz, pp. 63–70. Elsevier, Amsterdam.
2. Akil, H., Mayer, D. J., and Liebeskind, J. C. (1972): Comparaison chez le rat entre l'analgesie induite par stimulation de la substance grise peri-aqueducale et l'analgesie morphinique. *C. R. Acad. Sci. (Paris)*, 274:3603–3605.
3. Akil, H., Mayer, D. J., and Liebeskind, J. C. (1976): Antagonism of stimulation-produced analgesia by naloxone, a narcotic antagonist. *Science*, 191:961–962.
4. Akil, H., Richardson, D. E., Barchas, J. D., and Li, C. H. (1978): Appearance of beta-endorphin-like immunoreactivity in human ventricular cerebrospinal fluid upon analgesic electrical stimulation. *Proc. Natl. Acad. Sci. USA*, 75:5170–5172.
5. Akil, H., Watson, S. J., Berger, P. A., and Barchas, J. D. (1978): Endorphins, beta-LPH, and ACTH: Biochemical, pharmacological, and anatomical studies. In: *The Endorphins*, edited by E. Costa and M. Trabucchi, pp. 125–140. Raven Press, New York.
6. Amir, S., and Amit, Z. (1978): Endogenous opioid ligands may mediate stress-induced changes in the affective properties of pain related behavior in rats. *Life Sci.*, 23:1143–1152.
7. Basbaum, A. I., Marley, N. J., O'Keefe, J., and Clanton, C. H. (1977): Reversal of morphine and stimulus produced analgesia by subtotal spinal cord lesions. *Pain.*, 3:43–56.
8. Belluzzi, J. D., Grant, N., Garsky, V., Sarantakis, D., Wise, C. D., and Stein, L. (1976): Analgesia induced in vivo by central administration of enkephalin in rat. *Nature*, 260:625–626.
9. Berntson, G. G., and Walker, J. M. (1977): Effect of opiate receptor blockade on pain sensitivity in the rat. *Brain Res. Bull.*, 2:157–159.
10. Bodnar, R. J., Kelly, D. D., Spiaggia, A., Ehrenberg, C., and Glusman, M. (1978): Dose-dependent reductions by naloxone of analgesia induced by cold-water stress. *Pharmacol. Biochem. Behav.*, 8:667–672.
11. Bodnar, R. J., Kelly, D. D., Spiaggia, A., and Glusman, M. (1978): Biphasic alterations of nociceptive thresholds induced by food deprivation. *Physiol. Psych.*, 6:391–395.
12. Bluhme, R., Zsigmond, E. K., and Winnie, A. P. (1982): Potentiation of opioid analgesia by H_1 and H_2 antagonists. *Life Sci.*, 31:1229–1232.
13. Cannon, J. T., Lewis, J. W., Weinberg, V. E., and Liebeskind, J. C. (1983): Evidence for the independence of brain stem mechanisms mediating analgesia induced by morphine and two forms of stress. *Brain Res.*, 269:231–236.
14. Cannon, J. T., Prieto, G. J., Lee, A., and Liebeskind, J. C. (1982): Evidence for opioid and nonopioid forms of stimulation-produced analgesia in the rat. *Brain Res.*, 243:315–321.
15. Chance, W. T. and Rosecrans, J. A. (1979): Lack of effect of naloxone on autoanalgesia. *Pharmacol. Biochem. Behav.*, 11:643–646.
16. Chesher, G. B., and Chan, B. (1977): Footshock induced analgesia in mice: Its reversal by naloxone and cross-tolerance with morphine. *Life Sci.*, 21:1569–1574.
17. Crowley, W. R., Rodriguez-Sierra, J. F., and Komisaruk, B. R. (1977): Analgesia induced by vaginal stimulation in rats is apparently independent of a morphine-sensitive process. *Psychopharmacology (Berlin)*, 54:223–225.
18. Elde, R., Hokfelt, T., Johansson, O., and Terenius, L. (1976): Immunohistochemical studies using antibodies to leucine-enkephalin: Initial observations on the nervous system of the rat. *Neuroscience*, 1:349–351.
19. Fields, H. L., and Basbaum, A. I. (1979): Anatomy and physiology of a descending pain control system. In: *Advances in Pain Research and Therapy, Vol. 3.*, edited by J. J. Bonica, J. C. Liebeskind, and D. G. Albe-Fessard, pp. 427–440. Raven Press, New York.
20. Frederickson, R. C. A., Burgis, D., and Edwards, J. D. (1977): Hyperalgesia induced by naloxone follows diurnal rhythm in responsivity to painful stimuli. *Science*, 198:756–759.
21. Garbarg, M., Barbin, G., Rodergas, E., and Schwartz, J. C. (1980): Inhibition of histamine synthesis in brain by alpha-methylhistidine, a new irreversible inhibitor: In vitro and in vivo studies. *J. Neurochem.*, 35:1045–1052.
22. Giesler, G. J., Jr., and Liebeskind, J. C. (1976): Inhibition of visceral pain by electrical stimulation of the periaqueductal gray matter. *Pain*, 2:43–48.

23. Glick, S., and Crane, L. A. (1978): Opiate-like and abstinence-like effects of intracerebral histamine administration in rats. *Nature,* 273:547–549.
24. Goldstein, A., and Hilgard, E. R. (1975): Lack of influence of the morphine antagonist naloxone on hypnotic analgesia. *Proc. Natl. Acad. Sci. USA,* 72:2041–2043.
25. Goodman, S. J., and Holcombe, V. (1976): Selective and prolonged analgesia in monkey resulting from brain stimulation. In: *Advances in Pain Research and Therapy, Vol. 1,* edited by J. J. Bonica and D. Albe-Fessard, pp. 495–502. Raven Press, New York.
26. Grau, J. W., Hyson, R. L., Maier, S. F., Madden, J., IV, and Barchas, J. D. (1981): Long-term stress-induced analgesia and activation of the opiate system. *Science,* 213:1409–1410.
27. Hayes, R. L., Bennett, G. J., Newlon, P. G., and Mayer, D. J. (1976): Analgesic effects of certain noxious and stressful manipulations in the rat. *Soc. Neurosci. Abstr.,* 2:939.
28. Hayes, R. L., Bennett, G. J., Newlon, P. G., and Mayer, D. J. (1978): Behavioral and physiological studies of non-narcotic analgesia in the rat elicited by certain environmental stimuli. *Brain Res.,* 155:69–90.
29. Hokfelt, T., Ljungdahl, A., Terenius, L., Elde, R., and Nilson, G. (1977): Immunohisto-chemical analysis of peptide pathways possibly related to pain and analgesia: Enkephalin and substance P. *Proc. Natl. Acad. Sci. USA,* 74:3081–3085.
30. Hosobuchi, Y., Adams, J. E., and Linchitz, R. (1977): Pain relief by electrical stimulation of the central gray matter in humans and its reversal by naloxone. *Science,* 197:183–186.
31. Hosobuchi, Y., Rossier, J., Bloom, F. E., and Guillemin, R. (1979): Stimulation of human periaqueductal gray for pain relief increases immunoreactive beta-endorphin in ventricular fluid. *Science,* 203:279–281.
32. Howes, J. F., Harris, L. S., Dewey, W. L., and Voyda, C. (1969): Brain acetylcholine levels and inhibition of the tail-flick reflex in mice. *J. Pharmacol. Exp. Ther.,* 169:23–28.
33. Jacob, J. J., Tremblay, E. C., and Colombel, M. C. (1974): Facilitation de reactions nociceptives par la naloxone chez la souris et chez le rat. *Psychopharmacologie,* 37:217–223.
34. Jacquet, Y. F., and Lajtha, A. (1974): Paradoxical effects after microinjection of morphine in the periaqueductal grey matter in the rat. *Science,* 185:1055–1057.
35. Jensen, T. S., and Smith, D. F. (1981): The role of consciousness in stress-induced analgesia. *J. Neural Trans.,* 52:55–60.
36. Kollonitsch, J., Patchett, A. A., Marburg, S., Maycock, A. L., Perkins, L. M., Doldouras, G. A., Duggan, D. E., and Aster, S. D. (1978): Selective inhibitors of biosynthesis of aminergic neurotransmitters. *Nature,* 274:906–908.
37. Kosterlitz, H. W., and Hughes, J. (1978): Development of the concepts of opiate receptors and their ligands. In: *The Endorphins,* edited by E. Costa and M. Trabucchi, pp. 31–44. Raven Press, New York.
38. Levine, J. D., Gordon, N. C., and Fields, H. L. (1978): The mechanism of placebo analgesia. *Lancet,* 2:654–657.
39. Lewis, J. W., Cannon, J. T., and Liebeskind, J. C. (1980): Opioid and nonopioid mechanisms of stress analgesia. *Science,* 208:623–625.
40. Lewis, J. W., Cannon, J. T., and Liebeskind, J. C. (1983): Involvement of central muscarinic cholinergic mechanisms in opioid stress analgesia. *Brain Res.,* 270:289–293.
41. Lewis, J. W., Cannon, J. T., Liebeskind, J. C., and Akil, H. (1981): Alterations in brain β-endorphin immunoreactivity following acute and chronic stress. *Pain (Suppl. 1),* S263.
42. Lewis, J. W., Cannon, J. T., Ryan, S. M., and Liebeskind, J. C. (1980): Behavioral pharmacology of opioid peptides. In: *Role of Peptides in Neuronal Function,* edited by J. L. Barker, pp. 742–763. Marcel Dekker, Inc., New York.
43. Lewis, J. W., Chudler, E. H., Cannon, J. T., and Liebeskind, J. C. (1981): Hypophysectomy differentially affects morphine and stress analgesia. *Proc. West. Pharmacol. Soc.,* 24:323–326.
44. Lewis, J. W., Sherman, J. E., and Liebeskind, J. C. (1981): Opioid and nonopioid stress analgesia: Assessment of tolerance and cross-tolerance with morphine. *J. Neurosci.,* 1:358–363.
45. Lewis, J. W., Terman, G. W., Watkins, L. R., Mayer, D. J., and Liebeskind, J. C. (1983): Opioid and nonopioid mechanisms of footshock-induced analgesia: Role of the spinal dorsolateral funiculus. *Brain Res.,* 267:139–144.
46. Lewis, J. W., Tordoff, M. G., Liebeskind, J. C., and Viveros, O. H. (1982): Evidence for adrenal medullary opioid involvement in stress analgesia. *Soc. Neurosci. Abstr.,* 8:778.
47. Lewis, J. W. Tordoff, M. G. Sherman, J. E., and Liebeskind, J. C. (1982): Adrenal medullary enkephalin-like peptides may mediate opioid stress analgesia. *Science,* 217:557–559.

48. Liebeskind, J. C., Giesler, G. J., Jr., and Urca, G. (1976): Evidence pertaining to an endogenous mechanism of pain inhibition in the central nervous system. In: *Sensory Functions of the Skin in Primates*, edited by Y. Zotterman, pp. 561–573. Pergamon Press, Oxford.

49. Liebeskind, J. C., Guilbaud, G., Besson, J. M., and Oliveras, J. L. (1973): Analgesia from electrical stimulation of the periaqueductal gray matter in the cat: Behavioral observations and inhibitory effects on spinal cord interneurons. *Brain Res.*, 50:441–446.

50. MacLennan, A. J., Drugan, R. C., Hyson, R. L., Maier, S. F., Madden, J., and Barchas, J. D. (1982): Corticosterone: A critical factor in an opioid form of stress-induced analgesia. *Science*, 215:1530–1532.

51. Madden, J., Akil, H., Patrick, R. L., and Barchas, J. D. (1977): Stress-induced parallel changes in central opioid levels and pain responsiveness in the rat. *Nature*, 265:358–360.

52. Mayer, D. J., and Hayes, R. L. (1975): Stimulation-produced analgesia: Development of tolerance and cross-tolerance to morphine. *Science*, 188:941–943.

53. Mayer, D. J., and Liebeskind, J. C. (1974): Pain reduction by focal electrical stimulation of the brain: An anatomical and behavioral analysis. *Brain Res.*, 68:73–93.

54. Mayer, D. J., and Price, D. D. (1976): Central nervous system mechanisms of analgesia. *Pain*, 2:379–404.

55. Mayer, D. J., Price, D. D., Rafii, A., and Barber, J. (1976): Acupuncture hypalgesia: Evidence for activation of a central control system as a mechanism of action. In: *Advances in Pain Research and Therapy, Vol. 1*, edited by J. J. Bonica and D. Albe-Fessard, pp. 751–754. Raven Press, New York.

56. Mayer, D. J., Wolfle, T. L., Akil, H., Carder, B., and Liebeskind, J. C. (1971): Analgesia from electrical stimulation in the brainstem of the rat. *Science*, 174:1351–1354.

57. McGivern, R. F., and Berntson, G. G. (1980): Mediation of diurnal fluctuations in pain sensitivity in the rat by food intake patterns: Reversal by naloxone. *Science*, 210:210–211.

58. Melzack, R., and Melinkoff, D. F. (1974): Analgesia produced by brain stimulation: Evidence of a prolonged onset period. *Exp. Neurol.*, 43:369–374.

59. Miczek, K. A., Thompson, M. L., and Shuster, L. (1982): Opioid-like analgesia in defeated mice. *Science*, 215:1520–1522.

60. Morrow, T. J., and Casey, K. L. (1976): Analgesia produced by mesencephalic stimulation: Effect on bulboreticular neurons. In: *Advances in Pain Research and Therapy, Vol. 1*, edited by J. J. Bonica and D. Albe-Fessard, pp. 503–510. Raven Press, New York.

60a. Moskowitz, A. S., Breedlove, S. M., Arnold, A. P., and Liebeskind, J. C. (1982): Distribution of enkephalin-like immunoreactivity in the rat spinal cord: An immunohistochemical study. *Soc. Neurosci. Abstr.*, 8:100.

61. Oleson, T. D., Twombly, D. A., and Liebeskind, J. C. (1978): Effects of pain-attenuating brain stimulation and morphine on electrical activity in the raphe nuclei of the awake rat. *Pain*, 4:211–230.

62. Oliveras, J. L., Hosobuchi, Y., Redjemi, F., Guilbaud, G., and Besson, J. M. (1977): Opiate antagonist, naloxone, strongly reduces analgesia induced by stimulation of a raphe nucleus (centralis inferior). *Brain Res.*, 120:221–229.

63. Oliveras, J. L., Woda, A., Guilbaud, G., and Besson, J. M. (1974): Inhibition of the jaw opening reflex by electrical stimulation of the periaqueductal gray matter in the awake, unrestrained cat. *Brain Res.*, 72:328–331.

64. Penner, E. R., Terman, G. W., and Liebeskind, J. C. (1982): Cross-tolerance between opioid mediated stimulation-produced and stress-induced analgesia. *Soc. Neurosci. Abstr.*, 8:619.

65. Pert, A., and Walter, M. (1976): Comparison between naloxone reversal of morphine and electrical stimulation induced analgesia in the rat mesencephalon. *Life Sci.*, 19:1023–1032.

66. Pohorecky, L. A., and Wurtman, R. J. (1971): Adrenocortical control of epinephrine synthesis. *Pharmacol. Rev.*, 23:1–35.

67. Pomeranz, B., and Chiu, D. (1976): Naloxone blockade of acupuncture analgesia: Endorphins implicated. *Life Sci.*, 19:1757–1762.

68. Prieto, G. J., Cannon, J. T., and Liebeskind, J. C. (1983): N. raphe magnus lesions disrupt stimulation-produced analgesia from ventral but not dorsal midbrain areas in the rat. *Brain Res.*, 261:53–57.

69. Reynolds, D. V. (1969): Surgery in the rat during electrical analgesia induced by focal brain stimulation. *Science*, 164:444–445.

70. Richardson, D. E., and Akil, H. (1977): Pain reduction by electrical brain stimulation in man. Part 2: Chronic self-administration in the peri-ventricular gray matter. *J. Neurosurg.*, 47:184–189.

71. Rossier, J., French, E. D., Rivier, C., Ling, N., Guillemin, R., and Bloom, F. E. (1977): Foot-shock induced stress increases β-endorphin levels in blood but not brain. *Nature*, 270:618–620.

72. Rossier, J., Guillemin, R., and Bloom, F. E. (1978): Foot-shock induced stress decreases leu⁵-enkephalin immunoreactivity in rat hypothalamus. *Eur. J. Pharmacol.*, 48:465–466.

73. Sharpe, L. G., Garnett, J. E., and Cicero, T. J. (1974): Analgesia and hyperreactivity produced by intracranial microinjections of morphine into the periaqueductal gray matter of the rat. *Behav. Biol.*, 11:303–313.

74. Sherman, J. E., and Liebeskind, J. C. (1980): An endorphinergic, centrifugal substrate of pain modulation: Recent findings, current concepts, and complexities. In: *Pain*, edited by J. J. Bonica, pp. 191–204. Raven Press, New York.

75. Simantov, R., Kuhar, M. J., Uhl, G. R., and Snyder, S. H. (1977): Opioid peptide enkephalin: Immunohistochemical mapping in rat central nervous system. *Proc. Natl. Acad. Sci. USA* 74:2167–2171.

76. Snyder, S. H., and Childers, S. R. (1979): Beta-endorphin is a potent analgesic agent. *Ann. Rev. Neurosi.*, 2:35–64.

77. Stern, A. S., Lewis, R. V., Kimura, S., Rossier, J., Gerber, L. D., Brink, L., Stein, S., and Udenfriend, S. (1979): Isolation of the opioid heptapeptide Met-enkephalin from bovine adrenal medullary granules and striatum. *Proc. Natl. Acad. Sci. USA*, 76:6680–6683.

78. Terenius, L. (1978): Endogenous peptides and analgesia. *Proc. Natl. Acad. Sci. USA*, 73:2895–2898.

79. Terman, G. W., Lewis, J. W., and Liebeskind, J. C. (1981): Monoaminergic mechanisms of stress analgesia. *Soc. Neurosci. Abstr.*, 7:879.

80. Terman, G. W., Lewis, J. W., and Liebeskind, J. C. (1982): Role of the biogenic amines in stress analgesia. *Proc. West. Pharmacol. Soc.*, 25:7–10.

81. Terman, G. W., Lewis, J. W., and Liebeskind, J. C. (1982): Evidence for the involvement of histamine in stress analgesia. *Soc. Neurosci. Abstr.*, 8:619.

82. Terman, G. W., Lewis, J. W., and Liebeskind, J. C. (1983): Opioid and nonopioid mechanisms of stress analgesia: Lack of cross-tolerance between stressors. *Brain Res.*, 260:147–150.

83. Terman, G. W., Lewis, J. W., and Liebeskind, J. C. (1983): Parametric variations in foot-shock stress produce different forms of opioid mediated analgesia. *Proc. West. Pharmacol. Soc.*, 26:49–52.

83a. Terman, G. W., and Liebeskind, J. C. (1983): The role of current intensity in opioid and nonopioid stress-induced analgesia. *Soc. Neurosci. Abstr.*, 9:795.

84. Urca, G., Frenk, H., Liebeskind, J. C., and Taylor, A. N. (1977): Morphine and enkephalin: Analgesic and epileptic properties. *Science*, 197:83–86.

85. Viveros, O. H., Diliberto, E. J., Jr., Hazum, E., and Chang, K.-J. (1979): Opiate-like materials in the adrenal medulla: Evidence for storage and secretion with catecholamines. *Mol. Pharmacol.*, 16:1101–1108.

86. Viveros, O. H., Diliberto, E. J., Jr., Hazum, E., and Chang, K.-J. (1980): Enkephalins as possible adrenomedullary hormones: Storage, secretion, and regulation of synthesis. In: *Neural Peptides and Neuronal Communication*, edited by E. Costa and M. Trabucchi, pp. 191–204. Raven Press, New York.

87. Wamsley, J. K., Lewis, M. S., Young, S., III, and Kuhar, M. J. (1981): Autoradiographic localization of muscarinic cholinergic receptors in rat brainstem. *J. Neurosci.*, 1:176–191.

88. Watkins, L. R., Cobelli, D. A., Faris, P., Aceto, M. D., and Mayer, D. J. (1982): Opiate vs. non-opiate footshock induced analgesia (FSIA): The body region shocked is a critical factor. *Brain Res.*, 242:299–308.

89. Watkins, L. R., Cobelli, D. A., and Mayer, D. J. (1982): Opiate vs. non-opiate footshock analgesia (FSIA): Descending and intraspinal components. *Brain Res.*, 245:97–106.

90. Watkins, L. R., Cobelli, D. A. Newsome, H. H., and Mayer, D. J. (1982): Footshock induced analgesia is dependent neither on pituitary nor sympathetic activation. *Brain Res.*, 245:81–96.

91. Watkins, L. R., and Mayer, D. J. (1982): The organization of endogenous opiate and non-opiate pain control systems. *Science*, 216:1185–1192.

92. Yaksh, T. L., and Rudy, T. A. (1978): Narcotic analgetics: CNS sites and mechanisms of action as revealed by intracerebral injection techniques. *Pain*, 4:299–359.

93. Yaksh, T. L., Yeung, J. C., and Rudy, T. A. (1976): An inability to antagonize with naloxone the elevated thresholds resulting from electrical stimulation of the mesencephalic central gray. *Life Sci.*, 18:1193–1198.
94. Yang, H-Y. T., Hexum, T. D., Majane, E., and Costa, E. (1980): Opiate peptides in bovine adrenal gland. In: *Neural Peptides and Neuronal Communication*, edited by E. Costa and E. Trabucchi, pp. 181–190. Raven Press, New York.

*Advances in Pain Research
and Therapy, Vol. 7,*
edited by C. Benedetti et al.
Raven Press, New York © 1984.

Pharmacology of Spinal Pain Modulatory Systems

Tony L. Yaksh, James R. Howe, and Gail J. Harty

*Departments of Neurosurgery and Pharmacology, Mayo Clinic, Rochester,
Minnesota 55905*

Stimulation of the brainstem, either electrically (10) or by the local microinjection of morphine into various brainstem sites (20), will exert a powerful inhibitory influence over the discharge of neurons in the spinal cord in response to Aδ and C fiber stimulation. More importantly, brainstem sites from which such inhibition is evoked are also associated with changes in the animal's organized response to an otherwise noxious stimulus (45). Such observations clearly suggest that the effects of supraspinal manipulation on spinal activity have relevance to the pain behavior of the intact and unanesthetized animal. Similarly, activation of intrinsic spinal systems, such as the lateral tract of Lissauer, a fiber system thought to originate in part from gelatinosa neurons, will also exert a powerful modulatory influence over the discharge of nociceptive neurons (32,47). Such observations indicate that information processing in the spinal cord is subject to considerable modulation before its transmission to higher cognitive centers.

Characterization of some of these modulatory pathways has been undertaken by attempting to determine the identity of the neurotransmitter found in the several systems and the pharmacology of the synaptic connections (i.e., the receptors) through which the inhibition is derived. In the following sections, we will discuss briefly the pharmacologic characteristics of three systems that have spinal terminals, one that is intrinsic to the spinal cord and two that originate in the brainstem, all of which serve to modulate the discharge of nociceptive neurons as well as to elevate the pain threshold in the unanesthetized animal.

INTRINSIC OPIATE MODULATORY SYSTEM

Physiologic and Anatomic Substrates

Within the spinal cord, it is known that there are cell bodies that contain a variety of putative inhibitory transmitters, notably GABA and glycine. In the last 10 years, it has become apparent that there are other receptor systems in the spinal cord whose activity results in the relatively specific modulation of nociceptive transmission. Classically, for example, it has been known that the opiates exert a direct effect on the spinal cord. The systemic administration of morphine in spinal animals will at analgesic doses inhibit the discharge of neurons (16,17,21,37) and block reflexes (23,33) evoked by nociceptive stimuli.

Precise structure-activity relationships and the pharmacology of these effects clearly point to the presence of specific receptor systems. The characterization of opiate ligand binding in the dorsal horn of the spinal cord (2), in conjunction with studies of rhizotomies showing a loss of binding after nerve lesion (11,19), suggests the presence of opiate receptors on primary afferent terminals. In this region, high levels of the pentapeptides met- and leu-enkephalin have been demonstrated in cell bodies and terminals within the substantia gelatinosa (13). *In vivo* spinal superfusion experiments have demonstrated that both met-enkephalin (38) as well as leu-enkephalin opioid materials (15) are released, suggesting that these materials may be the natural ligand acting on these biochemically and pharmacologically defined receptor systems within the dorsal horn of the spinal cord.

That such opioid binding sites in the dorsal horn might have physiologic relevance is supported by studies that demonstrated that local microinjection (5) or microiontophoresis (3,7,50) of opiates into the substantia gelatinosa, i.e., the area where the afferent terminals that contain the opiate binding sites exist, exerted a powerful modulation of the discharge evoked in dorsal horn neurons by Aδ and C fiber input. Jurna and Grossman (16) demonstrated that this effect of opiates on nociceptive discharge was observed on cells that did project into the ventrolateral tract, suggesting that spinal opiates could alter the content of the ascending sensory message.

Despite all the evidence that clearly demonstrated an effect of opiates on the processing of information at the spinal cord level, none of these studies could indicate the relevance of this modulation to the pain behavior of the intact animal.

The development of the spinal catheter system permitted the reliable application of materials into the spinal space in the animal model (44). As a result, extensive investigations were carried out identifying the physiology and pharmacology of the spinal receptor systems associated with the change in the animal's response to strong stimuli. In brief, we have demonstrated that the intrathecal action of opiates produced a prolonged and dose-dependent elevation in the nociceptive threshold as measured in the human with verbal report and in a variety of species—including mouse, rat, cat, rabbit, and primate—on spinally mediated nociceptive reflex measures (e.g., tail flick, skin twitch) and on more complex operant pain tasks such as the hot plate and shock titration (34,43). Importantly, the physiologic characteristics of this effect indicated a surprising absence of influence on autonomic or motor function at analgesic doses. This selective "modulation" results from the fact that the opiate receptors, if any, associated with preganglionic sympathetic efferent or motor horn cell outflow were not reached by the superficially applied opiate.

Characteristics of Spinal Opiate Receptors

The effects produced by opiates administered intrathecally (see later), iontophoretically (3,7), or systemically (36) in spinalized animals have been shown to possess characteristics indicating an action mediated through pharmacologically definable receptors. Thus the effects of opiates with an action limited to the spinal cord by these diverse manipulations have been shown to be dose dependent, stereospecific, and antagonized by naloxone.

Although it is without question that opiates act at receptors in the spinal cord to alter the transmission of nociceptive information, the question of whether or not these receptor systems are homogeneous is controversial. To identify a class of receptors, one requires a ligand that is selective for that receptor or a ligand that acts on all classes of receptors, and antagonists that are specific for the several receptors. Although there is no instance of the former, the latter has been used with some success. Thus the classic studies of Martin et al. (23) suggested the existence of multiple receptors (mu, kappa, and sigma, for which morphine, ethylketocyclazocine, and SKF10047, respectively, are the putative agonists). Lord et al. (22) suggested the existence of mu and delta receptors associated with the guinea pig ileum and the mouse vas deferens, respectively. For the mu receptor, morphine was suggested as a prototypical ligand; for the delta receptor, the pentapeptide D-ala^2-D-leu^5-enkephalin was the putative agonist. Opiate-binding studies have demonstrated that there are mu- and delta-binding sites in the afferents of the spinal cord (11). Pharmacologic characterization of the receptors relevant to analgesia after intrathecal administration has been carried out by examining the structure-activity relationships, the quantitative antagonism of the agonist affected by naloxone, and the cross-tolerance that may exist between different classes of putative opiate receptor ligands.

Figure 1 presents intrathecal dose response curves for selected opioid alkaloids and peptides in the rat on the tail flick test. In this structure-activity series, there is nothing that discriminates the effect as being mediated by mu or delta receptors. The slopes of the dose-response curves do not differ statistically. D-ala^2-D-leu^5-enkephalin, while active on the mouse vas deferens (delta receptor), also possesses considerable activity on the guinea pig ileum. Similarly, in the present experiments, intrathecal D-ala^2-D-leu^5-enkephalin is only slightly more active on a molar basis than morphine in elevating the nociceptive threshold after intrathecal administration.

With regard to quantitative studies of naloxone antagonism, Fig. 1B (left) shows that the systemic administration of naloxone produces a parallel rightward shift in the agonist dose-response curve (for intrathecal morphine, D-ala^2-met-enkephalin amide and D-ala^2-D-leu^5-enkephalin and β-endorphin)

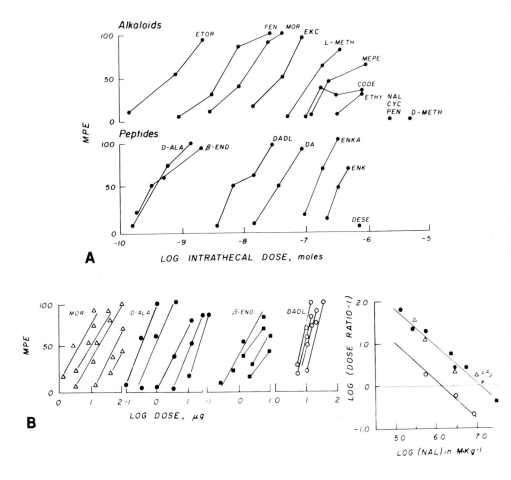

FIG. 1. A: Effect of intrathecally administered alkaloids (*upper half*) and peptides (*lower half*) on the tail flick. Ordinate indicates the maximum percentage effect; the doses of drugs are plotted as the log intrathecal dose in moles. Each point represents the mean of 4–15 animals. Drug abbreviations are: ETOR = Etorphine; FEN = fentanyl; MOR = morphine; EKC = ethylketocyclazocine; L-METH = L-methadone; MEPE = meperidine; CODE = codeine; ETHY = ethyl-morphine; NAL = nallorphine; CYC = cyclazocine; PEN = pentazocine; D-METH = D-methadone; D-ALA = D-ala²-met-enkephalin amide; β-END = β-endorphin; DADL = D-ala²-D-leu⁵-enkephalin; DA = D-ala²-met-enkephalin; ENKA = met-enkephalin amide; ENK = methionine-enkephalin; DESE = des-met-enkephalin. **B (left):** Dose-response curves for morphine, D-ala²-enkephalin amide, β-endorphin, and D-ala²-D-leu⁵-enkephalin carried out in the presence of increasing doses of intraperitoneally administered naloxone. **Right:** dose-ratio plot for naloxone carried out in the presence of intrathecally administered morphine, β-endorphin, D-ala²-met⁵-enkephalin amide, and D-ala²-D-leu⁵-enkephalin. The intersection of the plotted line with log (dose ratio = 1) = 0 is the pA₂ value for naloxone. The symbols of the dose-ratio plot are for the same drugs whose family of dose-response curves appears to the left. (From refs. 39,41,42,44a; *unpublished observations.*)

and the magnitude of this shift is dose dependent. Plotting the log [dose ratio − 1] (i.e., dose ratio = ED_{50} of agonist in the presence of naloxone ÷ ED_{50} of agonist in the absence of naloxone) versus the log dose of naloxone in moles/kg allows one to calculate the apparent pA_2 of naloxone. This analysis, described by Schild (28), provides an estimate of the affinity of naloxone for the relevant receptor acted on by the particular agonist. Of particular interest is the observation that the apparent pA_2 value of naloxone for the antagonism of intrathecally administered morphine and D-ala²-met-enkephalin amide are around 7, whereas the pA_2 of naloxone in the presence of D-ala²-D-leu⁵-enkephalin is 6.1. Similar studies carried out with intrathecally injected β-endorphin (41) and ethylketocyclazocine (31) also yield a naloxone pA_2 of around 7, whereas the pA_2 of naloxone with metkephamid is 6.3 (T. L. Yaksh and G. J. Harty, *unpublished data*). These results suggest that these opiate ligands fall into two classes: those that are morphine-like (naloxone pA_2 about 7) and those that are like D-ala²-D-leu⁵-enkephalin (naloxone pA_2 about 6). These data may be taken to suggest that naloxone interacts with two different classes of receptors as defined by the two different classes of opiate ligands. Similar results recently have been obtained in the primate on the shock titration task (38a).

The most descriptive experiments carried out to date regarding multiple receptors are the ones relating to cross-tolerance. The repeated administration of morphine results in a significant decrement in its effects day by day (i.e., tolerance). The daily intrathecal injection of morphine, the twice daily injection of morphine intraperitoneally (A. S. Tung, J.-Y. Wang, and T. L. Yaksh, *unpublished observations*), or the implantation of morphine-containing pellets will render the animal less responsive to morphine, such that at the end of each tolerance sequence, the ED_{50} for intrathecal morphine will be increased by a factor of about 7. Figure 2 presents the results of experiments carried out in catheter-implanted rats after a 5-day period where the rat received a 75-mg pellet followed at day 3 by two 75-mg pellets and tested on day 5. As shown, dose-response curves for D-ala²-D-leu⁵-enkephalin, metkephamid, or β-endorphin are then determined. In animals made so tolerant to morphine, it was found that there is no shift in the D-ala²-D-leu⁵-enkephalin dose-response curve in the morphine-tolerant animal, that is, it seems that animals made tolerant to morphine show normal responsiveness under these conditions to D-ala²-D-leu⁵-enkephalin.

In contrast, the dose-response curves for β-endorphin and morphine show an increasing rightward shift. Similar results were obtained in primate experiments. Figure 3 shows the shock titration records for a series of experiments carried out at 7-day intervals in a single macaque monkey. The animals were tested for their base-line responsiveness to doses of β-endorphin, D-ala²-D-leu⁵-enkephalin, and metkephamid, which had been previously determined to be about equally active. In the center panel of the top part, the effects of daily intrathecal administration of morphine (1200 μg) is shown for days 1, 3, and 5. As can be seen, by day 5, the animal ceases to respond

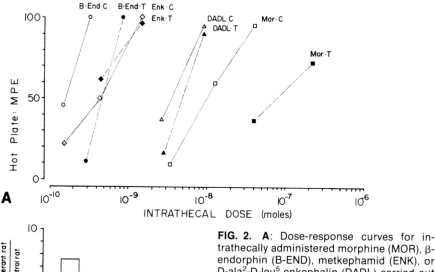

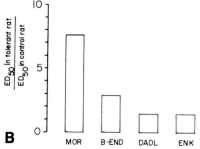

FIG. 2. A: Dose-response curves for intrathecally administered morphine (MOR), β-endorphin (B-END), metkephamid (ENK), or D-ala²-D-leu⁵-enkephalin (DADL) carried out in control rats (C) or tolerant rats previously implanted with morphine pellets (T). Each point represents the mean result observed on the hot plate in 6–8 animals. **B**: Histogram presents the ratio of the ED_{50} observed in the morphine-tolerant rat divided by the ED_{50} on the hot plate observed in nonmorphine-tolerant rats for morphine, β-endorphin, DADL, and metkephamid.

to the intrathecally administered opiates. This rapid loss of responsiveness to intrathecal morphine has been documented in previous studies from this laboratory. On the succeeding days, the animal received intrathecal injections of D-ala²-D-leu⁵-enkephalin, followed by 2 days of intrathecal morphine (data not shown), the intrathecal injection of metkephamid, followed by 2 days of intrathecal morphine (data not shown), and finally the injection of β-endorphin. As can be seen, neither metkephamid nor D-ala²-D-leu⁵-enkephalin seemed to show any diminution in effectiveness in an animal made tolerant to morphine. In contrast, β-endorphin showed a significant reduction in its apparent analgetic potency (38a).

Our interpretation of these accumulated data is that there are at least two populations of receptors in the spinal cord. First is one whose pharmacologic properties resemble those found in the guinea pig ileum, often referred to as the mu receptor, and for which morphine is a prototypical agonist. Second is a population of receptors whose pharmacologic profiles resemble those found in the mouse vas deferens, which are referred to as delta receptors, and for which D-ala²-D-leu⁵-enkephalin is a prototypical agonist. These observations are supported by the different pA_2 values observed and the lack of tolerance of D-ala²-D-leu⁵-enkephalin and metkephamid in morphine-tolerant animals.

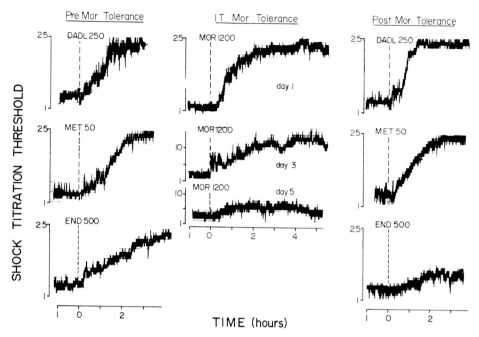

FIG. 3. Shock titration records obtained from one primate in a series of experiments. **Left**: records show the shock titration threshold after the intrathecal administration of 250 μg of D-ala²-D-leu⁵-enkephalin (DADL), 50 μg of metkephamid (MET 50), or the intrathecal administration of 500 μg of β-endorphin (END 500). Each figure presents the shock titration threshold (steps 1 through 25) plotted as a function of time after the intrathecal injection. **Middle**: selected records are shown which were obtained after the intrathecal administration of morphine (MOR 1200 μg) on days 1 through 5 (with records of 1, 3, and 5 presented). After the development of tolerance, the animal was tested on different days for its response to the same doses of D-ala²-D-leu⁵-enkephalin, metkephamid, and β-endorphin. **Right**: results from these series of intrathecal injections are shown. Other details of the injection procedure are as described in the text. (From ref. 38a.)

DESCENDING MONOAMINE MODULATORY SYSTEMS

Physiologic and Anatomic Substrates

It has long been known that the spinal reflex activity is subject to modulation by descending pathways. Classic work by Swedish investigators has clearly indicated the role of monoaminergic pathways in this effect (1,8). The observation by Dahlstrom and Fuxe (6) that descending monoamine pathways originate in brainstem nuclei and terminate in the spinal cord offered a neural substrate for these pharmacologic observations. That monoamines might, in fact, serve as modulatory transmitters in the spinal cord has been supported by a number of observations.

Microinjection of morphine into the periaqueductal gray (PAG) in a variety of species (25,28,49) or the nucleus reticulogigantocellularis (nGC) of the rodent (18) will block spinal reflex activity and elevate the animal's nociceptive threshold as defined by supraspinally mediated reflex tasks. These observations, taken jointly, indicate that these supraspinal manipulations have acted to alter not only the local reflex function of the spinal cord, but the content of the ascending sensory message generated by the otherwise noxious stimulus. In view of the considerable information that indicates that spinal reflex function is under a monoaminergic control, it seems reasonable to assume that the descending monoaminergic pathways might be activated by these several supraspinal manipulations. Thus although there are no monoamine cell bodies that descend to the spinal cord from the PAG, the demonstrated connections between the ventrolateral PAG and the caudal raphe system (27) provided a substrate whereby such modulatory influences could gain access to a descending link. Several lines of evidence support the behavioral relevance of the brainstem-mediated spinal inhibitions and indicate that the spinopetal pathways mediating these effects are monoaminergic in character.

First, if one assumes that the essential spinopetal link through which this descending influence is modulated is monoaminergic, then the physiologic manipulation should increase the release of monoamines in the spinal cord.

Using spinal superfusion procedures (see Chapter by T. L. Yaksh, P. E. Micevych, R. P. Elder, and V. L. W. Go, *this volume*), we have demonstrated that manipulations in the brainstem that give rise to the inhibition of spinal nociceptive reflexes are associated with an increased release of 5-HT or noradrenaline or both. The microinjection of morphine into the PAG results in a significant elevation in the nociceptive threshold and increases the levels of 5-HT in spinal superfusates (46), while systemic morphine increases the levels of the monoamine metabolites in spinal tissue (29,30) of the spinally intact animal. Electrical stimulation of the periraphe region of the caudal medulla also gives rise to an inhibition of spinal reflex activity and increases spinal monoamine terminal activity as evidenced by an increase in the release of 5-HT and noradrenaline in spinal superfusates (40). Thus supraspinal manipulations that increase spinal monoamine terminal activity also inhibit spinal reflex function and produce analgesia.

A second requirement to demonstrate that the descending pathways activated by these supraspinal manipulations are monoaminergic is to demonstrate that the antagonism of the appropriate receptor system will antagonize the physiologically measured effect. It should be noted here that these criteria deal implicitly with the monoamine terminals in the spinal cord. Systemic administration of the pharmacologic antagonists would be inappropriate, as drugs administered by such a route potentially would exert an effect through actions on supraspinal centers. In the first of such series of experiments, we demonstrated that the effects of PAG-morphine on spinal reflex activity were antagonized by the intrathecal administration of phentolamine (an α-adrenergic antagonist) and methysergide (a putative serotonergic antagonist) (35). Subsequent experiments by Kuriashi et al. (18)

indicated that the effects of morphine in the nGC were antagonized by α-adrenergic but not serotonergic antagonists. In recent experiments, we have observed that the system is considerably more complex than originally envisioned. The antinociceptive effects of stimulation at some periraphe sites are antagonized by the intrathecal administration of α-adrenergic or serotonergic antagonists, or at other periraphe sites by both (D. L. Hammond and T. L. Yaksh, *unpublished observations*). This reliable differentiation of certain brainstem sites with regard to the effects of the various intrathecal antagonists clearly points to the complex organization at the brainstem systems that give rise to activity in the several monoamine descending pathways.

Third, if the descending monoamine pathways mediate the spinopetal modulation, then increasing monoamine tone in the spinal cord should exert a modulatory influence over the nociceptive response measured both at the cellular and behavioral levels. The iontophoretic administration of 5-HT and noradrenaline into the dorsal horn, notably the substantia gelatinosa, has been shown to inhibit profoundly the discharge of nociceptive neurons (4,9,12). Importantly, cells showing a primary response to innocuous stimuli such as light brush or touch, or Aβ afferent activation, do not show a similar degree of inhibition. The relevance of this spinal monoamine effect on nociceptive neurons to the behavior of the intact animal is more directly assessed by increasing monoamine tone in the spinal cord in the unanesthetized animal. Thus we have demonstrated that the intrathecal administration of 5-HT (48) and α-adrenergic agonists (26,43) will produce a significant elevation in the nociceptive threshold in a variety of species, including the rat, cat, and primate. These effects with α-adrenergic and serotonergic agonists occur in the absence of any major effect on motor function and have been demonstrated on both reflexive tasks, such as tail flick and skin twitch, as well as more complex tasks requiring supraspinal mediation, such as the hot plate and the shock titration.

In sum, the above observations showing close correlations among the antinociceptive effects evoked by brainstem manipulation, the spinal release of monoamines, and the pharmacology of the synaptic system through which these descending pathways are activated strongly suggest that a powerful spinopetal modulation of spinal nociceptive processing occurs as a result of activation of spinal serotonergic and noradrenergic synapses.

Characteristics of Spinal Monoamine Receptors

An essential question in these investigations is what are the characteristics of the receptor through which these monoaminergic effects are mediated. To date, relatively little characterization has been done with serotonin in light of the controversial pharmacology associated with its receptor, although its intrathecal effects are antagonized by methysergide and cyproheptadine (48). We have, however, begun to detail the pharmacologic profile of the receptor through which the intrathecal action of adrenergic agonists are mediated. First, it is certain that the effect is mediated by an α-adrenergic receptor, i.e., antagonized by phentolamine but not by propranolol (26). Two classes of α-adrenergic receptors (α_1 and α_2) have been identified in a variety of tissues. In recent experiments, we have demonstrated that pharmacologically differentiable α_1 and α_2 receptors exist postsynaptically in the spinal cord to modulate the physiologic response to a strong stimulus. Evidence supporting this statement is as follows.

First, both traditional α_1 agonists, notably methoxamine and phenylephrine, and traditional α_2 agonists, such as clonidine and ST-91, will produce analgesia when administered intrathecally. As a group, α_2 agonists show less steep dose-response curves and a greater potency than α_1 agonists (14). That these different classes of α agonists are activating different populations of α-receptor subtypes when administered intrathecally is supported by intrathecal studies with subtype selective antagonists.

Second, the analgesic effects of α_1 agonists are more preferentially antagonized by prazosin than yohimbine (an α_1 and an α_2 antagonist, respectively). The converse is true for α_2 agonists (14).

Third, although both α_1 and α_2 agonists elevate the nociceptive threshold, α_1 agonists produce an enhanced motor tone as revealed by tremor and licking of the hindlimbs and serpentine movement of the tail; α_2 agonists in analgesic doses have no such effects.

Fourth, animals treated with intrathecal 6-hydroxydopamine show very low levels of cord norepinephrine, indicating the loss of noradrenergic terminals. The intrathecal administration of both α_1 and α_2 agonists in such animals continues to produce a measurable increase in the nociceptive threshold. This indicates that the effects of both α_1 and α_2 agonists can be mediated by receptors postsynaptic to the noradrenergic terminal (J. R. Howe and T. L. Yaksh, *unpublished observations*).

In sum, the above data clearly indicate the existence of physiologically defined pathways that originate in the brainstem and descend into the spinal cord, and that release monoamines when activated. This release after a variety of supraspinal manipulations is associated with elevations in the nociceptive threshold, and such elevations have a pharmacology that is clearly indicative of monoamine receptors. Importantly, it seems that the complexity of the spinal systems mediating this antinociceptive effect are even greater than originally thought, with populations of both α_1 and α_2 receptors mediating overlapping functions. Whether the descending pathways activated by supraspinal manipulations exert their effects through α_1 or α_2 receptors or both and whether subpopulations of descending systems interact with specific receptor populations are not currently known.

In the preceding discussion, we have outlined the data to indicate the modulatory substrates whose existence is defined by the pharmacology of the receptors through which the effects are mediated. Such basic investigations have revealed to us the potency and nature of opiates and α-adrenergic receptors in the spinal cord in mediating the response of the animal to a strong stimulus, that is, the intrathecal action of these agents produces analgesia.

Two questions naturally follow from the findings. First, if these receptors exert such a powerful modulatory control over spinal processing, what stimulus naturally activates the neuron from which the ligand for that receptor is released? As will be discussed in the Chapter by T. L. Yaksh, P. E. Micevych, R. P. Elde, and V. L. W. Go, *this volume*, we have shown that certain types of somatic stimulation will increase the release of monoamine and opiate ligands from the spinal cord. This suggests the likelihood that a reflex modulation of spinal processing may occur. Such information may lead to insights whereby somatic stimuli such as transcutaneous nerve stimulation or acupuncture may produce a suppression of nociceptive responses.

Second, do these findings regarding multiple spinal modulatory receptor systems promise any clinical relevance? That opiates act via specific membrane receptor systems has been appreciated for several decades, but the observation that multiple opiate receptors exist within the cord arose from systematic spinal studies with peptides that have only marginal activity when administered systemically. Similarly, the studies with agonists have advanced because it has been possible with intrathecal administration to produce effects on the spinal cord in the absence of peripheral autonomic receptor activation. Thus these contributions do not offer any particular insights into advances in systemic analgetic therapy. Nevertheless, the increasing clinical experience with spinal morphine has indicated the potential for such therapy. The development of implantable infusion pumps has led to the possibility of long-term analgetic therapy with low doses of the agent delivered over relatively long periods of time (24). The essential drawback thus far has *not* been the technology of infusion or surgery, but the likelihood that the morphine-sensitive receptor will become morphine-tolerant. The demonstration that there are populations of noncross-tolerant, naloxone-sensitive receptors suggests the possibility of increasing the duration of beneficial therapy by selective opiate receptor activation. Similarly, the existence of spinal α receptors associated with nociceptive processing offers yet other possible intrathecal therapeutic paradigms. Our observations that intrathecal α-adrenergic agonists will potentiate the effects of intrathecal opiates through a synergistic interaction (32a) suggest the possibility that combination therapy will reduce the amount of either agent required and therefore reduce the likelihood of observing side effects peculiar to either type of receptor (i.e., changes in blood pressure and respiratory depression for α-adrenergic and opiate agonists, respectively). The use of α-adrenergic or α-receptor agonists is not accepted currently as clinically useful analgetic therapy, and whether such therapy might in the future become clinically useful has not to date been examined.

The essential point to be made, however, is that these several potential advances in clinical therapy come about only through investigations that are aimed, not at better clinical techniques, but from a desire to understand the basic physiology and pharmacology of the spinal cord. Rational advances in pain therapy occur not because drugs are randomly selected from the shelves or random pathways are stimulated or inhibited, but because of a basic understanding in how the system functions.

ACKNOWLEDGMENTS

Support for work reported here is derived from Mayo Foundation grants NS 14629 and NS 16541. We would like to thank Ms. Gail Harty and Ms. Diane Weis for their collaboration in several of these experiments, and Ms. Ann Rockafellow for preparing the manuscript.

REFERENCES

1. Anden, N. E., Jukes, M. G. M., Lundberg, A., and Vyklicky, L. (1966): The effect of DOPA on the spinal cord. *Acta Physiol. Scand.*, 67:373–386.
2. Atweh, S. F., and Kuhar, M. J. (1977): Autoradiographic localization of opiate receptors in rat brain. I. Spinal cord and lower medulla. *Brain Res.*, 123:53–67.
3. Belcher, G., and Ryall, R. W. (1978): Differential excitatory and inhibitory effects of opiates on non-nociceptive neurones in the spinal cord of the cat. *Brain Res.*, 145:303–314.
4. Belcher, G., Ryall, R. W., and Schaffner, R. (1978): The differential effects of 5,6-hydroxytryptamine, noradrenaline and raphe stimulation on nociceptive and non-nociceptive dorsal horn interneurons in the cat. *Brain Res.*, 151:307–332.
5. Bell, J. A., Sharpe, L. G., and Berry, J. N. (1980): Depressant and excitant effect of intraspinal microinjections of morphine and methionine-enkephalin in the cat. *Brain Res.*, 196:455–465.
6. Dahlstrom, A., and Fuxe, K. (1965): Evidence for the existence of monoamine neurons in the central nervous system. II. Experimentally induced changes in the intraneuronal amine levels of bulbospinal neuron systems. *Acta Physiol. Scand. [Suppl.]* 247:1–36.
7. Duggan, A. W., Hall, J. G., and Headley, P. M. (1977): Suppression of transmission of nociceptive impulses by morphine: Selective effects of morphine administered in the region of the substantia gelatinosa. *Br. J. Pharmacol.*, 61:65–76.
8. Engberg, I., Lundberg, A., and Ryall, R. W. (1968): Is the tonic decerebrate inhibition of reflex paths mediated by monoaminergic pathways? *Acta Physiol. Scand.*, 72:123–133.
9. Engberg, I., and Ryall, R. W. (1966): The inhibitory action of noradrenaline and other monoamines on spinal neurones. *J. Physiol. (Lond.)*, 185:298–322.
10. Fields, H. L., and Basbaum, A. I. (1978): Brainstem control of spinal pain transmission neurons. *Annu. Rev. Physiol.*, 40:193–221.
11. Fields, H. L., Emson, P. C., Leigh, B. K., Gilbert, R. F. T., and Iversen, L. L. (1980): Multiple opiate receptors in primary afferent fibres. *Nature*, 214:351–352.
12. Griersmith, B. T., and Duggan, A. W. (1980): Prolonged depression of spinal transmission of nociceptive information by 5-HT administered in the substantia gelatinosa: antagonism by methysergide. *Brain Res.*, 187:231–236.
13. Hökfelt, T., Ljungdahl, A., Elde, R., Nilsson, G., and Terenius, L. (1977): Immunohistochemical analysis of peptide pathways possibly related to pain and analgesia: enkephalin and substance P. *Proc. Natl. Acad. Sci. USA*, 74:3081–3085.
14. Howe, J. R., Wang, J.-K., and Yaksh, T. L. (1983): Selective antagonism of the antinociceptive effect of intrathecally applied α-adrenergic agonists by intrathecal prazosin and intrathecal yohimbine. *J. Pharmacol. Exp. Ther.*, 224:552–558.

15. Jhamandas, K., Yaksh, T. L., Bergström, L., and Terenius, L. (1981): Release of endogenous opioids from spinal cord *in vivo* following sciatic nerve stimulation. I.N.R.C. Meeting, Kyoto, Japan, July 26–30.

16. Jurna, I., and Grossman, W. (1976): The effect of morphine on the activity evoked in ventrolateral tract axons of the cat spinal cord. *Exp. Brain Res.*, 24:473–484.

17. Kitahata, L. M., Yosaka, Y., Taub, A., Bonikos, A., and Hoffert, M. (1974): Lamina-specific suppression of dorsal horn activity by morphine sulfate. *Anesthesiology*, 41:39–48.

18. Kuriashi, Y., Harada, Y., Satoh, M., and Takagi, H. (1979): Antagonism by phenoxybenzamine of the analgesic effect of morphine injected into the n. reticulogigantocellularis of the rat. *Neuropharmacology*, 18:107–110.

19. LaMotte, C., Pert, C. B., and Snyder, S. H. (1976): Opiate receptor binding in primate spinal cord: Distribution and changes after dorsal root section. *Brain Res.*, 112:407–412.

20. LeBars, D., Dickenson, A. H., and Besson, J. M. (1980): Microinjection of morphine within nucleus raphe magnus and dorsal horn neurone activities related to nociception in the rat. *Brain Res.*, 189:467–481.

21. LeBars, D., Menetrey, D., Conseiller, C., and Besson, J. M. (1975): Depressive effects of morphine upon lamina V cells activities in the dorsal horn of the spinal cat. *Brain Res.*, 93:261–277.

22. Lord, J. A. H., Waterfield, A. A., Hughes, J., and Kosterlitz, H. W. (1977): Endogenous opioid peptides: multiple agonists and receptors. *Nature*, 267:495–499.

23. Martin, W. R., Eades, C. G., Thompson, J. A., Huppler, R., and Gilbert, P. E. (1976): The effects of morphine- and nalorphine-like drugs in the non-dependent and morphine dependent chronic spinal dog. *J. Pharmacol. Exp. Ther.*, 197:517–532.

24. Onofrio, B. M., Yaksh, T. L., and Arnold, P. G. (1981): Continuous low-dose intrathecal morphine administration in the treatment of chronic pain of malignant origin. *Mayo Clin. Proc.*, 56:516–520.

25. Pert, A., and Yaksh, T. L. (1975): Localization of the antinociceptive action of morphine in primate brain. *Pharmacol. Biochem. Behav.*, 3:133–138.

26. Reddy, S. V. R., and Yaksh, T. L. (1980): Spinal noradrenergic terminal system mediates antinociception. *Brain Res.*, 189:391–401.

27. Ruda, M. (1975): Autoradiographic study of the efferent projections of the midbrain central gray of the cat. Ph.D. Dissertation, University of Pennsylvania, Philadelphia.

28. Schild, H. O. (1957): Drug antagonism and pAx. *Pharmacol. Rev.*, 9:242–259.

29. Shiomi, H., Murakami, H., and Takagi, H. (1978): Morphine analgesia and the bulbospinal serotonergic system: increase in concentration of 5-hydroxyindoleacetic acid in the rat spinal cord with analgesics. *Eur. J. Pharmacol.*, 52:335–344.

30. Shiomi, H., and Takagi, H. (1974): Morphine analgesia and bulbospinal noradrenergic system: Increase in the concentration of 5-normetanephrine in the spinal cord of the rat caused by analgesia. *Br. J. Pharmacol.*, 52:519–526.

31. Tung, A. S., and Yaksh, T. L. (1982): *In vivo* evidence for multiple opiate receptors mediating analgesia in the rat spinal cord. *Brain Res.*, 247:75–83.

32. Wall, P. D., and Yaksh, T. L. (1978): The effect of Lissauer tract stimulation on activity in dorsal and ventral roots. *Exp. Neurol.*, 60:570–583.

32a. Wang, J.-Y., Yasuoka, S., and Yaksh, T. L. (1980): Studies on the analgetic effect of intrathecal ST-91 (2-[2,6-diethylphenylamine]-2-imidazoline): antagonism, tolerance and interaction with morphine. *Pharmacologist*, 22:302.

33. Wikler, A. (1950): Sites and mechanisms of action of morphine and related drugs in the central nervous system. *Pharmacol. Rev.*, 2:435–506.

34. Yaksh, T. L. (1978): Direct evidence that spinal serotonin and noradrenaline terminals mediate the spinal antinociceptive effects of morphine in the periaqueductal gray. *Brain Res.*, 160:180–185.

35. Yaksh, T. L. (1978): Opiate receptors for behavioral analgesia resemble those related to the depression of spinal nociceptive neurons. *Science*, 199:1231–1233.

36. Yaksh, T. L. (1978): Inhibition by etorphine of the discharge of dorsal horn neurons: Effects upon the neuronal response to both high- and low-threshold sensory input in the decerebrate spinal cat. *Exp. Neurol.*, 60:23–41.

37. Yaksh, T. L. (1981): Spinal opiate analgesia: Characteristics and principles of action. *Pain*, 11:293–346.

38. Yaksh, T. L., and Elde, R. P. (1981): Factors governing the release of methionine enkephalin-like immunoreactivity from the mesencephalon and spinal cord of the cat *in vivo*. *J. Neurophysiol.*, 46:1056–1075.

38a. Yaksh, T. L. (1983): *In vivo* studies on spinal opiate receptor systems mediating antinociception. I. Mu and delta receptor profiles in the primate. *J. Pharmacol. Exp. Ther.*, 226:303–316.

39. Yaksh, T. L., Frederickson, R. C. A., Huang, S. P., and Rudy, T. A. (1978): *In vivo* comparison of the receptor populations acted upon in the spinal cord by morphine and pentapeptides in the production of analgesia. *Brain Res.*, 148:516–520.

40. Yaksh, T. L., Hammond, D. L., and Tyce, G. M. (1981): Functional aspects of bulbospinal monoaminergic projections in modulating processing of somatosensory information. *Fed. Proc.*, 40:2786–2794.

41. Yaksh, T. L., and Henry, J. L. (1978): Antinociceptive effects of intrathecally administered human β-endorphin in the rat and cat. *Can. J. Physiol. Pharmacol.*, 56:754–760.

42. Yaksh, T. L., Huang, S. P., Rudy, T. A., and Frederickson, R. C. A. (1977): The direct and specific opiate-like effect of Met^5-enkephalin and analogues on the spinal cord. *Neuroscience*, 2:593–596.

43. Yaksh, T. L., and Reddy, S. V. R. (1981): Studies in the primate on the analgetic effects associated with intrathecal actions of opiates, α-adrenergic agonists and baclofen. *Anesthesiology*, 54:451–467.

44. Yaksh, T. L., and Rudy, T. A. (1976): Chronic catheterization of the spinal subarachnoid space. *Physiol. Behav.*, 17:1031–1036.

44a. Yaksh, T. L., and Rudy, T. A. (1977): Studies on the direct spinal action of narcotics in the production of analgesia in the rat. *J. Pharmacol. Exp. Ther.*, 202:411–428.

45. Yaksh, T. L., and Rudy, T. A. (1978): Narcotic analgesics: CNS sites and mechanisms of action as revealed by intracerebral injection techniques. *Pain*, 4:299–359.

46. Yaksh, T. L., and Tyce, G. M. (1979): Microinjection of morphine into the periaqueductal gray evokes the release of serotonin from the spinal cord. *Brain Res.*, 171:176–181.

47. Yaksh, T. L., and Wall, P. D. (1978): Activation of a local spinal inhibitory system by focal stimulation of the lateral Lissauer tract in cats. *Fed. Proc.*, 37:398.

48. Yaksh, T. L., and Wilson, P. R. (1979): Spinal serotonin terminal system mediates antinociception. *J. Pharmacol. Exp. Ther.*, 208:446–453.

49. Yaksh, T. L., Yeung, J. C., and Rudy, T. A. (1976): Systematic examination in the rat of brain sites sensitive to the direct application of morphine: Observation of differential effect within the periaqueductal gray. *Brain Res.*, 114:83–103.

50. Zieglgansberger, W., and Bayerl, H. (1976): The mechanism of inhibition of neuronal activity by opiates in the spinal cord of cat. *Brain Res.*, 115:111–128.

*Advances in Pain Research
and Therapy, Vol. 7,*
edited by C. Benedetti et al.
Raven Press, New York © 1984.

Measurement of Clinical Pain: A Review and Integration of Research Findings

Karen L. Syrjala and C. Richard Chapman

*Multidisciplinary Pain Center, Department of Anesthesiology, University of
Washington, Seattle, Washington 98195*

Sound methodology for measuring pain is of vital importance to clinicians,
researchers, and governmental agencies concerned with the evaluation of
pain interventions. Development of satisfactory procedures for pain assessment continue to depend on the evolution of knowledge about pain at
theoretic, neurophysiologic, and psychologic levels. The classic model of
pain as a purely sensory experience is clearly no longer tenable; comprehensive assessment must involve scaling of sensory, emotional, and behavioral factors. Consequently, many new testing instruments and methodol-
ogies have emerged. This chapter critically reviews these developments with
the goal of describing state-of-the-art methods for pain measurement. It first
provides an overview of the concepts, techniques, and issues in clinical pain
assessment. It then offers an integrated perspective for the clinician who
must deal with the challenge of measuring pain or pain relief in a patient
population.

THE CONCEPT OF PAIN

The first step in assessing pain is the formulation of a conceptual model
that identifies its important attributes and permits quantification of those
attributes. Historically, conceptual oversimplification has been a major limitation in the development of the field.

That pain is not a simple neurophysiologic event has been recognized for
decades. The influence of emotions and meaning on the extent of pain reported has long been appreciated (for a review, see ref. 10) and was especially
emphasized by Beecher (5) who noted that, in soldiers wounded during
World War II, pain expressions and reaction to injury were less than those
encountered in noncombat, surgical patients with similar injuries. For the
soldier, the injury meant survival with dignity and removal from the combat
situation. Beecher's later landmark review of pain measurement (6) emphasized the need to define pain not as a purely sensory dimension determined

by tissue injury, but as a two-dimensional experience consisting of sensory and emotional aspects.

The literature on pain measurement and treatment has since expanded, reflecting our increased recognition of the complexity of this area. Melzack and Casey (78) elaborated Beecher's model to include sensory, emotional, and evaluative aspects of pain. More recently, Casey (12) presented a neurophysiologic model with both sensory-discriminative and motivational-affective pathways. This model implies that physiologic explanations of pain must consider affective dimensions to the same extent that psychologic explanations must consider nociceptive inputs.

A greater understanding of the meaning of pain has developed since Beecher emphasized its importance, and this concept appears to warrant inclusion in a model of pain. The meaning of pain for the patient can be assessed through evaluation of cognitive processes. This requires more sophisticated psychologic assessment than simple judgment of the pain as "real" or "imagined." In a recent review of the effects of personal control on extent of pain experienced, Thompson (101) noted that pain report may be lower when an individual sees the painful event as being associated with a highly meaningful outcome, such as the reevaluation of life or the opportunity to escape from combat. Sternbach (99) observed that, for the chronic pain patient, this concept of meaning has been lost. Others have reported that, with some chronic pain patients, disability compensation may itself be a meaningful outcome that maintains high levels of pain report and pain behavior (26,56).

Since Beecher (6), Bonica (10), and others called attention to the error of construing pain as a purely sensory event, its subjective and variable nature has been fully recognized. Not only are psychologic, physiologic, and social reinforcement factors interrelated, but one may actively influence the other. For instance, when subjects in a laboratory study inhibited their facial expressions in response to painful stimuli, their autonomic and self-reported pain responses also were attenuated. This occurred when subjects were requested to inhibit their responses, but also extended to a situation in which they were not given instruction but were informed that they were being observed. Conversely, when subjects were asked to exaggerate their facial displays of pain, their subjective and autonomic responses increased (59,69). Thus it would appear that increasing the social influence on pain behavior can impact the subjective and physiologic expressions of pain as well. These results suggest that expressive responses serve a self-regulatory as well as a communicative function, and that acting has an effect on the actor as well as on the observers.

Chapman (13) has offered a model that emphasizes the active interrelationship of contributing factors. An elaboration of this concept is shown in Fig. 1. This model indicates that private experience and pain behavior are both complex phenomena. The bidirectional arrows emphasize that the components of the pain experience are interdependent.

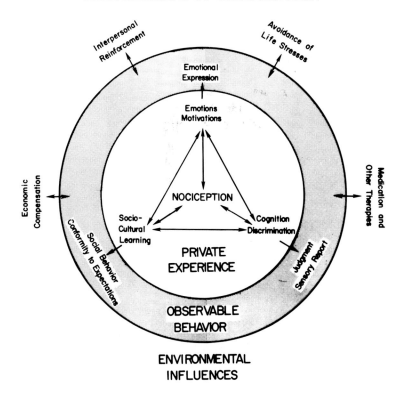

FIG. 1. Interactional model of pain. Nociception is incorporated into private experience, which is expressed in observed behavior. Environmental influences further interact with observed behavior. Pain measurement is necessarily limited to observed behaviors, including reports of private experience.

The measurement of clinical pain is a major challenge. This chapter cannot provide the reader with a definitive set of measurement rules or guidelines for pain research because decisions about pain measurement must depend on the purpose of the individual investigation and the nature of the pain problem being assessed. In the following section, contemporary approaches to measuring pain are reviewed and appraised.

METHODS OF MEASURING CLINICAL PAIN

There have been three major approaches to quantifying pain. The first centers on quantifying the subjective reports of patients. This can provide information on the cognitive and affective, as well as sensory, dimensions of the pain. The second approach attempts to quantify behaviors or patterns of activity that reflect the presence of pain or to document departures from normal behavior patterns that may be attributed to pain. These provide information on behavioral and performance dimensions, although they may also provide clues as to affective and cognitive state. For instance, sleep or appetite disturbance in the pain patient may be a sign of depression even without the self-reported affective experience of depression. Third, efforts have been made to define physiologic correlates of pain states. The most extensive of these attempts has been with electromyography, but thermography and other physiologic parameters also have been explored. These methods all consist of noninvasive means of observing the pain from external signs.

Self-Report Rating Scales: Simple Assessment of Subjective States

Although the multidimensional nature of pain has gained widespread recognition among pain specialists, the most common approach to pain assessment continues to be the unidimensional, self-report scale on which the patient provides a rating of pain intensity. Such measures are quick and easy to understand, both important considerations in a clinic setting. As the multidimensional nature of pain has been recognized, these scales are increasingly being used in repeated measures on a number of dimensions. The scales take several forms: words presented on a continuum of increasing value; numbers reflecting increasing values; or a line without markers other than endpoints of least-to-greatest value. Below, each type of scale will be considered.

Verbal and Nonverbal Category Rating Scales

With these scales, a group of adjectives with an ascending order of severity is given to the patient who is required to rate his or her pain state on the scale. Usually the scale is defined in terms of intensity, but aversiveness or some other aspect of pain can be scaled as easily. For example, a sensory scale might read: Faint Pain, Moderate Pain, Strong Pain, Very Strong Pain. In contrast, Melzack and Torgerson (79) have used the following categories to scale intensity of pain: Mild, Discomforting, Distressing, Horrible, Excruciating. Regardless of the pain dimension scaled, this method essentially classifies the pain experience. In most applications, the classifications are given numbers from 1 to 5 to permit use of higher-order statistical analyses. The use of parametric statistics with these, at best, rank-ordered numbers has given rise to problems that will be considered below.

An 8-point facial expression picture scale also has been developed recently; this might prove useful for those with language or mental capacity difficulties (29). This scale has been shown to correlate well with visual analog and numeric rating scales.

Visual Analog Scales and Numeric Rating Scales

The visual analog scale (VAS) consists usually of a 10-cm line anchored at one end by a label such as "no pain" and at the other end by a label such as "the worst pain imaginable." Theoretically, there are an infinite number of possible points on the line, but 10 to 100 points are usually scored. The numeric rating scale is an attempt to approximate the VAS in a form that allows the subject to respond orally. It usually consists of telling the patient to rate pain from 0 to 10 or 0 to 100, with similar anchors as are given with the VAS.

Critical appraisal

Since the VAS and verbal rating scales are perhaps the oldest and most commonly used pain measurements, they also have been evaluated extensively and comparisons have been made on a multitude of forms of presentation. Major findings indicate that the VAS and numeric scales correlate fairly well; the VAS and adjective or verbal scales cannot be assumed to be equivalent, however, even though they correlate significantly (53,65,75,81). The VAS has been found to be more sensitive, more reliable, and as valid as the verbal scales, although patient preference may vary for one or the other (53,65,81,110).

Some researchers have reported that 7 to 11% of the patients studied were not able to complete the VAS, or that the VAS can be confusing (22,65,91). In particular, it has been suggested that some older people, whose ability to think abstractly has diminished, may have difficulty with the VAS. Kremer et al. (65) found that the mean age for failure to complete the VAS was 75.3 years, whereas the mean age for successful completion was 54.4. In contrast, others have reported that the VAS was less often omitted, was preferred, or was considered closer to the patient's actual experience as long as it was explained carefully and practice was given if it was to be used outside of the clinic (50,53,81,96). Since the age of subjects was not always reported in these studies, it remains to be established whether some patients who can respond on the verbal scales are unable to complete the VAS, even after careful explanation, because of abstract thinking limitations. However, there is little controversy about the statistical superiority of the VAS over the adjective scales.

The number of points that may be meaningfully presented to the subject has been argued for many years. The VAS is preferred by some because of its theoretically infinite number of points. Indeed, one drawback of the adjective scales is that the fewer number of possible points may produce artificially augmented scores (81). Wolff (110) has contended that the VAS is superior because the average patient has difficulty conceptually managing more than five categories due to semantic rather than scaling limitations (e.g., what are the differences between "mild," "slight," and "moderate" categories?). Hardy et al. (43), however, found 21 noticeable differences between the perception of pain and pain tolerance, leading Scott and Huskisson (96) to argue for 20 divisions of the visual analogue scale and suggesting that a 0 to 20 numeric scale would also provide increased sensitivity over the 0 to 10 scale commonly used. A 0 to 100 scale has been advocated by those who prefer its greater range of scores and supposed greater sensitivity to change (65).

Although the most common form of presentation is "no pain" to "worst pain possible," certain writers have advocated a scale of "pain relief" or the use of previous scores to measure pain change rather than absolute pain. The argument in favor of this approach is that patients are then being compared with themselves on a scale that begins for everyone at a common level of "0" for "no change" and has the same potential for change within the range provided by the scale (50,96,97). In addition, it has been reported that patients overestimate their current pain severity when previous scores are not available and that this overestimate increases with increasing time between tests (97). Of course, providing previous scores could contribute to a response demand for reporting reduced pain, particularly when pre- and posttreatment comparisons are being made.

Scott and Huskisson (97) stated that memory for the initial state of pain faded over time and that since patients in natural settings report their pain as "the same," "better," or "worse," rather than on an absolute scale of no pain to extreme pain, this rating of pain change made more sense. The decay in pain memory over long periods of time has been reported by other investigators as well (82). Over short periods of time (5 days), memory for pain has been reported to be fairly accurate except for certain women who had high intensities of pain and affect when first measured (48). If the loss of memory for a previous pain is common, one could question the validity of requiring a patient to compare a current subjective state with the faded memory of a subjective state.

Response set has been of great concern to those who work toward effective comparisons of subjective pain reports. It has been noted that, with numeric scales, preferred numbers such as 0, 5, and 7 may appear too often to satisfy statistical needs for probability and homogeneous distribution (80). With repeated measures, VAS responders may tend to spread their responses over the entire scale (34). Errors in comparisons of patient scores may come from a "halo effect" or from "bias" (42). Halo effect refers to patients' tendencies to rate all subjective variables high or low, or their tendencies to respond similarly on one scale to the way they responded on a previous scale. This is of particular concern when multiple scales are given in an effort to provide a multidimensional measure. For example, a patient may first be asked to report how strong his or her pain is and then how unpleasant it is; a halo effect would be found in the tendency to rate the latter dimension similarly to the first dimension. Bias refers to the tendency to rate the pain as consistently high or low, probably in an effort to convey an affective rather than sensory condition. Efforts to avoid these confounding problems have included comparisons within the patient rather than between individuals (97,105).

That different types of rating scales, or scales with different anchors, do not correlate precisely has been used as evidence for different dimensions of pain report. Johnson and Rice (52) found that culture and ethnic origins did not effect sensory report but did correlate with distress report. Atkinson et al. (2) reported that the VAS was subject to confounding by the affective disturbance of patients; greater affective disturbance seemed to induce a response set for the report of greater intensity. However, they felt that, with these disturbed patients, it was necessary to include the VAS without intermediary verbal anchors as a validity check when adjective scales such as the McGill Pain Questionnaire (described later) are administered, because these patients reported a lower intensity on the VAS than on the adjectival intensity measures.

The importance of routinely establishing the correspondence between pain measures such as the McGill and the VAS was stressed by Reading (86) after he found that acute pain patients tested for pain changes sometimes scored higher on verbal scales of pain despite declaring their pain intensity diminished. The affective component of pain may be weighted more heavily in adjective scales than the sensory component, even when the sensory component purportedly is being measured. These results indicate that the adjective scales do not have the same meaning to the patient as the VAS has, and that to assign and compare numbers on one scale with numbers on another may lead to errors in conclusions.

A major problem in the use of these rating scales is choosing appropriate statistics for data analysis. The numbers obtained appear equally spaced, linear, and rank ordered, but it is not known whether they correspond in a one-to-one fashion with the attribute being measured. There is potential in these cases for great distortion. Many investigators apply parametric statistics to such data, and some have provided a rationale for this (4). However, this practice is still highly questionable unless it has been determined that patients use the numbers, categories, or line as though the points were equally spaced. The limitations for statistical manipulation of pain scores obtained from either verbal or VAS rating scales may vary, depending on the sampling procedure or on the sample population used.

If repeated measures are obtained with the same painful stimulus, responses can be scored as category-response probabilities (8). This frees the investigator from concerns about the direct scaling of a private experience and allows unlimited statistical treatment of the probability scores. Unfortunately, although repeated measures of the same experience are possible in the laboratory, clinical measures rarely are obtained repeatedly over many samplings without interventions. Even when many scores are obtained, as in a log of pain report, the pain state typically fluctuates over time even without intervention. This further confounds the interpretation of response probabilities.

Alternatively, rating scale responses may be tested for homogeneity of the distribution. If this testing is done and the distribution is homogeneous, there is some justification for the use of parametric statistics (53,81). However, homogeneity of the distribution cannot be assumed with these rating scales, and other investigators who have carefully considered the statistical questions strongly recommend the use of ordinal statistics (31,81,96). Cross-modality matching techniques have been developed, which may provide a sounder base for assuming interval or ratio scaling even with adjectival scales (37,104). These scales would allow the use of parametric statistics, and their consideration for substitution for the VAS or other verbal rating scales is recommended, particularly in research settings. They are reviewed more fully below.

Clinical considerations

Simple, unidimensional scaling methods can be used quickly, require only minimal instructions to patients, and are easily scored. Very sick patients are not taxed by giving category or VAS responses. Patients with limited language skills are not asked to respond to words that they do not understand. Moreover, these instruments have face validity for most clinicians, and clinical investigators do not have to familiarize themselves with the intricate and sometimes esoteric issues of scaling in order to use them. The VAS, in particular, has been shown to be a reliable and sensitive measure of the patient's subjective experience of his or her pain. Although the affective and sensory dimensions of the pain experience cannot be separated reliably in some patient reports, if the VAS is the only measure being used, it is probably useful to ask about both sensory/intensity and unpleasantness after telling the patient that both will be scaled. When treatment interventions are being evaluated, the use of pain change scores is possibly preferable to absolute pain, but measurement of both current pain and pain change would provide a more solid base of data for analysis.

A serious limitation of these devices is that they potentially oversimplify the experience of pain. Use of multiple VAS scales, each targeting a different aspect of pain, helps offset this limitation (e.g., 52). However, this is not a completely satisfactory solution because cognitive and affective judgments of pain do not fully capture the impact of pain on the patient's experience and because the effects of response sets cannot yet be validly measured and controlled for. More fundamentally, pain intensity (or some other dimension) may not represent itself in private experience in a linear fashion, and the forcing of judgments onto a length scale may be quite distorting. Although rank statistics can be performed on the data, clinical investigators typically think of the scales in interval terms. The pain change experienced between no pain and two divisions on the rating scale is probably not equal to the pain change experienced between the seventh and ninth divisions on the rating scale. The health care professional who interprets patient scores on these scales needs to consider this statistical limit when conclusions are being drawn.

Multidimensional Scales: Complex Assessment of Subjective States

Testing psychologists have devised many instruments that assess multiple dimensions of personality, affective state, and attitude. In each case a large pool of test items is used, and subjects must respond to each item. The items are drawn from subscales representing different dimensions of the factor being studied, and each subscale can be scored by evaluating the subject's performance on the respective subscale items. This type of measurement has been difficult to achieve for pain, but impressive progress has been made in the last decade by using word descriptors of pain as test items, with different items representing different dimensions of pain.

Melzack and Torgerson (79) called attention to the use of words representing several dimensions of experience for the scaling of pain. They noted that many words exist in English, and in nearly all languages, to describe pain. These words appear to represent different aspects of the subjective experience of pain, and patients choose them selectively to express sensory, emotional, or other aspects of a pain state. There have been a number of efforts to refine this language into a standardized form that can provide measurement of different dimensions. One involved the use of semantic differentials (27); most have involved attempts to define the independent factors that describe the various dimensions of pain (3,71). The most popular and most heavily used multifactor instrument of this kind is the McGill Pain Questionnaire (MPQ), which was introduced by Melzack (77) and has since been translated into several other languages, including Finnish (58). On the basis of work from the MPQ, this multidimensional language approach also has been extended by others into cross-modality matching techniques (37,103).

McGill Pain Questionnaire

This test instrument consists of 20 sets of words that describe pain. Patients are instructed to select those word sets that are relevant to their pain and to circle the word that best applies in each set. Each of the sets lists two to six words that are ranked in ascending order of intensity for the quality described by the set. Three purportedly distinct dimensions of pain are tapped by the word sets: sensory, affective, and evaluative, with a fourth miscellaneous group of words computed only in the total score. Sensory qualities are described most intensively with 10 of the sets devoted to them. Of those remaining word sets, five are affective descriptor sets and one set of words is evaluative. Presumably, this imbalance in test items across the dimensions occurs because the number of words in the English vocabulary that describe pain are not divided equally across the three categories.

Four types of scores are commonly computed from the MPQ. Scores are obtained for each of the three primary dimensions by either summing or averaging the word set scores in each dimension. Summing scores of all the word sets also gives a total score or Pain Rating Index. An investigator may count the Number of Words Chosen for a third type of score, and, finally, there is a Present Pain Intensity (PPI) score, which is the patient's rating on a verbally anchored 5-point scale for intensity of pain. The test instrument also gathers information about medications taken, the change in pain over time, and pain location, and it requires the patient to relate the present pain to previous, selected pain experiences such as headaches.

The measure may be administered either orally or in written form. Research has indicated that these forms are not entirely interchangeable, however. Although Graham et al. (39) found no difference between oral or written presentation, other researchers have reported higher scores on five of the six MPQ scales on the basis of oral versus written presentations (61). The primary difference in these two studies seems to have been providing the subject the opportunity to ask about the meaning of words, even if the administration was ultimately written. As Wolff (110) has noted, many words are too difficult for patients without college educations unless the words are defined for them. Walsh and Bowman (107) suggested that, for very sick patients, a combined visual and oral presentation was most effective.

Melzack (77) reported that the evaluative score correlated highly with the PPI. Because the PPI interpretation fluctuates considerably as a function of many individual factors, he suggested using change scores on the PPI rather than absolute scores when treatment comparisons are being made. Graham et al. (39) confirmed a close correlation between PPI and evaluative scores. The PPI score also has been shown to correlate with the VAS (108). Therefore, it may be preferable to use the VAS as a separate pain intensity score rather than the PPI, since the PPI contains all of the inherent difficulties discussed with the verbal rating scales and does not clearly provide additional information beyond that already contained in the other MPQ scales.

Critical evaluations of the MPQ have been largely supportive. The practice of grouping words into word sets was examined by Reading (88), who used a different methodology and statistical technique for this purpose. He found support for the grouping of words into semantically homogeneous subgroups with some comparatively small differences between his derived and the original MPQ formats. There was less consensus concerning the scaling of words which suggested that the range may vary across groups, or some of the subgroups may not lend themselves to description on a unitary dimension of intensity. Graham et al. (39) found that the response profiled by the test was replicable with repeated assessment.

The essential factor structure of the instrument also has been confirmed by a number of studies. The number of factors found for the words first delineated by Melzack and Torgerson (79) has varied from four to seven, depending on the population and the methods used. In sifting this evidence, it is clear that investigators consistently have reported a sensory dimension, an affective-evaluative dimension, and a mixed sensory-and-affective dimension (3,11,20,71,76,85,87). There does not appear to be definitive support for a separate evaluative dimension. Intensity has been reported to be affective-evaluative in nature rather than sensory, suggesting that asking patients to define their sensory experience will not provide intensity information (3).

The growing literature on the MPQ continues to yield generally supportive findings on its concurrent validity as well. Unique patterns of response have been obtained for different acute and chronic clinical pain syndromes including arthritis, labor and childbirth, pelvic pain, cancer pain, low back pain, and headaches (23,47,66,87,89). Reports have consistently indicated that increased use of affective descriptors is associated with higher levels of emotional disturbance in patients (2,70,76). Since chronic patients also may use more affective descriptors or a greater number of words, these factors may make diagnoses of chronic patients more difficult (2,27). However, scoring of the affective scale also may provide a measure of general emotional disturbance since this scale correlates well with other measures of affective states (64).

Taken together, these studies demonstrate impressive support for the basic structure of the MPQ, its reliability, and its validity. More studies are needed, of course, before strong conclusions can be achieved. It must be noted that this instrument's development has engendered a large number of investigations in the area of multidimensional pain scaling, and it has helped to sensitize clinical investigators to the multidimensional nature of pain.

Critical appraisal

The MPQ is an unconventional test instrument that is difficult to judge. It obtains data on both the quantitative and qualitative aspects of pain, and it achieves multidimensional scaling. Its factor structure appears sound, and it has wide applicability. More data are needed before its usefulness can be appraised properly. It is not yet certain whether the MPQ can provide refined discriminations within its dimensions. For example, the test should show reliably that a given clinical pain state changes after the patient is administered an opiate, and a different pattern of responses should be observed when a placebo is given. Patterns of pain description should change dramatically over days following surgery. The instrument may need refinement before it can achieve these criteria.

The work of defining replicable factors has not been completed, although the affective factor appears repeatedly strong. The sensory factor may need further refinement. These two dimensions have been the most useful in providing research results; however, it is not yet clear what other dimensions may be measured profitably with what word groupings. The MPQ, and all multidimensional subjective scaling techniques, assume that these pain dimensions are orthogonal. In fact, this is still a contested conclusion. Gracely et al. (38) provided support for this assumption with their ability to demonstrate that diazepam reduced affective but not sensory scores for subjects receiving experimentally induced pain. Atkinson et al. (2), on the other hand, found that mood change influenced the choice of both sensory and affective descriptors in a chronic pain patient population.

The scoring format for the MPQ also needs careful evaluation. Using ranked scores may distort the data, particularly since the word sets have unequal numbers of words and the dimensions have unequal numbers of word sets. Investigators have used both summed scores and averaged scores when computing the pain rating indices. Standardized scoring is greatly needed. The meaning of the total pain index, the number of words chosen, and the present pain intensity scores is still unclear. This issue of scoring format has received little attention yet is important for valid comparisons between research results. The statistical manipulation of the numbers obtained has received essentially no attention, yet the problems inherent in the data analysis are similar to those that have been so carefully enumerated in relation to the rating scales. The MPQ scores are best treated qualitatively but certainly do not merit use of parametric statistics.

One problem associated with the MPQ is that some patients, especially the poorly educated, have difficulty with the complexity of the vocabulary that it uses. Words such as *lancinating* are not commonly used to describe pain, even though they may be a part of the language. If the words presented to a patient are too demanding or unclear, compliance with the testing instructions cannot be assured. Moreover, patients may skip over words that they do not understand or that they never use, even though the words are strictly appropriate for the pain state. On the other hand, providing an opportunity to ask about the words in a set may place a response demand on the patient to choose a word in that set. The frequency of usage of words or word groups has not been taken into account in the construction of the instrument, and all groups and words are given equal weight in scoring. The preponderance of sensory descriptors in the test must certainly influence the test results. These issues require further research.

Clinical considerations

The MPQ is the most extensively tested multidimensional subjective scale available for pain measurement. It is therefore useful to clinical pain research. However, like any sophisticated test instrument, it is demanding and time consuming. It is difficult to use with very sick individuals as well as with patients who are poorly educated or whose native language is other than that used in the test. It requires strict assumptions about the ability of subjects to use and respond to its vocabulary. If a subject cannot handle the vocabulary fully, responses may be uninterpretable. A review of past research indicates that the sensory and affective scales would likely be most useful, that a VAS may be of greater value than the present pain intensity scale, and that, if written administration is planned, the words need to be gone over with the patient to clarify meanings that may not be understood. Plans for statistical analysis should be considered carefully before its use as a research tool.

Cross-Modality Matching: Objectifying Subjective Report?

These scales represent attempts to provide more objective, ratio scales for word descriptors that refer to subjective experiences of pain. They are based on magnitude estimation procedures developed for psychophysics by Stevens (100) and have been validated primarily in the laboratory. A unique power exponent is derived for each sensory experience being scaled, and the relation between the stimulus and response modalities is defined in terms of these exponents. This methodology has introduced a justified means of potentially matching clinical and experimental pain. Such a matching approach was used in pain measurement in the past and then dropped into disfavor (110). For instance, Sternbach (99) matched clinical pain with sub-maximum effort tourniquet pain and then measured submaximum tolerance to assess a ratio of current pain to pain tolerance. This ratio could then be compared with pain as rated by the patient on a numeric rating scale of pain tolerance. However, he eventually abandoned this method of matching pain.

The more recent psychophysical efforts have chosen words from the list by Melzack and Torgerson (79). These words have been ranked on two or three scales of sensation, affect, and intensity (37,104). The numeric magnitude of each word on the scale is determined through a cross-modality matching of psychophysical data. Handgrip, line length, or a similar objective measure is used repeatedly to establish magnitude standards, which may then be cross-matched with another variable such as experimental pain. These standards can be used by patients to rate their clinical pains. This procedure assures response consistency and is reportedly less sensitive to the response bias difficulties that effect category scales. The resulting data have been reliable across subjects, between groups, and within subjects (37,104). The advantage of matching techniques over the VAS, in addition to possible reduced response bias, lies in their quantification of verbal descriptors and clarification of dimension qualities. It has been reported that when subjects were requested to score intensity and unpleasantness separately, they tended to scale only intensity until verbal descriptors were provided. They then appeared able to judge the dimensions independently (36).

The ratio scales are treated without statistical limits, unlike the data from other rating scales or the MPQ. The validity and sensitivity of these scales has been supported primarily by experimental manipulations (36,37,103). However, there are some indications that these measurements will be equally relevant for clinical use (44,104).

Efforts to expand the usefulness of cross-modality matching into a clinical form have included development of the Pain Perception Profile by Tursky et al. (104). This instrument has four parts. The first measures sensation threshold; the second uses magnitude estimation procedures to judge induced pain; the third involves psychophysical scaling of the verbal pain descriptors, which are then used to measure pain on the three dimensions of intensity, reaction, and sensation; and the fourth allows the use of the psychophysically scaled descriptors in a diary format for repeated assessment over time.

Critical appraisal

This approach is of great potential value because it offers to bridge research in the clinical context with that carried out in the human subjects laboratory. Approval of these scales is not unanimous, however, and controversy centers on how complicated they are and whether they are bias-free, reliable, or valid as ratio rather than ranked data (35,41). They do appear to be at least as valid and reliable as the other subjective techniques available, and they have more valid justifications for the numeric distance between verbal anchors. However, the requirements for matching may well make them appear too complex for easy clinical use. With the level of agreement on the ranks of the word descriptors as well as the numeric magnitude of the descriptors, it may be possible to use the word scales with number equivalents without the cross-modality matching.

In support of this single scale approach, rather than the MPQ word set approach, Shapiro (98) argued that intensity of feeling can be least ambiguously measured by one scaled variable rather than by adding multiple questionnaire items that purport to test the same factor. If the adjectives on the MPQ prove useful in themselves for making diagnostic distinctions, that measure may justify itself. If only total scores on the affective and sensory dimensions of the MPQ are used, however, the Gracely or Tursky scales, even if used as ranked scores, may prove as valid and reliable as the MPQ.

Clinical considerations

The word scales provided by either the Gracely or Tursky techniques may be useful ultimately because they are shorter than the MPQ and may provide more reliable, valid information than simple rating scales. If the ratio scale values are reliable within subjects on repeated measures and between subjects, as they have been reported to be, it may be possible to use the scales with ratio values without the need to match handgrip or line length. However, before these scales will be advantageous for wide use in clinical settings, further research is needed on the extent of matching necessary and on their validity and reliability in clinical populations.

Behavioral Assessment: Objective Data

No matter how elegant and sophisticated the methods used, quantification of subjective states is problematic. The data obtained are always subject to affective influence and cognitive mediation, even in cases such as cross-modality matching, which appears to rely to a greater extent on performance. One assumes that the patient's report of pain experience includes components of nonpain states or traits such as anxiety, depression, social contingencies, and cognitive styles. These are important facets of the pain experience, but they do not give reliable information on what the patient's observable behavior will be. The importance of behavior in both the experience and treatment of pain is now an accepted fact (26). Thus an alternative approach, which can be used as an adjunct to subjective assessment, is the quantification of behavior. By relating behavior to documented tissue injury and to subjective report, the investigator can evaluate what patients actually *do* relative to how they say they *feel* and in conjunction with what they should be capable of doing.

Behavior has not always been seen as an important target for pain measurement. In large part this has been for the same reasons that it is now increasingly considered an essential component, that is, the lack of congruence between behavior and self-reported subjective measures. If a patient complained of pain, physicians felt an obligation to respond to the patient's request for help even if nonverbal indications of pain were not readily evident. Huskisson (49) recommended not using behavioral measures because volunteers in experimental studies were found to feel pain that was not visible in their facial expressions, and this disparity in report and expression increased over time. Other investigators also have documented that facial expression of pain can be manipulated by research subjects (19,69). Another study has reiterated that changes in pain relief among chronic arthritis sufferers did not relate to their ability to tie shoelaces or address envelopes (50). This points out a major issue of behavior measurement: the need to choose for measurement those dimensions of activity that are specific to pain rather than to other functional disabilities.

Behaviorists take an aggressive stance on pain measurement. They point out that self-report is highly obstrusive, sensitizes people to situational demands, and may be distorted; some people are unable to use language as a medium to communicate their thoughts and feelings (19). Furthermore, research has confirmed that nurses respond more to physiologic signs, nonverbal behaviors, or their own biases when self-report and nonverbal communication conflict (9,21,51). Most treatment programs for chronic pain sufferers work toward increasing the patient's functioning; thus it seems inconsistent to measure their results in terms of subjective experience of pain rather than increased rates of functioning. These considerations are used to support behavior analysis as a more valid form of pain assessment than subjective report.

Behavior patterns can be recorded in a number of ways. Self-report activity information is commonly collected from the patient. The use of activity diaries to document global activities on a daily basis is now common in treatment centers (e.g., 26). These not only provide information to clinicians but also serve to make the patient more aware of his or her patterns of pain-related behavior. Increasingly, observational methods such as video recording equipment, other instrumentation, or trained nurses can record the frequency of certain behaviors over time. Electrical or mechanical devices sometimes can provide additional information about the speed or force of certain actions, or they can record the patient's general level of activity over some unit of time. Most investigators study verbal behavior, postural changes, groaning, complaining, rest or withdrawal, and medication demand. Frequency or rate of occurrence is commonly scored. The discrepancy between the patient's actual pain behavior and expected behavior in view of their physical limitations defines the pain problem for the clinician in most instances.

Once the behavioral abnormalities of the patient are documented, the clinician may choose to discriminate which aspects of the behavioral aberrations are attributable to organic problems such as disease or injury, rewards for pain behavior in the patient's environment, or internal psychologic problems. For example, Craig and Prkachin (19), in a review of nonverbal pain behavior, reported that pain disorders with greater psychologic than organic components are characterized by more verbal complaints, acute reactions when changing position, and groaning as opposed to sucking in breath during pangs of distress. Studies also have documented that pain reports vary depending on the patient's perception of the observer (7). The patient whose spouse reinforces his or her pain behavior is more likely to complain of higher levels of pain.

The specific behaviors recorded in a given study vary according to the type of pain under investigation and the questions asked by the investigators. Measures used for acute pain studies are, in general, simpler than those examined in chronic pain research. Often basic data such as vocalization, withdrawal, or movement in bed will suffice for acute pain research, whereas chronic pain studies will be much more comprehensive, involving data from a number of social and medical settings rather than a single setting. Keefe (54) has reviewed behavioral assessment procedures for chronic pain. Among the common variables are: (a) measures of the amount of time spent standing, sitting, or reclining (uptime versus downtime); (b) patterns of sleep; (c) sexual activity; (d) performance of specified tasks such as stair climbing or situps, medication demand or intake; (e) food intake; (f) normal household activities such as meal preparation and gardening; and (g) engagement in recreational activity.

Behaviors Reported by Patients

The most efficient and economic way to obtain data from patients is to ask them what they do. A number of pencil and paper instruments have been designed to catalog patient activities. Among these are pain diaries in which patients record their activities and medications over 24-hr periods for days or weeks. Other data commonly collected are records of things the patient can currently do and things that the patient could do before the accident or disease but can no longer do.

Patients can be accurate and reliable observers, but the data available thus far indicate that they often are not. For example, Ready et al. (90) found that chronic pain patients reported medication use that was 50 to 60% less than actual drug intake. Kremer et al. (67) observed discrepant reports of patient activity and social behavior when comparing patient records with staff observations. Disability compensation has been noted to be associated most consistently with distortions in self-report. Sanders (95) found a moderate positive correlation between self-report and automated monitoring of uptime by normal controls, psychiatric inpatients, and chronic low back pain patients. All groups averaged less self-reported uptime than the automated report indicated, although the discrepancy was greatest for low back pain patients. Thus, although self-reports of activity are relatively easy to obtain from patients, the accuracy and reliability of such data are open to question. Testing devices that incorporate methods of assessing the proclivity of patients to respond untruthfully have not yet been developed for pain assessment, although these are commonly used in personality testing.

Observational Data

When patients can be observed or videotaped, behaviors can be scored. Such measures are usually quite specific to types of pain rather than general in nature. Kerner and Alexander (57) found that, when activities could be broken down into independent task components, the reliability of ratings increased when the behavior definitions were specific rather than gross. For highly interdependent tasks, a behaviorally anchored gross rating scale may be more effective. While self-report measures might be quite similar for headache and back pain patients (indeed, the same inventories could be used for each), behavioral observation data might be altogether different. Nevertheless, some general statements have been made about observational pain data. Fredericksen et al. (30) distinguished three general categories of pain behavior: (a) somatic interventions such as the use of medications or the seeking of surgery; (b) impaired functioning indicated by reduced mobility or range of movement, avoidance of occupational committment, or impaired interpersonal relationships; and (c) pain complaints, moaning, or contorted facial expression.

Most coding of facial expressions of pain has been done with gross judgments, such as "grimacing." More elaborate codes have been developed by Ekman and Friesen (25), but this system has been used rarely for assessing pain levels. The major research in this area has been by LeResche (72), who coded candid photographs of people in acute pain and isolated one prototypic pain expression, with some variations, which was characterized by "brow lowering with skin drawn in tightly around closed eyes, accompanied by a horizontally-stretched, open mouth, sometimes with deepening of the nasolabial furrow" (*p. 53*). This total pattern showed little overlap with prototypic expressions of fear, sadness, anger, or disgust. The usefulness of extensive work on facial expression likely will vary, depending on the pain location and duration, particularly since these expressions of pain are reportedly less frequent in chronic patients and can be so easily dissimulated. With acute facial pain, this work may be quite productive. The rigor and attention to coding detail is worth emulation in other methods of behavior assessment.

A specific schema for scoring back pain was introduced by Keefe and Block (55), who developed an observational system for scoring pain behavior in chronic back pain patients. Guarded movement, bracing, rubbing, and sighing were assessed in a series of studies. The investigators found that: (a) these behaviors could be observed reliably and their frequencies correlated with reports of pain; (b) both the frequencies of these behaviors and pain reports decreased with treatment; and (c) pain patients engaged in these behaviors more often than did normals or depressed controls. Bracing and rubbing were not significantly related to observers judgments of extent of pain; guarding was most highly related. Grimacing and sighing were infrequent behaviors in this chronic population.

Although Keefe and Block remarked that behaviors were correlated with pain self-report, none of these correlations reached 0.60; thus the two are clearly not equivalent. Guarding was most highly associated with observer and self-report, suggesting that, for low back pain, guarding may provide the best discriminator of pain behavior. These authors helped to validate their measures as indicators of back pain by comparing the behavior of patients with that of controls. Similar procedures will be needed by other investigators who attempt to develop behavioral indicators of pain. Since few, if any, behaviors are pain-specific, the validity of inferences based on behavioral data will require cleverly designed controls.

Other systems have been developed to measure pain behaviors similarly. These tend to be for low back pain. Fordyce et al. (28) reported a consistent negative relation between the amount of exercise performed and expressions of pain as measured by: (a) verbal statements of pain; (b) verbal statements about inability to perform; (c) gestures of holding, rubbing, or guarding; and

(d) audible gasps or moans. Cinciripini and Floreen (16) developed a system for evaluating treatment outcome that can be used in natural settings rather than requiring videotaping, thus reducing response demand characteristics. Their observation system incorporates both "pain- and well-behaviors," including pain talk, nonverbal pain behavior, nonpain complaints, pro-health talk, and assertive behaviors. In their sample, pro-health changes were less dramatic than decreases in pain-behaviors. These results suggest that well-behaviors may be supported by different contingencies, and therefore may require direct modeling and staff reinforcement.

The importance of well-behaviors has not often been recognized by pain psychometrists; however, its relevance was strikingly documented in a study of burn patients (60). When given equal weighting with pain behaviors, it was discovered that well-behaviors significantly outnumbered complaints even during intensely painful procedures. The observation system used in this study was derived from Lewinsohn (73) and targeted primarily the content of verbalizations. As a result, it allowed closer evaluation not only of coping behaviors but of probable cognitive coping styles as well. It may be useful for future work in discriminating which coping styles relate more to development of chronic pain in acute patients and in developing staff sensitivity to reinforcing well-behaviors.

A 0 to 10 scale has also been developed, which rates 10 behaviors from verbal complaints to medication use (92). The UAB Pain Behavior Scale is rated by an observer on each of the global functions as "none," "occasionally," or "frequent." This measurement has had some validity and reliabiity checking and has been shown to change from pre- to posttreatment. It does not show a consistent correlation with the MPQ or rated self-report of pain during pretreatment assessment; however, the correlation increased after treatment. Well-behaviors correlated negatively with pain-behaviors, although they were not mirror images. The advantage of this measure is that it can be completed quickly. As with the other behavioral rating systems, it requires further cross-validation and perhaps refinement before confirmation of its sensitivity and validity.

Mobility and quality of motion also may be measured. Two studies have reported objective systems for assessing low back pain based on responses to such directed tasks as lateral bending and leg raising (68,106). Lankhorst et al. (68) contrasted the patient's self-report of pain with his or her functional capacity and mobility of the lumbar spine. Waddell et al. (106) demonstrated that specific forms of physical examination can discriminate patients with non-organic physical signs from those with pathologic conditions.

One of the few studies of headache behaviors evaluated oversensitivity to, and avoidance of, stimuli such as noise and bright lights to distinguish headache and pain-free subjects (83). The subjects calibrated the stimuli on a scale from "comfortable" to "definitely unpleasant." Further investigation will be required to validate whether this tool can discriminate levels of pain reliably as well as pain versus pain-free states. It is evident that the significant behaviors that denote headache pain vary dramatically from many of those that denote low back pain. This limits the generalizability of the scales and substantially increases the development work required for this form of measurement.

There also have been efforts to record pain behavior technically. Sanders (94) developed a device that could be worn by patients. The device contains a timer activated by movement and it can be used to score uptime in chronic pain patients. Similar records can be obtained by a portable activity recorder developed commercially by Medilog, Inc.

Critical appraisal

The objective scales for counting behaviors and medications or the mechanical devices for timing posture changes and activities provide more sensitive measures and allow higher level statistical manipulation than scales that rate behaviors and therefore have the weaknesses of subjective scales. Consequently, they are preferable.

Observer-rated scales measure behavior rather than pain per se. As a result, they might be considered pain correlates rather than measurements of pain level. They are not able to separate dimensions of pain such as emotional or sensory components; however, they are also not potentially distorted by cognitive or affective mediation from the patient. They are able to take into account fluctuations based on external environmental or social contingencies. This benefit is also a limitation in that the data obtained by specific observation rather than global self-report are situation-specific. Therefore, variations by social setting or environment need to be considered in measurement and research conclusions. Investigators who undertake this form of measurement in the clinical context should be aware that behavioral and subjective report measures may yield inconsistent or even opposite outcomes in some chronic pain populations. This does not mean that one or the other is invalid. Rather, it reflects the tendency of certain patients to exaggerate their expressions of pain while at the same time showing none of the expected postural or activity indicators of severe pain. The opposite occurrence also may be observed in stoic patients: the report of moderate pain with severe behavioral indicators.

Clinical considerations

Behavioral assessment now seems an essential component of any treatment efficacy evaluation. The best form of this assessment is less clear, partially because the tools available that may be most objective are new and not extensively contrasted or validated. Activity diaries may provide useful qualitative information; however, their results must be evaluated with some skepticism. Observational data will provide more reliable information than self-report, and time or count data will be more statistically robust than subjective scaling even by observers. In regard to medication, it is essential that dosages be converted to a standardized scale of equivalents rather than being simply summed by number of pills or other such loose measurement systems. Rapid conversion tables are available (e.g., 90). Assessment of well-behaviors in addition to pain-behaviors is certainly of relevance. There is still much room to incorporate the elements from a number of the systems reviewed into a comprehensive program for objectively observing behaviors. This program ideally would not require an intrusive observer and could be done in a variety of natural settings for a representative sample of behavior. An evaluation of appropriate timing and places for assessment is still needed, and systems that would incorporate objective, observational data into follow-up as well as posttreatment outcome have not been discussed in the literature.

Physiologic Correlates of Pain States

Efforts to measure clinical pain through autonomic indicators or other physiologic tools have met with limited success (46). These measures have produced a large body of contradictory findings. They now serve primarily as supporting evidence for verbal pain reports in laboratory studies or are used as feedback adjuncts to treatment. The exception to this may be with headache pain, where physiologic recordings continue prevalent. Efforts have been made to correlate pain with muscle tension, autonomic indices, and central nervous system variables. Although all of these indicators have demonstrated fluctuations with changes in pain, no consistent associations have been found between individual pain report and these physiologic measurements. The usefulness of autonomic measures, particularly, is limited by their tendency to decrease over recording time irrespective of pain perception and their sensitivity to nonpain factors such as stress. Nonetheless, they may help to quantify emotional aspects of human pain experience, such as anxiety, which are currently ignored in much research.

Muscle Tension

Electromyographic (EMG) studies have been reported extensively, in part because biofeedback has been integrated into most chronic pain treatment programs for low back pain or myofascial pain. Studies have shown EMG differences between pain patients and normal controls, but these differences are not consistent across studies or patients even with the same pain location or diagnosis. Lower back pain (LBP) provides a good area for elucidation of the difficulties in using these measures to treat, much less quantify, clinical pain. Kraus and Raab (62) estimated that 80% of all LBP problems result from back muscle deficiencies or decreased mobility. Yet in a review of LBP and EMG studies, Wolf et al. (109) reported that a growing number of researchers have found that paraspinal EMG may be either elevated or reduced in LBP patients even with identical diagnoses. They noted that EMGs do not correlate with pain perception, and that methods of recording and placement of electrodes have varied greatly between investigations. Furthermore, data have not been available on patterns of normal EMGs to allow patient comparisons.

Wolf et al. (109) presented a case for more complex understanding and treatment of LBP with EMGs. It has been reported that more consistent paraspinal fluctuations from normal are evident in LBP patients when they are tensing muscles or active than when at rest (18,63). The study by Collins et al. (18) demonstrated that LBP patients generally were more aroused than controls during performance of stress tasks but not in their paraspinal muscles. Wolf et al. noted that their LBP patients had disproportionate activity from each side of the low back, with symmetrical patterns during rotation and asymmetrical patterns during movement. Normals responded in the reverse. These researchers noted that static and dynamic EMG measures are required with dual channel, bilateral feedback. With this design, they were then able to train internalized postural adjustments and to demonstrate changes in EMG recordings that corresponded to MPQ sensory pain report.

In a review of headache research and a study that attempted to control for previous methodologic shortcomings, Andrasik et al. (1) found no consistent patterns of physiologic measurement outcomes between types of headache or types of measurement. Contradictory findings were recorded with forehead and forearm EMG, temporal artery blood flow, hand surface temperature, heart rate, and skin resistance level. They concluded that headache pain is a complex phenomenon without a unidimensional physiologic response etiology. Nonetheless, physiologic measurement continues to receive attention particularly from headache investigators and treatment centers despite methodologic flaws and inconsistent results (e.g., 84).

Autonomic Indices

These measures now serve primarily as supporting evidence for verbal pain reports, although significant findings have been reported. For instance, Glynn et al. (33) found that chronic pain patients hyperventilated, and patients whose pain decreased with treatment showed drops in hyperventilation. Autonomic assessments are frequent in pain research; however, they may prove most useful as correlates of emotional dimensions of pain. Their greatest limitation is that with experimental pain they show decrements in response over time, and, in clinical populations, results have been inconsistent both with subjective reports and between studies (1). Common measures have included heart rate, skin temperature, finger pulse volume, skin conductance and resistance, and temporal artery blood flow.

An exception to the questionable value of autonomic measures seems to be thermography, which provides color change patterns reflecting skin tem-

behavioral measures, but this work needs extending into other pain areas. Until a quality comprehensive system is available for evaluating pain patients, clinicians and researchers must pick and choose among the scales and instruments available.

ACKNOWLEDGMENTS

We thank Patricia Kunz for word processing and editorial assistance. The first author was supported by NIH NRSA grant N507217 and the second author was supported by NIH grant NS16329 during the writing of this chapter.

REFERENCES

1. Andrasik, F., Blanchard, E. B., Arena, J. G., Saunders, N. L., and Barron, K. D. (1982): Psychophysiology of recurrent headache: Methodological issues and new empirical findings. *Behav. Ther.*, 13:407–429.
2. Atkinson, J. H., Kremer, E. F., and Ignelzi, R. J. (1982): Diffusion of pain language with affective disturbance confounds differential diagnosis. *Pain*, 12:375–384.
3. Bailey, C. A., and Davidson, P. O. (1976): The language of pain: Intensity. *Pain*, 2:319–324.
4. Beaver, W. T. (1983): Measurement of analgesic efficacy in man. In: *Advances in Pain Research and Therapy, Vol. 5*, edited by J. J. Bonica, U. Lindblom, and A. Iggo. Raven Press, New York.
5. Beecher, H. K. (1956): Relationship of significance of wound to pain experienced. *JAMA*, 161:1609–1613.
6. Beecher, H. K. (1957): The measurement of pain. *Pharmacol. Rev.*, 9:59–209.
7. Block, A. R., Kremer, E. G., and Gaylor, M. (1980): Behavioral treatment of chronic pain: The spouse as a discriminative cue for pain behavior. *Pain*, 9:243–252.
8. Bock, R. D., and Jones, L. V. (1968): *The Measurement and Prediction of Judgement and Choice*. Holden-Day, San Francisco.
9. Bond, M. R., and Pilowsky, I. (1966): Subjective assessment of pain and its relationship to the administration of analgesics in patients with advanced cancer. *Psychosom. Res.*, 10:203–208.
10. Bonica, J. J. (1953): *Management of Pain*. Lea and Febiger, Philadelphia.
11. Byrne, M., Troy, A., Bradley, L. A., Marchisello, P. J., Geisinger, K. F., Van der Keide, L. H., and Prieto, E. J. (1982): Cross validation of the factor structure of the McGill Pain Questionnaire. *Pain*, 13:193–201.
12. Casey, K. L. (1980): Supraspinal mechanisms in pain: The reticular formation. In: *Pain and Society*, edited by H. W. Kosterlitz and L. Y. Terenius, pp. 183–200. Verlag Chemie, Weinheim.
13. Chapman, C. R. (1978): Psychologic aspects of pain. (Special Report) *Hosp. Pract.* 13:15–19.
14. Chapman, C. R., Colpitts, Y. H., Mayeno, J. K., and Gagliardi, G. J. (1981): Rate of stimulus repetition changes evoked potential amplitude: Dental and auditory modalities compared. *Exp. Brain Res.*, 43:246–252.
15. Chudler, E. H., and Dong, W. K. (1983): The assessment of pain by cerebral evoked potentials. *Pain*, 16:221–244.
16. Cinciripini, P. M., and Floreen, A. (1982): An evaluation of a behavioral program for chronic pain. *J. Behav. Med.*, 5:375–389.
17. Coger, R. W., Kenton, B., Pinsky, J. J., Crue, B. L., Carmon, A., and Friedman, Y. (1980): Somatosensory evoked potentials and noxious stimulation in patients with intractable noncancer pain syndromes. *Psychiatr. Res.*, 2:279–294.

18. Collins, G. A., Cohen, M. J., Naliboff, B. D., and Schandler, S. L. (1982): Comparative analysis of paraspinal and frontalis EMG, heart rate and skin conductance in chronic low back pain patients and normals to various postures and stress. *Scand. J. Rehabil. Med.*, 14:39–46.
19. Craig, K. D., and Prkachin, K. M. (1983): Nonverbal measures of pain. In: *Pain Measurement and Assessment*, edited by R. Melzack, pp. 173–182. Raven Press, New York.
20. Crockett, D. J., Prkachin, K. M., and Craig, K. D. (1977): Factors of the language of pain in patient and volunteer groups. *Pain*, 4:175–182.
21. DePaulo, B. M., Rosenthal, R., Eisenstat, R. A., Rogers, P. L., and Finkelstein, S. (1978): Decoding discrepant nonverbal cues. *J. Pers. Soc. Psychol.*, 36:313–323.
22. Downie, W. W., Leatham, P. A., Rhind, V. M., Wright, V., Brancho, J. A., and Anderson, J. A. (1978): Studies with pain rating scales. *Ann. Rheum. Dis.*, 37:378–381.
23. Dubuisson, D., and Melzack, R. (1976): Classification of clinical pain descriptions by multiple group discriminant analysis. *Exp. Neurol.*, 51:480–487.
24. Duncan, G. H., Gregg, J. M., and Ghia, J. N. (1978): The pain profile: A computerized system for assessment of chronic pain. *Pain*, 5:275–284.
25. Ekman, P., and Friesen, W. V. (1978): *Manual for the Facial Action Coding System.* Consulting Psychologists Press, Palo Alto, Calif.
26. Fordyce, W. E. (1976): *Behavioral Methods for Chronic Pain and Illness.* C. V. Mosby, St. Louis.
27. Fordyce, W. E., Brena, S. F., Holcomb, R. J., DeLateur, B. J., and Loeser, J. D. (1978): Relationship of patient semantic pain descriptions to physician diagnostic judgments, activity level measures and MMPI. *Pain*, 5:293–303.
28. Fordyce W., McMahon, R., Rainwater, G., Jackins, S., Questad, K., Murphy. T., and DeLateur, B. (1981): Pain complaint–exercise performance relationship in chronic pain. *Pain*, 10:311–321.
29. Frank, A. J. M., Moll, J. M. H., and Hort, J. F. (1982): A comparison of three ways of measuring pain. *Rheumatol. Rehabil.*, 21:211–217.
30. Fredericksen, L. W., Lynd, R. S., and Ross, J. (1977): Methodology in the measurement of pain. *Behav. Ther.*, 9:486–488.
31. Fuccella, L. M., Corvi, G., Gorini, F., Mandelli, V., Mascellani, G., Nobili, F., Pedronetto, S., Ragni, N., and Vandelli, I. (1977): Application of nonparametric procedure for bioassay data to the evaluation of analgesics in man. *J. Clin. Pharmacol.*, 17:177–185.
32. Gandhavadi, B., Rosen J. S., and Addison, R. G. (1982): Autonomic pain: Features and methods of assessment. *Postgrad. Med. J.*, 71:85–90.
33. Glynn, C. J., Lloyd, J. W., and Folkhard, S. (1981): Ventilatory responses to chronic pain. *Pain*, 11:201–212.
34. Gracely, R. H. (1980): Pain measurement in man. In: *Pain, Discomfort and Humanitarian Care*, edited by L. K. Y. Ng and J. J. Bonica. Elsevier/North Holland, New York.
35. Gracely, R. H., and Dubner, R. (1981): Pain assessment in humans: A reply to Hall. *Pain*, 11:109–120.
36. Gracely, R. H., Dubner, R., and McGrath, P. (1979): Narcotic analgesia: Fentanyl reduces the intensity but not the unpleasantness of painful tooth pulp sensations. *Science*, 203:1261–1263.
37. Gracely, R. H., McGrath, P., and Dubner, R. (1978): Ratio scales of sensory and affective verbal pain descriptions. *Pain*, 5:5–18.
38. Gracely, R. H., McGrath, P., and Dubner, R. (1978): Validity and sensitivity of ratio scales of sensory and affective verbal pain descriptors: Manipulation of affect by diazepam. *Pain*, 5:19–29.
39. Graham, C., Bond, S. S., Gerkovich, M. M., and Cook, M. R. (1980): Use of the McGill Pain Questionnaire in the assessment of cancer pain: Replicability and consistency. *Pain*, 8:377–387.
40. Grennan, D. M., and Caygill, L. (1982): Infra-red thermography in the assessment of sacroiliac inflammation. *Rheumatol. Rehabil.*, 21:81–87.
41. Hall, W. (1981): On "Ratio scales of sensory and affective verbal pain descriptors." *Pain*, 11:101–107.
42. Hamilton, M. (1968): Some notes of rating scales. *Statistician*, 18:11–17.
43. Hardy, J. D., Wolff, H. G., and Goodell, H. (1952): *Pain Sensation and Reaction.* Williams & Wilkins, Baltimore.

44. Heft, M. W., Gracely, R. H., Dubner, R., and McGrath, P. A. (1980): A validation model for verbal descriptor scaling of human clinical pain. *Pain*, 9:363–373.
45. Hendler, N., Uematesu, S., and Long, D. (1982): Thermographic validation of physical complaints in 'psychogenic pain' patients. *Thermogr. Psychosom*, 23:283–287.
46. Hilgard, E. R., and Hilgard, J. R. (1975): *Hypnosis in the Relief of Pain*. William Kaufmann, Inc., Los Altos, Calif.
47. Hunter, M., and Philips C. (1981): The experience of headache: An assessment of the qualities of tension headache pain. *Pain*, 10:209–219.
48. Hunter, M., Philips, C., and Rachman, S. (1979): Memory for pain. *Pain*, 6:35–46.
49. Huskisson, E. C. (1974): Measurement of pain. *Lancet*, 2:1127-1131.
50. Huskisson, E. C., Jones, J., and Scott, P. J. (1976): Application of visual-analogue scales to the measurement of functional capacity. *Rheumatol. Rehabil.*, 15:185–187.
51. Jacox, A. K. (1980): The assessment of pain. In: *Pain: Meaning and Management*, edited by W. L. Smith, H. Merskey, and S. C. Cross, pp. 75–88. Spectrum Publications, New York.
52. Johnson, E., and Rice, H. (1974): Sensory and distress components of pain: Implications for the study of clinical pain. *Nurs. Res.*, 23:203–209.
53. Joyce, C. R. B., Zutish, D. W., Hrubes, V., and Mason, R. M. (1975): Comparison of fixed interval and visual analogue scales for rating chronic pain. *Eur. J. Clin. Pharmacol.*, 18:415–420.
54. Keefe, F. J. (1982): Behavioral assessment and treatment of chronic pain: Current status and future directions. *J. Consult. Clin. Psychol.*, 50:896–911.
55. Keefe, F. J., and Block, A. R. (1982): Development of an observation method for assessing pain behavior in chronic low back pain patients. *Behav. Ther.*, 13:363–375.
56. Keefe, F. J., Block, A. R., Williams, R. B., Jr., and Surwit, R. S. (1981): Behavioral treatment of chronic low back pain: Clinical outcome and individual differences in pain relief. *Pain*, 11:221–231.
57. Kerner, J. F., and Alexander, J. (1981): Activities of daily living: Reliability and validity of gross vs. specific ratings. *Arch. Phys. Med. Rehabil.*, 62:161–166.
58. Ketovuori, H., and Pontinen, P. J. (1981): A pain vocabulary in Finnish: The Finnish Pain Questionnaire. *Pain*, 11:247–253.
59. Kleck, R. E., Vaughan, R. C., Cartwright-Smith, J., Vaughan, K. B., Colby, C. Z., and Lanzetta, J. T. (1976): Effects of being observed on expressive, subjective, and physiological responses to painful stimuli. *J. Pers. Soc. Psychol.*, 34:1211–1218.
60. Klein, R. M., and Charlton, J. E. (1980): Behavioral observation and analysis of pain behavior in critically burned patients. *Pain*, 9:27–40.
61. Klepac, R. K., Dowling, J., Rokke, P., Dodge, L., and Schafer, L. (1981): Interview vs. paper-and-pencil administration of the McGill Pain Questionnaire. *Pain*, 11:241–246.
62. Kraus, H., and Raab, W. (1961): *Hypokinetic Disease*. Charles C Thomas, Springfield, Ill.
63. Kravitz, E., Moore, M. E., and Glaros, A. (1981): Paralumbar muscle activity in chronic low back pain. *Arch. Phys. Med. Rehabil.*, 62:172–176.
64. Kremer, E., and Atkinson, J. H., Jr. (1981): Pain measurement: Construct validity of the affective dimension of the McGill Pain Questionnaire with chronic benign pain patients. *Pain*, 11:93–100.
65. Kremer, E., Atkinson, J. H., and Ignelzi, R. J. (1981): Measurement of pain: Patient preference does not confound pain measurement. *Pain*, 10:241–248.
66. Kremer, E. F., Atkinson, J. H., Jr., and Ignelzi, R. J. (1982): Pain measurement: The affective dimensional measure of the McGill Pain Questionnaire with a cancer pain population. *Pain*, 12:153–163.
67. Kremer, E. F., Block, A., and Gaylor, M. S. (1981): Behavioral approaches to treatment of chronic pain: The inaccuracy of patient self-report measures. *Arch. Phys. Med. Rehabil.*, 62:188–191.
68. Lankhorst, G. J., van de Stadt, R. J., Vogelaar, T. W., van der Korst, J. K., and Prevo, A. J. H. (1982): Objectivity and repeatability of measurements in low back pain. *Scand. J. Rehabil. Med.*, 14:21–26.
69. Lanzetta, J. T., Cartwright-Smith, J., and Kleck, R. E. (1976): Effects of nonverbal dissimulation on emotional experience and autonomic arousal. *J. Pers. Soc. Psychol.*, 33:354–370.

70. Leavitt, R., and Garron, D. C. (1979): Psychological disturbances and pain report differences in both organic and nonorganic low back pain patients. *Pain*, 7:187–195.

71. Leavitt, F., Garron, D. C., Whisler, W. W., and Sheinkop, M. B. (1978): Affective and sensory dimensions of back pain. *Pain*, 4:273–281.

72. LeResche, L. (1982): Facial expression of pain: A study of candid photographs. *J. Nonverb. Behav.*, 7:46–56.

73. Lewinsohn, P. (1976): Manual of instructions for the behavior ratings used for the observation of interpersonal behavior. In: *Behavior Therapy Assessment: Diagnosis, Design and Evaluation*, edited by E. Mash, and L. Tendal, pp. 335–343. Springer, New York.

74. Lewith, G. T., and Machin, D. (1981): A method of assessing the clinical effects of acupuncture. *Acupunct. Electrothera. Res.*, 6:265–276.

75. Matyas, T. A. (1982): Letter to the editor. *Pain*, 13:203–204.

76. McCreary, C., Turner, J., and Dawson, E. (1981): Principal dimensions of the pain experience and psychological disturbance in chronic low back pain patients. *Pain*, 11:85–92.

77. Melzack, R. (1975): The McGill Pain Questionnaire: Major properties and scoring methods. *Pain*, 1:277–299.

78. Melzack, R., and Casey, K. L. (1968): Sensory, motivational and central control determinants of pain: A new conceptual model. In: *The Skin Senses*, edited by D. Kenshalo, pp. 423-443. Charles C Thomas, Springfield.

79. Melzack, R., and Torgerson, W. S. (1971): On the language of pain. *Anesthesiology* 34(1): 50–59.

80. Murrin, K. R., and Rosen, M. (1981): Measurement of pain. In: *Persistent Pain. Modern Methods of Treatment, Vol. 3*, edited by S. Lipton and J. Miles, pp. 17-38. Academic Press, London.

81. Ohnhaus, E. E., and Adler, R. (1975): Methodological problems in the measurement of pain: A comparison between the verbal rating scale and the visual analogue scale. *Pain*, 1:379–384.

82. Pakula, A., and Milvidaite, I. (1983): Memory for acute coronary pain: Decay with time versus reliability of measures. In: *Advances in Pain Research and Therapy, Vol. 5*, edited by J. J. Bonica, U. Lindblom, and A. Iggo, pp. 877–885. Raven Press, New York.

83. Philips, H. C., and Hunter, M. (1982): A laboratory technique for the assessment of pain behavior. *J. Behav. Med.*, 5:283–294.

84. Raczynski, J. M., and Thompson, J. K. (1983): Methodological guidelines for clinical headache research. *Pain*, 15:1–18.

85. Reading, A. E. (1979): The internal structure of the McGill Pain Questionnaire in dysmenorrhea patients. *Pain*, 7:353–358.

86. Reading, A. E. (1980): A comparison of pain rating scales. *J. Psychosom. Res.*, 24:119–124.

87. Reading, A. E. (1982): A comparison of the McGill Pain Questionnaire in chronic and acute pain. *Pain*, 13:185–192.

88. Reading, A. E. (1983): The McGill Pain Questionnaire: An Appraisal. In: *Pain Measurement and Assessment*, edited by R. Melzack, pp. 55–62. Raven Press, New York.

89. Reading, A. E., and Newton, J. R. (1977): A comparison of primary dysmenorrhoea and intrauterine device related pain. *Pain*, 3:165–176.

90. Ready, L. B., Sarkis, E., and Turner, J. A. (1982): Self-reported vs. actual use of medications in chronic pain patients. *Pain*, 12:285–294.

91. Revill, S. I., Robinson, J. O., Rosen, M., and Hogg, M. I. J. (1976): The reliability of a linear analogue for evaluating pain. *Anaesthesia*, 31:1191–1198.

92. Richards, J. S., Nepomuceno, C., Riles, M., and Suer, Z. (1982): Assessing pain behavior: The UAB Pain Behavior Scale. *Pain*, 14:393–398.

93. Rubal, B. J., Traycoff, R. B., and Ewing, K. L. (1982): Liquid crystal thermography. A new tool for evaluating low back pain. *Phys. Ther.*, 62:1593–1596.

94. Sanders, S. H. (1980): Toward a practical instrument system for the automatic measurement of "up-time" in chronic pain patients. *Pain*, 9:103–109.

95. Sanders, S. H. (1983): Automated versus self-monitoring of "up-time" in chronic low-back pain patients: A comparative study. *Pain*, 15:399–405.

96. Scott, J., and Huskisson, E. C. (1976): Graphic representation of pain. *Pain*, 2:175–184.

97. Scott, J., and Huskisson, E. C. (1979): Accuracy of subjective measurements made with or without previous scores: An important source of error in serial measurement of subjective states. *Ann. Rheum. Dis.*, 38:558–559.

98. Shapiro, M. B. (1975): The single variable approach to assessing the intensity of the feeling of depression. *Eur. J. Behav. Anal. Modif.*, 1:62–70.
99. Sternbach, R. (1974): *Pain Patients: Traits and Treatment.* Academic Press, London.
100. Stevens, S. S. (1975): *Psychophysics.* Wiley, New York.
101. Thompson, S. C. (1981): Will it hurt less if I can control it? A complex answer to a simple question. *Psychol. Bull.*, 90:89–101.
102. Toomey, T. C., Taylor, A. G., Skelton, J. A., and Carron, H. (1982): Stability of self-report measures of improvement in chronic pain: A five-year follow-up. *Pain*, 12:273–283.
103. Tursky, B. (1976): The development of a pain perception profile: A psychophysical approach. In: *Pain: New Perspectives in Therapy and Research*, edited by M. Weisenberg and B. Tursky, pp. 171–194. Plenum Press, New York.
104. Tursky, B., Jamner, L. D., and Friedman, R. (1982): The pain perception profile: A psychophysical approach to the assessment of pain report. *Behav. Ther.*, 13:376–394.
105. Twycross, R. G. (1976): The measurement of pain in terminal carcinoma. *J. Int. Med. Res.*, 4:58–67.
106. Waddell, G., McCulloch, J. A., Kummer, E., and Venner, R. M. (1980): Nonorganic physical signs in low-back pain. *Spine*, 5:117–125.
107. Walsh, T. D., and Bowman, K. (1982): Letter to the editor. *Pain*, 14:75.
108. Walsh, T. D., and Leber, B. (1983): Measurement of chronic pain: Visual Analog Scales and McGill Melzack Pain Questionnaire compared. In: *Advances in Pain Research and Therapy, Vol. 5*, edited by J. J. Bonica, U. Lindblom, and A. Iggo, pp. 897–899. Raven Press, New York.
109. Wolf, S. L., Nacht, M., and Kelly, J. L. (1982): EMG feedback training during dynamic movement for low back pain patients. *Behav. Ther.*, 13:395–406.
110. Wolff, B. B. (1978): Behavioural measurement of human pain. In: *The Psychology of Pain*, edited by R. A. Sternbach, pp. 129–168. Raven Press, New York.

Advances in Pain Research and Therapy, Vol. 7,
edited by C. Benedetti et al.
Raven Press, New York © 1984.

Pain and the Elderly

*S. W. Harkins, **Joseph Kwentus, and †Donald D. Price

*Departments of *Gerontology, Psychiatric and Psychology, **Psychiatry, and
†Anesthesiology, Medical College of Virginia, Virginia Commonwealth
University, Richmond, Virginia 23298*

The population of most industrialized countries including the United States is growing older. Estimates for 1983 indicated Americans over 65 years of age (approximately 27 million) outnumbered teenagers (approximately 26 million) for the first time in American history. The rising number of elderly in our society brings increasing awareness of the importance of quality of life in the later years. For many elderly people, pain is a constant companion with many forms. In a recent announcement, the National Institute on Aging, in considering the psychosocial needs of the elderly, included pain as a problem area worth warranting further research funding. The purpose of this chapter is to review current knowledge about age-related changes in pain perception and reporting. The laboratory study of pain in the elderly will be considered along with clinical and chronic pain.

LABORATORY STUDY OF AGE DIFFERENCES IN PAIN PERCEPTION

Age and Bioculture History

Knowledge about age-related changes in pain can be obtained through descriptive, developmental studies aimed at identification of intraindividual change across the lifespan or interindividual comparisons between young and old people. Chronological age is the primary organizational variable (4). The longitudinal study design examines lifespan changes or intraindividual change across time, allowing inferences about individual adaptation to the aging process. Unfortunately, there are no longitudinal studies of age-related responses to laboratory pain. All experimental studies of the relationship of pain to age compare younger and older groups. These cross-sectional studies allow inferences about interindividual differences, but it is impossible to determine whether observed group differences are due to age or confounding factors because such cross-sectional studies evaluate subjects at only one time point. Cross-sectional studies do not control for effects of biocultural history (3,53) because they involve groups born many years apart. Generational effects, or birth cohort differences between groups born many years apart, cannot be controlled. Thus all available studies of the relationship between pain and age are limited by confounding actual age-related intraindividual change with interindividual differences due to biocultural history.

Although all sensory experience is extremely personal, pain is especially difficult to assess in terms of stimulus-response functions alone because the affective dimension is critically influenced by contextual factors and meanings. Stimuli used to study the major senses, such as sight or hearing, can be specified as to their physical properties. This is more difficult, but not impossible, for stimuli giving rise to pain. Nevertheless, pain and discomfort are open to measurement whether due to a pathological state or induced in the laboratory.

Presbycusis, Presbyopia, and Presbyalgos

The later years are associated with a loss of auditory and visual function. These losses have been well characterized. Presbycusis (*presby*–old; *cusis*–hearing), is a gradual, symmetrical, progressive hearing loss, preferentially affecting high frequency sounds (19). Presbyopia (*opia*–sight) is an age-related visual loss characterized by loss of accommodation, slowing of dark-light adaptation, and loss of depth perception (19). Both presbycusis and presbyopia are characterized by changes in receptor anatomy and, to a lesser degree, by changes in the central nervous system (CNS). Etiology of these age-related sensory losses is unknown, but humoral, genetic, environmental, and disease processes are implicated to various degrees.

Although the effect of age on vision and hearing are well documented, it is unclear if systematic age-related changes in pain sensibility exist. Laboratory studies of the effects of aging on pain are ambiguous. There are studies that indicate that pain sensitivity may increase, decrease, or remain unchanged in the later years of life. Such varying results probably reflect differences between studies in behavioral endpoints, psychophysical procedures, methods employed to induce pain, criteria employed in subject selection, and training procedures. As a result, it is unclear if presbyalgos (*algos*–pain) exists.

Table 1 summarizes the literature comparing pain sensitivity in elderly and young volunteers. There are important differences in the methods for pain induction employed in these studies. Methods used in these studies include radiant heat, electrical stimulation, and mechanical stimulation. Additional variation between these studies occur because different dependent measures were employed. Several focused on pain threshold; others used pain reaction (reflexive behavior), and some studied pain tolerance. Such different behavioral endpoints may be differentially affected by bioculture history, age, or age-related pathology. For example, threshold and tolerance for noxious stimuli are measures of pain "sensitivity" that are independently influenced by differences in biocultural history.

TABLE 1. *Effects of age on pain sensitivity*

Investigators (ref.)	Modality/ method	Measurements of pain sensitivity in elderly compared to young groups				
		Pain threshold	Pain reaction threshold	Pain tolerance	Discrimination of suprathreshold painful stimuli	Response criterion for pain
Schumacher et al. (57)	Cutaneous/ thermal	Similar	—	—	—	—
Hardy et al. (26)	Cutaneous/ thermal	Similar	—	—	—	—
Chapman and Jones (16)	Cutaneous/ thermal	Higher	Higher	—	—	—
Birren et al. (7)	Cutaneous/ thermal	Similar	Similar	—	—	—
Sherman and Robillard (60,61)	Cutaneous/ thermal	Higher	Higher	—	—	—
Schludermann and Zubek (56)	Cutaneous/ thermal	Higher	Higher	—	—	—
Collins and Stone (18)	Cutaneous/ shock	Lower	—	Lower	—	—
Procacci et al. (50)	Cutaneous/ thermal	Higher	—	—	—	—
Clark and Mehl (17)	Cutaneous/ thermal	Higher[a]	—	—	Men: Similar[a,b] Women: Poorer	Higher[a]
Woodrow et al. (68)	Achilles tendon/ pressure	—	—	Lower	—	—
Harkins and Chapman (28,29)	Tooth/ shock	Similar	—	—	Poorer	Intensity dependent

[a] Middle-aged subjects.
[b] Young and older men, no difference in discrimination; older women, lower discrimination than younger.
From Harkins and Warner (32), with permission.

Thermal Pain Sensitivity

All studies of age and thermal pain have used the projection lamp technique, which focuses radiant energy on skin blackened with ink. Both the intensity of the heat stimulus and duration of exposure are controlled. Pain threshold is best defined as the point at which the subject verbally reports a sharp pricking or stinging sensation (27).

Studies employing radiant heat have generally found that pain threshold increases 12 to 20% in elderly compared to younger subjects. Chapman and Jones (16) evaluated threshold to noxious thermal stimuli delivered to blackened spots on the forehead in 200 volunteers between the ages of 12 and 85 years. In addition to verbal report, they included a "pain reaction threshold," defined as the smallest stimulus intensity necessary to produce a contraction of the eye muscles at the outer cantus as determined by the experimenter's visual inspection. The authors considered verbal report to be a more subjective and variable measure of pain sensitivity than pain reaction threshold. Cutaneous heat-pain sensitivity, as indexed by both pain (verbal report) and reaction thresholds, was found to decrease with age. Sherman and Robillard (59–61) also reported elevations of thermal pain and reaction thresholds in normal elderly subjects. Similar results were reported by Schluderman and Zubek (56), who evaluated radiant heat-pain sensitivity by verbal report at forearm, upper arm, forehead, thigh, and leg in 171 male volunteers ranging in age from 12 to 83 years. Their results indicated that pain threshold to noxious thermal stimuli remained constant during adolescence and middle-age but increased after the late 50s. These results can be interpreted to reflect a loss of cutaneous pain sensitivity in senescence (see Table 1).

Thus the studies reviewed so far indicate a loss of sensitivity to noxious cutaneous-heat stimulation during the later years of life. These results have been interpreted to reflect a change with age in CNS processes subserving pain perception. Such results are consistent with the generally accepted view that a decrease in the information processing capacity of the CNS occurs with aging. However, increases in thresholds for pure tones (presbycusis) and changes in vision (presbyopia) are more often due to changing receptor function than to changes with age in CNS processes (19). Changes with age in the skin senses of humans may be the result of subclinical peripheral neuropathies secondary to disease or injury, the probability of which increase with age (37). Thus the results reviewed above are not informative as to whether age-pain differences are due to peripheral factors, central factors, or some combination of both.

Procacci et al. (50) also employed radiant heat techniques and also found a decrease in cutaneous pain sensitivity with advancing age (see Table 1). They recognized, however, that increased radiant-heat pain thresholds in the elderly may be due to changes in the skin with age. This factor was not considered in earlier research. Procacci and his colleagues evaluated the thermal-energy dispersal properties of skin and found a significant increase in energy dispersion in senescent compared to younger skin. They concluded that age differences in thermal pain thresholds were due to (a) changes in skin thickness with age, which resulted in increased thermal dispersion and (b) increased nociceptor thresholds. They discounted CNS processes as the source of age differences in thermal nociceptors (50,51).

While Procacci's results regarding increased thermal dispersion properties of senescent skin are of great importance, there is no direct evidence for changes in receptor function with age. Peripheral receptor organs of human dermis are dynamic structures that undergo continuous transformation throughout the individual's lifespan. This is, however, more true of corpuscular receptor organs than of "free" nerve endings. Cauna (15) evaluated age-related changes in the human skin receptors in 200 individuals ranging in age from birth to 93 years. Pacinian corpuscles increased in size and appeared to remodel or reform on the axons of absolute corpuscles. Meissner's corpuscles decreased in number and increased in length from birth to old age. Free nerve endings, on the other hand, underwent little change. The histological development of corpuscular receptors is consistent with recent behavioral findings showing a logical, age-dependent change in vibrotactile thresholds for stimuli between 50 and 1,000 Hz but no age-related changes for lower frequencies (67). Such findings, although consistent with a duplex theory of mechanoreception, add little to the understanding of age-related changes in pain perception. Morphological study of "free" nerve endings and physiological study of A^{δ}- and C-fiber activity are necessary before conclusions about the peripheral mechanisms of age-related differences in nociception can be drawn.

In contrast to studies reporting increases in thermal pain threshold with aging, several studies have reported no age-related differences in thermal pain sensitivity (see Table 1). As early as 1943, Hardy et al. (26) noted the importance of separating attitudinal and judgmental factors from other interindividual factors influencing pain threshold. They reported that thermal pain threshold did not differ as a function of age when subjects were well instructed to maintain an unprejudiced and detached attitude. Attitudinal and judgmental issues are important in aging research in general (48). For example, Botwinick (10) suggests that reaction time slowing, a ubiquitous finding in geriatic research (31), may be due to increased "cautiousness" or general unwillingness to respond, rather than slowing in CNS information processes. Attitudinal and judgmental variables are particularly important in studies of pain perception. Age-related differences in pain threshold may well be due to attitudinal variables or response bias differences in cohorts rather than age-related differences in sensory/perceptual processes.

The introduction of Signal Detection Theory (SDT) (25) procedures to pain and aging research has aided in separation of individual differences in sensory processing from differences in attitudinal motivational and cognitive factors. Two SDT parameters, d' and response bias, differentiate efficiency of sensory processing from the willingness to group stimuli as belonging to a particular class of events (i.e., painful or not painful). In pain studies, high values of d', the index of "acuity," indicate efficiency in detecting an event or discriminating between events. High values of response bias indicate a reticence to report stimuli as being painful. High bias values could, therefore, be interpreted as stoicism. The methodology of SDT has been successfully applied to the study of pain in middle-age subjects by Clark and Mehl (17) and in elderly subjects by Harkins and Chapman (28,29).

Clark and Mehl (17) employed SDT procedures in their study of the effects of age on pain sensitivity. Using the radiant heat technique, they found that elevated pain thresholds in middle-aged subjects (mean age, 44 years) were accompanied by a stringent response bias. They suggested that the elevated pain threshold in their middle-aged subjects was due to a higher criterion for pain report, rather than age differences in sensory processes. These results are consistent with those of Rees and Botwinick (52) for pure tone thresholds. Rees and Botwinick's findings suggest that age differences in response bias are not limited to noxious stimuli. The elderly may withhold a response at low levels of stimulation to allow time to formulate a more certain response. This "cautious" approach in the elderly may result in a spuriously higher value of threshold measures.

Electrical Shock Sensitivity

Electrical stimulation of the teeth has been used in several laboratories to study the effects of age on pain. This technique has several advantages over radiant heat stimulation, including: (a) a relatively pure pain sensation; (b) consistent pain experience without tissue damage or irritation on repeated trials; and (c) a sensation similar to clinical pain and to pain elicited by natural stimuli.

The data from the tooth shock studies do not support the view that pain thresholds increase with age (see Table 1). Mumford (47), used electrical dental stimulation to study pain thresholds in subjects between 10 and 71 years of age and found no differences in pain threshold. He stated that "it seems reasonable to conclude that the pain perception threshold is not affected by age." Harkins and Chapman (28,29) confirmed Mumford's findings. Thus, although aging impairs some senses, this may not be the case for dental pain, despite age-related changes in dentin deposition, size of the pulp canal, retrogressive nerve changes, decreases in tooth nerve populations, and decreases in vascularity (66). Considering such intradental changes, the stability of dental pain thresholds with increasing age is all the more surprising.

Harkins and Chapman (28,29) evaluated the ability to distinguish between suprathreshold shocks using SDT methodology. Although their results indicated no effect of age on pain threshold, elderly subjects did display a deficit in discriminating among shocks (i.e., lower d'). Since thresholds for dental pain did not change with age for healthy, unfilled teeth, it is unlikely that the age-related discrimination deficit was due to peripheral changes and suggests that the age deficit in suprathreshold tooth-shock discrimination results from CNS factors.

Harkins and Chapman (28,29) also found an interaction between age, subjective estimation of shock intensity, and response bias. When compared to young subjects, elderly subjects were less likely to label low levels of perceived stimulus intensity as painful. This finding is consistent with those of Clark and Mehl (17) and Rees and Botwinick (52), who used near-threshold stimuli and found similar results. At higher levels of perceived stimulus intensity, elderly individuals were more likely to respond "moderate pain" than were young individuals. These data indicate that perceptual or response biases interact with age so that, when compared to the young, the elderly are inclined to label faint, vaguely noxious stimuli as nonnoxious sensations, while they are significantly more willing to label the stimuli as painful at higher levels of tooth shock.

Collins and Stone (18) studied 56 men between 18 and 75 years of age and demonstrated increased pain sensitivity in older compared to younger subjects. Shocks were delivered to electrodes placed over the dorsal surface of the second and fourth fingers of the subject's right hand. The experimenters determined sensory threshold, pain threshold, and pain tolerance. Sensory threshold was defined as the point at which the subject reported a sensation. Pain threshold was defined as the subject's first report of the stimulation as painful. Tolerance was defined as that level at which the pain became too intense to be further tolerated. Tests were repeated at weekly intervals for 5 weeks, but within- and between-sessions variability was not reported. Although sensory threshold was not related to age, significant and negative relationships between age and pain threshold and pain tolerance were observed. These results indicate an increase in pain sensitivity with age. Woodrow et al. (68) reported similar findings when they applied mechanical pressure to the Achilles tendon and found a decrease in pain tolerance with age. The age-related decrease in tolerance was greater for women than men, but women were less tolerant than men at all ages.

Studies evaluating cutaneous pain thresholds may deal with discomfort rather than frank pain. Pressure and ischemic techniques evoke a diffuse pain or dull ache that tends to be poorly localized. Such pain may have a more meaningful relationship to clinical or chronic pain. Suffering is important in management of acute and chronic pain and is related to pain tolerance rather than pain threshold. Pain tolerance is influenced by psychological factors, including response biases and probably biocultural history. The effects of age on response criterion have not been evaluated in relation to pain tolerance. The psychologic factors influencing pain tolerance also have not been systematically evaluated in relation to aging.

The interaction between age, perceived pain intensity, and response bias observed by Harkins and Chapman (28,29) sheds some light on these important issues. Elderly individuals labeled stronger shocks to teeth as more painful than did young subjects. Woodrow et al. (68) observed increased sensitivity to deep pain in elderly subjects. It is not clear if this was due to age differences in sensory processes of nociception or differences in willingness to label the noxious pressure as painful. Consideration of such psychological factors influencing pain reporting may explain why some elderly have an increased frequency of subjective pain report yet tolerate minor surgery and even dental extractions with little apparent discomfort (20).

The relationship between the pain experience and aging is complex. It appears that pain threshold may not change dramatically with normal aging. Where elevated pain thresholds do occur with age, integrity of receptor function and first-order neurons mediating nociception must be considered. Much of the apparent increase in pain thresholds, like the skin senses in general, may reflect peripheral rather than CNS changes with age (37). The ability to discriminate between suprathreshold stimuli does decrease with age and this is probably due to CNS age-change in processing nociception (17,28–30). The effect of psychologic factors on pain tolerance or pain sensitivity range in the elderly is not known.

In summary, the results of laboratory study of experimental pain suggest no major age differences in pain sensitivity. Assertions of changes in pain sensation with age should be viewed with extreme caution, particularly considering the difficulties in defining and assessing pain (44). The fact that no age differences in density or morphology of nociceptor endings has been found (15,34) supports the view that basic processes of nociception are probably not influenced by age. This lack of a direct effect of aging on pain perception is also supported by recent animal research. Krauter et al. (39) evaluated startle reflex threshold and startle amplitude in rats ranging in age from 10 to 31 months and observed no age effect for the startle reflex threshold. There was, however, a significantly reduced startle reflex amplitude in the oldest rats. These results can be interpreted to indicate that sensitivity to electric shock develops early in life and remains invariant throughout the lifespan of the rat. Reduction in startle reflex amplitude reflects a reduction in reactivity to shock in the oldest group of rats. The finding of Krauter et al. (39) that age had no effect on electric shock sensitivity is consistent with the findings of Mumford (47) and Harkins and Chapman (28–30). Thus the literature on experimental pain and age strongly suggests there is little age-related difference in pain sensation among mature adults compared with younger persons. Intraindividual changes in pain sensitivity may exist. However, no longitudinal studies of this question exist.

ACUTE PATHOLOGIC PAIN

Pain related to specific, brief clinical events that terminate relatively soon after resolution of the pathological insult is regarded as acute. Under this rubric, we would include pain associated with myocardial infarct (MI), burn, trauma, and surgery as well as pain due to various somatic and visceral disorders. Pain persistent a month or so beyond the expected resolution of an acute disease or a reasonable period for an injury to heal should be considered chronic pain (9). Chronic pain in the elderly is treated in the next section of this chapter. The observation that the elderly often experience minor surgical procedures and dental extractions with little or no discomfort (20) implies there is a change in response to acute pain with age. The nature of any age-related change in acute pain perception is difficult to determine because there are no systematic studies of this issue.

Some painful conditions, such as acute appendicitis, present similarly regardless of the patient's age (1,63). Myths held by some about change in pain perception with age have led to misdiagnosis of appendicitis in the elderly (1,63). On the other hand, there is evidence that pain associated with acute MI may change with increasing age. In a study of residential care patients, MI episodes in 52 patients were evaluated with regard to pain reported (55). Approximately 40% did not report pain as the major complaint and an additional 16% suffered a painless MI. Based on these and other data, Caird and Dall (12) point out that "absence of cardiac pain is a relatively frequent phenomenon in the elderly with cardiac infarction." More recently, in a survey of 1,474 middle-aged and elderly MI patients (criteria according to the World Health Organization), MacDonald (43) found that approximately 30% of the 317 patients over 70 years of age did not have acute pain as the major presenting symptom. Surprisingly, in the 296 patients under 60 years of age, 23% did not have acute pain as the presenting symptom. The increase in atypical or painless MI in the older group was statistically significant.

MacDonald's (43) sample is more representative of the general MI population than those of earlier studies. Samples based on residential care or nursing home patients include a significant number of patients suffering from dementia. Elderly MI patients who suffer from communication disorders or confusion could be expected to present with atypical MI symptomatology. This factor may have biased earlier findings based on samples from long-term care settings where prevalence of cognitive dysfunction is high. Future research on clinical pain in the elderly population must explicitly control for cognitive status. The degree to which the slight (i.e., 7%) increase in atypical MI (43) represents a pure age-related phenomenon or individual differences in end-organ and referred pain mechanisms due to disease is unknown.

While it is unclear if age influences the presentation of acute pain, there is no doubt that age influences pain relief obtained from analgesics. In postoperative patients, age is highly related to analgesic pain relief (6). The increased sensitivity of the elderly to narcotics depends on multiple factors, including alteration of receptors, changes in plasma protein binding, and prolonged clearance (35). Thus narcotics should be used in smaller doses in the elderly than in young patients not only because of the factors noted above, but also because elderly patients are sensitive to narcotic side effects, including respiratory depression, cough suppression, and, most importantly, clouding of mental functions. The dose of narcotic analgesic should be adjusted for each individual patient by gradually increasing the dose until the patient has obtained good pain relief. The dose of morphine should provide good relief for 3 to 4 hr, and the frequency of administration should be at such intervals that the dose is given before the recurrence of pain, thus avoiding anticipatory anxiety and the behavioral reinforcement of drug use. Mental status should be closely monitored to avoid narcotic-induced delirium. If possible, oral agents are preferred to parenteral agents and carry less risk of side effects. Ellison (21) has reviewed many of these issues in detail.

In many acute pain situations, the clinician will use nonnarcotic analgesics and anti-inflammatory agents. The backbone of analgesic therapy is nonsteroidal anti-inflammatory drugs. The safety margin between therapeutic

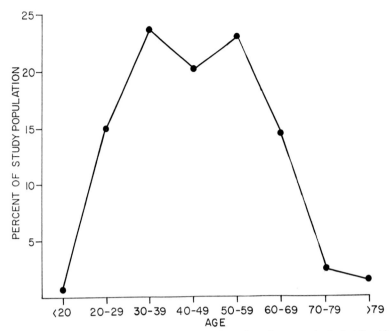

FIG. 1. Percentage of chronic pain patients as a function of age evaluated at the Medical College of Virginia Chronic Pain Clinic.

and toxic levels of these agents is reduced in the elderly. In addition, the elderly frequently make errors in the self-administration of their medicines. Since the elderly often have multiple-system disease and require polypharmacy, there is an increased potential for drug-drug interaction. Finally, the elderly are more prone to CNS side effects.

CHRONIC PAIN

Bonica (9) has estimated that between 50 and 60 million individuals in the United States suffer from chronic pain, resulting in an annual cost between 60 and 65 billion dollars for health care, compensation, and loss of work productivity. Considering that 80% of the elderly have at least one chronic ailment, it might be expected they should constitute a large proportion of those treated in pain centers. This does not appear to be the case.

Figure 1 presents the age profile of 174 consecutive patients seen at the Medical College of Virginia Pain Clinic. Age approximates a normal distribution in this population, with those over 70 years of age representing less than 5% of the total population. Recent data from the Pain Clinic at the University of Washington indicate that the patient population over 65 seen there is on a percentage-basis larger than that represented in Figure 1. At the University of Washington, over a 2-month period, 20% of the patients seen were 65 years of age or older (C. Benedetti, *personal communication*). Informal inquiry to directors of other pain clinics at major medical centers suggests the percentage of elderly (over 65) seen in their clinics ranges between 7 and 10%, which is consistent with the data in Fig. 1. It would appear the elderly are underrepresented as a group in the chronic pain clinic setting where only complex chronic pain problems are seen. Most of these facilities do not manage persistent pain, which is present in some 24 of the 35 million patients with chronic arthritis, or 20 million patients who have recurrent moderate to severe migraine headaches, or some 2 ½ million patients who have angina pectoris. Moreover, only a small percentage of patients with chronic low back pain and other chronic musculoskeletal painful disorders usually managed by family physicians, orthopedists, and physiatrists and only about 10 to 15% with chronic cancer pain who are cared for by oncologists or family physicians are referred to pain control clinics.

No formal demographic data exist to support the possible underutilization of pain clinics by the elderly. Considering the fact that the elderly underutilize health care opportunities in general, it would not be surprising to find them underrepresented in pain clinics.

Butler and Gastel (11) point out that pain in the elderly demands diagnosis and treatment no different from pain in younger individuals. They describe the case of Morris Rocklin, a volunteer in a longitudinal study of aging who complained to his physician that his left leg hurt. The doctor's response, that Mr. Rocklin was 101 years old and should expect some discomfort, was met with Mr. Rocklin's rejoinder, then why didn't his right leg hurt? Pain, discomfort, and suffering are not natural consequences of growing old.

No epidemiologic data exist concerning age differences in chronic pain with regard to cause, treatment, or outcome. Those illnesses that increase in frequency and severity in the later years of life certainly produce suffering. There are no precise epidemiologic data to support a widely held belief that pain, discomfort, and suffering associated with low back pain, postherpetic neuralgia, cancer, trigeminal neuralgia, arthritis, and other pain-producing conditions are more frequent in elderly patients. However, the incidence of pain among patients with these conditions seen by experienced clinical algologists is higher than is seen in younger persons. If anything, the negative social and psychologic accompaniments of aging may decrease the elderly individual's capacity to respond successfully to the negative consequences of chronic pain. When pain in the elderly is due to degenerative disease or cancer, no single treatment is likely to provide lasting relief (11). In such cases the multidisciplinary treatment approach, provided by some pain clinics, becomes increasingly necessary.

In our survey, the patients were asked questions concerning the nature of their pain complaint, including their concern for the future, expectancies of treatment outcome, ability to control pain, and the degree to which their pain interferes with activities of daily living. Responses to these concerns were recorded using visual analog scales. No consistent age-related finding was observed, with only one exception. There was a significant inverse relationship between age and concern for the future ($r = 0.32$; 139 df; $p \leq 0.01$). This preliminary result is consistent with a model of acceptance by the elderly of pain as an expected companion of old age.

Patients are also requested to rate their pain at its most severe level on a visual analog scale. Neither the ratings for intensity nor unpleasantness of the chronic pain varied with age. These results are consistent with laboratory studies showing little change in experimental pain sensitivity with increased age (see Table 1).

Depression and Chronic Pain

Clinically, chronic pain is a psychobiologic disorder with characteristic physiologic, biochemical, psychodynamic, behavioral, and biographic features. In some, but not all quarters, there has been a recent shift in emphasis from peripheral aspects of pain to central and psychologic aspects of pain, which has resulted in renewed interest in the interplay between chronic pain and a variety of psychiatric disorders, notably depression (8). The incidence of both chronic stress and depression is high in the elderly population (36). Because the elderly are subject to a higher prevalence of pain-producing illnesses, the opportunity for pain to intensify the experience of stress and depression is even greater than in the general population. Not only do the elderly have more pain-producing illnesses, but they also have increased pain-related psychosomatic complaints. Nowlin and Busse (49) and Angle et al. (2) point out that psychophysiologic symptoms such as chronic musculoskeletal pain may be regarded as a depressive equivalent in some individuals. In other patients, chronic psychogenic pain may represent a type of depressive illness with somatized pain as the prime expression of mental agony (8). The relationship between pain, stress, and depression is sufficiently complex that therapeutic formulations should be made on a case-by-case basis to be clinically effective.

The naturally occurring amines of norepinephrine, dopamine, and serotonin are important in the central modulation of pain perception (5,65) and in the etiology of affective disorders (42). These biologic amines undergo oxidative deamination to biologically inactive compounds by the enzyme monamine oxidase (MAO). Monamine oxidase enzyme activity increases at about age 45 and continues to increase steadily with age (54). The greater activity of MAO in elderly individuals could reduce available neurotransmitters at postsynaptic sites and thus affect mood and pain perception concurrently.

At the present time, there is considerable data that serotonergic neurons in the periaqueductal grey area of the midbrain, and in the nucleus raphe magnus and nucleus reticularis magnocellularis of the medulla, exert a negative feedback effect on nociceptive transmission and pain perception (5).

Antidepressants such as amitriptyline, doxepin, and clomipramine act on serotonergic systems and therefore may have analgesic properties that are independent of their antidepressant properties. Effects on pain may actually have a more rapid onset of action than effects on depression (33).

Antidepressants such as desipramine and maprotiline, which affect primarily norepinephrine systems, are not effective analgesics (33). On the other hand, opiates that are the most powerful analgesics also have mood-enhancing capabilities. Unfortunately, euphoria produced by opiates is not useful clinically because of physiological and psychologic side effects. Nevertheless, the physiologic and pharmacologic interdependence of pain and depression appears obvious. The importance of this interdependence may be enhanced in the elderly because of the frequency of pain-producing peripheral pathologies and because of the increased incidence of depression in the elderly.

In addition to changes in basic physiologic functions and biologic changes produced by age, the elderly patient with pain is subject to age-related psychologic stress. These stresses derive not only from the loss of physical health, but also from the loss of loved ones, loss of economic resources, and loss of social status. There may be little support available to help the individual cope with these stresses. Complaining about pain may represent a socially acceptable behavior whereby the elderly adult may attempt to elicit caretaking from another person. According to Kolb (38), pain complaints may be a form of attachment behavior.

Increases in questioning, demands, and anger may signal separation anxiety. If the patient is unable to establish a trusting and secure attachment to replace some of the accumulated losses, he or she becomes depressed. In some elderly individuals, symptoms of depression are similar to those observed in younger individuals with depression. In old age, however, depression is more often characterized by dysphoria, loss of interest in outside matters, and somatic illness and fatigue (64). This form of depression increases the probability of pain-related behaviors. Thus pain complaints may increase with age. The extent to which any elevation of frequency of pain reporting by the aged stems from nociception or depression is unknown (14). However, it is clear that depression may mask as pain.

If the patient denies depression and acknowledges only pain, the hallmarks of depression may still be present. Symptoms depend on severity and whether the depression is autonomous and endogenous, or purely reactive. The endogenously depressed patients complains of sleep-disturbance with characteristic early morning wakening, psychomotor retardation or agitation, and anorexia or weight loss. There is loss of interest, low energy, poor concentration, and inappropriate guilt that may be expressed by pain complaints. Since severe pain without coexisting endogenous depression can cause similar symptoms, the clinical laboratory is useful in differentiating the truly depressed patient. In about 50% of depressed patients, a test dose of dexamethasone is followed by a rise of plasma cortisol above critical levels (13).

In 25% of depressed patients, the thyroid stimulating hormone (TSH) response following the administration of thyrotropic releasing hormone (TRH) is blunted (41). Electroencephalogram (EEG) changes associated with depression include shortened rapid eye movement (REM) latency, increased REM activity, and increased REM density (40). Electroencephalogram sleep studies are positive for depression in 65% of patients with endogenous depression. If dexamethasone supression, TRH stimulation, and EEG sleep studies are used sequentially, about 85% of patients with endogenous depression can be identified (24). Since both age and chronic pain states are associated with a tendency to minimize feelings of depression, these laboratory tests may be of considerable significance in elderly pain patients. Patients requiring aggressive treatment for depression can be identified. If the depressive symptoms of the elderly pain patient is viewed as the consequence of a physical suffering for which there is no relief, proper evaluation will not be undertaken and successful therapy precluded.

Pain and Dementia

Although depression and pain are frequently associated, pain complaints may occasionally be the earliest manifestation of cognitive impairment. Since the cognitively impaired elderly have reduced capacity to complain of psychologic phenomena, pain from accompanying physical illnesses may be exaggerated and used to explain or hide increasing psychologic disability. Symptoms of poor concentration, poor attention, and memory dysfunction may be ascribed to pain. Often the patient with early symptoms of a progressive dementia complains of head pain or other vague discomfort.

Of course, the treatment of pain in a patient who is cognitively impaired requires an initial evaluation of the organic mental syndrome. Computed tomography, EEG, and neuropsychologic testing help determine the severity of the cognitive changes and whether there are underlying treatable causes stemming from metabolic, toxic, infectious, vascular, or inflammatory disorders. If the brain syndrome is mild, treatment may be similar to that undertaken for any pain patient. But often interventions must be tailored so that excessive demands are avoided. In cases of more severe dementia, treatment is symptomatic at best. Sometimes merely confronting the patient and his or her family with the diagnosis of organic brain syndrome reduces anxiety about some more bizarre pain complaints and provides support. Neuroleptic medication such as haloperidol (Haldol®) may be of some help but antidepressants should be given with caution because anticholinergic effects may worsen the underlying dementia.

Personality and Chronic Pain

Not only does chronic pain influence the personality of the patient, but certain personalities are more susceptible to pain than others (22,45). Some elderly patients had a personality disorder before the onset of pain. Although once there may have been an organic basis for the pain, the symptom proved so useful that it continued after resolution of the pathologic condition. Pain complaints are frequently employed by patients with personality disorders to manipulate friends and relatives. Unfortunately, there have been no detailed studies of the effects of aging on personality disorders. An individual's personality patterns probably continue throughout life. A complete psychiatric examination and history should probably be sufficient to establish their existence. The features of personality disorders may change in accordance with well-known personality changes that take place with aging. As the older person turns inward and withdraws from outward concerns, there may be a preoccupation with bodily functions. Obsessive-compulsive, dependent, and narcissistic traits may be accentuated. Acting-out behavior may decrease (62).

The personality structure predetermines the presentation of a pain syndrome. The dependent person may use pain complaints as a substitute for separation anxiety; a narcissistic person may be more concerned with body-image changes. Since there is a high incidence of both pain and depression in the elderly, pain should be considered a manifestation of personality disorder *only* if the disorder is well established throughout life and other etiologies are ruled out. Although patients may develop pain complaints for purely unconscious reasons, pain as a pure conversion symptom is uncommon at any age, and probably rare in the elderly. In patients with personality disorder, every effort should be made to avoid narcotic medication because medication abuse among these patients is a significant problem. The risk of iatrogenic drug addiction is high in patients with personality disorders, even in older age groups.

Social Environment and Chronic Pain

Another important consideration in the management of the chronic pain patient is the patient's environment and the people involved with the patient. Since the behavioral responses associated with chronic pain persist over a long period of time, there are many opportunities for these behaviors to be systematically and positively reinforced. Fordyce (23) points out that pain behavior may be operantly conditioned in the elderly, as in younger patients, by the positive reinforcing consequences of those behaviors to the individual. As pain behaviors and pain talk are reinforced, the frequency of occurrence increases (23).

15. Cauna, N. (1965): The effects of aging on receptor organs of the human dermis. In: *Advances in Biology of Skin, Vol. VI: Aging*, edited by W. Montagna, pp. 63–96. Pergamon Press, New York.
16. Chapman, W. P., and Jones, C. M. (1944): Variations in cutaneous and visceral pain sensitivity in normal subjects. *J. Clin. Invest.*, 23:81–91.
17. Clark, W. C., and Mehl, L. (1971): Thermal pain: A sensory decision theory analysis of the effect of age and sex on d', various response criteria, and 50% pain threshold. *J. Abnorm. Psychol.*, 78:202–212.
18. Collins, G., and Stone, L. A. (1965): Pain sensitivity, age and activity level in chronic schizophrenics and in normals. *Br. J. Psychiatry*, 112:33–35.
19. Corso, J. F. (1981): *Aging Sensory Systems and Perception*. Praeger, New York.
20. Critchley, M. (1931): The neurology of old age. *Lancet*, 1:225:1221–1230.
21. Ellison, N. (1975): Problems in geriatric anesthesiology. *Surg. Clin. North Am.*, 55:919–945.
22. Engle, G. (1959): Psychogenic pain and the pain prone patient. *Am. J. Med.*, pp. 899–918.
23. Fordyce, W. E. (1978): Evaluating and managing chronic pain. *Geriatrics*, 33:59–62.
24. Friedel, R. O. (1982): Sleep and laboratory measurements in autonomous depression. *J. Clin. Psychiatry*, 43:28–30.
25. Green, D. M., and Swets, J. A. (1966): *Signal Detection Theory and Psychophysics*. Wiley, New York.
26. Hardy, J. D., Wolff, H. G., and Goodell, H. (1943): The pain threshold in man. *Ann. J. Psychiat.*, 99:744–751.
27. Hardy, J. D., Wolff, H. G., and Goodell, H. (1952): *Pain Sensation and Reactions*. Williams & Wilkins, Baltimore.
28. Harkins, S. W., and Chapman, C. R. (1976): Detection and decision factors in pain perception in young and elderly men. *Pain*, 2:253–264.
29. Harkins, S. W., and Chapman, C. R. (1977): The perception of induced dental pain in young and elderly women. *J. Gerontol.*, 32:428–435.
30. Harkins, S. W., and Chapman, C. R. (1977): Age and sex differences in pain perception. In: *Pain in the Trigeminal Region*, edited by B. Anderson and B. Mathews, pp. 435–441. Elsevier, Amsterdam.
31. Harkins, S. W., Nowlin, J. B., Ramm, D., and Schroeder, S. (1974): Effects of age, sex and time-on-watch on a brief continuous performance task. In: *Normal Aging II*, edited by E. Palmore, pp. 140–150. Duke University Press, Durham.
32. Harkins, S. W., and Warner, M. (1980): Age and pain. In: *Annual Review of Gerontology and Geriatrics, Vol. 1*, edited by C. Eisdorfer, pp. 121–131. Verlag Springer, New York.
33. Hendler, N. (1982): The anatomy and psychopharmacology of chronic pain. *J. Clin. Psychiatry*, 43:15–20.
34. Hunter, R., Ridley, A., and Malleson, A. (1969): Meissner corpuscles in skin biopsies of patients with presenile dementia: A quantitative study. *Br. J. Psychiatry*, 115:347–349.
35. Kaiko, R. F., Wallenstein, S. L., Rogers, A. G., Brabinski, P. Y., and Houda, R. W. (1982): Narcotics in the elderly. *Med. Clin. North Am.*, 66:1079–1089.
36. Kay, D. W. K., Beamish, P., and Roth, M. (1964): Old age mental disorders in Newcastle-Upon-Tyne, Part 1. A study of prevalence. *Br. J. Psychiatry*, 110:146–158.
37. Kenshalo, D. R. (1977): Age changes in touch, vibration, temperature, kinesthesis, and pain sensitivity. In: *Handbook of the Psychology of Aging*, edited by E. Birren and K. W. Schaie, pp. 562–601. Von Nostrand Reinhold, New York.
38. Kolb, L. C. (1982): Attachment behavior and pain complaints. *Psychosomatics*, 23:413–429.
39. Krauter, E. E., Wallace, J. E., and Campbell, B. A. (1981): Sensory-motor function in the aging rat. *Behav. Neural. Biol.*, 31:367–392.
40. Kupfer, D. J., Foster, F. G., Coble, P., McPartland, R. J., and Ulrich, R. F. (1978): The application of EEG sleep for the differential diagnosis of affective disorders. *Am. J. Psychiatry*, 135:69–74.
41. Lossen, P. T., and Prange, A. J. (1982): Serum thyrotropic response to thyrotropic releasing hormone in psychiatric patients: A review. *Am. J. Psychiatry*, 139:405–416.
42. Maas, J. W. (1975): Biogenic amines and depression: Biochemical pharmacological separation of two types of depression. *Arch. Gen. Psychiatry*, 32:1357–1361.
43. MacDonald, J. B. (1983): Coronary care in the elderly. *Age Ageing* 12:17–20.
44. Melzack, R. (1973): *The Puzzle of Pain*. Basic Books, New York.

45. Merskey, H. (1978): *The Physiology of Pain*, edited by R. A. Sternbach, pp. 111–128. Raven Press, New York.
46. Miller, C., and Lelieuvre, R. B. (1982): A method to reduce chronic pain in the elderly nursing home resident. *Gerontologist*, 22:324.
47. Mumford, J. M. (1965): Pain perception threshold and adaptation of normal human teeth. *Arch. Oral Biol.*, 10:957–968.
48. Nesselroade, J. R., and Harkins, S. W. (1980): Methods for studying behavioral aging: An overview. In: *Aging in the 1980s: Psychological Issues*, edited by L. W. Poon, pp. 485–491. American Psychological Association Press, Washington, D.C.
49. Nowlin, J. B., and Busse, E. (1977): Psychosomatic problems in the older person. In: *Psychosomatic Medicine*, edited by E. D. Witkower and H. Warnes. Harper & Row, New York.
50. Procacci, P., Bozza, G., Buzzelli, G., and Della Corte, M. (1970): The cutaneous pricking pain threshold in old age. *Gerontol. Clin.*, 12:213–218.
51. Procacci, P., Della Corte, M., Zoppi, M., Romano, S., Maresca, M., and Voegelin, M. (1974): Pain threshold measurement in man. In: *Recent Advances on Pain: Pathophysiology and Clinical Aspects*, edited by J. J. Bonica, P. Procacci, and C. Pagoni, pp. 105–147. Charles C Thomas, Springfield, Ill.
52. Rees, J., and Botwinick, J. (1971): Detection and decision factors in auditory behavior of the elderly. *J. Gerontol.*, 26:133–147.
53. Riley, M. W. (1976): Age strata in social systems. In: *Handbook of Aging and the Social Sciences*, edited by R. Binstock and E. Shanas, pp. 189–217. Van Nostrand Reinhold, New York.
54. Robinson, D., Davis, J., Niles, A., Rauaris, C., and Sylvester, D. (1971): Relation of sex and aging to monoamine oxidase activity on human brain plasma and platelets. *Arch. Gen. Psychiatry*, 24:536–537.
55. Rodstein, M. (1956): The characteristics of non-fatal myocardial infarction in the aged. *Arch. Intern. Med.*, 98:684–690.
56. Schludermann, E., and Zubek, J. P. (1962): Effects of age on pain sensitivity. *Percept. Mot. Skills*, 14:295–301.
57. Schumacher, G. A., Goodell, H., Hardy, J. D., and Wolff, H. G. (1940): Uniformity of the pain threshold in man. *Science*, 92:110–112.
58. Shader, R. I., and Greenblatt, D. J. (1979): Pharmacokinetics and clinical drug effects in the elderly. *Psychopharmacol. Bull.*, 15:8–14.
59. Sherman, E. D., and Robillard, E. (1960): Sensitivity to pain in the aged. *Can. Med. Assoc. J.*, 83:944–947.
60. Sherman, E. D., and Robillard, E. (1964): Sensitivity to pain in relationship to age. In: *Age with a Future: Proceedings of the Sixth International Congress of Gerontology*, edited by P. F. Hansen, pp. 325–333. Davis, Philadelphia.
61. Sherman, E. D., and Robillard, E. (1964): Sensitivity to pain in relationship to age. *J. Am. Geriatr. Soc.*, 12:1037–1044.
62. Simon, A. (1980): The neuroses, personality disorders, alcoholism, drug abuse, and crime in the aged. In: *Handbook of Mental Health and Aging*, edited by A. E. Birren and R. B. Stone, pp. 654–670. Prentice-Hall, Englewood Cliffs, N.J.
63. Stair, T., and Corlett, M. B. (1980): Appendicitis over forty. *Ann. Emerg. Med.*, 9:76–78.
64. Stenbach, A. (1980): Depression and suicidal behavior in old age. In: *Handbook of Mental Health and Aging*, edited by A. E. Birren and R. B. Sloane, pp. 616–652. Prentice-Hall, Englewood Cliffs, N.J.
65. Sternbach, R. A., Janowsky, D. S., and Hirey, L. Y. (1976): Effects of altering brain serotonin activity on human chronic pain. In: *Advances in Pain Research and Therapy*, Vol. 1, edited by J. J. Bonica and D. Albe-Fessard. Raven Press, New York.
66. Tomma, E. A. (1977): Aging of skeletal-dental systems and supporting tissue. In: *Handbook of the Biology of Aging*, edited by C. E. Finchand and L. Hayflick, pp. 470–495. Van Nostrand Reinhold, New York.
67. Verillo, R. T. (1980): Age-related changes in the sensitivity to vibrations. *J. Gerontol.*, 35:185–193.
68. Woodrow, K. M., Friedman, G. D., Siegelaub, A. B., and Collen, M. F. (1972): Pain tolerance: Differences according to age, sex, and race. *Psychosom. Med.*, 34:548–556.

*Advances in Pain Research
and Therapy, Vol. 7,*
edited by C. Benedetti et al.
Raven Press, New York © 1984.

Review of Prevalence of Coexisting Chronic Pain and Depression

Judith A. Turner and Joan M. Romano

*Pain Center, Department of Psychiatry and Behavioral Sciences, University of
Washington, Seattle, Washington 98195*

Patients with chronic pain represent both an individual and societal problem in terms of their suffering, stress experienced by their families, time lost from employment, costs associated with litigation and disability compensation, and overuse of health care resources. The recognition that many people experience persistent pain that is refractory to standard medical treatments, and that their functional disability is often in excess of that expected on the basis of identified physical pathology, has led clinical investigators to examine factors other than physiologic ones that may contribute to these problems. It has long been recognized that subjectively experienced pain and pain-related behaviors are not solely dependent on tissue damage or organic dysfunction (11). The intensity of pain reported and amount of pain behavior displayed seem to be influenced by a wide range of factors such as social, financial, and environmental contingencies; attention; anxiety; and cultural background. Thus the role of psychologic processes, especially dysfunctional ones, in the etiology and maintenance of chronic pain has received increasing attention (11).

One of the primary psychologic problems commonly observed to accompany chronic pain is depression. A number of published studies have reported high rates of depression in chronic pain patients, and many have found antidepressant medications to be helpful in managing patients with chronic pain (13,16,20,33). Some authors have even suggested that chronic pain without identified organic pathology is a form of "masked" depression (4). However, the wide range of rates of prevalence of depression in chronic pain populations that have been published has led to differences of opinion and controversy regarding this issue.

In this chapter, we will focus on this issue by critically examining empirical studies of the combined prevalence of depression and chronic pain, with attention to methodologic concerns. Some general conclusions then will be presented, along with suggestions for future research.

PREVALENCE OF DEPRESSION IN CHRONIC PAIN PATIENTS

The most basic question researchers have attempted to address is the extent to which depression occurs in conjunction with chronic pain. Studies that have assessed the prevalence of depression in chronic pain populations have yielded widely varying results. Most often these investigators have drawn subjects from psychiatric settings. In pain patients referred for psychiatric evaluation, depression has been diagnosed with frequencies ranging from 22% of ''nonorganic'' abdominal pain patients (15) to 78% of hospitalized patients with pain of varying types (34). Other studies have reported intermediate rates of depression in inpatients and outpatients with pain seen for psychiatric evaluation or treatment (17,22,24–26,29).

Only a few studies have used populations of pain patients other than those specifically referred for psychiatric care. Two groups (20,27) assessed patients from general pain clinic populations, and even though they drew some of their subjects from the same pain clinic, they found highly disparate results. Pilowsky et al. (27) reported that only 10% of 100 patients could be classified as depressed on the basis of a self-report measure, whereas Lindsay and Wyckoff (20) diagnosed 87% as depressed using Research Diagnostic Criteria (30). In one study of hospital neurosurgery service patients (3), depression was found in 83% of the patients. In two studies of patients with specific types of pain, depression was found in 100% of the patients with nonorganic face and head pain (18) and in 100% of the patients with painful lower-extremity diabetic neuropathy (31).

These wide discrepancies in the rates of depression reported in patients with chronic pain seem to be due to several factors. First, as described, there has been considerable diversity in subjects studied. Most investigators have used psychiatric patients or patients referred for psychiatric evaluation. It is not surprising to find a high rate of depression in such populations, as many of these patients probably were recommended for psychiatric care because of depression, which may or may not have been recognized as such by the referring physician. Thus results from studies of such patients may not be applicable to the general population of chronic pain sufferers. Further, given that subjects in various investigations were drawn from such different settings as psychiatric wards, private practices, pain clinics, and psychiatry consultation services, it is highly likely that they also varied on a number of other characteristics. These may include severity and chronicity of pain, medication use, employment and compensation status, and severity of psychologic problems, all of which could affect the development of depressive symptoms.

A second factor quite probably contributing to the inconsistency of research findings has been the lack of application of a standard methodology for diagnosing depression. Many studies (15,17,24,25,29) did not even specify how depression was assessed. Others (18,22,26,31,34) reported only that assessment was conducted by psychiatric interviews, and apparently specific, operationally defined criteria were not used to make diagnoses. One study (20) did use Research Diagnostic Criteria but did not report interrater reliability of diagnoses. Some researchers (3,26,27,31) relied solely on self-report measures of depression or used psychologic tests in conjunction with psychiatric interviews. Given this variety of assessment techniques, it seems likely that different criteria were used in these studies to diagnose "depression." Different classes of assessment instruments (such as self-reports and external observations) have not been found to correspond highly in many cases (14). Thus differences in reported rates of depression may be due in part to variation in assessment techniques. Further, the validity of some of the measures (e.g., Rorschach, Thematic Apperception Test) used for diagnosing depression in these studies is questionable.

Prevalence of Depression in Individuals With and Without Chronic Pain

A basic question that must be asked is how the prevalence of depression in patients with chronic pain compares to that in pain-free control subjects. Lower rates of depression have been found in psychiatric patients with non-organic pain compared to pain-free psychiatric patients (24); in medical-surgical outpatients with pain referred for psychiatric consultation versus similar patients without pain (26); and in Canadian Indians and Inuits with versus without pain referred for psychiatric evaluation (25). However, Spear (29) reported depression to be more common in psychiatric outpatients with pain than in those without and about equally common in psychiatric inpatients with and without pain.

All of these investigators found substantial rates of depression (43–65%) in chronic pain sufferers drawn from different populations. However, once again, in most of these studies subjects were either psychiatric patients (24) or pain patients referred for psychiatric evaluation (25,26). This presents the same problems of selection bias noted in the uncontrolled studies reviewed previously.

Several studies have compared nonpsychiatric groups with and without chronic pain on self-report measures of depression. For example, Ziegler et al. (35) administered the Zung Self-Rating Depression Scale to community residents and found a higher mean score in the group who suffered from disabling, severe headaches than in those without headaches. Crisp et al. (8) obtained similar results using the Middlesex Hospital Questionnaire, but only for women. Another study (21) examined depression in patients with facial pain compared to a control group of patients with no pain and found no difference between these two groups using the Institute of Personality and Ability Testing depression scale.

Thus there is conflicting evidence as to whether higher depression scores are found in patients with pain compared to those who are pain-free. One difficulty with these studies is that the use of mean scores may obscure differences between these groups in the frequency with which clinically significant depression occurs. For example, one study (26) that used both diagnostic interviews and a self-report depression measure found that patients with pain compared to patients without pain differed in the frequency of clinically diagnosed depression, but the mean self-report scores of these groups did not differ significantly.

Temporal Relation Between the Onset of Pain and Depression

Another question that arises with respect to the relationship between chronic pain and depression concerns the temporal relation between the onset of the two syndromes. To our knowledge, only two groups of investigators (5,20) have examined this issue, and both found that the majority (50–54%) of patients with pain and depression reported the pain and depressive symptoms developed at the same time. Slightly fewer patients (38–46%) reported they became depressed after the onset of pain, and relatively few (0–12%) stated that pain developed after the onset of depression. However, these studies relied solely on patients' retrospective self-reports, and thus results may have been influenced by inaccurate recall of events.

Prevalence of Pain in Depressed Patients

The relation between depression and chronic pain also has been examined by assessing the frequency of pain complaints in depressed patients. Again, varying results have been obtained across studies. Most often, the frequency with which depressed patients in a particular sample acknowledge pain has been reported, with rates of 30 to 100% being found (10,12,20,33). The only study to use Research Diagnostic Criteria for diagnosing subjects as depressed reported that 59% of these patients reported pain of greater than 3 months' duration (20). Ward et al. (33) used subjects with scores on self-report measures indicating moderate depression and anxiety and found that 100% acknowledged persistent pain problems.

Only two studies could be found in the literature in which the frequency of pain in patients diagnosed as having different subtypes of depression was compared. Delaplaine et al. (9) found significant complaints of pain in 40% of patients with "endogenous depression" and in 58% of "neurotic/mixed depression" patients. However, these sample sizes were small and reliability of diagnostic category uncertain. VonKnorring et al. (32) found that 57% of 161 depressed psychiatric patients reported pain. Pain was more often acknowledged by patients with neurotic-reactive depressions than by those with unipolar, bipolar, or other depressive disorders. Pain also was more commonly acknowledged by women and by highly tense, anxious patients.

Only two studies were found that compared the frequency of pain complaints in depressed patients versus a control group. An early report (7) observed that 100 bipolar patients had more headaches but less chest pain and roughly similar rates of back, abdominal, and extremity pain than medically ill patients. This study was flawed by failure to specify the affective status of the bipolar patients at the time of assessment and the use of medically ill "controls" rather than matched healthy controls.

In a more methodologically sophisticated investigation, Mathew et al. (23) compared 51 patients diagnosed as depressed by a psychiatrist to 51 age- and gender-matched healthy controls. On a physical symptom questionnaire, headaches were reported by 76.5% of the depressed patients and by 39.2% of subjects in the control group. Chest pain was acknowledged by 37.3% of the depressed patients, but only by 5.9% of the subjects in the control group. Unfortunately, other types of pain were not assessed.

In summary, studies have revealed that 30 to 100% of various groups of depressed patients acknowledge some kind of persistent pain. There is some evidence that certain types of depressed patients may be more likely to report pain, including women (32), patients with "neurotic/reactive" depressions (9,32), and patients with high levels of tension and anxiety (32,33). However, in only one investigation (23) were nondepressed, healthy subjects included as a control group. Although this study showed headaches and chest pain to be more frequent in the depressed group, further research is needed to replicate these findings and to compare depressed with nondepressed individuals on other types of pain.

A further problem is that many studies did not specify the basis for diagnosing pain complaints (e.g., spontaneous report of patient, response to interview questions, or questionnaires). In some cases, only certain pain problems were assessed (23), whereas others inquired about all types of pain (20). Finally, the severity and duration of pain complaints often were not reported. Thus the comparability of findings across studies is questionable.

SUMMARY AND CONCLUSIONS

The weight of clinical and empirical evidence reviewed in this chapter indicates that a substantial proportion of chronic pain patients are likely to be significantly depressed, although many others are not. Research findings also suggest that pain, especially headache, is a common symptom of depression, with some evidence that this is particularly common in patients who are tense and anxious as well.

It also seems that the coexistence of chronic pain and depression can take different forms. Neither depression nor chronic pain is a homogeneous disorder, but rather both are complex phenomena involving biologic, psychologic, and social dimensions. There exists a considerable body of literature describing various subtypes of depression (e.g., endogenous versus reactive, agitated versus retarded, unipolar versus bipolar, and primary versus secondary) (2). Several studies (1,6,19) have indicated that subgroups of chronic pain patients differing in type and degree of psychologic problems can be identified as well. Thus interactions between chronic pain and depressive syndromes could be expected to vary in their manifestations.

There may be at least two major forms of the coexistence of chronic pain and depression. In some patients who have a primary depression, pain seems to develop as one of a constellation of psychologic and somatic symptoms. One cause of pain (especially headache and myofascial pain) in such cases may well be tension and anxiety, and identifiable organic pathology other than elevated levels of muscle tension may be absent. In other individuals, depression may develop secondary to persistent pain caused by other factors. These two depression-pain syndromes may share, to some extent, a "final common pathway" and thus present similarities in clinical symptoms and physiologic abnormalities.

Nevertheless, drawing definitive conclusions about either the epidemiology or etiology of coexisting chronic pain and depression is impeded by a number of methodologic problems in studies to date. The most noteworthy of these relates to inadequate techniques for assessing pain and depression. In general, studies have not specified clearly how these disorders were diagnosed and by what criteria patients were categorized. Reliability data for assessment techniques used have been lacking. A second major problem has been the absence in most studies of appropriate age- and gender-matched healthy control groups, so that the prevalence of pain complaints and depressive symptoms in the target sample could be compared to general population base rates.

Research clearly is needed to resolve a number of basic issues. First, the frequency of depression and type and severity of depressive symptoms need to be assessed in well-specified samples of chronic pain patients and matched healthy controls. Research Diagnostic Criteria or other standard diagnostic criteria with demonstrated interrater reliability should be used in diagnosing depression.

Second, studies are needed to assess the frequency, type, severity, and chronicity of pain symptoms in depressed patients, again using standardized criteria.

Third, ideally, prospective longitudinal studies could begin to clarify the temporal relation(s) between persistent pain and depression by monitoring patients from the time of diagnosis of one of the syndromes. Patients' self-reports could be corroborated by data from family or health care professionals. Factors associated with the presence of pain in patients diagnosed as having a primary depression and with the presence of depression in patients with a primary pain complaint need to be identified.

Fourth, an important goal of future research will be to identify factors predictive of response to different psychologic and somatic treatments for coexisting pain and depression. Currently, the results from a number of studies support the use of antidepressant medications for some depression/chronic pain syndromes (13,16), but in others (28) these drugs have not been superior to placebos. Additional well-designed investigations are needed to determine which types of patients benefit from such treatments and which alternative approaches are indicated for others.

ACKNOWLEDGMENT

During the writing of this chapter, J. M. Romano was supported by NIH #NS07217.

REFERENCES

1. Armentrout, D. P., Moore, J. E., Parker, J. C., Hewett, J. E., and Feltz, C. (1982): Pain-patient MMPI subgroups: The psychological dimensions of pain. *J. Behav. Med.*, 5:201–211.
2. Beck, A. T. (1973): *The Diagnosis and Management of Depression.* University of Pennsylvania Press, Philadelphia.
3. Blumer, D., and Heilbronn, M. (1981): The pain-prone disorder: A clinical and psychological profile. *Psychosomatics,* 22:395–402.
4. Blumer, D., and Heilbronn, M. (1982): Chronic pain as a variant of depressive disease: The pain-prone disorder. *J. Nerv. Ment. Dis.*, 170:381–406.
5. Bradley, J. J. (1963): Severe localized pain associated with the depressive syndrome. *Br. J. Psychiatry*, 109:741–745.
6. Bradley, L. A., Prokop, C. K., Margolis, R., and Gentry, W. D. (1978): Multivariate analyses of the MMPI profiles of low back pain patients. *J. Behav. Med.*, 1:253–272.
7. Cassidy, W. L., Flanagan, N. B., Spellman, M., and Cohen, M. E. (1957): Clinical observations in manic-depressive disease: A quantitative study of 100 manic-depressive patients and fifty medically sick controls. *JAMA,* 164:1535–1546.
8. Crisp, A. H., McGuiness, B., and Kalney, R. S. (1977): Some clinical, social, and psychological characteristics of migraine subjects in the general population. *Postgrad. Med. J.*, 53:691–697.
9. Delaplaine, R., Ifabumuji, D. I., Merskey, H., and Zarfas, D. (1978): Significance of pain in psychiatric hospital patients. *Pain,* 4:361–366.
10. Diamond, S. (1964): Depressive headache. *Headache,* 4:255–258.
11. Fordyce, W. E. (1976): *Behavioral Methods for Control of Chronic Pain and Illness.* C. V. Mosby, St. Louis.
12. Gallemore, J. L., and Wilson, W. P. (1969): The complaint of pain in the clinical setting of affective disorders. *South Med. J.*, 62:551–555.
13. Hameroff, S. R., Cork, R. C., Scherer, K., Crago, B. R., Neuman, C., Womble, J. R., and Davis, T. P. (1982): Doxepin effects on chronic pain, depression and plasma opioids. *J. Clin. Psychiatry,* 43:22–27.
14. Hersen, M. (1976): Historical perspectives in behavioral assessment. In: *Behavioral Assessment: A Practical Handbook,* edited by M. Hersen and A. S. Bellack, pp. 3–22. Pergamon Press, New York.
15. Hill, O. W., and Blendis, L. (1967): Physical and psychological evaluation of "non-organic" abdominal pain. *Gut,* 8:221–229.
16. Johansson, F., and VonKnorring, L. (1979): A double-blind controlled study of a serotonin uptake inhibitor (Zimelidine) versus placebo in chronic pain patients. *Pain,* 7:69–78.
17. Large, R. (1980): The psychiatrist and the chronic pain patient: 172 anecdotes. *Pain,* 9:253–263.
18. Lascelles, R. G. (1966): Atypical facial pain and depression. *Br. J. Psychiatry,* 112:651–659.
19. Leavitt, F., and Garron, D. C. (1982): Patterns of psychological disturbance and pain report in patients with low back pain. *J. Psychosom. Res.*, 26:301–307.
20. Lindsay, P., and Wyckoff, M. (1981): The depression-pain syndrome and its response to antidepressants. *Psychosomatics,* 22:571–577.
21. Marbach, J. J., and Lund, P. (1981): Depression, anhedonia, and anxiety in temporomandibular joint and other facial pain. *Pain,* 11:73–84.
22. Maruta, T., Swanson, D. W., and Swenson, W. M. (1976): Low back pain patients in a psychiatric population. *Mayo Clin. Proc.*, 51:57–61.
23. Mathew, R., Weinman, M., and Mirabi, M. (1981): Physical symptoms of depression. *Br. J. Psychiatry,* 139:293–296.

24. Merskey, H. (1965): The characteristics of persistent pain in psychological illness. *J. Psychosom. Res.*, 9:291–298.
25. Pelz, M., Merskey, H., Brant, C., and Haselting, G. (1981): A note on the occurrence of pain in psychiatric patients from a Canadian Indian and Inuit population. *Pain*, 10:75–78.
26. Pilling, L. F., Brannien, T. L., and Swenson, W. M. (1967): Psychologic characteristics of psychiatric patients having pain as a presenting symptom. *Can. Med. Assoc. J.*, 97:387–394.
27. Pilowsky, I., Chapman, C. R., and Bonica, J. J. (1977): Pain, depression, and illness behavior in a pain clinic population. *Pain*, 4:183–192.
28. Pilowsky, I., Hallett, E. C., Bassett, D. L., Thomas, P. C., and Penhall, R. K. (1982): A controlled study of amitryptyline in the treatment of chronic pain. *Pain*, 14:169–179.
29. Spear, F. G. (1967): Pain in psychiatric patients. *J. Psychosom. Res.*, 11:187–193.
30. Spitzer, R. L., Endicott, J., and Robins, E. (1978): Research diagnostic criteria: Rationale and reliability. *Arch. Gen. Psychiatry*, 35:773–782.
31. Turkington, R. W. (1980): Depression masquerading as diabetic neuropathy. *JAMA*, 243:1147–1150.
32. VonKnorring, L., Perris, C., Eisemann, M., Eriksson, U., and Perris, H. (1983): Pain as a symptom in depressive disorders. I. Relationship to diagnostic subgroup and depressive symptomatology. *Pain*, 15:19–26.
33. Ward, N. G., Bloom, V. L., and Friedel, R. O. (1979): The effectiveness of tricyclic antidepressants in the treatment of coexisting pain and depression. *Pain*, 7:331–341.
34. Wilson, W. P., Blazer, D. G., and Nashold, B. S. (1976): Observations on pain and suffering. *Psychosomatics*, 17:73–76.
35. Ziegler, D. K., Rhodes, R. J., and Hassenein, R. S. (1978): Association of psychological measurements of anxiety and depression with headache history in a non-clinic population. *Res. Clin. Stud. Headache*, 6:123–135.

Advances in Pain Research
and Therapy, Vol. 7,
edited by C. Benedetti et al.
Raven Press, New York © 1984.

Chronic Pain States and Compensable Disability: An Algorithmic Approach

Steven F. Brena and Stanley L. Chapman

Emory University Pain Control Center, Atlanta, Georgia 30322

Chronic pain syndromes are often labeled "intractable" when they fail to respond successfully to traditional medical interventions. A state of chronicity implies a time factor (*chronos*–time) across which the individual learns to cope with health problems. A breakdown of coping skills usually causes additional suffering through mutually reinforcing physiological and psychosocial malfunctions. This breakdown, the so-called learned pain syndrome, can be independent from any co-existing pathological condition (8). In the past, and even currently, lack of appreciation of this issue by the medical profession has led to ineffective therapy and, at times, iatrogenic complications. In this chapter we will discuss: (a) some of the difficulties in the diagnosis and treatment of chronic pain; (b) the Emory Pain Estimate Model, proven to be a useful tool for the quantification and classification of chronic pain states; (c) the problems of defining impairment and disability; and (d) rating impairment and evaluating disability.

DIFFICULTIES WITH DIAGNOSIS AND TREATMENT

In medicine, a correct diagnosis is essential for proper treatment; successful outcome of treatment should be expected if the diagnosis is correct. Present-day technology has progressed to the point that some physiologic abnormality could be found in almost any person (27). To expect remission of a complex chronic pain syndrome following correction of a minor pathological defect may be a risky oversimplification. Among other important factors, the present "epidemic" of chronic pain may well be related to deficiencies in diagnostic procedures applied to chronic sufferers, whereby the endless search for biologic abnormalities may become in itself an iatrogenic stressor.

Chronic pain states cannot be diagnosed solely within this unidimensional framework of traditional medicine. Every diagnostic process is a form of measurement; invalid methods of measurement may lead to random rather than scientifically predictable results. In clinical practice, the quantification of pain relies on the rather crude postulate that patients' verbal reports are a reliable index of the intensity of their discomfort and an accurate symptom of an underlying pathology; several reports have emphasized that in some patients pain complaints may be indeed a "learned language" dependent on variables other than nociceptive perceptions (3,6,25). The diagnostic complexity in chronic pain states is demonstrated by the findings of Fordyce et al. (22), who showed that medical judgments as to organic versus nonorganic pain have only a moderate level of reliability across raters.

The diagnostic deficiencies in assessing chronic pain states are reflected in present legislation governing compensation and disability benefits for injury. Judicial acceptance of proof to establish entitlement in individual cases is based on "objective clinical findings," "medical diagnoses," and "subjective evidence of pain and disability" as testified to by the claimant and corroborated by the spouse, family members, neighbors, and others who have observed the claimant. Of course, testimonial responses vary according to the identity of the declarant and the circumstances in which the statements are made. Legal professionals approach the diagnostic problem with a single question: "Is the claimant telling the truth?" In disability cases, "the truth" almost invariably concerns whether the perception called pain is severe enough to prevent normal productivity.

Perceptions cannot be described accurately by one person in terms understandable by another, nor can they be assessed or denied objectively. In the absence of an accepted method for the diagnosis of chronic pain states, issues of pain are usually settled in a court of law within the cultural framework of the "disease model" that views pain as a mere symptom of disease. In cases where clear pathologic conditions cannot be demonstrated, claimants are kept idle with pending disability claims, while the needless search for more medical diagnoses as "proof" of disability goes on. In behavioral language, these delays act as major reinforcers of learned idleness (21); the longer the delay, the greater the damage to the claimant's capability to function socially and the deeper the suffering.

QUANTIFICATION AND CLASSIFICATION OF CHRONIC PAIN STATES

In the absence of a valid, reliable biologic indicator for pain perception, a diagnostic evaluation of patients with chronic pain is best obtained by a cross-matched, multilevel analysis of medical, psychologic, and social factors. So far, few attempts have been made to obtain a quantified assessment of nociceptive stimulation (defined in terms of documented pathologic findings or systemic dysfunctions), of pain behaviors, and of correlates between these two sets of data (7,19). In 1975, Brena and Koch (14) proposed a model for quantification and classification of chronic pain states that has stood the test of time and subsequent research.

The Emory Pain Estimate Model (EPEM) is designed to evaluate chronic pain states by analysis of three quantifiable sets of data: data relating to tissue pathology and systemic dysfunctions, data relating to pain behaviors, and assessment of the relationship between the medical-behavior correlates. Measurement of pathological and dysfunctional factors is depicted graphically on a 0 to 10 horizontal scale and assessed through a traditional medical, diagnostic process: physical examination, neurologic examination, radiologic studies, and laboratory studies. A value from 0 to 2.5 points is assigned for the degree of abnormality in each of the four different components. Similarly, the measurement of pain behavior is depicted on a 0 to 10 vertical scale. Again, a value from 0 to 2.5 points is assigned for each of the following data: pain intensity measured from a visual-analog scale or similar semantic inventory; activities of daily living (ADL) measured as the amount of "uptime," that is, time spent in activities requiring standing, walking, or sitting with both feet on the floor; drug use scale; and Minnesota Multiphasic Personality Inventory (MMPI). "Medical" scores are based on the physician's assessment of all medical data judged relevant to the presenting complaint; "behavioral" scores are based on information generated by the patients through a paper-and-pencil testing packet (see Table 1). The horizontal medical scale is intersected midway by the vertical behavior scale to yield four quadrants (Fig. 1).

Based on these scores, patients can be assigned to one of four quadrants. Each quadrant represents a separate pain state or class, describes a distinctly different clinical profile, and indicates variations in treatment strategies.

Class 1

Class 1 pain patients have a pathology score below 5 and a behavior score above 5, and display pain behavior in excess of documented medical findings. They score low in activity levels, high in pain verbalization, and show prominent social and psychologic malfunctions, with frequent misuse of several drugs. They demonstrate primary "learned pain," that is, they are incapacitated not by a pathologic disorder, but by conditioned factors such as musculoskeletal inactivity, incompetent coping with psychosocial stressors, and drug dependence. In Class 1 patients, successful treatment outcome may be expected by structured rehabilitation programs based on behavior modification, not by drug therapy or surgery for pain.

Class 2

Class 2 patients have pathology and behavior scores below 5. These patients are still functional despite the pain complaints. They demonstrate close to normal range of ADL, no misuse of habit-forming medications, and various problems in coping with pain. Actually, many of these patients are overdoers, with poor skills in self-pacing. Their pain complaints are often responses to periods of disordered activity without appropriate rest. Treatment should

TABLE 1. *Emory Pain Estimate Model Guidelines for Scoring*

A. Pathology ratings: (0–10)
  1. Physical examination: (0–5 points)
    Joint mobility: (Restricted)
      Cervical spine   Above midrange of motion: 0.5
      Lumbar spine   Below midrange of motion: 1
      Each of the four extremities
    Muscle strength:
      For each group of muscles   Movement against some resistance:
                                      0.5
                                Movement against gravity only: 1
                                Loss of movement: 2
    Trigger points and/or splinting (for each anatomic location): 0.5
    Enlarged organ or abnormal mass: 0.5–1 (depending on size)
    Systemic functions: Abnormality in each parameter: 0.5–1 (depending on
      severity)
    Loss of reflexes: 0.5 each
    Sensory abnormality   Segmental: 1
                               Nonsegmental: 0.5
    Loss of vibration: 1
    Motor abnormality (muscle atrophy, dystrophy, spasticity): 0.5–1 for each
      (depending on severity)
    Loss of coordination: 1
    Other abnormality: 0.5–1 (depending
      on severity)
  2. Diagnostic procedures: (0.5 points)
    Radiologic studies: For each   Severity: 0.5–2
      abnormality   Diffusion: 0.5–2
    Other studies: For each abnormality   Severity: 0.5–2
                                  Diffusion: 0.5–2

B. Behavior ratings: (0–10 points)
  1. Activity profile: (0–2.5 points)   10–14 hr: 0.5
    Uptime: (Feet on the floor while   8–10 hr: 1
      sitting or walking. Normal value: 6–8 hr: 1.5
      above 14 hr daily[a])   4–6 hr: 2
                                 Below 4 hr: 2–5

  2. Pain verbalization (0–2.5 points)
    Pain density: (intensity × frequency   10–29: 0.5
      × duration)[b]   30–49: 1.0
                                 50–69: 1.5
                                 70–89: 2.0
                                 90–100: 2.5

  3. Drug profile: (0–2.5 points)
    Drug dependence: 2.5
    Drug dosage (for each drug): Within suggested doses: 0.5
                           Above clinically suggested doses: 2.5
  4. Personality profile: (MMPI) (0–2.5
      points)
    For each clinical scale with a T-score between 70 and 84: 0.5
    For each clinical scale with a T-score of 85 or above: 1.0

---

    [a] Uptime measures may be obtained through the use of a daily diary.
    [b] Density is defined as mean subjective pain intensity at any moment in time. It can be
calculated by multiplying the proportion of the time the person reports pain by the mean
pain intensity rating when pain is present. Example: 12 hr of pain experience daily and
mean intensity = 60, density = ½ of 60 = 30.

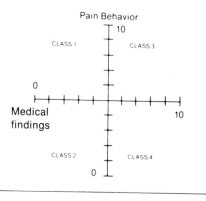

FIG. 1. Emory University Pain Clinic pain estimate model.

RATING

Medical examination

Physical Examination
Neurological Examination
Radiological Studies
Laboratory Studies

Pain Behavior

Verbal Inventory
Activity Levels
Drugs Intake
Psychometric Testing

be targeted to proper pacing of ADL, relaxation, and training in self-control. Iatrogenic displacement of these patients from Class 2 to Class 1 is likely to follow medical management based on overprescription of medication or counseling the patient to be inactive.

Class 3

Class 3 patients have pathology and behavior scores above 5. These patients demonstrate secondary learned pain; they are incapacitated both by a pathologic disorder and by conditioned factors. Competent coping with the difficulties created by the chronic illness is lost. Because pathologic conditions and illness behaviors are independent variables, resolution of the biological disorder is not necessarily followed by extinction of the conditioned pain behavior. Proper treatment strategy in these patients should include medical intervention targeted at the pathologic condition, matched with a rehabilitation program for adequate reactivation and competent coping.

Class 4

Class 4 patients have a pathology score above 5 and behavior score below 5, and demonstrate adequate skills of self-management in the presence of a

TABLE 2. *Percentages of low back pain and headache patients in pain classes according to disability status*

Pain classification	Pending disability[a]	No pending disability[b]
Low back pain (N = 207)		
1	66.7	36.0
2	12.5	32.4
3	20.8	27.9
4	0.0	3.6
Headache (N = 45)		
1	75.0	17.1
2	0.0	82.9
3	25.0	0.0
4	0.0	0.0

[a] 96 low back pain patients; 4 headache patients.
[b] 111 low back pain patients; 41 headache patients.

demonstrable pathologic condition. Long-term medical treatment of their disease process should be careful and restrained, so as not to interfere any more than necessary with their coping ability. As in Class 2 patients, relaxation training and improved self-pacing skills may be quite successful in Class 4 patients. Overtreatment with drugs or other traditional medical interventions may displace them from Class 4 to Class 3. Actually, patients in Class 4 fit remarkably well into the description of "Group 1" of illness behavior syndromes reported by Pilowsky and Spence (26).

Assignment of 15 case histories to classes of pain states by five independent physicians yielded a Pearson product-moment correlation of 0.85, indicating high reliability of the EPEM (15). This agreement in the evaluation of pain patients is possible because the EPEM provides a standard method to weigh traditional medical data and compare them with standard measures of pain behaviors. Three validity studies have also shown the ability of the EPEM to predict empirical data (9).

Table 2 demonstrates distribution by classes in a population of 207 patients with chronic low back pain and of 45 patients with chronic headaches.

Table 3 demonstrates changes in pain intensity in patients with low back pain following lumbar sympathetic blocks with either 0.25% bupivacaine or normal saline (16). As predicted, the data show that prolonged pain relief following one single treatment modality is least likely in patients with high levels of pain behaviors, defined as Classes 1 and 3.

In summary, the EPEM is a simple, quantified, and multidimensional clinical judgment; it results in an operational definition of pain patient groups that any health professional can clearly understand and communicate. Wide use of the EPEM would significantly improve management of patients with chronic pain by allowing targeting of treatment to the main problems manifested by the patient.

TABLE 3. *Percentage of patients reporting significant[a] 24-hr pain relief after bupivacaine and saline injections according to pain classification*

Pain classification	N	Bupivacaine	Saline
1	34	21	9
2	17	41	24
3	15	7	13
4	1	100	100

[a] At least 25% mean reduction in subjective pain intensity.

IMPAIRMENT AND DISABILITY

One of the massive health problems facing society today is the individual with temporary or permanent partial or total disability. Data from the World Health Organization (WHO) indicate that in industrialized countries the most important causes of impairment and disability are chronic somatic diseases and chronic pain. On the other hand, in developing countries, about 70% of all disability is caused by malnutrition, communicable disease, and low quality of prenatal care (1). A United Nations expert group has estimated that at least 25% of any population in the world are people whose time and energy are deflected by requirements of impaired individuals (1).

The same confusion that hinders assessment of chronic pain patients also cripples evaluation of their impairment and disability. When assessing disability claims in chronic sufferers, health and legal professionals, insurance companies, industry, government, and the clients themselves are faced with a chaotic system. All parties involved are forced to make judgments on an inadequate information base; because of this, the claim is often settled in favor of the party who has chosen the best attorney rather than the party with the most substantial claim. Disability benefits are often granted to those who have learned to play the best "pain game" rather than those who have objective data.

Few institutions are prepared to provide a total systematic approach to problems of chronic pain, impairment, and disability. Such an approach would (a) assess pathologic and functional conditions; (b) evaluate illness behaviors; (c) establish a pain classification; (d) provide an impairment rating; (e) match the degree of impairment with the ability to perform a specific job so as to reach an objective, job-related disability judgment; and (f) perform a vocational evaluation to establish vocational potential for productivity. If performed at all, these various tasks are usually done through different and independent agencies, operating without systematic coordination.

A major problem in disability determinations is the fact that the concept of "disability" is viewed quite differently by the various disciplines that participate in its formulation. Physicians see it as inability to work primarily due to a physical or mental illness. Rehabilitation counselors see it in terms of the availability and requirements of jobs. Legal professionals see it as an administrative decision as to the client's entitlement.

Rehabilitation International and WHO have defined impairment as the "loss or limitation of an organ of the body or mind" that is stable after maximum medical rehabilitation and nonprogressive at the time of evaluation (28). When an individual, because of an impairment, has a loss or limitation of a specific function, the individual is considered to be "disabled" so far as that function is concerned. "Handicapped" is also used if the disabling status creates a socioeconomic disadvantage for the person. On the other hand, the statutory definition of disability by the Social Security Act reads: "inability to engage in substantial gainful activity by reason of any medically determined physical or mental impairment which can be expected to result in death or which has lasted or can be expected to last for a continuous period of not less than 12 months" (Section 223-d-1).

A physical or mental impairment is defined as one "that results from an anatomic, physiologic, or psychologic abnormality which is demonstrable by medically acceptable clinical and laboratory diagnostic techniques" (Section 223-d-3). An applicant for Social Security disability must be incapable of engaging in any kind of "substantial gainful work which exists in the national economy" (Section 223-d-2-A). State workers' compensation laws generally define compensable disability as "inability to perform or obtain suitable work as a result of a work-connected injury." Total and partial disability are recognized in these state compensation laws; however, if the injured worker is still able to perform his or her job or a lesser but comparable work, then the worker is not entitled to disability compensation.

To avoid collusion with other agencies involved in the disability determination process, the Committee on Rating of Mental and Physical Impairment of the American Medical Association has determined that rating an impairment is a physician's responsibility, while a disability evaluation is an administrative task (2). This has resulted in disability decisions being made by people less expert than the physicians themselves. In many cases, these individuals do not know how to interpret the confusing array of available medical data. The Honorable Howard Grossman, former Administrative Judge of the Social Security Administration, has written that physicians, by "washing their hands" of the disability issue and leaving it to the attorneys, have failed to realize the human, social, and economic wastage involved in cases of people who have been granted unjustified disability benefits and have been condemned to spend the rest of their lives unemployable and in idleness, except to have periodic, expensive medical treatment to substantiate their disability claims continually (23).

Impairment Rating

The evaluation of impairment is an appraisal of the nature and extent to which an injury or disease limits a person's ability to carry out normal ADL, such as self-care, communication, standing and walking, housekeeping, shopping, and traveling. Functional assessment is central to environmental functioning and adaptation; in its broadest sense, it refers to measurement of the interaction between an impaired individual and the environment. A usable, if not entirely accurate, impairment rating can be constructed following the AMA "Guides to the Evaluation of Permanent Impairment" (2). A general medical examination and pertinent, systemic functional assessment are required. For instance, in cases of musculoskeletal pain syndromes involving the back, adequate radiologic and electromyographic documentation must be obtained and matched with assessment of joint mobility, muscle strength, and sensory abnormality; in cases of chest pain with dyspnea, exercise electrocardiogram, pulmonary function tests, and blood gases will also be required. Whole body impairment is expressed as percentage determined according to specific guidelines relating to individual body parts.

While the AMA guidelines for impairment are imperfect, they are a widely used standard in the United States today. However, interest in the measurement of physical functioning has evolved over the past 30 years from the measurement of single body functions to measurements of the composite functioning of the whole person. For this purpose, several multidimensional indices, inventories, scales—such as the Katz Index, the Functional Assessment Inventory (FAI), and the Longitudinal Functional Assessment System (LFAS)—have been recently developed and tested for their relative usefulness (18).

Disability Evaluation

The WHO definition of disability involves a multitude of factors, such as age, education, motor performance, motivation, economic and social environments, and vocational skills. One may be disabled for a given task but capable of performing other tasks. For example, a patient with left upper extremity neuralgic pain may be totally disabled if he were a violinist, but scarcely disabled at all for a job as a radio announcer. In patients disabled by pain, a disability rating is constructed by estimating the effects of the person's impairment on ability to perform social roles and job requirements. Pain classification, impairment rating, and a vocational evaluation are required to assess disability.

Several systems are presently available to assess vocational abilities, including the Singer, Valpar, and Hester systems. The usefulness of each system depends on the amount of time available for testing and the expected use of the information obtained, such as job placement, training, and settlement of pending disability claims.

The Singer Evaluation System is basically a job sample that limits itself to the skills and abilities involved in specific jobs. The system consists of approximately 26 carrels having all the tools necessary to perform a job. The subject receives instructions from a cassette and filmstrips. The evaluator checks the subject's progress at various points. The overall quality of work is assessed using the Singer Group Norms. The testing requires from one to several hours for each work sample.

The Valpar Evaluation System uses several different types of physical capacity tests and work samples. The aptitudes assessed include manual dexterity, size discrimination, sorting, gross body movements, mechanical aptitude, right and left arm-hand motor coordination, and form perception. The job samples include clerical tests, assembly work, and electronic assembly tasks. For most of the tests, an evaluator must observe the subject while he or she works and time responses with a stopwatch. The evaluator collects information about the subject's aptitudes and skills compared to the average worker. It requires from a few minutes to several hours to administer the majority of the tests.

With both the Singer and Valpar evaluation systems, the evaluator compiles the data and uses judgment to make specific job recommendations. In contrast, the Hester Evaluation System is a computerized method of assessing a person's vocational abilities. The system consists of 27 factor-pure vocational tests that measure 28 independent ability factors. After testing, the raw scores, plus some additional demographic data about the individual, are fed into a computer that analyzes the scores to determine how the subject's abilities relate to jobs contained in the Dictionary of Occupational Titles. The resulting printout provides scaled scores for ability factors, various job families, and a list of specific, feasible jobs in various industries that the patient has demonstrated the ability to perform. It usually requires 4 to 6 hr to administer the Hester test. The higher the number of vocational alternatives and job skills available to an impaired person, the less likely the person is to be a candidate for disability benefits, according to the Social Security definition. In cases of injured workers on Workers' Compensation benefits, a vocational evaluation is not only useful to determine the patient's capability to return to the previous occupation, but also to help the patient eventually obtain another suitable occupation.

A study of the Emory group has shown significant relationships among classes of chronic pain states, impairment, and disability (12). Class 3 pain patients demonstrated the highest impairment and disability ratings, whereas Class 1 patients showed significantly higher ratings of impairment and disability than Class 2 patients (Fig. 2).

Fifty-nine percent of the patients in this study demonstrated higher disability than impairment ratings, indicating the presence of feasible job alternatives. In many cases, these ratings also reflect conditioned pain behaviors that can be reversed through proper rehabilitation (4,11,24).

Problem of Malingering

The possibility of malingering in cases of compensable disability is difficult to assess. In patients with chronic pain, malingering may be defined as a

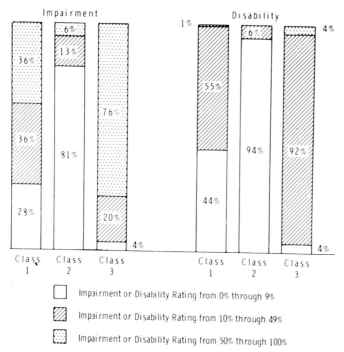

FIG. 2. Impairment and disability ratings for patients in different pain classes. [Reprinted from S. F. Brena et al. (12), with permission.]

conscious playing of the sick role. Legally, malingering cannot be proved. However, evidence of documented inconsistencies may be introduced before a jury, leading to a judgment of likely malingering. Independently from each other, Ellard (20) and the Emory group (11) have developed an "Inconsistency Profile," showing remarkable similarities in the documentation of likely malingering. The Emory Inconsistency Profile, presented in Table 4, describes several pieces of evidence that may suggest malingering *if* combined with other indices. No single measure should be used to indicate likely malingering.

CONCLUSION

No evaluation system can avoid controversy, but the better the information on which decisions are made, the fairer they will be. The problem of evaluating compensable disability in patients incapacitated by chronic pain is mammoth, but the challenge can be met by using presently available multidisciplinary tools and by continuous efforts to test and improve them. The process requires a Sherlock Holmes-like attitude, where all pertinent data must be assembled, analyzed, and put into perspective following a systematic, algorithmic approach (10). Figure 3 presents a step-by-step procedure for evaluating pain-disabled patients.

TABLE 4. *"Inconsistency Profile"*

1. Complete absence of objective findings for organic pathology.
2. Over-dramatized complaints which do not fit any anatomical nor physiological pattern.
3. Logical inconsistencies between statements or between statements and behaviors (examples: a patient who is observed to sit for a long period of time, yet claims that he is unable to do so; patient who claims he cannot bend more than a few degrees, but is observed picking up objects off the floor easily).
4. The patient is resistive to be evaluated for his ability to work or for a complete assessment of his medical difficulties, while claiming that he wants "to find the cause of his pain."
5. Responses to diagnostic nerve blocks do not fit any predictable physiological, pharmacological, and anatomic pattern (example: a patient who claims to be "paralyzed" in both lower extremities 24 hours after receiving a unilateral lumbar sympathetic block with 0.25 percent bupivacaine).
6. Increase in pain complaints while patient reports improvement in other aspects of a pain rehabilitation program.
7. Rewards for malingering compare favorably with alternative rewards.
8. History of manipulative behaviors.
9. Discrepancies between reports of patient and the spouse regarding pain behavior at home.
10. Unprompted expression of desire to work, inconsistent with behavior.
11. Unprompted denial of malingering.
12. Inappropriately flat or histrionic affect.
13. The following MMPI patterns may occur:
    a. Extreme elevations on the following scales: Lie (L), Defensiveness (K), Hypochondriasis (Hs).
    b. Extreme number of bizarre psychological complaints, as measured by high score on scale F.
    c. High Psychopathic Deviance scale score (scale Pd).
    d. Inconsistencies in responses to repeated items on the MMPI.
    e. All scores are well within normal limits despite reports of continuing, severe, and disabling pain.

The National Council on the Handicapped estimates that approximately 14 billion dollars are spent each year in the United States for treatment or compensation for low back pain alone. Impairment of the back and spine are the most frequent chronic conditions causing limitations of activity among people between the ages of 20 and 60 years; it ultimately affects more than half of the labor force in the United States (13). As is shown in Table 1, 66.7% of patients with chronic low back pain and pending disability claims belong to Class 1. Many of these patients have been out of work more than 2 years, literally floating through the health care system in search of "diagnoses" to secure an administrative decision granting them continuing disability benefits. To grant a blanket disability status to Class 1 pain patients is socially irresponsible and medically wrong, as it provides incentives for lack of productivity and misuses taxpayers' funds. It also condemns these unfortunate sufferers to a lifestyle dominated by their sick roles and an image of hopelessness and worthlessness. On the other hand, proper multidimensional evaluation of chronic pain patients can lead to appropriate medical and vocational treatment strategies that may restore workers to former or new occupations, to the enormous benefit of society. Return to productivity

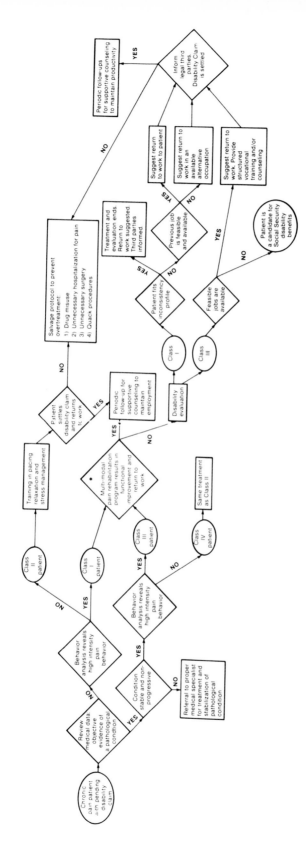

FIG. 3. Chronic pain states and compensable disability: An algorithm for management. *For Program Quality Control see Standards Manual for Facilities Serving People with Disabilities: Chronic Management Programs published by the Commission on Accreditation of Rehabilitation Facilities, 2500 North Pantano Road, Tucson, Arizona 85715.

is an essential variable in the assessment of treatment outcome in pain-disabled patients (5,17).

REFERENCES

1. Acton, N. (1982): The world response to disability: Evolution of a philosophy. *Arch. Phys. Med. Rehabil.*, 63:145–149.
2. American Medical Association (1958): Committee on Rating of Mental and Physical Impairment. "Guides to the Evaluation of Permanent Impairment." Special Edition.
3. Agnew, D. C., and Meskey, H. (1976): Words of chronic pain. *Pain*, 2:73–82.
4. Ahlmen, J., and Olander, R. (1973): Influence of pre-operative tension on vocational rehabilitation following renal transplantation. *Acta Med. Scand.*, 194:13–16.
5. Aronoff, G. M., Evans, W. O., and Enders, P. L. (1983): A review of follow-up studies of multidisciplinary pain units. *Pain*, 16:1–11.
6. Bailey, C., and Davidson, P. (1976): The language of pain intensity. *Pain*, 2:319–394.
7. Black, R. G., and Chapman, C. R. (1976): The SAD Index for clinical assessment of pain. In: *Advances in Pain Research and Therapy, Vol. 1*, edited by J. J. Bonica and D. Albe-Fessard. Raven Press, New York.
8. Brena, S. F., and Chapman, S. L. (1981): The learned pain syndrome. *Postgrad. Med.*, 69:53–64.
9. Brena, S. F., and Chapman, S. L. (1982): Validity of the Emory pain estimate model. *Anesthesiol. Rev.*, 9:42–45.
10. Brena, S. F., and Chapman, S. L. (1982): Chronic pain: An algorithm for management. *Postgrad. Med.*, 72:111–117.
11. Brena, S. F., and Chapman, S. L. (1983): Pain and litigation. In: *Textbook of Pain*, edited by P. D. Wall. Churchill-Livingstone, London.
12. Brena, S. F., Chapman, S. L., Stegall, P. G., and Chyatte, S. B. (1979): Chronic pain states: Their relationship to impairment and disability. *Arch. Phys. Med. Rehabil.*, 60:387–389.
13. Brena, S. F., Johnson, S. J., Fordyce, W. E., and White, A. A. (1982): Annual Report of the National Council of the Handicapped. Topic 2: Chronic Back Pain. U.S. Department of Education, March.
14. Brena, S. F., and Koch, D. L. (1975): The "Pain Estimate" for quantification and classification of chronic pain state. *Anesthesiol. Rev.*, 2:8–13.
15. Brena, S. F., Koch, D. L., and Moss, R. M. (1976): Reliability of the pain estimate model. *Anesthesiol. Rev.*, 3:28–29.
16. Chapman, S. L., and Brena, S. F. (1982): Learned helplessness and responses to nerve blocks in chronic low back pain patients. *Pain*, 14:355–364.
17. Chapman, S. L., Brena, S. F., and Bradford, L. A. (1981): Treatment outcome in a chronic pain rehabilitation program. *Pain*, 11:255–268.
18. Diller, L., Granger, C. V., Katz, S., and Nagi, S. (1982): Annual Report of the National Council on the Handicapped. Topic 1: Functional Assessment. U.S. Department of Education, March.
19. Duncan, G. H., Gregg, J. M., and Ghia, J. N. (1978): The pain profile: A computerized system for assessment of chronic pain. *Pain*, 5:275–284.
20. Ellard, J. (1970): Psychological reaction to compensable injury. *Med. J. Aust.*, 8:349–355.
21. Engberg, L. A., Hansen, G., and Welker, R. L. (1973): Acquisition of key-pecking via auto-shaping as a function of prior experience. *Science*, 178:1002–1004.
22. Fordyce, W. E., Brena, S. F., and Holcomb, R. (1978): Relationship of semantic pain descriptions to physician diagnostic judgments, activity level measures, and MMPI. *Pain*, 5:293–303.
23. Grossman, H. I. (1983): Legal aspects of pain and disability. In: *Management of Patients with Chronic Pain*, edited by S. F. Brena and S. L. Chapman, pp. 225–229. Spectrum Publications, New York.
24. Hammonds, W., Brena, S. F., and Unikel, I. P. (1978): Compensation for work-related injuries and rehabilitation of patients with chronic pain. *South. Med. J.*, 71:664–666.
25. Melzack, R., and Torgerson, W. S. (1971): On the language of pain. *Anesthesiology*, 34:50–59.

26. Pilowsky, I., and Spence, N. D. (1976): Illness behavior syndromes associated with intractable pain. *Pain*, 2:61–71.
27. Robin, E. D. (1978): Determinism and humanism in modern medicine. *JAMA*, 240:2273–2275.
28. World Health Organization (1980): International Classification of Impairments, Disabilities and Handicaps. Geneva, World Health Organization.

*Advances in Pain Research
and Therapy, Vol. 7,*
edited by C. Benedetti et al.
Raven Press, New York © 1984.

Drugs in the Management of Pain: Pharmacology and Appropriate Strategies for Clinical Utilization

Lawrence M. Halpern

*University of Washington, Department of Pharmacology, Seattle, Washington
98195*

I am very pleased and feel privileged to have been invited to write this paper as part of a volume prepared to honor Dr. John J. Bonica for his outstanding leadership, contributions and encouragement to the further development of pain research and therapy throughout the world, and for his critical role in founding, developing, and directing the University of Washington Pain Center during the past quarter century. My association with Dr. Bonica has been very rewarding both from a standpoint of our personal and productive interaction, and for the encouragement and help he has given me and so many others.

During the past decade and a half, there has been an unprecedented surge of interest and work in pain research. Consequently we have acquired a vast amount of new and scientific information on the neurophysiologic, biochemical, and psychologic substrates of pain. This has markedly enhanced our knowledge of sensory coding and sensory modulation.

Enkephalin and endorphin have come to explain everything from endogenous relief of pain to acupuncture-induced analgesia, "runner's high," and the physiologic/psychologic basis for drug dependence of both the opiate and alcohol type. What we have learned about the scientific basis of pain is paralleled by the information derived from records of patients treated by members of the Clinical Pain Service at our own center over the last quarter century.

All of these have brought about a change in our conceptualization of clinical pain and the management of patients with acute, chronic, and cancer pain. These advances would not have been possible, nor would they have been so quickly disseminated and adopted, without the foresight, energy, and guidance of Dr. John J. Bonica.

This chapter concerns basic principles and current practices in the use of systemic analgesia for the relief of pain. To appreciate the significant changes in our concepts of the use of these drugs, it is desirable to discuss some basic premises first.

BASIC CONSIDERATIONS

In considering the proper application of analgesics or any other therapeutic modality for pain relief, it is essential to determine various characteristics of the pain and, specifically, whether pain is acute or chronic. If it is chronic, it is important to determine the underlying mechanism. One of the early and very important contributions by Bonica (4,6–9) to this field was the emphasis on the differences between acute pain, chronic pain, and cancer pain, and the systematic classification of pain syndromes. The differences between these types of pain pertain to etiology, mechanisms, pathophysiology, symptomatology, diagnosis and treatment, and biologic function. Despite repeated efforts by Bonica and others, these differences were virtually ignored by the medical profession until the past decade, when studies by Sternbach (34), Fordyce (16), Merskey (24), Pilowsky (25), and others defined them more precisely, more clearly, and more convincingly. Sternbach (35) not only emphasized the contrasting characteristics of acute and chronic pain, but developed in a very intriguing way and in an impressively logical sequence convincing evidence that the pain in acute pain is a symptom of disease, whereas the pain itself in chronic pain is the disease.

Acute Pain

Bonica has defined acute pain as a constellation of unpleasant sensory, perceptual, and emotional experiences, of certain associated autonomic (reflex) responses, and of psychologic and behavioral reactions provoked by injury or acute disease (6,7). The tissue injury provokes a series of noxious stimuli, which are transduced by nociceptors to impulses that are transmitted to the spinal cord and then to the upper part of the central nervous system (CNS). These responses to nociceptive stimulation are enhanced by bradykinin, histamine, and prostaglandin formation from biosynthesis of arachidonic acid and other by-products of cellular damage.

These nociceptive impulses from the periphery are transmitted via slowly conductive A delta and C fibers to the substantia gelatinosa of the spinal cord, where substance P, an 11-amino-acid peptide, activates postsynaptic neuronal elements. Some of these are interneurons that connect with the anterolateral and anterior horn cells, which become involved in segmental reflex responses; others are transmitted to cell bodies of neurons whose axons pass to the opposite anterolateral quadrant and constitute the paleo and neospinothalamic pathways. These transmit the nociceptive impulses to the brainstem to produce suprasegmental responses and impulses to the cortex, where they are perceived and experienced as pain and initiate psychodynamic mechanisms and motor responses. (See Chapter by C. Benedetti and J. J. Bonica, *this volume*, for descriptions of responses to tissue injury.)

These multidimensional factors and responses are inextricably interrelated and all contribute to the total subjective pain experience and the pain behavior. Although psychologic factors influence acute pain, it is rare that it is caused primarily by operant (environmental) factors or psychopathology. As a result of effective therapy or the self-limiting nature of the disease or injury, the pain and associated responses usually disappear within days, or at most, a few weeks.

It has long been appreciated that acute pain of disease has the important biologic function of warning the individual that something is wrong. In certain injuries it enforces stillness, which promotes healing and recuperation. Moreover, the physiologic and neuroendocrine responses and the usual psychologic reaction of anxiety initially prepare the organism for an emergency response and help it cope with the disease or injury. However, what is not generally appreciated by many health professionals is that acute pain and segmental, suprasegmental, and neuroendocrine reflex responses that develop in the postoperative period or after massive injury or burns have no useful function. If not promptly and effectively relieved, these responses produce progressively serious pathophysiologic responses. These consist of excessive adrenergic activity and abnormal neuroendocrine stress response, that is, increased secretion of catabolically-acting hormones and decrease of anabolically-acting hormones.

These persistent pathophysiologic responses, in turn, produce marked increases in the workload of the heart, excessive increase in metabolism and oxygen consumption, and inhibition of gastrointestinal and genitourinary function, with consequent ileus and oligurea. The neuroendocrine stress response invariably leads to substrate mobilization from storage to the central organs and the traumatized tissue, and ultimately to a catabolic state with negative nitrogen balance. Persistent skeletal muscle spasm, together with the fear of aggravating the pain and bronchial spasm induced by cutaneovisceral and viscerovisceral reflexes, results in decreased chest wall compliance, vital capacity (VC), and functional residual capacity (FRC), which lead to atalectasis, hypoxemia, and to pneumonitis if not relieved. Moreover, in cases of severe trauma, pain and the associated reflex responses, especially excessive splachnic vasoconstriction, are likely to initiate and sustain shock (7).

Similar deleterious effects occur if, after they have served their biologic function, the severe pain and the associated responses of myocardial infarction, pancreatitis, renal colic, pulmonary embolism, and other acute pathologic processes are not effectively relieved. There is experimental evidence that persistent pain and the associated sympathetic hyperactivity increase the discrepancy between myocardial oxygen demand and oxygen supply and consequently increase the size of infarction and risk of death (see Chapter by V. Pasqualucci, *this volume*). Acute pancreatitis causes excruciating pain reflex spasm of the abdominal and chest wall, which often produces severe hypoventilation that may progress to death unless promptly corrected (4). Even severe pain and the associated reflex responses inherent in human parturition, if allowed to persist, will produce serious deleterious effects on the mother and the fetus (10). Finally, and most relevant, is the fact that if acute painful processes are not effectively treated, they may and often do progress to a chronic pain state.

Chronic Pain

Chronic pain is defined as pain that persists beyond the usual course of an acute disease or beyond a reasonable time for an injury to heal (6,7). Although some clinicians use the arbitrary figure of 6 months to designate pain as chronic, this is not appropriate because there are many acute diseases or injuries that heal in 2, 3, or 4 weeks. In such conditions, if pain is still present 3 to 4 weeks after cure should have been achieved, it must be considered chronic pain.

Chronic pain is the result of persistent dysfunction of the nociceptive pain system. Its mechanisms have been classified by Bonica (6) into four mechanisms. First is peripheral mechanisms, in which chronic tissue pathology produces persistent and prolonged (chronic) stimulation and/or sensitization of nociceptors, as occurs in arthritis, chronic pancreatitis, and certain types of cancer. The second is peripheral-central mechanisms, in which there is peripheral nerve injury that produces pathophysiologic changes in the spinal cord and other parts of the neuraxis, as exemplified by causalgia, postamputation pain, and cancer-related damage to peripheral nerves. Third is central pain mechanisms which is pain arising within the central nervous system as a result of surgery, accidental injury, tumor of hemorrhage (thalamic syndrome), or demyelinating diseases of the neuraxis. Pain produced by these conditions is usually chronic, severe, and debilitating, and accompanied by bouts of episodic, severe, lancinating pain. Examples are tic douloureaux, postherpetic neuralgia and the thalamic syndrome (4,6). The fourth consists of psychologic mechanisms, which can be further subdivided into operant (environmental) and psychophysiologic (psychosomatic) mechanisms.

Operant pain is a complex behavior occurring months or years after the initial injury. It is characterized by persistent pain disproportionate to or completely without underlying pathology, undue suffering, depression, anxiety, and, frequently, inappropriate or excessive use of analgesics, sedatives, and other medications (16,19). Pain behavior is a result of the learning process, predominantly environmental and interpersonal factors. It is often associated with predisposing emotional disorders or secondary gain. Although operant pain is responsible for chronic illness behavior in many patients complaining of pain, it deserves emphasis that this group constitutes only a fraction of the chronic pain population. Therefore, the suggestion of some clinicians (3) that the term *chronic pain syndrome* is limited to persistent pain caused by operant or psychologic mechanisms is inappropriate and confusing and should be avoided. Similarly, the use of the term *benign* chronic pain to differentiate it from cancer pain is also inappropriate because chronic pain is never benign, and it is best to use the term *nonneoplastic* chronic pain.

Chronic pain caused by peripheral, peripheral-central, or central mechanisms may be continuous with minimal changes in severity, or it may vary in intensity on a daily or weekly basis, or it may recur in bouts lasting hours, days or weeks. For the latter, some writers use the term *recurrent acute pain of malignant origin* or *recurrent acute pain of nonneoplastic origin*. Although the periodicity is an important characteristic to be ascertained in patients with chronic pain, Bonica insists that the use of *recurrent acute pain* as a classification of pain is inappropriate and leads to further confusion.

One final and important point about chronic pain: in contrast to acute pain, in its chronic, persistent form, pain *never* has a biologic function, but is a malific force that often imposes severe emotional, physical, economic and social stresses on the patient, and on the family, and is one of the most costly health problems for society (4,7).

Multidisciplinary Pain Management

Experience has emphasized that patients with complex pain problems can be managed more successfully by a multidisciplinary team, each member contributing individual knowledge and skill to the common cause of making a correct diagnosis and developing the most appropriate strategy. This approach, discussed in detail by T. Murphy and S. Anderson (*this volume*), was conceived and first practiced by Bonica nearly 40 years ago in a large military hospital (4,5,11). Subsequently, he put the concept to a test in civilian practice in a private community hospital during the 14-year period following the war. In 1961, he initiated a similar program at the University of Washington (4). In the ensuing decade, the program evolved into a group of some 25 persons from 14 different disciplines. The members of the group participated in patient care, teaching, and research in varying degrees, and devoted varying amounts of time.

Since the formation of the multidisciplinary pain program a quarter century ago, much has been learned about the complexity of dealing with pain in its variety of manifestations. The recognition of two phases in the progression of pain and suffering in malignant disease quickly brought the entire body of experience with chronic pain management to bear on the problem of treating cancer pain. An understanding of the roles of anxiety and depression, and their relation to all types of pain, has changed the way our group approaches preoperative anxiety, postoperative pain, and, if it occurs, postoperative depression (38). Through the leadership and efforts of Professor Bonica, and the active participation and collaboration of scientists from various biologic sciences and clinical disciplines, a pain research center evolved that currently has one of the foremost and largest programs of pain investigation in the world.

PHARMACOLOGIC AND CLINICAL CONSIDERATIONS

The various aspects of drug management in pain control will now be considered. The opiates and nonsteroidal anti-inflammatory agents are still the mainstay of pain relief. They are simple to use and relatively inexpensive. Unfortunately, it is precisely these attributes that cause imprecise application of these agents. Before discussing each specific drug, general comments are in order.

General Considerations

Drug Selection

Is there an opiate of choice for use in pain management or is the technique of application more important? Candidate agents now being examined include heroin (21), morphine, methadone (2), nalbuphine (33), and buprenorphine (20,27). At equianalgesic doses, all opiates have the same ability to reduce pain and, unfortunately, the same ability to induce physiologic dependence. Thus far, no one drug provides superior pain relief to another, although some show a remarkably lower incidence of use in drug dependency situations.

Usually failures to respond to analgesic drugs with reduction in pain are not idiosyncratic reactions to the narcotic, and can be traced to inadequate dosage repeated less frequently than required to produce stable analgesic blood levels of the drug (12,22,23). This, in turn, has been due to inadequate knowledge of the clinical pharmacology of narcotics, with consequent prescription and administration of insufficient amounts at less than optimal frequency. An important factor is the unwarranted fear of addiction—a phenomenon that is rare following the use of narcotics for acute pain and for cancer pain (15,27).

The correction of this problem in most cases lies in the administration of larger doses at shorter time intervals so the blood level of the drug is high enough to produce analgesia. Unfortunately, the usual course of events is for the physician to abandon the original drug that seemed ineffective in favor of another of the same type. This hit or miss approach causes needless suffering and the dose-effect information learned about the patient's response to the original drug at the dosage originally provided is lost. The systematic approach is for the physician to increase the dose stepwise to the endpoint of effective analgesia, or to depression of the respiratory rate to levels of about 16, or to the endpoint of pinpoint pupil. If analgesia fails to occur with a respiratory rate at 16 or just under, this approach must be abandoned if one is unprepared to deal with respiratory arrest in the patient. Should severe respiratory depression or arrest occur due to narcotic overdosage, naloxone may provide total reversal of respiratory depression due to opiates. This reversal does not occur after overdoses with another drug type, e.g., sedatives such as benzodiazepines.

How are drugs selected if all narcotics have equal ability to alleviate pain or to produce dependence? For pharmacokinetic reasons discussed below, one may choose narcotic analgesics on the basis of their known duration of action, or from patient care considerations on the basis of their routes of administration.

Adjunct analgesics may be used in certain situations (1,12). In other situations, weaning to a lower dose of narcotic while substituting psychotropic drugs may reduce fear, anxiety, and depression, and may provide better pain control than existed with higher doses of narcotics alone.

Route of Administration

What is the most appropriate route of administration of opiates for the management of pain? Routes suggested and currently being debated include oral, intravenous, intramuscular, and, recently, indwelling spinal epidural catheter. Depending on the drug, each route seems to be of value in appropriate circumstances. Oral administration of narcotics may be desirable in the management of patients with cancer pain and where health care professionals are not readily available to administer drugs parenterally. To use orally administered narcotics safely, one must keep in mind the parenteral-to-oral dose conversion for each drug, as described below (15,17).

Parenteral medication may be used when oral medications cannot be used, when the enteric tract has been surgically interrupted, or when close medical supervision is not available. When rapid changes in dose facilitate maintaining analgesia or when other soluble agents are to be given concomitantly, the intravenous route may be very useful. Some situations may require doses of narcotic be given continuously by pump via indwelling intravenous catheters.

Epidural morphine is currently being provided for cancer patients and acute pain patients in research settings as a dramatic new therapy devoid of problems of systemic administration of opiates (for details see Chapter by L. Jacobson, *this volume*). When administered epidurally, morphine does not produce dizziness, nausea and vomiting, constipation, or other adverse side effects of opiate administration. Opiate dependence has not been reported after this route of administration, and tolerance when it occurs is of a lesser order of magnitude than that occurring following systemic administration. Interestingly, plasma levels of morphine shortly after epidural administration of morphine are the equivalent of those after administration by the oral route. The epidural route of administration is not without potential lethal consequences; fatal respiratory depression has occurred two to three days after administration of 2 to 3 mg morphine. Why delayed respiratory depression occurs when other effects anatomically linked to the same region of the CNS as control of respiration occurs immediately after epidural administration is not clearly understood, but may be related to parenteral use of morphine prior to epidural use. Agents that provide analgesia yet cannot get through the blood-brain barrier, such as beta-endorphin or some of the D-substituted enkephalines, have been tried. Another approach to this problem is the future development of a pure kappa agonist, a drug that will produce segmental analgesia but not be capable of producing respiratory depression.

Time Contingent versus P.R.N. Medication

Another way of describing pain with underlying pathology but with behavioral overtones is operant or respondent pain. Operant pain is pain resulting from its behavioral consequences. Respondent pain results primarily from nociception. Thus having pain may result in attention, provision of medication, or some other satisfying outcome. When patients find an outcome desirable, they may, inadvertently or consciously, need to have pain to produce the desired response of attention, desired medication effects, or reduction of fear and loneliness. Providing time contingent medication, e.g., adequate doses at time intervals frequent enough so the patient does not have to request them nor frequently enough to produce toxicity, reduces that component of pain controlled by its consequences (16).

Pharmacokinetic Considerations

Pharmacokinetic considerations relate specifically to time of drug concentrations in blood serum and plasma as a result of simultaneous absorption, distribution, and elimination. These considerations aid in drug, dosage, and dosage schedule selection but are not a substitute for astute clinical judgment, nor do they eliminate the absolute requirement for careful clinical monitoring of degree of drug effect.

For the purpose of this discussion, pharmacokinetic principles may be based on the simple model of the body as a single compartment. Distribution of a drug in this model occurs rapidly with respect to absorption or elimination. In this situation, absorption and elimination of the drug follow first-order kinetics, that is, a constant fraction of the drug is either absorbed or eliminated in a given unit of time. Narcotics follow exponential elimination curves. This is fortunate because drug concentrations required for saturation of these mechanisms would be lethal.

A single dose of narcotic administered parenterally might be assumed to rise at latency fixed by the absorption characteristics of the individual drug to a peak of drug concentration. Thereafter, a linear fall in plasma concentration occurs over time. The effect of the dose can be characterized by latency, time of peak effect, magnitude of peak effect, and duration of therapeutic action. Four biologic half-times are required for almost complete elimination of a drug. A shorter dosage interval leads to drug accumulation in plasma.

During repeated administration of a drug, its plasma concentration is described by the time course of its accumulation, the maximal amount accumulated, the fluctuations that result from the dose interval, and the half-time for excretion of the drug. When a drug is given repeatedly, the total body store of the drug increases exponentially with a half-time for increase equal to the half-time for elimination of the agent. Thus 50% of the maximal plateau is achieved in one elimination half-time, 75% in two, 87.5% in three, and so on. Maximal accumulation is generally considered to have occurred after about four half-times. When this occurs, the rate of elimination is equal to the rate of administration. The dosage interval chosen on the basis of the above considerations would be based on the drug concentration that can be tolerated without excess loss of efficacy or toxicity.

In patients with acute pain treated with narcotics for several days or even 1 or 2 weeks, it is rare for tolerance, loss of efficacy, or abstinence syndrome precipitated by inappropriate use of antagonist analgesics to occur. In cancer patients, loss of efficacy or reversal with antagonist agents may not only cause exposure to the discomfort of abstinence syndrome, but also further exposure to needless pain. The apparent benefits from fixed-time interval dosage with narcotics are plateau concentrations that can be maintained over longer time intervals, uninterrupted analgesia, protection of patients from abstinence syndrome, and analgesia at doses lower than those that would obtund patients at peak effect.

Is There a Narcotic Drug or Mixture "of Choice" for Management of Cancer Pain?

Over the last few years, several drugs have been championed as "drug of choice" for cancer pain management. Oral heroin was promoted for this use until a controlled clinical trial failed to demonstrate significant differences in patient acceptability between drugs (21). Moreover, heroin in equianalgesic doses has been shown to be indistinguishable from morphine by cancer patients with postoperative pain and ongoing pain due to cancer.

Brompton's cocktail containing heroin, cocaine, and alcohol has been used frequently for cancer pain control. Clinical trials demonstrated no difference between Brompton's with and without cocaine, indicating the concentration of cocaine used in the mixture is ineffective. A controlled clinical study failed to find differences between a simple solution of oral morphine and Brompton's cocktail by cancer patients who could not distinguish between the two (21,39,40,41). This study casts doubt on the wisdom of using a mixture of agents when adequate oral doses of morphine or methadone given often enough, or in quantities large enough for self-administration, provide adequate relief (15,29).

TABLE 1. *Summary of guidelines for rational pain relief*

Specific guidelines that can help provide state-of-the-art pain relief can be stated succinctly.

1. Choose the drug type to match the pain type: centrally acting if necessary, for severe pain; peripherally acting for mild to moderate pain.
2. Choose the drug duration of action to match the duration of the pain being treated.
3. Choose the route of administration with patient comfort and safety in mind, but be sure to provide rapid onset of analgesic activity.
4. Know the detailed pharmacology of the drug to be prescribed. It is better to use a drug you know well than to use a newer drug about which little is known.
5. If the drug chosen fails to provide adequate pain relief, do not switch drugs. Try increased doses but do not proceed to the point of toxicity.
6. Administer analgesics on a fixed-time interval basis to take advantage of kinetic factors leading to improved analgesia.
7. Administer analgesics on a fixed-time interval basis to avoid or minimize the development of chronic phase pain.
8. Treat side effects appropriately or provide a drug that has fewer side effects and is more acceptable to the patient.
9. Remember the development of tolerance cannot be avoided. Increase medication to provide adequate analgesia necessary as time progresses.
10. Medication levels must be changed slowly to avoid precipitating withdrawal or increased respiratory depression and other overdose complications.
11. There is no place for placebo medication in the management of pain.
12. Most physicians undermedicate their patients postsurgically because of irrational fears of addiction, and overmedicate their patients chronically because they do not realize that, in chronic pain situations, it may be the medicine itself that is responsible for the increased pain. The development of chronic pain in many cases comes from inappropriate and ineffective undertreatment of acute pain.

The discussion above has encouraged the reader to attempt to understand that beyond knowing the basic pharmacology of the drugs involved (the science of rational drug use), there must be an awareness of degrees of effect using the patient's response to drug type and dose selection as feedback to make midstream course corrections continuously. This can be thought of as the "art" of pain relief. Physicians are like music students in the respect that they are frequently expected to give virtuoso performances before mastery of the fundamentals. Fundmentals to improve performance in the fine art of pain relief are listed in Table 1. Patients and their loved ones are considered to be our most important critics. Experience has shown that physicians as patients are actually the most informed critics, quick to point out the drug choice and timing errors of their peers.

Peripherally Acting Analgesics

The substances in this heterogeneous group all possess the ability to inhibit the biosynthesis of prostaglandins (14). Since prostaglandins are involved in amplification of pain due to tissue injury and as messengers in inflammation inhibitors of the synthesizing enzyme, they reduce pain by direct action in desensitizing nociceptors and indirectly by reducing inflammatory pain. These drugs also possess an antipyretic action based on their ability to inhibit prostaglandin biosynthesis. It has been suggested these agents may have an antitumor effect and may help reduce the inflammatory tissue response to tumor invasion in some patients with bony metastases.

Aspirin and Congeners

Aspirin is the prototype agent in this class. It is useful to characterize the potency and side effects of each drug class and to compare these to aspirin (17,31,32). As with aspirin, these drugs are usually administered orally for the treatment of mild to moderate pain. In the management of pain, it is important to continue aspirin-like agents as required and as long as possible into the period when narcotics are used. There is some evidence that antagonism of central prostaglandins by these drugs increases the analgesic action of the narcotic analgesics. Tolerance and physical dependence do not develop to these agents but there is a ceiling past which increasing doses increase side effects and toxicity, which outweighs the benefits of their use.

As is well understood in the management of the arthritides, the choice of drug must be individualized for each patient (31,32). This may be done on the basis of efficacy, side effects and toxicity, and patient acceptability. Each patient must receive adequate trial of an agent before it is abandoned in favor of a new drug that, if used inexpertly, may be of no more benefit than the first. An adequate trial consists of administration of the drug at fixed time intervals, increasing the dosage up to maximum levels tolerated and acceptable to the patient. Should the drug prove to be toxic or not to produce adequate analgesia, the patient should be switched to an anti-inflammatory agent of another chemical class. Use of aspirin concomitantly with other members of this group lowers available concentrations of the second drug by displacing it from plasma protein.

If pain control after an adequate trial of nonnarcotic analgesics is inadequate or obtained at a level where toxicity adds to patient discomfort, these agents should be abandoned and the patient should be switched to narcotic analgesics. Despite biases to the contrary, narcotic analgesics have fewer metabolic consequences and are often more easily tolerated than nonsteroidal anti-inflammatory agents.

Pyrazoles

Phenylbutazone and oxyphenbutazone, derivatives of phenacetin, are potent inhibitors of prostaglandin synthesis. For acute musculoskeletal inflammatory conditions, e.g. acute gout, tendonitis, and traumatic myopathy, doses up to 600 mg/day are tolerated in short courses of up to a week. For anklylosing spondylitis, juvenile rheumatoid arthritisides, and some forms of Reiter's syndrome, 200 mg/day are almost specific. Side effects include gastrointestinal and renal problems, and bone marrow depression, including agranulocytosis. Because of their ability to retain salt, these compounds are contraindicated in patients with peptic ulcer, congestive heart failure, or hypertension, as well as in patients with a reduction in granulocytes.

Pyroles

Indomethacin (Indocin), tolmetin (Tolectin), sulindac (Clinoril), and zomepirac (Zomax[1]) comprise this group and are potent prostaglandin synthetase inhibitors.

Proprionic Acid Derivatives

Ibuprofen (Motrin), fenoprophen (Nalfon), naproxen (Naprosyn), and benoxaprophen (Oroflex[1]) comprise this group and are potent prostaglandin synthetase inhibitors.

Anthranilic Acids

Mefanamic acid (Ponstel) and meclofenamic acid (meclomen) are the only members of this group of prostaglandin synthetase inhibitors currently available. The frequent occurrence of side effects, including diarrhea, rash, elevation of blood urea nitrogen, and bone marrow toxicity, make these agents somewhat less than ideal for use for long periods. Mefanamic acid is heavily promoted for use in patients with dysmenorrhea; however, other peripherally acting analgesics work as well and are less toxic.

Oxicams

Piroxicam (Feldene) is a new chemical entity unrelated to other chemical families. It is a potent inhibitor of prostaglandin synthetases and has a half-life of 44 hr, permitting once a day dosage regimens. Doses above 20 mg/day for prolonged periods lead to a high incidence of peptic ulcer. For short-term therapy, 60 mg/day for 2 weeks appears to be safe in this regard.

Centrally Acting Analgesics

The tendency of physicians to undermedicate patients requiring narcotic analgesic drugs has been well documented; reasons for this are described above (12,22,23). Needless suffering by inadequate pain treatment approaches brutality, exceeded only by failure to prevent the patient from

---

[1] Withdrawn from clinical use because of side effects.

experiencing the added discomfort of the syndrome. It is incumbent on the physician to recognize that, as tolerance and physical dependence to narcotics develop, doses must slowly increase to provide adequate analgesia; plasma levels must be maintained to prevent abstinence syndrome in an already overburdened patient. The recent recognition of ineffective medication in chronic nonmalignant pain may have its roots in undermedication in acute pain situations.

No patient should have to beg for pain relief because of a health professional's unfounded worry about development of potential drug abuse or addiction (19). Similarly, no patient should wish for death, or be forced to consider or actually commit suicide because of a physician's inability or unwillingness to provide pain relief.

A patient's primary fears are of excruciating pain or, worse, of dying an excruciatingly painful death with no one caring to alleviate the pain. A physician's primary concern in diagnosis and treatment of disease needs to be matched with attention to the patient's concerns for adequate palliative care as well. Maintaining optimum quality of life, even in the dying process, is and should be a realistic treatment goal. At issue here is the difference between curing a patient's ills and of caring for a patient, even when nothing more can be done.

Narcotic analgesics are a class of drugs with heterogeneous structures that possess minimal structural resemblance to one another. These agents vary in intrinsic potency, efficacy, and adverse side effects. Potency describes the intrinsic analgesic properties of a drug, using morphine as the standard for comparison. Efficacy describes the analgesic effect of a given drug. Equianalgesic dose describes the dose of a narcotic required to provide the same degree of analgesia as another narcotic. At equianalgesic doses, all narcotics have the same ability to alleviate pain. With special exceptions noted below, all narcotics also have the ability to induce tolerance and physical dependence. Thus 10 mg i.m. of morphine produces the same degree of analgesia as 100 to 150 mg i.m. of meperidine, 2 mg of levorphanol i.m., or 2 mg hydromorphine i.m. Tolerance begins to develop after 30 days of administration of 60 mg i.m. morphine sulfate, 600 to 900 mg i.m. of meperidine, 12 mg i.m. levorphanol, and so on. In general, narcotic analgesics share the properties of inducing tolerance and physical and psychologic dependence, which lessen their desirability for chronic nonmalignant pain management. The incidence of addiction among medical patients is extremely low (26).

At present, our understanding of the mechanisms underlying analgesia describes narcotics binding to discrete opiate receptors within the central and peripheral nervous systems (29,30,37). A pathway in the dorsolateral funiculus carries descending antinociceptive information to segmental levels after activation of the central opiate receptors. Activation of narcotic receptors in the spinal cord causes segmental limitations on nociceptive transmission to the spinothalamic tract and other ascending systems, thereby reducing afferent impulse flow. Other receptor sites within the CNS alter mood, reduce fear and anxiety, produce sedation, and cause nausea and vomiting.

Additional pathways that parallel opiate receptor pathways but do not involve opiate receptors are thought to exist. These produce analgesic responses that are not naloxone reversible. Recently, it has been shown that analgesia occurs after doses of certain GABA agonists such as Baclofen, THIP, and kadotic acid (13). Analgesia produced by these agents is not clearly understood and is not naloxone reversible. Several other classes of drugs produce analgesia that is clinically useful but does not seem to involve opiate receptors.

Morphine is the prototype drug of a group of agents characterized as agonists because of the way they occupy and activate opiate receptors. The narcotic antagonists are drugs that block opiate receptors. These agents may block or reverse the actions of morphine or other agonist drugs. Antagonists may be naloxone-like and may simply block the opiate receptor, or they may be nalorphine-like and produce analgesia while they block the opiate receptor. This latter property of the nalorphine-like agents has given rise to a series of antagonist analgesic drugs such as pentazocine, nalbuphine, and butorphanol. These agents have a somewhat lower rate of development of narcotic dependence. They also have the disturbing property of producing hallucinations and dysphoria in a significant percentage of patients; this has been disturbing enough to cause discontinuation of these agents, with a change to more conventional narcotic agonists.

Two fundamentally different classes of agonists are now described on the basis of their pharmacologic effects and the character of their withdrawal syndrome. One of these classes is morphine-like and the other is nalorphine-like. It is the nalorphine-like drugs that produce the disturbing psychotomimetic effects.

To explain the variety of actions that distinguish these two groups of agents, it has been hypothesized that at least three subgroups of opiate receptors exist. A mu receptor is thought to mediate supraspinal analgesia, respiratory depression, euphoria, and physical dependence. A kappa receptor mediates spinal analgesia, meiosis, and sedation. A sigma receptor mediates dysphoria, hallucinations, and respiratory and vasomotor stimulation. Phencyclidine and ketamine produce a peculiar type of dissociative analgesia/anesthesia and seem to work selectively by activating the sigma receptor. These receptor subgroups need to be kept in mind during initial choice of an agent so that undesirable characteristics may be avoided; they are also used to evaluate the risks and benefits of new agents as they appear.

NARCOTIC AGONISTS

Morphine Congeners

Since the isolation of morphine from opium 175 years ago, the analgesic effectiveness of 10 mg of morphine i.m. has become the standard against which all other drugs are compared. It is quite useful in advanced pain management to describe the doses of all narcotics in terms of the number of morphine-equivalent doses they represent. In Table 2 these values are provided to facilitate this comparison.

Morphine

Morphine is still the drug of choice for moderate to severe pain; a dose of 55 to 60 mg of morphine orally produces the same degree of analgesia as 10 mg morphine i.m. For reasons such as rapidity of onset of action, parenteral administration is most commonly used. Despite poor oral efficacy, morphine has been used orally (Brompton's cocktail and other oral preparations). Oral morphine produces effective analgesia as long as the concentration in the solution is appropriate.

Heroin

Heroin is the diacetylated derivative of morphine and 3 to 5 mg i.m. produces the same analgesia as 10 mg of morphine i.m. The drug is not available in the United States, but has been widely used in Great Britain for pain control in terminal cancer patients. Heroin is similar to morphine in analgesic and mood-altering actions (21). Cancer patients were unable to discern which drug was being used for pain control. The drug has better oral efficacy than morphine. Its onset of action is slightly faster, but its duration of action is somewhat shorter. Side effects are similar to those of morphine at equianalgesic doses, and recent studies failed to substantiate that heroin offers special advantages in the management of cancer pain (21). Periodically there is movement toward the legalization of heroin for use in terminal patients. Since the drug offers no special advantages and has shorter duration of action than morphine, its use in the management of terminal pain is not advocated by this author. Consistency with our current philosophy requires consideration of longer-acting drugs as more advantageous for the patient with relentless pain.

Hydromorphine

Hydromorphine is a potent analgesic congener of morphine. Its onset of action is rapid, similar to that of heroin. Its short duration of action makes it less than ideal for general use, but it is useful for titrating analgesia in patients with diminished renal or hepatic function. It is also useful in elderly patients to avoid the confusion and sedation that may be observed with longer-acting drugs. Thus it may be considered an alternative to morphine that offers advantages only in special situations. Preparations are available for all portals of entry.

TABLE 2.

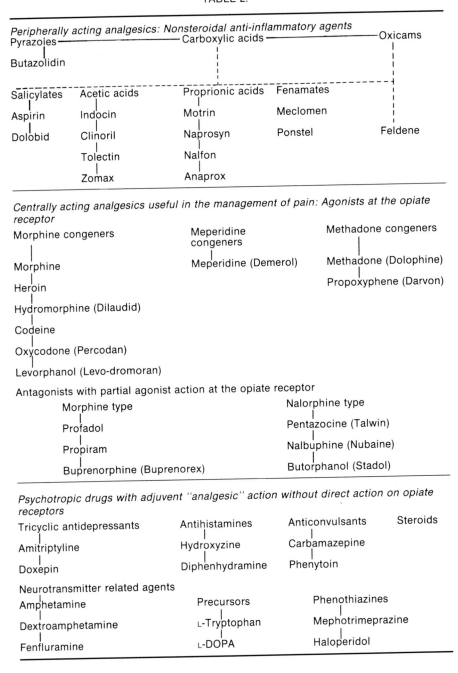

Peripherally acting analgesics: Nonsteroidal anti-inflammatory agents

Pyrazoles		Carboxylic acids		Oxicams
Butazolidin				
Salicylates	Acetic acids	Proprionic acids	Fenamates	
Aspirin	Indocin	Motrin	Meclomen	
Dolobid	Clinoril	Naprosyn	Ponstel	Feldene
	Tolectin	Nalfon		
	Zomax	Anaprox		

Centrally acting analgesics useful in the management of pain: Agonists at the opiate receptor

Morphine congeners	Meperidine congeners	Methadone congeners
Morphine	Meperidine (Demerol)	Methadone (Dolophine)
Heroin		Propoxyphene (Darvon)
Hydromorphine (Dilaudid)		
Codeine		
Oxycodone (Percodan)		
Levorphanol (Levo-dromoran)		

Antagonists with partial agonist action at the opiate receptor

Morphine type	Nalorphine type
Profadol	Pentazocine (Talwin)
Propiram	Nalbuphine (Nubaine)
Buprenorphine (Buprenorex)	Butorphanol (Stadol)

Psychotropic drugs with adjuvent "analgesic" action without direct action on opiate receptors

Tricyclic antidepressants	Antihistamines	Anticonvulsants	Steroids
Amitriptyline	Hydroxyzine	Carbamazepine	
Doxepin	Diphenhydramine	Phenytoin	

Neurotransmitter related agents

Amphetamine	Precursors	Phenothiazines
Dextroamphetamine	L-Tryptophan	Mephotrimeprazine
Fenfluramine	L-DOPA	Haloperidol

Codeine

Codeine is a low ceiling analgesic useful to patients who cannot tolerate nonnarcotic agents. Side effects such as dizziness, nausea and vomiting, and constipation often limit protracted use of this drug at doses high enough to produce analgesia. The analgesic effects produced by 30 mg of codeine p.o. is roughly equivalent to those produced by 600 mg of aspirin p.o.

Oxycodone

Oxycodone is available as the sole agent or in combination with 325 mg of aspirin or 325 mg of acetaminophen. It is a short-acting, orally effective agent. Oral administration of 30 mg of oxycodone is equivalent to 10 mg i.m. of morphine. Because of the combination of ingredients, 30 mg of the mixture only contains 5 mg of oxycodone. The full narcotic potency of this agent is generally not appreciated, and physical dependence commonly occurs in chronic nonmalignant pain situations where drug use is not generally desirable. Care must be exercised in elevating the dose of oxycodone lest side effects from nonnarcotic drugs in the mixture lead to undue toxicity. The potency and relatively insidious development of dependence on this agent call for a special caveat that this agent, in combination or alone, is more like morphine than codeine.

Levorphanol

Levorphanol is a narcotic with high potency, good oral efficacy, and a long duration of action. It is a useful alternative to morphine or methadone because it is active by a parenteral and oral route. Analgesia equal to 10 mg i.m. of morphine was produced by 4 mg p.o. When used at fixed time intervals, the drug tends to be more sedating than morphine. After 5 days, however, the duration of action approaches that of methadone. The half-lives are as follows: levorphanol, 12 to 16 hr; methadone, 17 to 24 hr; and morphine, 3 to 4 hr.

Meperidine

Meperidine is a short-acting narcotic used for moderate to severe pain but with poor oral efficacy. Absorption via the gastrointestinal route is unpredictable and it is rare that patients are afforded adequate analgesia when the drug is administered orally. Parenterally, 100 to 125 mg i.m. produces analgesic effects equal to 10 mg i.m. of morphine. In fact, analgesic threshold is not reached until at least 70 mg have been administered. Analgesic action of the drug peaks at 90 min and is virtually gone after 2 to 2.5 hr. This relatively short duration of action is not generally well appreciated. Much needless suffering occurs because the drug is given in homeopathic quantities and at infrequent time intervals, and patients are without adequate relief. Chronic pain states may occur as a result of undertreatment of acute pain.

Central nervous system excitation can occur and multifocal myoclonus and major seizures have been observed. When this occurs, it is cause to abandon the drug and to choose another narcotic. Treating the seizures with diazepam or clonazepam, then switching to phenobarbital is usually recommended. Phenytoin given in parenteral loading doses, followed by oral phenytoin may be considered because oral phenytoin alone may take up to 4 days for useful antiseizure activity to develop. Meperidine is contraindicated in patients with compromised renal function.

Methadone Congeners

Propoxyphene

This is an optical enantiomorph of methadone that cannot be distinguished from placebo in some studies. It is frequently dispensed in combination with either acetaminophen or aspirin. Because it has clearly defined analgesic effects separate from placebo or aspirin alone when combined with aspirin, it may be useful in certain clinical situations. Respiratory depression, tolerance, and physical dependence may develop, and abstinence syndrome occurs if the drug is suddenly discontinued. However, drug dependence has not been the major problem with its use. Escalated doses of propoxyphene carry either aspirin or acetaminophen that may be in the toxic range. Seizures, tinnitus, and gastrointestinal hemorrhage have been observed in patients taking as many as 40 propoxyphene capsules containing aspirin each day. Acetaminophen toxicity includes direct hepatotoxicity. Patients have been observed to have elevated transaminases after long-term use of high doses of propoxyphene with acetaminophen. The drug represents a first approach to the management of patients who cannot tolerate nonnarcotics or codeine and should not be escalated past the point where low doses of narcotic would produce analgesia with less risk of disturbing side effects.

Methadone

Methadone is a potent, long-acting narcotic analgesic with good oral efficacy. Methadone at 15 to 20 mg p.o. is equivalent to 10 mg morphine i.m., or 60 mg of morphine p.o. (2,17). Due to its long half-life (17 to 24 hr), it provides long plateau analgesia after 4 days of regular doses at fixed time intervals. Methadone is one of the drugs of choice for acute and chronic cancer pain.

Methadone is probably not best used for early cancer pain management. However, when doses of short-acting, rapid-onset analgesics have approached the point where the patient has been receiving the equivalent of 60 to 100 mg of morphine i.m., it is appropriate to switch the patient to oral methadone. Care must be taken to switch to the correct equivalent dose so as to not overdose, nor precipitate abstinence syndrome.

Caveats to the use of methadone include the warning that, because of its long half-life, it may tend to cumulate in elderly patients, or in patients with decreased hepatic or renal function. In these cases, excess sedation or respiratory depression may occur. To prevent excess sedation or toxicity, the dosage regimen must be decreased to ensure effective pain relief without excess side effects. Patients may have doses of methadone reduced as much as 10 to 20% per day without serious withdrawal symptoms to compensate between excess sedation and adequacy of pain relief. The appropriate rate of withdrawal can be gauged by observing decreased sedation and increased respiratory rate. The long half-life of methadone with plateau analgesia makes valuable management strategies possible for cancer patients with pain. Methadone at fixed time intervals produces sedation and long-duration analgesia. Doses are easily adjusted downward to compensate for increased sedation.

Patients may be stabilized at much lower doses than originally anticipated from observation of responses to shorter-acting agents previously used. Several reasons for this effect have been proposed. First, patients do not experience periodic episodes of pain or abstinence effects, and therefore do not complain as the dose is systematically lowered. Second, medication requests in anticipation of pain are reduced by protracted analgesia. Patients are less debilitated and feel better as a result of lowering the narcotic dose, and pay more attention to their social and physical environments.

Methadone doses may be lowered to the point where some pain may recur. If the pain can be localized to peripheral sources, regional or local block with local anesthetic may reveal a peripheral nociceptive source that can be eliminated by means of permanent neurolytic procedures. If this is the case, following elimination of peripheral nociceptive sources, dosages of methadone may be further reduced to the endpoint of the reappearance of pain, then elevated slightly.

Methadone is an ideal agent for substitution-detoxification protocols. It has long been known that methadone withdrawal produces less undesirable side effects during abstinence syndrome than the symptoms after withdrawal from morphine or other agonist agents. Use of this agent has provided a stable and reliable method for detoxifying chronic nonmalignant pain patients with long histories on nonbeneficial use of high-dose opiate agonist agents.

Drug Combinations

Combination of methadone and hydroxyzine provides additional analgesia without increased exposure to narcotic agents. Hydroxyzine 100 mg deep i.m. is the equivalent of 10 mg i.m. morphine; however, analgesia from hydroxyzine is not naloxone-reversible, indicating it produces analgesia by other than opiate receptor mechanisms. When hydroxyzine is added by either oral or parenteral route, sedation increase may again be experienced. Should this happen, further reduction of methadone to the point of reduced sedation with adequate pain control is possible. Further discussion of the antianxiety and sedative components of the action of this useful antihistamine appear below.

Tricyclic antidepressants may be combined with methadone for even more pain control. Amitriptyline and doxepin 50 to 150 mg p.o. at HS provide increased comfort and reduced pain, even when other drugs have failed. This effect occurs within 24 to 48 hr of onset and is apparently unrelated to the effect these agents have on depression. When sedation occurs after introduction of antidepressants in patients receiving methadone and hydroxyzine, further reduction of the opiate agent may be accomplished.

The use of these techniques, much as the use of small doses of epidural morphine, facilitates less restrictions on patients, who may be followed or cared for at home or in less threatening, less expensive environments than the hospital. Visiting nurse services and hospice nurses have become expert at medication management of the terminally ill and provide daily or more frequent feedback on the success or failure of analgesia, and the treatment of other symptoms.

NARCOTIC AGONISTS/ANTAGONISTS

Most of these drugs have only recently become available for clinical use; extensive experience with them is lacking. The available information suggests that antagonist analgesics of the morphine type possess major advantages over the antagonist analgesic of the nalorphine type. Nalorphine derivatives induce sigma receptor stimulation, producing severe psychotomimetic reactions, and are relatively more deleterious in cardiac patients.

Agonist/Antagonists of the Morphine Type

Buprenorphine

Buprenorphine is the first member of this drug class to be released for clinical use and has been used for several years in Great Britain (27). Although clinical experience with this agent is limited, several of its properties are unusual enough to create great excitement about its potential availability.

Buprenorphine is a semisynthetic derivative of thebaine closely related to etorphine. It is highly lipophilic and binds strongly to mu-class opiate receptors. Theoretically, it is this unusually strong binding that gives this drug several unique features.

Buprenorphine is 20 to 30 times as potent as morphine; 0.3 to 0.4 mg i.m. is equivalent to morphine 10 mg i.m. Onset of action is from 15 to 60 min, but the duration of action is anywhere from 6 to 12 hr after a single dose (20,27). Data from over 9,000 patients indicate the mean duration of action is 8.4 hr. The drug has proven effective in postoperative myocardial infarction pain, pain of neoplastic and orthopedic origin, labor pain, and as an adjunct to anesthesia. Generally, the drug is as effective as morphine, meperidine, and pentazocine; however, it has side effects much like morphine. Incidence of euphoria has been reported at less than 0.3% and psychotomimetic reactions at 0.09%. In only 5 of 9,000 patients did systolic blood pressure fall to under 100 mm Hg, and no instances of respiratory depression requiring treatment were reported.

Respiratory depressant activity is slow in onset but has been reported as being equal to that after equianalgesic doses of morphine. Peak respiratory depression occurs at about 3 hr and lasts for 7 hr following a single dose. There has been discussion of a plateau or ceiling of respiratory depression occurring at 0.6 to 1.2 mg buprenorphine, but the degree of respiratory depression does seem to vary directly with the dose.

Buprenorphine has been used as an analgesic after open-heart surgery, with minimal effects on the cardiovascular system. Small decreases in heart rate and systolic blood pressure were noted and were of the same magnitude as those seen after morphine. Unlike other narcotics, the respiratory depressant effect of buprenorphine is only partially reversible even after high doses of naloxone. Paradoxically, buprenorphine has been used as an antagonist of the respiratory depressant effects of fentanyl.

Buprenorphine may induce abstinence syndrome in dependent patients or may block development of abstinence syndrome. Addicts state the effects of buprenorphine are like those of morphine. However, buprenorphine can block the effect of injected morphine for up to 30 hr.

Chronic pain patients who received buprenorphine by sublingual administration for weeks or months did not require elevation of the dosage, indicating failure of development of tolerance to the analgesic effects of buprenorphine. Some patients elected to discontinue the drug because of nausea and sedation, not because of any failure of the analgesic effect. Abrupt withdrawal of buprenorphine in dependent patients resulted in a mild to moderate abstinence syndrome described as half as severe as after morphine withdrawal. The abstinence syndrome is delayed, peaking at 2 weeks after discontinuation of buprenorphine and lasting for over a week.

Buprenorphine is a useful potent narcotic with high intrinsic potency, available for parenteral or sublingual routes of administration and possessing an extremely long duration of action. It has a low abuse potential, and tolerance to the analgesia does not appear to develop; abstinence syndrome is, however, observed after sudden discontinuation of the drug. Side effects are mainly drowsiness, nausea and vomiting, constipation, diaphresis, respiratory depression, bradycardia, and a lowering of systolic blood pressure; 70% of an administered dose of buprenorphine is excreted unchanged via the fecal route.

Buprenorphine may be given 0.3 to 0.6 or 0.4 to 0.8 mg every 6 to 8 hr parenterally, or by sublingual administration. Major drawbacks in ambulatory patients are sedation and nausea. It should be used with caution in the presence of CNS depressants, head injury, respiratory problems, and biliary stasis. Cancer patients already receiving doses of agonist analgesics may develop precipitated abstinence syndrome when given buprenorphine.

Agonist Antagonists of the Nalorphine Type

Pentazocine, nalbuphine, and butorphanol are the agents of this class, generally available for clinical use.

Pentazocine

Pentazocine has been used for the past decade as an analgesic; however, the appearance of psychomimetic effects with increasing frequency at increasing doses mars the clinical use of this agent. Pentazocine 50 mg i.m. is equivalent to morphine 10 mg i.m. Abstinence syndrome can be precipitated by introduction of pentazocine to a patient dependent on agonist analgesics such as morphine or methadone. The use of pentazocine to treat headache in an opiate-dependent patient receiving regular doses of agonist agents such as morphine, methadone, or levodromoran is to be deplored. This agent as well as the other commercially available antagonist agents may precipitate an uncomfortable abstinence syndrome, including nausea and vomiting. In cancer patients this is extremely unfortunate because, in addition to abstinence syndrome, these patients may reexperience the pain of their primary and/or metastatic lesions, forcing them to lose whatever psychologic gain they have made. Tolerance and physical dependence to pentazocine have been observed regularly. Although this and other antagonist agents are generally less of an addiction problem, chronic pain patients may differ from the norm if they become dependent on analgesic or sedative drugs.

Nalbuphine

Nalbuphine is an antagonist analgesic with roughly the same potency as morphine, but with a lesser degree of respiratory depression per dose (27,28). Nalbuphine 10 mg i.m. induces as much respiratory depression as morphine 10 mg i.m.; however, there seems to be no further increase in respiratory depression after 30 mg of nalbuphine (28).

The drug has been successfully used in the management of cancer patients and seems more like morphine than pentazocine in this respect (27). Euphoria is observed at 8 mg i.m., and dysphoria and psychotomimetic reactions have generally not been problematical until doses of 75 mg are used.

Nalbuphine is metabolized in the liver and has a plasma half-life of 5 hr. Tolerance and physical dependence have been described but addicts report that, after a week of daily doses of 140 mg/day, irritability, inability to concentrate, strange thoughts and dreams, depression, and headaches are experienced. Nalbuphine may precipitate abstinence syndrome and should be avoided in patients receiving doses of agonist analgesic drugs. The usual analgesic dose of nalbuphine is 10 mg i.m., i.v., or s.c. every 3 to 4 hr.

Butorphanol

Butorphanol is only available for parenteral administration and is 3 to 5 times as potent as morphine. Use of this agent for the management of cancer pain is limited because there is a correlation between the frequency of psychotomimetic reactions and the cumulative dose used. Since every attempt should be made to use oral medication in treating cancer patients, recommendations for use of this agent should be reserved for provision of analgesia preoperatively, intraoperatively, and for a short time during the postoperative period. For patients who must receive parenteral medication for physical reasons, 2 to 4 mg every 3 to 4 hr for up to 8 months provided effective analgesia in 70% of patients with neoplastic disease.

Psychotropic Drugs and Related Agents

Tricyclic antidepressant drugs such as amitriptyline and doxepin have been used for some time as adjuncts in the management of chronic pain (18,36). These agents reduce patient complaints and discomfort soon after onset of their use, an action apparently separate from their antidepressant action. Use of these agents in conjunction with narcotics has been described in the discussion on methadone and is covered in detail by S. Butler (*this volume*).

Antihistamines have been used in chronic pain management for some time. Particularly useful is the analgesic effect of hydroxyzine, which is not due to opiate receptor mechanisms and is not naloxone reversible; 400 to 500 mg/day p.o. may be used without observing myoclonus or other seizure activity. Below that dose the drug provides analgesia, effective antianxiety action, and nighttime sedation. The drug is also a useful antiemetic. Usual doses are 50 mg p.o. and 100 mg p.o. HS. The drug is irritating when given parenterally and Z-track injection technique is recommended. Use of this agent in combination with methadone is very helpful and is discussed fully in the section on methadone above.

Mephotrimeprazine is a phenothiazine that produces potent analgesia and is appropriate for use in certain situations. The compound causes orthostatic hypotension and sedation. Situations where this compound is useful include (a) when patients are not ambulatory; (b) when pain does not respond to further use of nonnarcotics; (c) when nonnarcotic use gives rise to intolerable side effects; and (d) when it is not yet desirable to start the patient on narcotic analgesics.

Carbamazepine is a major anticonvulsant drug that may be of use when pharmacologic intervention in central pain states, e.g., postherpetic neuralgia, is desirable (18). An adequate trial in each patient in whom the drug is used is important before any decision is made to discontinue the drug. In most instances, inadequate doses are tried and the drug abandoned. Doses from 1,400 to 1,600 mg/day p.o. are necessary for optimum effect and these must be given for at least 6 weeks or until side effects limit further use. Hematological consequences are relatively rare but severe when they occur. Hematologic monitoring frequently during the onset of use and periodically during the use of the drug is advised.

Should carbamazepine prove ineffective, the combination of an antidepressant and depot phenothiazine may be useful. Doses of amitriptyline or doxepin up to 150 to 200 p.o. HS in conjunction with perphenazine 1 to 6 mg may provide relief of central pain when other drugs do not (36). At onset, 50 mg of antidepressant and 1 mg phenothiazine are started, and the doses incremented at 3-day intervals until the doses suggested above are achieved.

Phenytoin may also be tried as a third-order drug for relief of central pain states. The frequency of positive response to this agent is not as great as for others recommended, but for patients not responsive to other therapies, this provides an additional alternative.

Amphetamine may be used for short periods in patients on doses of narcotic analgesics. This drug potentiates the analgesic action of narcotics while antagonizing sedation induced by high doses of these agents. Tolerance and physical dependence develops rapidly to sympathomimetic amines and this factor limits the duration of use of this agent; 5 mg and 10 mg have been shown to increase analgesia 1.5 and 2 times, respectively. Fenfluramine, an amphetamine analog, may be used to potentiate the action of narcotics.

L-tryptophane, the dietary precursor of serotonin, is sometimes of use as a mild sedative and antidepressant. More importantly, since serotonin is required for proper function of the descending anti-nociceptive pathway, serotonin depletion may cause failure of this system. Providing dietary precursor is thought to elevate systemic serotonin and restore the function of anti-nociceptive neurons. Similarly, *l*-dihydroxyphenylalanine precursor to brain dopamine may be required to restore depleted dopamine and endogenously facilitate catecholamine potentiation of narcotic analgesia.

REFERENCES

1. Beaver, W. T. (1979): Comparison of analgesic effects of morphine sulphate, hydroxyzine and their combination in patients with postoperative pain. In: *Advances in Pain Research and Therapy, Vol. 2*, edited by J. J. Bonica and V. Ventafridda. Raven Press, New York.
2. Beaver, W. T., Wallenstein, S. L., and Houde, R. W. (1967): A clinical comparison of the analgesic effects of morphine and methadon administered intramuscularly and of orally and parenterally administered methadon. *Clin. Pharmacol. Ther.*, 8:415–426.
3. Black, R. G. (1975): Chronic pain syndrome. *Surg. Clin. North Am.*, 55:999–1011.
4. Bonica, J. J. (1953): *The Management of Pain*. Lea & Febiger, Philadelphia.
5. Bonica, J. J. (1974): Organization and function of a pain clinic. In: *International Symposium on Pain, Advances in Neurology, Vol. 4*, edited by J. J. Bonica, pp. 433–443. Raven Press, New York.
6. Bonica, J. J. (ed.) (1977): Symposium on Pain, Parts I and II. *Arch. Surg.*, 112:749–788, 861–902.
7. Bonica, J. J. (1979): Important clinical aspects of acute and chronic pain. In: *Mechanisms of Pain and Analgesic Compounds*, edited by R. F. Beers and E. J. Bassett, pp. 13–31. Raven Press, New York.
8. Bonica, J. J. (1980): Pain research and therapy: Past and current status and future needs. In: *Pain, Discomfort and Humanitarian Care*, edited by J. J. Bonica and L K. Y. Ng. Elsevier/North Holland, Amsterdam.
9. Bonica, J. J. (1984): Pain research and therapy: Achievements of the past and challenges of the future. In: *Neural Mechanisms of Pain*, edited by J. C. Liebeskind and L. Kruger. Raven Press, New York.
10. Bonica, J. J. (1984): Labour pain. In: *Textbook of Pain*, edited by P. D. Wall and R. Melzack. Churchill Livingstone, London.
11. Bonica, J. J., Benedetti, C., and Murphy, T. M. (1983): Functions of pain clinics and pain centres. In: *Relief of Intractable Pain, 3rd Ed.*, edited by M. Swerdlow. Elsevier/North Holland, Amsterdam.
12. Cohen, F. L. (1980): Postsurgical pain relief: Patients' status and nurses' medication choices. *Pain*, 9:265–274.
13. Defeudis, F. V. (1982): GABAergic analgesia: A naloxone insensitive system. *Pharmacol. Res. Commun.*, 14:383–390.
14. Ferreria, S. H., Moncada, S., and Vane, J. R. (1973): Prostaglandins and the mechanism of analgesia produced by aspirin-like drugs. *Br. J. Pharmacol.*, 49:86–97.
15. Foley, K. (1982): Practical use of narcotic analgesics. *Med. Clin. North Am.*, 66:1091.
16. Fordyce, W. F. (1976): *Behavioral Methods for Chronic Pain and Illness*. C. V. Mosby, St. Louis.
17. Gilman, A. G., Goodman, L. S., and Gilman, A. (1980): *Goodman and Gilman's The Pharmacological Basis of Therapeutics, 6th Ed.* Macmillan, New York.
18. Halpern, L. M. (1979): Psychotropics, ataractics and related drugs. In: *Advances in Pain Research and Therapy, Vol. 2*, edited by J. J. Bonica and V. Ventafridda. Raven Press, New York.
19. Heaton, R. K., Getto, C. J., Lehman, R. A. W., Fordyce, W. F., Brauer, E., and Groban, S. E. (1982): A standardized evaluation of psychosocial factors in chronic pain. *Pain*, 12:165–174.
20. Jasinski, D., Pernich, J. S., and Griffith, J. D. (1978): Human pharmacology and abuse potential of the analgesic buprenorphine. *Arch. Gen. Psychiatry*, 35:501–516.
21. Kaiko, R. F., Wallenstein, S. L., and Rogers, A. (1981): Analgesic and mood effects of heroin and morphine in cancer patients with postoperative pain. *N. Engl. J. Med.*, 304:1501–1505.
22. Marks, R. M., and Sachar, E. J. (1973): Undertreatment of medical patients with narcotic analgesics. *Ann. Intern. Med.*, 78:173–181.
23. Mather, L., and Mackie, J. (1983): The incidence of postoperative pain in children. *Pain*, 15:271–282.
24. Merskey, H. (1980): Psychiatry and the treatment of pain. *Br. J. Psychiatry*, 136:600–602.
25. Pilowsky, I. (1980): Abnormal illness behavior and social cultural aspects of pain. In: *Pain and Society*, edited by H. W. Kosterlitz and L. Y. Terenius. Verlag-Chemie, Weinheim.

26. Porter, J., and Jicks, H. (1980): Addiction rate in patients treated with narcotics. *N. Engl. J. Med.*, 302:123.
27. Robbie, D. S. (1979): Trial of sublingual buprenorphine in cancer pain. *Br. J. Clin. Pharmacol.*, 7:3155–3185.
28. Romagnoli, S., and Keats, A. S. (1980): Ceiling effect for respiratory depression by Nalbuphine. *Clin Pharmacol. Ther.*, 27:478–485.
29. Sawe, J., Hansen, J., and Ginman, C. (1981): Patient-controlled dosage regimen of methadon for chronic cancer pain. *Br. Med. J.*, 282:771–773.
30. Simon, E. J., and Hiller, J. M. (1978): Opiate receptors. *Annu. Rev. Pharmacol. Toxicol.*, 18:371–394.
31. Simon, L. S., and Mills, J. A. (1980): Drug therapy: Non-steroidal anti-inflammatory agents: Part I. *N. Engl. J. Med.*, 302:1179–1185.
32. Simon, L. S., and Mills, J. A. (1980): Drug therapy: Non-steroidal anti-inflammatory agents: Part II. *N. Engl. J. Med.*, 302:1237–1243.
33. Stambauh, J. E. (1982): Evaluation of Nalbuphine: Efficacy and safety in the management of chronic pain associated with advanced malignancy. *Curr. Ther. Res.*, 31:393–401.
34. Sternbach, R. (1974): *Pain Patients: Traits and Treatments.* Academic Press, New York.
35. Sternbach, R. (1981): Chronic pain as a disease entity. *Triangle*, 20:27–33.
36. Taub, A. (1973): Relief of postherpetic neuralgia with psychotropic drugs. *J. Neurosurg.*, 39:235–241.
37. Terenius, L. (1978): Endogenous peptides and analgesia. *Annu. Rev. Pharmacol. Toxicol.*, 18:189–204.
38. Turner, J. A., and Chapman, C. R. (1982): Psychological Interventions for chronic pain: A critical review. 2. Operant conditioning, hypnosis, and cognitive-behavioral therapy. *Pain*, 12:23–46.
39. Twycross, R. G. (1974): Clinical experience with diamorphine in advanced malignant disease. *Int. J. Clin. Pharmacol.*, 9:184–198.
40. Twycross, R. G. (1977): A comparison of diamorphine-with-cocaine and methadon. *Br. J. Pharmacol.*, 4:691–693.
41. Twycross, R. G. (1977): Value of cocaine in opiate containing elixers. *Br. Med. J.*, 23:1348.

Advances in Pain Research
and Therapy, Vol. 7,
edited by C. Benedetti et al.
Raven Press, New York © 1984.

Present Status of Tricyclic Antidepressants in Chronic Pain Therapy

Stephen Butler

University of Washington School of Medicine, Seattle, Washington 98195

During the past three decades, tricyclic antidepressants (TCAs) have been used widely for treatment of a variety of clinical chronic pain states. This use has provoked numerous laboratory and clinical studies to identify their mode(s) of action and appropriate clinical application. In this chapter, I will (a) discuss the historical development of these drugs, (b) examine some of the neurophysiologic and pharmacologic data published to date, and (c) review the use and results of TCA therapy in patients with various chronic pain syndromes.

BACKGROUND

Historical Development

The structural chemical base for all TCA drugs, iminodibenzyl, was synthesized originally in 1889 by Thiele and Holzinger, who described this chemical in detail. It remained unexplored pharmacologically until 1948 when Haflinger synthesized and tested more than 40 analogs. Animal studies for possible sedative, analgesic, and antiparkinsonian effects led to a few compounds, including imipramine, being selected for human studies because of promising sedative properties. Since these iminodibenzyl compounds have structural similarities to the phenothiazines, they were used initially in clinical trials on psychiatric patients. Fortuitously, Kuhn (52) found them to be effective in treating depression in some patients, and specific antidepressant trials were begun. These trials led to the emergence of the large group of TCAs presently available and actively used in psychiatry for the treatment of depression.

Not long after this, reports appeared, mainly in the European literature, about the use of this class of drugs in the treatment of a variety of pain states. An early, often-quoted article by Paoli et al. (72) anecdotally describes imipramine for treating chronic pain. Saunders (80) discussed TCAs for pain associated with cancer. The literature has grown steadily since that time and consists of a few animal studies, a few well-controlled double-blind clinical trials, but mainly anecdotal collections of case histories without much solid scientific data on mechanisms of action, dosage, interdrug variability, or long-term efficacy. Many reports illustrate the use of TCAs in combination with other agents without adequate comparisons against these drugs separately or against the combination. We are left with some hazy guidelines from these data, these needing careful scrutiny and demanding further controlled studies, both human and animal, to investigate closely their mechanisms of action in chronic pain states so that TCA therapy can be based on empirical findings.

The biochemical activity of the TCAs directs us primarily to the central nervous system (CNS), where we must review the pain-modulating systems, most importantly the bulbospinal system, where serotonin acts as a neurotransmitter. While some alternate pathways and chemical mediators will be discussed, the most impressive data to date substantiate the importance of this restricted neuroanatomical focus.

There is a great wealth of evidence on the importance of the bulbospinal system as a prime modulator of pain transmission, much of it coming from the work on stimulation-induced analgesia and the neuropharmacology of the endogenous and exogenous opioid compounds. The reader is directed to two reviews by Besson et al. (9,10) and Basbaum and Fields (6,31). Some specific discussion of the neurophysiology and neuropharmacology is necessary to highlight the basis for TCA therapy in the context of recent more detailed knowledge of nociception.

Neurophysiology

Oliveras et al. (70) showed that there are descending unmyelinated fibers from the raphe nuclei to the spinal cord that are pain inhibitory in function and have serotonin as their neurotransmitter. They descend via the lateral columns of the dorsal spinal cord to terminate in the superficial laminae of the dorsal horn. It would appear that some serotonergic myelinated fibers descend from the raphe nuclei to the spinal cord as well (77,101). There is also evidence that other neurotransmitters might be active in these pathways (75), among them norepinephrine (90), which has a bearing on the TCA activity. Serotonin (and norepinephrine) applied directly to the substantia gelatinosa of the dorsal spinal cord in animals produces a strong antinociceptive effect (46). Serotonin injected into the cerebrospinal fluid (CSF) in animals and humans has antinociceptive and analgesic effects (96,104). Behavioral studies pinpoint serotonin as the mediator in stimulation-induced analgesia as well (71). It would appear from the anatomic, electrophysiologic, and behavioral data that serotonergic pathways descending from the raphe nuclei and periaquaductal grey matter of the brainstem to the dorsal horn of the spinal cord significantly modify transmission of nociceptive impulses. This is true of studies using both stimulation-induced analgesia and opiate analgesia.

Other animal studies have shown that sectioning of serotonergic ascending pathways from the midbrain to the forebrain (medial forebrain bundle of the hypothalamus) produced hyperalgesia (44). The effects were accompanied by a delayed decrease of forebrain serotonin content, which was mirrored in delay of nociception-response change. It was implied that this was specifically a serotonin-depletion effect. However, it must be pointed out that there were changes in dopaminergic and noradrenergic systems as well, although these were not as profound as the serotonergic changes. In contrast, mesencephalic lesions affecting solely serotonergic systems did not have this effect. Injection of a serotonin precursor, L-5-hydroxytryptophan, into median forebrain bundle-lesioned rats would reverse the hyperalgesic state. Several other biochemical manipulations have been performed to indicate a serotonin-forebrain link to nociceptive responses. More sophisticated neurotoxin experiments substantiate these effects.

More global studies relating hyperalgesia to decreased CNS availability of serotonin have been done using dietary manipulation (57), systemic toxins (85), and experimental allergic encephalomyelitis (102). In many studies, manipulations to restore serotonin availability specifically were able to reverse this. This same protocol has been explored in humans with some success as well (89).

There is conflicting evidence with regard to the role of noradrenergic activity in pain modulation. There is neurophysiological evidence for a descending bulbospinal pathway with noradrenaline as the neurotransmitter (75), which may function as a nociceptive suppression system (79). Stimulation of this system locally within the spinal cord produces decreased sensitivity to thermal stimulation in animals (105), but other studies have shown that analgesia produced by stimulation of periaquaductal grey is decreased by noradrenaline (2). More evidence has appeared recently to support this; the use of two noradrenergic reuptake inhibitors, nisoxetine and desipramine, appeared to decrease the tonic inhibition of dorsal horn nociceptive neurons (87).

The conflicting data may have a neurophysiological basis that is currently being investigated. Those studies supporting the serotonergic hypothesis for antinociception in animals have, in general, used electric footshock and flinch-jump latencies to measure nociception. The research supporting the noradrenergic hypothesis has used heat and tail-flick latencies. The Soja and Sinclair (87) studies are important in that they used heat as well as footshock and flinch-jump latencies as a nociceptive stimulus, but showed an antianalgesic effect of noradrenaline at the dorsal horn level.

The preceeding data briefly review the expanding knowledge of the neurophysiology of nociception and aid in the understanding of the pharmacological interventions made to understand TCA activity. One should note carefully that the majority of the information reviewed is from nonhuman, nonprimate animal research. It is also evident that most of the studies deal with an acute pain model rather than a chronic pain model; the information derived is difficult to transpose to chronic pain in humans, but it does indicate directions to explore. The present knowledge of the pharmacological effects of TCAs and their use in the treatment of chronic pain fits well into this background. However, the TCAs have not proven so effective in the treatment of chronic pain that they can replace other forms of therapy. Perhaps scrutiny of the data available will reveal why.

Pharmacology

In humans, other primates, and subprimate animals, the TCAs, when given acutely, inhibit the reuptake of serotonin and/or norepinephrine by the nerve terminal that releases them, thereby increasing the concentration of the neurotransmitter in the synapse and increasing tone or activity in the neural pathways where these substances act as neurotransmitters (41). The difficulty in accepting this action as the sole explanation of the effects of TCAs in chronic pain is one of timing. Acute administration of the agents leads to uptake inhibition of the neurotransmitter within minutes (76). However, the clinical effect on chronic pain is usually not seen for 2 to 4 weeks, although in one study results appeared in 2 to 5 days (27). This makes one uneasy in assuming that reuptake inhibition is the only mechanism of action. Some indirect support for the reuptake inhibition explanation comes from animal and human studies with a new class of antidepressants, the drugs such as alaproclate, fluoxetine (Trazadone), and zimelidine (84), which are pure uptake inhibitors of serotonin. They appear to be effective in altering the response to experimental pain in animals (62,68), and also decreasing chronic pain in humans (14). It has also been shown that nomifensine, a specific reuptake inhibitor of noradrenaline, is analgesic in animals (40), although norepinephrine was not implicated in analgesia. Therefore, we have some indirect evidence that separate or combined reuptake inhibition of serotonin and norepinephrine could account for the efficacy of the TCAs in chronic pain states.

There is a second mechanism of action of the TCAs that has been explored within the context of the forebrain serotonergic system in rats (64). Given chronically, the TCAs produce a hypersensitivity to serotonin in forebrain areas, a process not evident until after 1 to 2 weeks of therapy. This hypersensitivity to serotonin is not seen with fluoxetine, one of the antidepressants with specific serotonin reuptake inhibition properties. Although pain responses were not investigated in this model, the time course of this effect leads to speculation that this may be an important mechanism of pain control by the TCAs, and mimics the delay seen clinically in their activity on chronic pain. Results of studies of the brainstem and spinal cord serotonin receptors are not available and would be essential before pursuing this hypothesis further.

A third effect of TCA administration chronically in animals is the reduction of forebrain serotonin and norepinephrine receptors with the effect more pronounced for the serotonin-2 receptors than the serotonin-1 or the beta-adrenergic receptors (86). Investigators speculate that this is related to the antidepressant effect of the TCAs because it also occurs with monoamine oxidase inhibitors. Reduction of receptor number may simply be a consequence of increased receptor sensitivity and/or increased neurotransmitter availability acting in a biofeedback loop. No work has been done to implicate this activity in the TCA effect on chronic pain as yet, but this may play a part.

How do we apply the preceeding information to the efficacy of the TCAs in treating chronic pain? The obvious explanation is that this class of medications has an analgesic effect and this has been proposed by some (59,88). Antinociception has been shown in various animal studies previously referred to, but investigation of this possibility in human volunteers (20) did not show an analgesic effect. Administration of TCAs increases neurotransmitter and the sensitivity of some receptors to neurotransmitters, which are implicated in modulation of nociceptive input to the CNS. Therefore, one would expect analgesia to be part of the TCA's action, but no reports have been published demonstrating this effect in humans.

Another explanation of the effectiveness of TCAs in treating chronic pain is the interplay of pain and depression. The coexistence of these two entities has been discussed for some time (15,83,95), and Sternbach et al. (89) directly implicated decreased serotonin as the cause of both the depression and chronic pain. Many clinical studies (3,11–13,93) support this, but in many others TCA efficacy was shown in patients who were not depressed (38,55,58,74). It would appear that this simple explanation cannot account for the usefullness of the TCAs in chronic pain alone but may be an adequate explanation where pain and depression coexist (98). There are some investigators who believe the pain complaints are related to depression and not to any specific peripheral nociceptive source, and that relieving the depression is what improves the pain (93).

This brief review of laboratory data presents but one aspect of the TCA story. The discussion of possible analgesic activity and the pain/depression interrelationship have begun to introduce clinical data. There is a wealth of clinical data on the use of TCAs in the treatment of chronic pain, but it is somewhat inconclusive and difficult to organize. There are six general areas of application of the TCAs that show promise for continued help in chronic pain: (a) headache, (b) facial pain, (c) arthritis, (d) denervation states, (e) low back pain, and (f) pain associated with cancer. Each area will be discussed. An effort will be made to link the results of clinical reports to possible mechanisms of action based on the preceeding data and other information available. The aim is to guide clinicians in rational use of TCAs and to point out areas where clinical and basic research should be rigorously applied to further our understanding of chronic pain and its appropriate treatment.

CLINICAL USE OF TCAs IN PAIN SYNDROMES

Headache (Table 1)

The TCAs have been advocated for the treatment of headache of various, often overlapping etiologies. In the literature, they are categorized under the following headings: migraine, tension, mixed vascular and tension, psychogenic, and headache with depression. Tricyclic antidepressants alone or in combination with phenothiazines have been used in protocols of varying sophistication.

Migraine headache is the subject of two anecdotal reports (23,67) and two well-controlled double-blind studies with crossover (24,39). All demonstrated efficacy for amitriptyline or clomipramine; however, the controlled studies both used low-dose amitriptyline with 55 and 80% improvement rates, respectively. Couch and his colleagues (23,24) found the nondepressed patients with severe headache to be most benefitted; Gomersall and Stuart (39), found those patients with short prodromes in headache of short duration without known precipitating causes to be most benefitted. It is difficult to compare the predictors because the studies did not cover the same areas in evaluating headache. A repeat study with a similar design looking at both depression and headache characteristics might be more illuminating.

There are three good studies using double-blind comparison of amitriptyline versus placebo or amitriptyline versus clomipramine in tension headache. Diamond and Bates (29) showed low-dose amitriptyline to be slightly better than high-dose amitriptyline, and both significantly better than placebo. Lance and Curran (55), in a preliminary study, showed amitriptyline to be superior to imipramine; in a more refined controlled study, they showed that low-dose amitriptyline was better than placebo in a crossover design. The clomipramine versus amitriptyline study by Carasso et al. (18) showed a slight advantage of clomipramine, although the dosage here was lower than the dosage of amitriptyline. This amitriptyline dosage exceeded that of the other two tension headache studies, a fact that may suggest an influence of the "therapeutic window" phenomenon to be discussed later. Diamond and Bates (29) suggest that depression and anxiety, when associated with headache, are predictors of success, whereas Lance and Curran (55) found patients over 60 years of age to be better responders.

In the remainder of the studies of mixed headache, psychogenic headache, or headache with depression, doxepin was shown to be effective and slightly better than amitriptyline (69), with anxiety and depression as good indicators for benefit. The study by Sherwin (82) uses perphenazine along with high-dose amitriptyline in depressed patients, with an impressive 100% success rate long-term, although the study was uncontrolled and does not attempt to distinguish between separate effects of the two drugs. Added to this could be the good results of Ward et al. (97,98) with doxepin in headache associated with depression.

It would appear that many TCAs are beneficial in headache prophylaxis, with conflicting reasons having been proposed for their success. Co-existing depression is a predominant factor in six studies, but must be interpreted cautiously in migraine from Couch's careful work (23,24). It may be that the depression/pain correlation, either by the proposed biochemical link or the behavioral link, is supported by these results. Great efforts are made (39,55) to explain the results in terms of altered vascular dynamics for migraine and tension headaches, respectively, by both serotonergic and noradrenergic effects. A low serum serotonin has been reported in migraine (25), and it is thought that this may lead to intracranial vasodilatation causing headache. Increasing serotonin by blocking reuptake in varying tissues and increasing norepinephrine by the same mechanism, with the TCAs, could possibly prevent this vasodilatation and account for the migraine prophylactic effect. In tension headache, the vascular effect is somewhat different. Vasoconstriction of muscular vessels by chronic muscle tension may be a source of pain. It has been shown (17) that amitriptyline, acutely, can increase muscle blood flow; perhaps this is the analgesic mechanism.

In conclusion, a variety of TCAs are claimed to be beneficial for headache of varying etiologies. The choice of drug is difficult to make, with amitriptyline, clomipramine, doxepin, and imipramine all producing good results. Interstudy differences in effect may be related to dose, study duration, and/or patient population. The trend is toward low-dose TCA therapy, even when concomitant depression and pain confuse the issue of mechanism of action of these drugs. Future double-blind studies of clearly defined headache syndromes using depression, vascular flow studies, and serum TCA levels could prove illuminating.

Facial Pain (Table 2)

The literature is somewhat spotty in documenting TCA efficacy in facial pain. There are indicators suggesting that more studies should be done with closer controls to isolate a group of patients that could be saved from inappropriate surgery in whom tricyclics might be successful. The association of depression with facial pain and an incidence of 30% failure for oral surgical interventions should caution those treating this symptom.

The first association of depression with atypical facial pain was made by Webb and Lascelles (100), who treated 31 patients with monoamine oxidase (MAO) inhibitors in an uncontrolled trial. This protocol was refined by using depression and atypical facial pain as intake requirements for a further study (56) where the primary treatment was again an MAO inhibitor coupled with

TABLE 1. *Tricyclic antidepressant treatment for headache*

Author (ref.)	Headache type	Drug(s)	Dose (mg)	Control	Efficacy	Predictors	Value
Okasha-Ghales (69)	"Psychogenic"	doxepin amitriptyline diazepam placebo	30–50 30–50 6–10	double-blind no crossover	doxepin > amitriptyline ≫ diazepam > placebo	doxepin best with anxiety and depression	yes
Sherwin (82)	?	amitriptyline and perphenazine	100–200 8–64	no	100% in those followed	depression	?
Gomersall and Stuart (39)	Migraine	amitriptyline placebo	60	double-blind crossover	amitriptyline 80%	no or short prodrome short H/A no cause	yes
Diamond and Bates (29)	Tension	amitriptyline amitriptyline placebo	50–150 20–60 (not given)	double-blind no crossover	amitriptyline > low amitriptyline high ≫ placebo	depression and anxiety	? difficult to interpret

Study	Headache type	Drug	Dose	Design	Results	Comments	
Morland et al. (66)	Mixed	doxepin placebo	100	double-blind crossover	doxepin > placebo	none	yes
Carasso et al. (18)	Tension	clomipramine amitriptyline	20–75 30–110	double-blind no crossover	chlomipramine > amitriptyline both effective	none	yes
Lance and Curran (55)	Tension	amitriptyline placebo	30–75	double-blind crossover	amitriptyline > placebo (in preliminary study amitriptyline > imipramine > placebo)	elderly (>60 years) responded better	yes
Couch et al. (23)	Migraine	amitriptyline	25–175	no	55–60% improvement	depression (weak)	?
Couch and Hassanen (24)	Migraine	amitriptyline placebo	50–100	double-blind partial crossover	55%	nondepression with severe H/A > depression with mild H/A no response in depression with severe H/A	yes
Noone (67)	Migraine	clomipramine	30–75	no	improved	high frequency H/A	?

TABLE 2. *Tricyclic antidepressant treatment for facial pain*

Author (ref.)	Diagnosis	Drug(s)	Dose (mg)	Control	Efficacy	Predictors	Value
Lascelles (56)	atypical facial pain	imipramine and chlordiazepoxide	?	no	50% in a skewed population	depression obsessiveness short illness	some
Moore and Nally (65)	atypical facial pain	amitriptyline and chlordiazepoxide	? ?	no	71% "cure"	anxiety and depression	yes
Gessel (35)	myofascial pain	amitriptyline	10–100	no (patients failed biofeedback)	50% significant improvement	depression "hypermobilization" younger	yes
Carasso et al. (18)	trigeminal neuralgia	clomipramine amitriptyline	20–75 30–110	single-blind no crossover	80 vs 30% clomipramine vs amitriptyline	none	yes

a benzodiazepine. However, when this treatment was ineffective, a trial of the TCA imipramine with or without a benzodiazepine was used and proved effective in 50% of cases refractory to the first regimen. Predictive factors were depression, obsessiveness, and a short illness course in those with "good premorbid personalities."

A subsequent trial without controls (65) used a combination of amitriptyline and a benzodiazepine to produce a 71% "cure" rate in atypical facial pain where anxiety and depression were predictors of this successful outcome.

In looking at facial pain from myofascial sources (35), amitriptyline alone was used in a group of patients who failed electromyographic biofeedback therapy, a group with more depression and "hypermobilization" than the biofeedback responders. Successful treatment occurred in 50%, but failed in a questionably older group with severe depression who were all dysfunctional in the normal social settings of home and work.

A final study (18) addressed trigeminal neuralgia without identifying how the patients fit this diagnosis. It is a single-blind random comparison of two TCAs, clomipramine and amitriptyline, both being effective but with clomipramine more so with fewer side effects. No predictive factors were isolated.

It would appear that the TCAs are effective in facial pain from several causes, especially in those individuals where depression and anxiety are factors. It is implied that the pain is a depressive equivalent in the atypical facial pain studies, but muscle tension related to anxiety may also be a factor. Better double-blind crossover studies with single drugs versus combinations versus placebo are needed to clarify this issue. Simultaneous monitoring of muscle tension, depression, and anxiety would complete this protocol.

Low Back Pain (Table 3)

There are few clinical studies concerned with this problem, although the TCAs are frequently used on an empirical basis in refractory cases of low back pain. Those studies available are controlled prospective studies with mixed results. Two contrasting studies use imipramine versus placebo in a double-blind fashion (3,47). Although not overwhelming, the Alcoff et al. study (3) showed a statistically significant improvement with imipramine, compared to placebo, over 8 weeks (although correlations between imipramine, TCA levels, depression, or physical findings were reported). The earlier study (47) did not show a difference between imipramine and placebo. However, this study used a lower TCA dose over a shorter time, 4 weeks, and this could account for the conflicting results. Hameroff et al. (42) examined the effect of doxepin against placebo double-blind in low back pain and found doxepin in antidepressant doses to be superior to placebo. They found this effect related to TCA serum levels. Interestingly, the more active

TABLE 3. *Tricyclic antidepressant treatment for low back pain*

Author (ref.)	Diagnosis	Drug(s)	Dose (mg)	Control	Efficacy	Predictors	Value
Alcoff et al. (3)	low back pain	imipramine or placebo	150	double-blind no crossover	52% improvement with imipramine imipramine > placebo	change in depression score not absolute score; not blood levels; not physical findings	yes
Jenkins et al. (47)	low back pain	imipramine or placebo (with exercise)	75	double-blind no crossover	yes imipramine = placebo	none	?
Hameroff et al. (42)	low back pain	doxepin or placebo	50–300	double-blind no crossover	doxepin > placebo	TCA serum levels more active less sleep disturbance	yes } improved
Ward (*in preparation*)	low back pain with depression	doxepin or placebo	50–300	double-blind crossover	≈60% with doxepin less with placebo	?	yes

subjects and those with less sleep disturbance responded better. These results would seem to be supported by an ongoing study by Ward comparing doxepin, clomipramine, and placebo double-blind in a crossover paradigm in low back pain subjects with depression. Although incomplete, about 60% of the doxepin group responded; at this time no information is available on predictors.

The data available suggest that TCAs in antidepressant doses over a minimum of 4 weeks will improve low back pain symptoms. Depression and its improvement are not necessarily related to efficacy but adequate TCA serum levels may be. This information does not help in elucidating a mechanism of action but gives one cautious optimism for the use of TCAs in low back pain. This diagnosis encompasses a variety of clinical conditions, ranging from myofascial strain to the multiply operated back with neural damage and arachnoiditis. These varying etiologies make studies difficult unless one can separate carefully the subjects presenting for evaluation.

Arthritis (Table 4)

It is surprising that this area has not been further explored. Dudley Hart (30) discussed encouraging studies but deplored the implication by Geist (33) that rheumatoid diseases are a manifestation of psychopathology. This "labeling" may have discouraged rheumatologists and their patients from continued use of TCAs in the treatment of pain associated with the arthritides.

The first reported work with TCAs and arthritis was an open study from Holland (53), where imipramine was used in patients having mainly "nonarticular rheumatism" but classic rheumatoid arthritis as well. This showed a 60 to 70% response improvement rate.

To test this, McDonald Scott (58) conducted a single-center double-blind study with crossover of patients with rheumatoid arthritis and no history of psychiatric disorder. Subjects were given imipramine or placebo. Superior improvement on imipramine was appreciated by the patients and the blinded physicians. The results were validated objectively by improvements in grip strength. This study was tested in a multicenter study (36) using an identical protocol, although with longer drug periods (1 month versus 3 weeks), with similar results in a much larger population. The objective measures of function, morning stiffness, and grip strength were all improved in this study.

Two further studies have been done using low-dose clomipramine with conflicting results. The first (74) was an open study using low-dose clomipramine for treatment of "arthralgia" and indicated improvement by a decrease in analgesic intake, a decrease in stiffness, and an increase in activity. Both subjects and physicians felt an improvement in 57 and 60% of those involved, respectively. This was tested by a multicenter study (32) using low-dose clomipramine versus placebo in a double-blind fashion without crossover, which did not show a difference between the active drug and

TABLE 4. *Tricyclic antidepressants for arthritis*

Author (ref.)	Diagnosis	Drug(s)	Dose (mg)	Control	Efficacy	Predictors	Value
Kuipers (53)	non-articular rheumatism (some rheumatoids)	imipramine	20–40	no	60–70% improvement	none	yes
McDonald Scott (58)	rheumatoid	imipramine placebo	75	double-blind crossover	58% improvement	? grip strength	yes
Gingras (36)	rheumatoid osteo	imipramine placebo	50–75	double-blind crossover	imipramine/ placebo pain 48% function 60%		yes
Regalado (74)	arthralgia	clomipramine clomipramine	10 25	no	57–60% (P.T. vs M.D.) improvement no difference with dosage	none	?
Ganvir et al. (32)	arthralgia	clomipramine placebo lithium amitriptyline physiotherapy	25 serum levels 0.5–1.0 75	double-blind no crossover	none demonstrated		?
Tyber (94)	frozen shoulder		75	double-blind no crossover	100% with meds	depression	yes
Glick and Fowler (38)	osteo	imipramine placebo	75	double-blind crossover	↓ rest pain visual analogue imip ↓ 27% placebo →→	none (nondepressed)	yes

placebo. It would appear from reviewing the results (74) that trends toward significance appear in both groups (drug and placebo) for morning stiffness, pain, and joint tenderness. A crossover of the patient groups would have helped here.

Another view of arthritis and the TCAs is shown in a study by Tyber (94), where he looked specifically at arthritis of the shoulder. He found a high incidence of depression (76%) and found treatment with a combination of lithium and amitriptyline to control pain and to reverse radiographic changes in 100% of his patients. In a follow-up, he compared prolonged physiotherapy with medication by crossover, and reported success in 100% of cases with the medication combination where physiotherapy had failed. He examined arthralgia (excepting the shoulder) in his practice and found a low incidence of depression (12%) but did not give these patients a trial of the lithium/amitriptyline combination. Tyber felt that, despite the physical findings in painful shoulder syndrome, this was a "psychogenic" disorder.

How can the conflicting results be explained? One group demonstrates by well-controlled studies the efficacy of low-dose imipramine in rheumatoid disorders where all patients with a psychiatric history have been excluded. A second is a mixed group of arthralgias with a questionable response to low-dose clomipramine, again where overt psychiatric problems act as exclusion criteria. The last group is a combination of depression and a monoarthritis, with spectacular success using antidepressant medications in combination.

Can the differences in responses be explained? Let us consider the depression/pain explanation for results with TCAs first. Although those with psychiatric histories were excluded in the imipramine and clomipramine groups, specific testing for depression was not done. Subgroups of depressed responders identified by testing may have been found to show high success rates of treatment similar to Tyber's patients. In that instance, one would like to compare the results of amitriptyline and lithium separately in this group to understand the treatment better.

There is some evidence for a biochemical similarity between the rheumatoid disorders and depression on two fronts. It has been demonstrated that serum-free L-tryptophan is decreased, but the total of the free and bound forms is raised in rheumatoid disease (4,5) and "nonarticular rheumatism" (63). Although there are conflicting reports, there is evidence indicating abnormalities of plasma L-tryptophan in patients with depressive illness (for a review, see 28) in some studies returning to normal with treatment (22). It has been shown that antirheumatic medications (salicylates, indomethacin, butazolidine) change the L-tryptophan levels to normal (5).

There are two theories on how this phenomenon is involved in pain. One states that serum-free L-tryptophan mirrors brain metabolism of serotonin for which it is a precursor. Low free plasma L-tryptophan indicates low brain serotonin and a hyperalgesic state (60). The second theory states that serum-free serum L-tryptophan levels are similar to those of an endogenous anti-inflammatory substance that normally protects tissues. Low levels of this substance lead to rheumatoid disease and a low free serum L-tryptophan indicates this state. Reversal with antirheumatic agents gives remission of arthritis and decreased pain (5). Therefore, any medications that return serum L-tryptophan levels to normal would decrease pain. No specific studies have been done in humans with arthritic diseases being treated with TCAs. However, this author and colleagues have shown that abnormalities of plasma L-tryptophan binding in rats with adjuvant-induced arthritis are returned toward normal with chronic TCA administration (16).

As a final note, the TCAs have been shown to have mild anti-inflammatory effects by an inhibition of prostaglandin synthetase (51); this may account for some of their benefit. This is not the full story, however. The studies of MacDonald Scott (58) and Gingras (36) showed improvement in subjects given TCAs who had already received maximum benefit from a variety of prostaglandin synthetase inhibitors with much stronger activity than that of the TCAs.

It is obvious that more animal and human data are necessary to clarify the role of TCAs in the arthritides. The roles of depression, serum L-tryptophan, anti-inflammatory effects, and central serotonin metabolism must all be explored in closely controlled studies for a better understanding of the appropriate use of this class of drugs in treatment.

Denervation States (Table 5)

The use of TCAs in chronic pain secondary to nerve damage, whether traumatic (accidental or surgical), metabolic, infective, invasive or toxic, is probably one of the areas of use most familiar to physicians in general. The literature is extensive, although still largely anecdotal.

Use of TCAs for pain control has a longer history in the European literature, as witnessed by Kocher's (50) brief review of the extensive German and French literature. This catalogues TCA therapy with and without major tranquilizers for a variety of pain problems, including peripheral denervation states. Dalessio (26) reported on TCA use in North America for a variety of problems as well.

The most frequently reported denervation problem to respond to TCA therapy is postherpetic neuralgia (e.g., 18,21,34,43,45,91,92,99,103). Unfortunately, these are primarily anecdotal collections of case reports utilizing various TCAs (amitriptyline, clomipramine, nortriptyline) with or without phenothiazine, carbamazepine, or phenytoin. The drug doses for the TCAs vary, but again are consistently low, usually 25 to 100 mg/day.

Efficacy varies from a low of 27% for imipramine (18) to 100% for amitriptyline plus various phenothiazines (91,92). Few studies comment on concomitant depression, serum-drug levels, or interdrug comparisons when two drugs are used together. In contrast to this is the study by Watson et al.

(99), which is a double-blind crossover comparison of amitriptyline and placebo, which addresses problems of age, symptom duration, depression, and drug-serum levels in relation to efficacy. They found that patients' age and symptom duration did not relate to effectiveness and that depressed subjects responded better than nondepressed, although no change in their depression could be documented. Drug dose and blood level of amitriptyline related to age were of some importance. Apropos of this, it was shown that three subjects in the study had a possible therapeutic window in that as doses increased, the antinociceptive effect diminished only to increase again with lowering the dosage.

In light of this study, it seems that further studies should be done to compare more carefully in a double-blind manner the effects of the phenothiazines (alone or in combination with TCAs) to this well-documented effect of amitriptyline on postherpetic neuralgia. It would also seem indicated to pursue the possible phenomenon of a therapeutic window with the TCAs in chronic pain as has been proposed for depression in the psychiatric literature.

The other area of peripheral nerve damage that has been studied is diabetic neuropathy (27,93). The open study by Davis et al. (27) is remarkable for the fact that amitriptyline singly or in combination with fluphenazine was 100% successful in treating pain associated with postherpetic neuralgia within 2 to 5 days.

Turkington's well-controlled study (93) had an equally remarkable success rate. All patients were initially challenged with phenytoin therapy for 2 weeks, then carbamazepine therapy for 1 week prior to a double-blind treatment with imipramine, amitriptyline, or diazepam. Nerve conduction studies and depression levels were measured prior to and following the 10-week treatment. There was a 100% success rate for abolishing pain in the imipramine and amitriptyline groups. The diazepam group did not show change in pain symptoms but had 100% relief on imipramine 75 to 150 mg/day. This study indicates that the primary problem was depression, reversed by TCA therapy, which brought pain relief.

The results of these varying studies are difficult to explain. On the one hand, cautious, long-term therapy with low-dose TCAs proves very successful, especially for postherpetic neuralgia in depressed patients (99,103); on the other, the TCAs alone do not give relief (43,45,91,92) and phenothiazines must be added and are felt to have the major antinociceptive effect (91,92). Despite depression being a claimed predictor of success, an antidepressant effect was not seen in one study (99), but felt to be essential in another (93). The improvement in experimental design in TCA studies on denervation states only appears to complicate attempts to explain a single mechanism of action. The anecdotal evidence for a therapeutic window (99) would indicate that postherpetic neuralgia may require a different drug effect than diabetic neuropathy. One would like to see Watson et al.'s (99) protocol applied to diabetic neuropathy to test this point.

TABLE 5. *Tricyclic antidepressant therapy for postherpetic neuralgia*

Author (ref.)	Diagnosis	Drug(s)	Dose (mg)	Control	Efficacy	Predictors	Value
Taub (91)	postherpetic	amitriptyline and fluphenazine/ or perphenazine/ or thioridazine/	75–100 3–4 12–16 50–100	none	100%	none	small series of 5 only
Taub and Collins (92)	postherpetic denervation	amitriptyline and fluphenazine	75 3	none	82%	not successful after neurosurgery interventions	yes good follow-up
Clarke (21)	postherpetic	amitriptyline and perphenazine	75 6	none	54%	none	slight
Woodforde et al. (103)	postherpetic	amitriptyline	40–100	none	78%	all depressed	slight
Gerson et al. (34)	postherpetic	clomipramine and carbamazepine or TCNS	150–1000 10–75 inadequate	none partial crossover	≈60%	none	slight
Hatangdi	postherpetic	nortriptyline and carbamazepine	50–100 600–1600	none	79%	shorter duration responded at lower dosage	slight

Study	Condition	Drug	Dose	Design	Results	Comments	Effective?
Carasso et al. (18)	postherpetic	clomipramine or amitriptyline	20–75 30–110	single-blind no crossover	clomipramine 27% amitriptyline 50% ?	none	yes
Hanks (43)	postherpetic	amitriptyline or nomifensine or placebo	25–100 50–200	single-blind no crossover	no difference between antidepressants and placebo	?	incomplete report
Watson et al. (99)	postherpetic	amitriptyline or placebo	25–137.5	double-blind crossover	amitriptyline 67% placebo 4%	100% in depression (no antidepressant effect seen) ? blood level ?therapeutic window	yes
Davis et al. (27)	diabetic neuropathy	amitriptyline and fluphenazine (drugs used singly and in combination)	? ?	no	100%	none	slight
Turkington (93)	diabetic neuropathy	imipramine or amitriptyline or diazepam	100 100 15	double-blind crossover with diazepam group to TCA	100%	depression which responded to TCA	yes

Cancer Pain

Although very important and with a long history (7,80), this use for TCAs has been documented by anecdotal reports only in the literature to date. The bulk of the information is European and it would seem that in North America their use is not as widespread and is relegated to ancillary status in conjunction with the phenothiazines, contrary to the European experience (for review, see 1,50). Another facet of their use in Europe is by the parenteral route (54), which offers a more rapid onset of action (under 2 days), which is so essential in this patient population. This could possibly be used in a prospective way on an inpatient population to improve our treatment approach to a wide variety of chronic pain problems.

The lack of controlled clinical studies in patients with cancer is understandable given the ethical conflicts inherent in producing long-term double-blind trials comparing TCAs to placebo or even to narcotics. Another problem is the heterogeneity of pain sources in advanced cancer, which makes careful studies to delineate the site or mechanism(s) of action difficult to structure. This information is necessary to optimize pharmacological therapies for pain associated with cancer.

FURTHER OBSERVATIONS

The literature cited has generally been supportive for the use of TCAs in the treatment of chronic pain. Those studies that do not demonstrate improvement or where improvement is not statistically different from that on placebo can usually be faulted on methodology. One is left with the impression that any chronic pain problem unresponsive to other forms of treatment should be given a trial of TCAs. This approach has faults. A study to assess the results of just this approach (73) shows little difference between the results with TCA and placebo in a double-blind crossover protocol. Although problems with patient compliance and the possibility of a therapeutic window are raised as possible contaminating factors, this study indicates pitfalls in a "shotgun" approach to pain treatment. Careful use of TCAs with regard to specific indications is important.

Pilowsky et al. (73) also introduce a facet of TCA use mentioned but not prominent in the literature just reviewed: the problem of side effects. These appear, although thankfully in mild form, in close to 100% of subjects taking these medications. The precautions listed from the British Monthly Information Medical Services (MIMS) and quoted by Dudley Hart (30) are worth repeating:

> They [TCA] should be used with extreme caution in cardiovascular disease, liver disorders, epilepsy, patients with known suicidal tendencies, conditions where an anticholinergic agent would be undesirable, for example, glaucoma, urinary retention and pyloric stenosis; prostatic hypertrophy, pregnancy. Bar-

biturates alter the pharmacological effects of tricyclic antidepressants, which can in turn alter the action of other drugs administered concurrently including other antidepressants (especially MAOI's); alcohol; some antihypertensives, for example methyldopa and guanethidine; anticholinergics and local anaesthetics with noradrenaline.

As many of the medical conditions proposed for treatment by the tricyclics are more prevalent in the elderly, side effects are extremely important considerations with this quote in mind.

A related issue is that of drug dosage. The psychiatric literature discusses optimum doses of 150 mg or more of TCAs for a favorable antidepressant response. This is often monitored with serum-drug levels. A therapeutic window has also been mentioned in the psychiatric literature, but usually at higher dose levels than reported in the pain literature (29,74,99). With this therapeutic window, keeping patient age and side effects in mind, it seems wise to follow the advice of several authors to begin TCAs at the 10- to 25-mg/day level with increments by unit dose every 3 days to 1 week, closely monitoring side effects and efficacy. It is to be expected that this controlled dosing would increase the success rates in contrast to many studies, which rapidly escalate dosage to antidepressant levels. Increased patient compliance through a lower incidence of side effects and better assessment of a therapeutic window should help accomplish this.

CONCLUSIONS

The current literature supports the use of the TCAs in the treatment of a wide variety of chronic pain syndromes, including headache, facial pain, arthritis, denervation states, low back pain, and pain in cancer. Although the early clinical studies were mainly anecdotal, more recent reports are better controlled, with attempts at stricter entry criteria and with efforts to identify predictors of efficacy and to correlate treatment effects with serum-drug levels.

Most of the basic approach to date has focused on central mechanisms of action, primarily related to the bulbospinal nociception inhibition systems or to the biochemical links of pain and depression, which may also act at this level. Some indications exist for an effect of TCAs being involved at more rostral structures than the brainstem or spinal cord. The evidence available for a peripheral activity of the TCAs may also account for some of their efficacy in chronic pain.

The gap between clinical and basic research is closing. Further studies on both levels are obviously needed. Results of these will hopefully pinpoint the mode or modes of action of the TCAs for the many clinical pain problems presently being treated and will indicate more appropriate drug choice and drug dosing to optimize their pain-relieving effects in this most difficult group of patients.

REFERENCES

1. Adler, R. H. (1978): Psychotropic agents in the management of chronic pain. *J. Human Stress*, June, p. 18.
2. Akil, H., and Liebeskind, J. C. (1975): Monoaminergic mechanisms of stimulation produced analgesia. *Brain Res.*, 94:279–296.
3. Alcoff, J., et al. (1982): Controlled trial of imipramine for chronic low back pain. *J. Fam. Pract.*, 14:841–846.
4. Aylward, M., and Maddock, J. (1973): Total free plasma tryptophan concentrations in rheumatoid disease. *J. Pharm. Pharmacol.*, 25:570–572.
5. Aylward, M., and Maddock, J. (1974): Plasma L-tryptophan concentrations in chronic rheumatic diseases and the effects of some antirheumatic drugs on the binding of the aminoacid to plasma protein in vivo and in vitro. *Rheumatol. Rehabil.*, 13:62–74.
6. Basbaum, A. I., and Fields, H. L. (1978): Endogenous pain control mechanisms: Review and hypothesis. *Ann. Neurol.*, 4:451–462.
7. Bergouignan, M., and Force, L. (1960): Effects of cliniques de l'imipramine dans certains syndromes douloureux d'origine organique. Congres de psychiatrie et de neurologie de Langue Francaise. Lille 1960. Masson Edit, Paris, pp. 912–916.
8. Rivot, J. P., Weil-Fugazza, J., Godefroy, F., Bineau-Thurotte, M., Ory-Lavollee, L., and Besson, J. M. (1984): Involvement of serotinin in both morphine and stimulation-produced analgesia: Electrochemical and biochemical approaches. In: *Neural Mechanisms of Pain (Advances in Pain Research and Therapy Vol. 6)*, edited by L. Kruger, and J. C. Liebeskind, pp. 135–150. Raven Press, New York.
9. Besson, J.-M. et al. (1979): Opiate analgesia: The physiology and pharmacology of spinal pain systems in advance in pharmacology and therapeutics. In: *Neuropharmacology, Vol 5*, edited by C. Dumont. Pergamon Press, Elmsford, N.Y.
10. Besson, J.-M. et al. (1982): Physiologie de la nociception. *Journal De Physiologie*, 78:7–107.
11. Blumer, D. et al. (1980): Systemic treatment of chronic pain with antidepressants. *Henry Ford Hosp. Med. J.*, 28:15–21.
12. Blumer, D., et al. (1980): Systemic treatment of chronic pain with antidepressants. *Henry Ford Hosp. Med. J.*, 28:15–21.
13. Blumer, D., and Heilbronn, M. (1981): Second year follow-up study on systematic treatment of chronic pain with antidepressants. *Henry Ford Hosp. Med. J.*, 29:67–68.
14. Bobruff, A. (1980): Effect of tricyclics. *JAMA*, 244:1093.
15. Bradley, J. J. (1963): Severe localized pain associated with the depressive syndrome. *Br. J. Psychiatry*, 109:741–745.
16. Butler, S. et al. (1982): Comparison of the effects of the tricyclic antidepressant amitriptyline on "control" and "arthritic" rats as demonstrated by behaviour, physical signs of arthritis and tone in the bulbospinal serotonergic system. *Neurosci. Lett.*, Suppl. IV:97.
17. Cairncross, K. D. (1965): On the peripheral pharmacology of amitriptyline. *Arch. Int. Pharmacodyn.*, 154:438–448.
18. Carasso, R. L. et al. (1979): Clomipramine and amitriptyline in the treatment of severe pain. *Int. J. Neurosci.*, 9:191–194.
19. Castagna, A. M. A. (1967): New therapeutic approach to rheumatic pain in rheumatic disorders. *Excerpta Medica*, 143:1100.
20. Chapman, C. R., and Butler, S. H. (1978): Effects of doxepin on laboratory induced pain in man. *Pain*, 5:802–807.
21. Clarke, I. M. C. (1981): Amitriptyline and perfenazine in chronic pain. *Anaesthesia*, 36:210–212.
22. Coppen, A. et al. (1978): Amitriptyline plasma-concentration and clinical effect. *Lancet*, 1:63–66.
23. Couch, J. R. et al. (1976): Amitriptyline in the prophylaxis of migraine. *Neurology*, 26:121–127.
24. Couch, M. R., and Hassanein, R. (1979): Amitriptyline in migraine prophylaxis. *Arch. Neurol.*, 36:695–699.
25. Curran, D. A., Hinterberger, H. et al. (1967): Methysergide. In: *Research and Clinical Studies in Headache, Vol. 1*, edited by A. P. Friedman, pp.74–122. Karger, Basel.

26. Dalessio, D. J. (1967): Chronic pain syndromes and disordered cortical inhibition: Effects of tricyclic compounds. *Dis. Nerv. Syst.*, 28:325–328.
27. Davis, J. L., Lewis, S. B., Gerich, J. E. et al. (1977): Peripheral diabetic neuropathy treated with amitriptyline and fluphenazine. *JAMA*, 238:2291–2292.
28. DeMyer, M. K., Shea, P. A. et al. (1981): Plasma tryptophan and five other amino acids in depressed and normal subjects. *Arch. Gen. Psychiatry*, 28:642–646.
29. Diamond, S., and Bates, B. J. (1971): Chronic tension headache treated with amitriptyline-a double blind study. *Headache*, 11:110–116.
30. Dudley Hart, F. (1976): The use of psychotropic drugs in rheumatology. *J. Int. Med. Res.* 4(Suppl. 2):15–19.
31. Fields, H. L., and Basbaum, A. I. (1978): Brainstem control of spinal pain transmission neurons. *Annu. Rev. Physiol.*, 40:217–248.
32. Ganvir, P. et al. (1980): A comparative trial of clomipramine and placebo as adjunctive therapy in arthralgia. *J. Int. Med. Res.*, 8(Suppl. 3):60–66.
33. Geist, H. (1966): The psychological aspect of rheumatoid arthritis. Charles C Thomas, Springfield, Ill. p. 63.
34. Gerson, C. R. et al. (1977): Studies on the concomitant use of carbamazepine and clomipramine for the relief of post herpetic neuralgia. *Postgrad. Med. J. (Suppl.)*, 4:104–109.
35. Gessel, A. H. (1975): Electromyographic biofeedback and tricyclic antidepressants in myofascial pain-dysfunction syndrome, psychological predictors of outcome. *J. Am. Dent. Assoc.*, 9:1052.
36. Gingras, M. (1976): A clinical trial of Tofranil in rheumatic pain in general practice. *J. Int. Med. Res.*, 4(Suppl 2):41–49.
37. Glick, E. N. (1976): A clinical trial of Tofranil in osteo-arthritis. *J. Int. Med. Res.*, 4(Suppl. 2):20.
38. Glick, E. N., and Fowler, P. D. (1979): Imipramine in chronic arthritis. *Pharm. Med.*, 1:94–96.
39. Gomersall, J. D., and Stuart, A. (1973): Amitriptyline in migraine prophylaxis. *J. Neurol. Neurosurg. Psychiatry*, 36:684–690.
40. Gonzales, J. P. et al. (1980): Antinociceptive activity of opiates in the presence of the antidepressant agent nomifensine. *Neuropharmacology*, 19:613.
41. Goodman, L. S., Gilman, A. G., and Gilman, A. (1980): *The Pharmacological Basis of Therapeutics*, 6th ed. Macmillan, Cleveland.
42. Hameroff, S. R. et al. (1982): Doxepin effects on chronic pain, depression and serum opioids. *Anesth. Analg.*, 61:187.
43. Hanks, G. W. (1981): Antidepressants in postherpetic neuralgia: A double-blind study to investigate efficacy and possible mode of action. *Pain (Suppl.)*, 1:596.
44. Harvey, J. A., and Lints, C. E. (1965): Lesions in the medial forebrain bundle: Delayed effects on sensitivity to electrical shock. *Science*, 148:250–252.
45. Hatangdi, V. S. et al. (1976): Management of postherpetic neuralgia with antiepileptic and tricyclic antidepressant drugs. In: *Advances in Pain Research and Therapy, Vol 1*, edited by J. J. Bonica and D. Albe-Fessard. Raven Press, New York.
46. Headley, P. M. et al. (1978): Selective reduction by noradrenaline and 5-hydroxytryptamine of nociceptive responses of cat dorsal horn neurons. *Brain Res.*, 145:185–189.
47. Jenkins, D. G. et al. (1976): Tofranil in the treatment of low back pain. *J. Int. Med. Res.*, 4:28–40.
48. Johansson, F. and Von Knorring, L. (1979): A double-blind controlled study of a serotonin uptake inhibitor (Zimelidine) versus placebo in chronic pain patients. *Pain*, 7:69–78.
49. Katon, W., Kleinman, A., and Rosen, G. (1982): Depression and somatization: A review. Parts I and II. *Am. J. Med.*, 71/72:241–247.
50. Kocher, R. (1979): Use of psychotropic drugs for the treatment of chronic severe pains. *Int. Rehabil. Med.*, 1:116–120.
51. Krupp, P., and Wesp, M. (1975): Inhibition of prostaglandin synthetase by psychotropic drugs. *Experientia*, 31:330–331.
52. Kuhn, R. (1958): The treatment of depressant states with 622355 (imipramine hydrochloride). *Am. J. Psychiatry*, 115:459–464.
53. Kuipers, R. K. (1962): Imipramine in the treatment of rheumatic patients. *Acta Rheumatol. Scand.*, 8:45.
54. Laine, C., Linquette, M. and Fossati, P. (1962): Action de l'imipramine injectable dans les syndromes douloureux. Lille Medical, 3ᵉserie, annee tome VII, N.8 pp. 711–716.

55. Lance, J. W., and Curran, D. A. (1964): Treatment of chronic tension headache. *Lancet*, 1:1236–1239.
56. Lascelles, R. G. (1966): Atypical facial pain and depression. *Br. J. Psychiatry*, 112:651–659.
57. Lytle, L. D. et al. (1975): Effects of long-term corn consumption on brain serotonin and the response to electrical shock. *Science*, 190:691–694.
58. MacDonald Scott, W. A. (1969): The relief of pain with an antidepressant in arthritis. *Practitioner*, 202:802–807.
59. Malseed, R. T., and Goldstein, F. J. (1979): Enhancement of morphine analgesia by tricyclic antidepressants. *Neuropharmacology*, 18:827–829.
60. McArthur, J. N. et al. (1971): The displacement of L-tryptophan and dipeptides from bovine serum albumin in vitro and from human plasma in vivo by antirheumatic drugs. *J. Pharm. Pharmacol.*, 23:393.
61. Merskey, H., and Hester, R. N. (1972): The treatment of chronic pain with psychotropic drugs. *Postgrad. Med. J.*, 48:594–598.
62. Messing, R. B., Phebus, L., and Fisher, L. et al. (1975): Analgesic effect of fluoxetine HCl (Lilly 110140): A specific uptake inhibitor for serotonergic neurons. *Psychopharmacol. Commun.*, 1:511–521.
63. Moldofsky, H., and Warsh, J. J. (1978): Plasma tryptophan and muscoloskeletal pain in non-articular rheumatism ("Fibrositis Syndrome"). *Pain*, 5:65–71.
64. Montigny, C. De, and Aghajanian, G. K. (1978): Tricyclic antidepressants: Long-term treatment increases responsivity of rat forebrain neurons to serotonin. *Science*, 22:1303–1305.
65. Moore, D. S., and Nally, F. F. (1975): Atypical facial pain: An analysis of 100 patients with discussion. *J. Can. Dent. Assoc.*, 7:396–401.
66. Mørland, T. J. et al. (1979): Doxepin in the treatment of mixed vascular and tension headache. *Headache*, 19:382–383.
67. Noone, J. F. (1977): Psychotropic drugs and migraine. *J. Int. Med. Res. (Suppl.)*, 5:66–71.
68. Ogren, S.-O., and Holm, H. C. (1980): Test-specific effects of the 5-HT reuptake inhibitors alaproclate and zimelidine on pain. *J. Neural. Transm.*, 47:253–271.
69. Okasha-Ghales, H. A., and Sadek, A. (1973): A double-blind trial for the clinical management of psychogenic headache. *Br. J. Psychiatry*, 122:181–183.
70. Oliveras, J. L. et al. (1977): The topographical distribution of serotonergic terminals in the spinal cord of the cat: Biochemical mapping by the combined use of microdissection and microassay procedures. *Brain Res.*, 138:393–406.
71. Oliveras, J. L. et al. (1981): Implication des systemes serotonergiques dans l'analgesie induite par stimulation electrique de certaines structures du tronc cerebral. *J. Physiol. (Paris)*, 77:473–482.
72. Paoli, F. et al. (1960): Sur l'action de l'imipramine dans les etats douloureux. *Congress Psychiat. Neurol.*, pp. 908–911.
73. Pilowsky, I. et al. (1982): A controlled study of amitriptyline in the treatment of chronic pain. *Pain*, 14:169–179.
74. Regalado, R. G. (1977): Clomipramine (anafranil) and muscoloskeletal pain in general practice. *J. Int. Med. Res.*, 5(Suppl.):72–77.
75. Rivot, J.-P. et al. (1980): Nucleus raphe magnus modulation of response of rat dorsal horn neurons to unmyelinated fiber inputs: Partial involvement of serotonergic pathways. *J. Neurophysiol.*, 44:1039–1057.
76. Ross, S. B., and Reny, A. L. (1975): Tricyclic antidepressant agents I II. *Acta Pharmacol. Toxicol. (Copenh.)*, 36:382–408.
77. Ruda, M. A., and Gobel, S. (1977): Ultrastructural characterization of axonal endings in the substantia gelatinosa which take up (^{3}H) serotonin. *Brain Res.*, 138:393–406.
78. Saarnivaara, L., and Mattila, M. J. (1974): Comparison of tricyclic antidepressants in rabbits: Antinociception and potentiation of the noradrenaline pressor responses. *Psychopharmacology (Berlin)*, 35:221–236.
79. Sasa, M. et al. (1974): Noradrenalin-mediated inhibitions by locus coeruleus of spinal trigeminal neurons. *Brain Res.*, 80:443–460.
80. Saunders, C. (1963): The treatment of intractable pain in terminal cancer. *Proc. R. Soc. Med.*, 56:195–198.
81. Reference deleted.

82. Sherwin, D. (1979): A new method for treating headaches. *Am. J. Psychiatry*, 136:1181–1183.

83. Singh, G. (1968): The diagnosis of depression. *Punjab. Med. J.*, 18:53–59.

84. Siwers, B., Ringberger, V., Tuck, J. R. et al. (1977): Initial clinical trial based on biochemical methodology of zimelidine (a serotonin uptake inhibitor) in depressed patients. *Clin. Pharmacol. Ther.*, 21:194–200.

85. Smith, R. F. (1979): Mediation of foot shock sensitivity by serotonergic projection to hypocampus. *Pharmacol. Biochem. Behav.*, 10:381–388.

86. Snyder, S. H., and Peroutka, S. J. (1982): A possible role of serotonin receptors in antidepressant drug action. *Pharmacopsychiat.*, 15:131–134.

87. Soja, P. J., and Sinclair, J. G. (1983): Evidence that noradrenaline reduces tonic descending inhibition of cat spinal cord nociceptor-driven neurones. *Pain*, 15:71–81.

88. Sternbach, R. A. (1974): *Pain Patients: Traits and Treatment.* Academic Press, New York.

89. Sternbach, R. A. et al. (1976): Effects of altering brain serotonin activity on human chronic pain. In: *Advances in Pain Research and Therapy, Vol. 1*, edited by J. J. Bonica and D. Albe-Fessard, pp. 601–606. Raven Press, New York.

90. Takagi, H. (1980): The nucleus reticularis paragigantocellularis as a site of analgesic action of morphine and enkephalin. *Trends Pharmacol. Sci.*, 1:182–184.

91. Taub, A. (1973): Relief of post-herpetic neuralgia with psychotropic drugs. *J. Neurosurg.*, 39:235–239.

92. Taub, A., and Collins, W. F. (1974): Observations on the treatment of denervation dysesthesia with psychotropic drugs: Post-herpetic neuralgia, anesthesia dolorosa, peripheral neuropathy. In: *Advances in Neurology*, edited by J. J. Bonica, pp. 309–315. Raven Press, New York.

93. Turkington, R. W. (1980): Depression masquerading as diabetic neuropathy. *JAMA*, 243:1147–1150.

94. Tyber, M. A. (1974): Treatment of the painful shoulder syndrome with amitriptyline and lithium carbonate. *Can. Med. Assoc. J.*, 111:137–139.

95. von Knorring, L. (1975): The experience of pain in depressed patients. *Neuropsychology*, 1:155.

96. Wang, J. K. (1977): Antinociceptive effect of intrathecally administered serotonin. *Anesthesiology*, 47:269–271.

97. Ward, N. G. et al. (1979): The effectiveness of tricyclic antidepressants in the treatment of co-existing pain and depression. *Pain*, 7:331–339.

98. Ward, N. G. et al. (1982): Psychobiological markers in co-existing pain and depression: Toward a unified theory. *J. Clin. Psychiatry*, 43:32–38.

99. Watson, C. P. N. et al. (1982): Amitriptyline versus placebo in post-herpetic neuralgia. *Neurology (NY)*, 32:671–673.

100. Webb, H. E., and Lascelles, R. G. (1962): Treatment of facial and head pain associated with depression. *Lancet*, 1:355–356.

101. Wessendorf, M. W. et al. (1981): The identification of serotonergic neurons in the nucleus raphe magnus by conduction velocity. *Brain Res.*, 214:168–173.

102. White, S. R. et al. (1973): Increased shock sensitivity in rats with experimental allergic encephalomyelitis and reversal by 5-hydroxytryptophan. *Brain Res.*, 58:251–254.

103. Woodforde, J. M. et al. (1965): Treatment of post-herpetic neuralgia. *Med. J. Aust.*, 869–872.

104. Yaksh, T. L., and Wilson, P. R. (1979): Spinal serotonin terminal system mediates analgesia. *J. Pharmacol. Exp. Ther.*, 208:446–453.

105. Yaksh, T. L. et al. (1979): Intrathecal capsaicin depletes substance P in the rat spinal cord and produces prolonged thermal analgesia. *Science*, 206:481–483.

Advances in Pain Research and Therapy, Vol. 7,
edited by C. Benedetti et al.
Raven Press, New York © 1984.

Intrathecal and Extradural Narcotics

Louis Jacobson

University of Washington, Department of Anesthesiology,
Seattle, Washington 98195

In the past decade there have been major advances in understanding the mode of action of opiates and opioids. Opiate receptors were identified and localized in the central nervous system (CNS) (87), including the spinal cord (5). Since it would be unlikely there would exist in the CNS a set of receptors specific for a class of compounds not normally present, attention was turned toward finding naturally occurring opioids. As a result enkephalins (52), β-lipotrophin (36), and endorphins (103) were identified and their analgesic properties shown. With the demonstration of opiate analgesic drug effects in the spinal cord isolated from rostral brain input by cord transection (11) as well as the identification of opiate receptors in the spinal cord (5), it became apparent that spinal sites were important in mediating analgesic effects (113). Narcotics administered intrathecally acted directly on the spinal cord to modify nociceptive input and not centrally through either intrathecal spread or vascular absorption and subsequent systemic actions. Gross and microscopic studies of the spinal cord in rats (106) demonstrated no adverse reaction to intrathecal opiates. The way was secured for clinical studies with spinal opiates.

In this chapter I shall deal initially with the principles underlying the local effect of opiates at the spinal level. This will provide a framework for selecting the intrathecal or extradural route, the choice of drug, and understanding side effects. Thereafter, I shall survey the clinical evidence and the importance of side effects in affecting the practical choice of drug and route of administration. Finally the direction of future developments is considered. The generic term *intraspinal* has been used to cover both intrathecal (subarachnoid) and extradural (epidural) routes when considering them simultaneously. This chapter is also intended to update the excellent review of the subject by Yaksh in 1981 (112).

FUNDAMENTAL CONSIDERATIONS

Physiology of Spinal Opiates

Physiological and Anatomical Substrates and Spinal Opiate Receptors

This aspect is considered by T. L. Yaksh et al. (*this volume*) and will only briefly be alluded to here. A large body of neurophysiologic evidence exists which indicates that narcotics can act directly on the spinal cord to modify nociceptive input arriving predominantly via Aδ and C fibers (62,112). The principal site of action of opiates in impairing transmission of impulses in the spinal cord is in the substantia gelatinosa of the dorsal horn where the greatest concentration of opiate receptors is present (5,62). Nociceptive discharge from cells projecting to the ventrolateral tracts is also suppressed by narcotics, suggesting that spinal opiates can alter the content of the ascending sensory message (58).

Subarachnoid injections of narcotics exert a powerful action on the substantia gelatinosa area to produce profound and prolonged segmental analgesia free from other sensory, motor, or sympathetic changes (113). The receptor systems on which spinal opiates act are not related to somatic motor neurons or sympathetic preganglionic neurons or to a general effect on nonnoxious sensory input.

Multiple populations of noncross-tolerant, naloxone sensitive receptors exist both within the cord and elsewhere (112). The spinal action of opiates appears to be mediated by a specific population of opiate receptors (112). Morphine interacts preferentially with the Mu receptor but will also attach to the delta, both of which are central to the analgesic action of narcotic analgesics and are especially dense in the substantia gelatinosa of the spinal cord.

Mechanisms of Action

Intrathecal (subarachnoid)

Narcotics are injected into the cerebrospinal fluid (CSF) and thus a reservoir of drug is created which passively diffuses into the spinal cord to reach the receptors in the dorsal horn. The blood-brain barrier is bypassed and the narcotic effects, in the doses used, are confined to the lower CNS, hopefully the spinal cord. High levels of drug localized to the cord are produced and the agents exert a powerful action on this area to produce profound and prolonged segmental analgesia free from other sensory, motor, or sympathetic changes (23,112,113). Evidence exists that opiates may act presynaptically to block the release of the primary afferent nociceptive neurotransmitter substance P, thereby producing their analgesic effects (114).

Extradural opiates

The basis for the extradural use of narcotics lies in the spinal action of neuraxial opiates as well as the prior observation that drugs instilled into the extradural space reach the spinal cord (20). Extradural administration creates a large depot outside the dura. Regional pharmacologic effect will depend on the efficacy of drug transfer across dura and arachnoid into the CSF; the system then behaves as for intrathecal dosing. The CSF levels are never very high compared to those observed following intrathecal injection.

Systemic absorption of the extradural bolus begins immediately and the plasma profile resembles intramuscular injection (77,80,108). The substantial systemic levels of narcotics make a contribution to the analgesia as the drug is distributed to both the brain and spinal cord (23,62). Specific spinal and supraspinal systems with opiate receptors exert a potent influence over the response to aversive stimuli (113). Evidence exists for a spinal component of action of systemically administered opioids through a receptor system functionally similar to that acted on by intrathecal narcotics (62). The net analgesic effect produced by extradural narcotics results from a combined spinal and supraspinal action (23). The relative proportion that each component provides is uncertain. Absorbed drug leads to therapeutic cerebral levels and, hence, activation of the supraspinal limb of opiate action. Therefore, the effect of this at the cord level is probably synergistic (23).

Comparison of intrathecal and extradural routes

The basis of success with the intrathecal route is to inject a small opiate dose into the CSF, creating a reservoir of drug that will provide high, local spinal cord levels of drug beyond those seen in normal pharmacologic practice. The effects are confined to the spinal cord. By comparison, the extradural route requires the injection of much larger amounts that create a large depot outside the dura. The CSF levels are low and may resemble those achieved following systemic administration. This is contentious and a number of reports have emerged describing high CSF/blood concentration ratios of opiates exceeding those observed following intramuscular administration (16,46,99). Unfortunately, CSF sampling, confined by the constraints of ethics, has been erratic and none of these observations were conducted in a controlled fashion. Furthermore, the lumbar CSF may behave as a sump, thereby resulting in spuriously elevated levels of opioids sampled from this region. Substantial systemic levels are necessary to activate the supraspinal limb of the opiate analgesic mechanism, so as to produce synergism with the local opiate effect.

Comments

Spinal narcotics may provide significant advantages over local anesthetic agents used to produce analgesia. Local anesthetic drugs by the spinal route produce motor block that is unwanted in the postoperative period, during labor, and in chronic pain patients. Their cardiovascular and CNS toxicity cannot be reversed by a readily available antagonist. Furthermore, the sympathetic block they produce may result in arterial hypotension.

The use of intrathecal narcotics to provide effective analgesia without muscle paralysis/weakness permits the postsurgical patient to mobilize early and breathe freely, thereby avoiding the compromise of pulmonary function that develops when the pain of chest expansion prevents deep inhalation. This increased mobility is also of advantage to chronic pain patients and parturient females. The absence of sympathetic block circumvents the problem of postural hypotension so prevalent following local anesthetic administration and thus further facilitates early ambulation. There is no profound sensory deficit associated with the use of intrathecal narcotics. This accompaniment of local anesthetics can be distressing and the availability of an effective alternative is welcome.

Intrathecal opiates provide effective and prolonged analgesia when given in low dosage. Systemic effects are diminished resulting in alert subjects and fewer narcotic effects on the gastrointestinal tract. The effect is specific without other impairment of sensation and autonomic features or loss of motor power. A specific and safe opioid antagonist is available should the need arise.

Intrathecal doses far lower than when given by other routes provide superior analgesia in acute postoperative and posttraumatic pain, and chronic pain with few if any systemic effects. However, the purely local administration of an opiate only acts through the spinal limb of the opioid analgesic mechanism, and the supraspinal component is not involved. Loss of either system, spinal or supraspinal, theoretically requires an increased degree of opiate receptor activation and this is easily attained with the high local tissue concentrations following intrathecal injection. Supraspinal sites can depress spinal cord neuronal activity via descending pathways and the spinal element alone is unable to supply the degree of reflex suppression to the intense nociceptive stimulation inherent in the surgical operation. Simultaneous cerebral and spinal opiate action is required to provide the response-free conditions necessary during an operative procedure. This agrees with the general clinical experience that the sole use of regional opiate intraoperatively produces inadequate surgical anesthesia although postoperative administration in the same patient may produce adequate pain relief.

Pharmacokinetics and Pharmacology

Uptake of Intrathecal Opiates

Intrathecal (subarachnoid) narcotics probably have no significant analgesic effect outside the neuraxis. The antinociceptive effects of agents applied superficially to the spinal cord depend on movement of the agent from the surface to receptors associated with the activity; that is, specific interaction with the opiate receptors in the CNS must occur to produce analgesia.

Subarachnoid narcotics bypass the blood-brain barrier, enter the CSF in high concentration, and mix with CSF. The CSF protein concentration is low and, consequently, protein binding of the opiate in the CSF is insignificant. Hence, the majority of the drug is present in its free form. The agent in the CSF passively diffuses from the water phase into the lipid phase of the spinal cord tissues and reaches the receptors in the tip of the dorsal horn. During this process, opiate drug is nonspecifically bound by all the proteins and lipids of the nervous tissue. Spinal cord concentrations may be reached that are many times greater than those associated with normal clinical parenteral use.

The ability of the drug to penetrate into CNS tissue is closely correlated with its lipid partition coefficient, and entry into the neuraxis is a matter of balance between solubility in water and solubility in lipids (112). The time of onset of analgesia following intrathecal opioid administration corresponds to the lipid partition coefficient of the agent. A more rapid uptake and consequently a more rapid effect is observed with highly lipophilic agents, e.g., fentanyl and meperidine, than those that are poorly lipid soluble, e.g., morphine. White matter surrounds the gray and this lipid barrier must be penetrated by the narcotic before receptor association can occur.

Uptake of Extradural Opiates

By comparison with the intrathecal route, analysis of uptake following extradural administration is more complicated. Three additional factors play an important role: dural transfer, systemic absorption into the circulation, and uptake by the extradural fat.

Dural transfer

The dura mater forms a relatively thick barrier when compared with biological lipid membranes and therefore displays low rates of diffusion. Drug transfer across the dura into the CSF will depend on molecular weight and rate of absorption into the blood (78). Low molecular weight and slow absorption produce high dural transfers. When applied to narcotics, these factors could produce a difference of up to an order of magnitude in the amount transferred directly across the dura. Less lipophilic, small molecular weight drugs, such as morphine, will have the most efficient dural transfer, which could result in a significant spinal component of analgesic action. Conversely, lipid soluble, high molecular weight agents, such as buprenorphine, may find the dura an inert thick barrier, resulting in negligible drug transfer across to the CSF. Furthermore, unlike local anesthetic drugs, opiates have no proven regional action in the concentrations used clinically. Therefore, until the narcotic has traversed the dural barrier and combined with specific receptors in the spinal cord, no analgesic effect should be noted.

Systemic absorption

Systemic absorption of the extradural bolus begins immediately and the plasma profile resembles that following intramuscular injection (77,80,108). The absorption rate will depend on the rate of blood flow in the extradural venous plexus. This route of entry has two important consequences. First, it must contribute to the analgesia—the extent of this contribution is a matter of some dispute. Second, as drug is absorbed from the extradural site, the concentration gradient across the dura into the CSF decreases. Therefore, the more rapid the absorption into the circulation, the less opiate will be transferred regionally across to the neuraxis. In proportion to the dose given, the total amounts of directly transferred drug are small but may be elevated by judicious choice of agent, particularly morphine.

Uptake into extradural fat

Diffusion into extradural fat will vary with the amount of adipose tissue present and the lipophilicity of the drug. The more lipophilic drugs will show the fastest and greatest uptake by fat. The depot of drug in fat will persist for some time and could provide a sustained release mechanism for continued transfer of drug at low levels across the dura and/or into the vasculature. It will also complicate the results of repeated doses.

Distribution of Intraspinal Opiates

Intrathecal

The more lipophilic agents, such as fentanyl and meperidine, have higher concentrations in the neuraxis than the CSF and rapidly move out of the CSF as they are absorbed by the lipid tissues of the spinal cord. A short transit time in the CSF will leave little opportunity for the drug to move away from its original injection site and analgesia will tend to be rapid, intense, and segmental as the agent tends to be distributed mainly to the region of its deposition. In contrast, morphine, which is poorly lipid soluble, exhibits a very low brain/plasma ratio exactly opposite to fentanyl. This leads to concentrations much higher in CSF than in the neuraxis with slow drug removal, low tissue fixation, and the possibility of continued rostral spread of morphine. Drug levels at the receptor sites are maintained with consequent prolonged duration of action.

The rostral movement of CSF from the spinal space is an unimpeded process. Solutes placed in the CSF will gradually redistribute according to the CSF flow as demonstrated by radiographic contrast media and intrathecal local anesthetics. Consequently, a water soluble, lipid insoluble narcotic (e.g., morphine) may reach the fourth ventricle in a dose-dependent concentration. Penetration to subependymal nuclei may gradually occur and central depression manifest after an interval related to the lipid insolubility and slow penetration of the drug.

Extradural

The regional pharmacologic effect and distribution following extradural administration will depend on the efficacy of drug transfer into the CSF. Thereafter, the system behaves as for intrathecal dosing. The uptake and distribution of the systemically absorbed component will follow the pattern already described for other routes of parenteral narcotic administration (72).

Metabolism

The contribution of metabolism to the termination of spinal action of opiate alkaloids following intrathecal or extradural injection has yet to be firmly established. The extent of metabolism is likely to be small compared to the concentrations present after a bolus intrathecal injection.

Clearance

The termination of analgesia following intrathecal opiate administration results from clearance from the site of action. Combination of the opiate with the receptor is reversible. Specific receptor binding plays an important role with strong binding contributing to a prolonged duration of action. The more lipophilic opiates, such as fentanyl, show a more rapid rate of dissociation from the receptor and shorter action than more polar agents, such as morphine. In general, the rate of removal of opiate from the site of administration will be the major determinant of duration and speed of offset of analgesia (23).

Intrathecal

The two routes of removal of intrathecal narcotics are diffusion up the neuraxis and vascular absorption. The dura mater is a thick dense membrane and drug transfer across this barrier from the CSF to the extradural space will be negligible. There exists a drug concentration gradient from the CSF into the depths of the cord and the agent is continually removed by blood flow through the cord. Most of the intrathecal opiate will be removed by diffusion into the spinal cord and absorption into the blood flowing through the cord.

The rate-determining step for drug removal is likely to be the rate constant for drug transfer from CSF to spinal cord (23). This is directly related to lipophilicity; low lipophilicity will give a low rate constant, a long elimination half-life, and a long duration of action. Morphine has a drug characteristic which implies retention of the majority of the drug within the CSF in solution, increased mobility, and the potential for rostral migration.

Extradural

In contradistinction, drug clearance following extradural narcotic administration is predominantly from the site of administration rather than the site of action. Vascular absorption of the extradural narcotic may occur as a result of movement into the epidural venous system. High lipid solubility facilitates passage of the drug into the vasculature. Enhanced blood flow through the extradural venous plexus serves to promote clearance of drug from the epidural space (112). Thus epidural venous plexus blood flow and the physical characteristics of the agent employed are important in controlling the clearance of opiates from the extradural space.

The same mechanism of removal of intrathecal opiate will occur as before following extradural administration. The arterial cord blood now, however, contains appreciable concentrations of the opiate derived from systemic absorption. This reduces the concentration gradient for diffusion of drug from CSF to cord so that CSF levels will persist longer and maintain the analgesic effect.

Tolerance to Intraspinal Opiates

The development of tolerance, i.e., a loss of effect with a given dose of narcotic, is a problem associated with the opiate receptor mechanism, which has implications for the therapy of chronic pain. Repeated intrathecal administration of morphine in animals shows the rapid loss of effectiveness of a fixed dose (112). Intrathecal morphine in primates loses almost total effectiveness after 5 days of injection at 24-hr intervals. Cross tolerance between intrathecal and systemically administered morphine was shown (115). However, there was minimal evidence of naloxone-precipitated withdrawal.

In humans, the effect of repeated spinal administration has given rise to conflicting observations. Some workers have noted the development of tolerance over a time course that corresponds closely with that observed in animal experiments (105). Conversely, others have observed little change even at periods ranging from 30 to 50 days (65).

The mechanism of tolerance development is not known and several hypotheses have been presented (112). The rate of onset of tolerance seems to be proportional to the concentration of the agonist at the receptor, i.e., degree of receptor activation. Therefore, the lower the necessary dose of opiate, the slower the onset of tolerance.

Tolerance development may differ between "normal" animals/volunteer subjects and animals/humans under conditions of chronic pain. Animals exposed to strong stimuli failed to show significant tolerance development to systemically administered opiates, in contrast to normal controls (112).

There is a possibility that the rapid tolerance development to intrathecal opiates thus far reported in animals may, in part, be the consequence of opiate actions in nonstressed animals. Such observations may also account for the differential rates of tolerance development observed following multiple spinal injections or infusion in clinical studies that examined patients suffering from metastatic carcinoma.

Toxicology

The toxicology of spinally administered opiates has been examined in a number of animal and clinical situations. Repeated intrathecal and extradural injections of analgesic doses of narcotics revealed no deleterious effect on spinal cord cells or fibers even after prolonged administration (106,112).

An assessment of the compatibility of CSF and a number of opiate alkaloids showed no effect on CSF turbidity with morphine, methadone, and meperidine at doses normally employed for intrathecal administration (112). Heroin, however, caused increased turbidity, suggesting precipitation of protein.

With due consideration to the compatibility of the agent and CSF, pH, and osmolarity, the administration of spinal narcotics appears to be safe. Moreover, the ability to administer repeatedly significant concentrations in animal models over prolonged periods of time, as well as the extensive clinical experience now accrued without untoward effect on neurological function, supports the lack of toxicity occurring with the dose ranges required to produce profound analgesia.

CLINICAL CONSIDERATIONS AND APPLICATIONS

The clinical use of intrathecal morphine was initially reported in 1979 (107), and shortly thereafter extradural morphine was administered to humans (9). Extradural narcotics provided an alternative for clinicians reluctant to use the intrathecal route; by depositing the opiate epidurally it was proposed that high local concentrations would reach the appropriate spinal receptors by diffusion across the meninges.

Effective analgesia of prolonged duration without alteration of other neurologic functions was noted after low doses of spinal narcotics. Subsequently, many cases utilizing these techniques have been reported and widespread use continues by clinicians who have satisfied themselves that the technique works without formally documenting and/or presenting their results. There have been numerous reports of the spectacular efficacy of these methods with claims of complete analgesia of many hours duration. These were uncontrolled observations and the possibility of bias cannot be eliminated. In the scramble for analgesia free from undesirable effects, these substances have been indiscriminantly used and an early plea for controlled investigations has gone unheeded (4). Among the welter of favorable reports on the use of extradural narcotics, isolated cautious, skeptical, and dissenting views were recorded (4,26,37,51,56,75), but little attention has been paid to them.

Acute Postoperative Pain

Spinal opiates have been extensively employed in the treatment of acute postoperative pain following a variety of thoracic, abdominal, and peripheral procedures. The data on the dose, volume, and vehicle of injection as well as those pertaining to onset, duration, and efficacy are summarized in Table 1.

Intrathecal

A number of reports on the use of intrathecal narcotics for acute postoperative pain have been forthcoming (see Table 1). Paterson et al. (85) used morphine 0.625, 1.25, or 2.5 mg or diamorphine 1.25 or 2.5 mg with cinchocaine intrathecally in 81 patients having major orthopedic surgery. Both morphine and diamorphine produced consistent postoperative analgesia of long duration. They suggest that an intradural dose of between 0.625 and 1.25 mg of either morphine or diamorphine used with cinchocaine (dibucaine, Nupercaine®) and without parenteral opiate may be appropriate.

Plasma levels of morphine were measured in 17 patients following the intrathecal, intramuscular, and extradural administration of morphine 0.2 mg/kg (10–15 mg) for postoperative analgesia (28). While providing superb analgesia, the intrathecal route was associated with significantly lower plasma concentrations of morphine than either the extradural or intramuscular routes, which were similar.

Mathews and Abrams (73) reported on the use of intrathecal morphine in describing 40 patients undergoing major cardiac surgery. Morphine from 1.5 to 4 mg was given prior to the surgical incision and following the conclusion of the procedure, and discontinuation of anesthesia provided analgesia that extended well into the postoperative period. All the patients were free of pain and 17 required no further analgesia. Thirty-six were breathing spontaneously and extubated in the operating room.

Results of two recent studies suggest that hitherto excessive doses of narcotic have been given intrathecally and less would suffice and cause fewer side effects. Lofstrom and associates (69) reported the results of spinal anesthesia given to 40 patients for major hip surgery using bupivacaine plus either morphine 0.3 mg or saline in a double-blind randomized fashion. In the morpine group 17 of 23 patients (75%) required no postoperative analgesics and had excellent pain relief exceeding 24 hrs. All 17 patients in the placebo (saline) group had inferior analgesia requiring intravenous morphine postoperatively. In the other study spinal anesthesia was given to 280 patients having abdominal or vaginal hysterectomy (98). Either tetracaine alone or tetracaine plus morphine from 0.03 to 0.60 mg was instilled into the subarachnoid space. Tetracaine plus morphine provided outstanding postoperative analgesia more than three times longer than tetracaine alone (> 20 hrs). Increasing the dose beyond 0.2 mg did not prolong duration but increased side effects. Conversely, doses less than 0.1 mg produced inferior analgesia. Consequently, intrathecal morphine from 0.1 to 0.2 mg seems appropriate for adult use.

Extradural Opiates

The initial clinical description of the use of extradural narcotic analgesia involved 10 patients with acute and chronic pain. With morphine 2 mg epidurally, excellent analgesia of rapid onset (3–5 min) and prolonged duration were noted (9). Subsequently, there has been a profusion of clinical reports on the use of extradural narcotics (Table 1).

In a series involving 66 patients after major body cavity surgery, epidural methadone 1 mg, hydromorphine 1 mg, and morphine 5 mg were instilled (21). Narcotic requirements for satisfactory analgesia were approximately the same by the intravenous and epidural routes. Morphine 2 mg was inadequate for analgesia in the early postoperative period and at least 5 mg was required. Following thoracic and abdominal operations to 24 patients, effective postoperative analgesia was provided by epidural morphine 6 mg, methadone 6 mg, meperidine 60 mg, or fentanyl 60 μg (101). A controlled study was conducted on 18 patients who received either epidural morphine 2 mg or placebo (saline) via epidural in 60 post-caesarian-section patients (37). The results were disappointing in that epidural morphine was only associated with mild diminution of postoperative discomfort when compared with saline. However, when epidural morphine 5 mg was compared in a double-blind manner with placebo (saline), it was demonstrated to be superior to the placebo for pain relief, duration, and diminished parenteral narcotic requirements (12).

Morphine 10 mg either extradurally or intramuscularly was administered to 40 patients following major gynecological surgery (26). Both routes failed to provide useful analgesia when given at a time when the subject was already in discomfort. They were, however, far more effective if given prior to the onset of pain. Extradural morphine had a slower onset but longer duration than intramuscular morphine. In a double-blind study on 35 patients after caesarian section, morphine 4 mg was given either extradurally or intramuscularly (116). Extradural morphine proved superior to morphine given intramuscularly in both quality and duration of analgesia (20 hr). Epidural morphine 0.05 mg/kg (2.5–5 mg) provided more pronounced and prolonged pain relief than intramuscular morphine 0.1 mg/kg (5–10 mg) in 20 patients undergoing arthrotomy (49).

TABLE 1. Spinal opiate analgesia in postoperative pain

Drug	No. of Patients	Dose (mg)	Volume (ml); Type of solution	Injection site	Latency of onset (min)	Duration[a] (hr)	Success rate	Author (ref.)
Intrathecal Morphine	32	0.8–2	4–10; Saline	Lumbar	?	24	Good	Gjessing and Tomlin (44)
Morphine	280	0.03–0.63	2–3; Dextrose, tetracaine	Lumbar	?	27	Good	Takasaki and Asano (98)
Morphine	10	20	?; Dextrose	Lumbar	26	27	Good	Samii et al. (92)
Morphine	30	1–1.5	<2; Dextrose	Lumbar	10–15	26	Good	Samii et al. (91)
Morphine	30	10–15	<2; Dextrose	Lumbar	10–15	33	Good	Samii et al. (91)
Morphine	40	1.5–4	7.5–20; ?	?	?	>27	Good	Mathews and Abrams (73)
Morphine	40	0.3	0.3; Bupivacaine	Lumbar	?	24	Good	Lofstrom et al. (69)
Morphine	21	0.625	1–1.5; Dibucaine[b]	Lumbar	?	15	Good	Paterson et al. (85)
Morphine	17	1.25	1–1.5; Dibucaine	Lumbar	?	23	Good	Paterson et al. (85)
Morphine	14	2.5	1–1.5; Dibucaine	Lumbar	?	20	Good	Paterson et al. (85)
Diamorphine	9	1.25	1–1.5; Dibucaine	Lumbar	?	22	Good	Paterson et al. (85)
Diamorphine	20	2.5	1–1.5; Dibucaine	Lumbar	?	19	Good	Paterson et al. (85)

Extradural

Drug								
Morphine	15	2–3	10; Dextrose	Lumbar & Thoracic	10	4–36(8)	Good	Magora et al. (70)
Morphine	40	2	10; Saline	Lumbar & Thoracic	6	16–24	Good	Chayen et al. (29)
Morphine	20	2–6	20; Saline	Lumbar	?	8–16	Good	Nordberg et al. (80)
Morphine	35	4	10; Saline	Lumbar	?	20	Good	Youngstrom et al. (116)
Morphine	29	4–8	10; Saline	Lumbar	?	23–27	Good	Carmichael et al. (25)
Morphine	37	5	8–20; Saline	Lumbar & Thoracic	36	16	Partial	Bromage et al. (21)
Morphine	30	2–5	10; Saline	Lumbar	>20	?	Partial	McClure et al. (75)
Morphine	18	2	10; Saline	Lumbar	?	?	Partial	Crawford (37)
Morphine	40	10	10; Saline	Lumbar	>20	11	Partial	Chambers et al. (26)
Meperidine	7	100	10; Saline	Lumbar & Thoracic	5	4–20(6)	Good	Cousins et al. (35)
Meperidine	8	100	10; Saline	Lumbar & Thoracic	5	4–20(6)	Good	Glynn et al. (46)
Diamorphine	39	5–7	10; Saline	Lumbar & Thoracic	5	10–12	Partial	Jacobson et al. (56)
Methadone	11	5	8–20; Saline	Lumbar & Thoracic	17	6	Partial	Bromage et al. (21)
Hydromorphone	19	1	8–20; Saline	Lumbar & Thoracic	23	10	Partial	Bromage et al. (21)
Fentanyl	60	0.1	8; Saline	Lumbar & Thoracic	4–10	3–4	Good	Wolfe and Davies (110)
Alfentanil	18	0.75–2	?; Dextrose	Lumbar	10–15	1.5	Good	Chauvin et al. (27)
Pentazocine	20	15–30	10; Saline	Lumbar	1–5	4–24(11)	Good	Kalia et al. (61)
Buprenorphine	12	0.06	10; Saline	Thoracic	?	12	Good	Cahill et al. (24)

a Mean given in parenthesis.
b Cinchocaine (Nupercaine®).

Controlled studies using opiates other than morphine have been conducted. Following thoracotomy or lower abdominal laparotomy, 39 patients were given diamorphine 0.1 mg/kg (5–10 mg) in a double-blind fashion either extradurally or intramuscularly (56). There was no significant difference in the quality of analgesia between the intramuscular and epidural groups. Diamorphine by either route provided safe and effective analgesia of rapid onset, with no specific undesirable side effects attributable to the epidural route. Analgesia was more prolonged following extradural administration. Six patients received epidural meperidine 20 or 60 mg following total hip replacement with both regimes providing effective analgesia (50). When comparing the effect of intramuscular meperidine 1 mg/kg (50–80 mg), the authors were unable to exclude the possibility that the analgesic effect was at least partially systemically mediated. A number of other narcotic analgesics have been administered extradurally (24,27,61,109,110) (see Table 1).

Trauma pain, such as that deriving from multiple rib and lower limb fractures, has also been managed effectively using spinal opiates (9,29,57,70).

Labor Pain

Intrathecal narcotics have been reported to abolish the pain of both spontaneous and induced labor (2,6,14,84,94). The data on the characteristics of the solution and the results obtained are summarized in Table 2. Spinal opiates do not delay the onset of parturition, have no effect on the strength or frequency of uterine contractions, and do not delay the progress of labor. In view of the low dose of narcotic given and the small amount of the drug available for redistribution, the Apgar scores of infants delivered following intrathecal opiate administration have been good. The ability to control pain in the obstetric patient, without the problems of local anesthetics (i.e., motor block, loss of sensation, and sympathetic blockade) or the behavioral depression and sedation in both mother and fetus that is associated with parenterally administered narcotics, is of value. Extradural opiates have been disappointing when used for labor pains (15,29,37,53,55,70,86,111) (see Table 1).

Cancer Pain and Nonmalignant Chronic Pain

Pain associated with the metastases of cancer, low back pain, or ischemic pain associated with peripheral vascular disease has been shown to be reduced significantly by spinal opiates. Table 3 contains a summary of data on the techniques used and results obtained.

In their report on the pioneering use of intrathecal narcotics in clinical practice, Wang et al. (107) described 8 patients with chronic pain secondary to malignancy who were given morphine from 0.5 to 1 mg intrathecally with dramatic and long-lasting results. Cousins et al. (35) injected meperidine from 10 to 30 mg or morphine from 1 to 3 mg intrathecally in 5 patients and

TABLE 2. Spinal opiate analgesia labor pain

Drug	No. of Patients	Dose (mg)	Volume (ml); Type of solution	Injection site	Latency of onset (min)	Duration[a] (hr)	Success rate	Author (ref.)
Intrathecal								
Morphine	12	1.5	0.15; Saline	Lumbar	?	>8	Good	Scott et al. (94)
Morphine	25	1–1.75	1–1.75; Saline	Lumbar	?	18–22	Good	Bonnardot et al. (14)
Morphine	20	1–2	1–2; Saline	Lumbar	15–60	8–11	Good	Baraka et al. (6)
Morphine	30	0.5–1	?; Dextrose	Lumbar	<60	8	Good	Abboud et al. (1)
β-Endorphin	14	1	1; Saline	Lumbar	2–9	12–32	Good	Oyama et al. (84)
Extradural								
Morphine	10	2	8; Saline	Lumbar	?	?	Partial	Husemeyer et al. (53)
Morphine	25	2.5–4	5–8; Saline	Lumbar	15–50	3–11	Partial	Booker et al. (15)
Morphine	8	2–5	10; Saline	Lumbar	?	?	Partial	Crawford (37)
Morphine	16	2.5–3.5	10–15; Dextrose	Lumbar	?	?	Partial	Writer et al. (111)
Morphine	30	2–3	10; Dextrose	Lumbar	10	4–	Partial	Magora et al. (70)
Morphine	15	2	10; Saline	Lumbar	6	36(8) 16–24	Partial	Chayen et al. (29)
Meperidine	12	25–100	10–15; Saline	Lumbar	?	1–2.5	Partial	Perris (86)
Meperidine	10	100	10; Saline	Lumbar	5	?	Partial	Husemeyer et al. (54)

[a] Mean given in parenthesis.

TABLE 3. Spinal opiate analgesia in cancer pain and nonmalignant chronic pain

Drug	No. of patients	Dose (mg)	Volume (ml); Type of solution	Injection site	Latency of onset (min)	Duration[a] (hr)	Success rate	Comment	Author (ref.)
Intrathecal									
Morphine	8	0.5–1	0.5; Saline	Lumbar	<15	24–48	Good	Cancer	Wang et al. (107)
Morphine	?	1	1; ?	Lumbar	<30	12–24	Good	Cancer	Ventafridda et al. (105)
Morphine	5	1–3	?; Saline	Lumbar & Thoracic	?	≤48	Good	Cancer	Cousins et al. (35)
Meperidine	5	10–30	?; Saline	Lumbar & Thoracic	?	≤48	Good	Cancer	Cousins et al. (35)
β-Endorphin	14	3	3; Saline	Lumbar	1–16	23–74(33)	Good	Cancer	Oyama et al. (83)
Extradural									
Morphine	16	2–3	10; Dextrose	Lumbar & Thoracic	10	4–36(8)	Good	Cancer	Magora et al. (70)
Morphine	21	2–3	10; Dextrose	Lumbar	10	4–36(8)	Partial	Chronic low back pain	Magora et al. (70)
Morphine	4	2–3	10; Dextrose	Lumbar	10	4–36(8)	Partial	Causalgia	Magora et al. (70)
Morphine	7	2	10; Saline	Lumbar & Thoracic	6	16–24	Good	Cancer	Chayten et al. (29)
Meperidine	6	30	6; Saline	Lumbar & Thoracic	5	5–18(8)	Good	Cancer	Cousins et al. (35)
Meperidine	8	30–100	10; Saline	Lumbar & Thoracic	5	4–25(8)	Good	Cancer	Glynn et al. (46)

[a] Mean given in parenthesis.

produced complete analgesia for 48 hr. Continuous, low-dose intrathecal morphine administration in the treatment of chronic pain has been described (81). Repeated administration of intrathecal morphine through indwelling catheters has been used in an effort to achieve a prolonged pain-free period. Lazorthes et al. (66) observed extended analgesia after multiple injections delivered via an indwelling intrathecal catheter in 3 cancer patients over 30 to 50 days. Long-term pain relief (> 60 days) has been reported (112) in a single patient after implantation of an infusion system for intrathecal morphine. Oyama et al. (83) describe the use of β-endorphin 3 mg and its provision of profound prolonged analgesia in patients with chronic intractable pain secondary to metastatic malignancies. A multicenter study incorporating 8 departments in Denmark assessed 105 patients treated for longer than 7 days with extradural opiates (38). Ninety-four patients had malignant disease and 11 various nonneoplastic painful conditions, such as herpes zoster and phantom limb pain. The mean period of therapy was 65 days (range 7–283 days) and the average daily dose of morphine was 12.5 mg (range 4–30 mg) in about 3 injections (4 mg each), giving a duration of approximately 8 hr. Satisfactory analgesia was noted in 70 patients (67%) with extradural narcotics as the sole analgesic. No serious side effects, such as respiratory depression, were reported. Six patients suffering from intractable cancer pain received extradural morphine from 2 to 5 mg and all had complete pain relief within 20 min (43). They received 2 injections per day for 4 to 5 months and all 6 regained daily activities, abandoned oral medications and sleeping pills, and displayed marked mood improvement. No serious side effects, such as respiratory depression, neurological damage, tolerance, or addiction, occurred. Therefore, they concluded that close supervision was unnecessary and home care would be suitable.

Zenz et al. (117) reported on 40 patients (12 outpatients) with terminal cancer who received epidural morphine. The catheter was in place an average 23 days (range 1–118 days) with the patients usually getting morphine 9 mg per day in divided doses every 12 hr. No need for other analgesics existed. No severe side effects were apparent.

Twenty patients with intractable cancer pain have been treated both as in- and outpatients with epidural morphine at the University of Washington Pain Center (T. M. Murphy, *personal communication*). The results have been encouraging. Morphine 2 mg as a bolus is used initially but may be increased to 5 mg. The usual requirement is from 5 to 12 mg/day of morphine with a duration of from 8 to 24 hr.

Continuous epidural narcotic analgesia has been administered via a totally implanted system to 2 patients with metastatic cancer (32), who were sustained very well on low doses of morphine from 1 to 6 mg/day. Both patients resumed normal sleep patterns, appetite, and activity, and diminished their analgesic use. Subsequent observations on this technique have confirmed its early promise (33). Oyama et al. (82) administered synthetic β-endorphin

3 mg epidurally to 10 patients with disseminated cancer and observed good analgesia of prolonged duration.

Summary

Severe acute pain is more difficult to control than chronic pain. Consequently, analgesia for cancer pain is achieved with very small doses of extradural narcotics. Postoperative abdominal pain requires larger doses, with upper abdominal discomfort needing greater quantities than pain arising from the lower regions (21). Although labor pain is effectively relieved with intrathecal narcotics, it is poorly controlled by epidural opiates.

Controlled investigations on extradural opiates in postoperative pain revealed results nowhere near as satisfactory as the original claims suggested, and in some instances the technique has been of dubious value (26,37,51,53,56,75). To support their argument skeptics point out that the dose of extradural narcotics has been gradually increased because the low doses initially recommended were ineffective in the early postoperative period (21). The dose currently recommended to provide effective analgesia is approximately the same as that which must be given intravenously. Labor pains are poorly controlled by extradural narcotics, whereas intrathecal opiates are reported to be effective. These observations cast doubt on the assertion that extradural narcotics have an exclusive spinal action and lend credence to the contention that central effects contribute significantly to the analgesia.

Optimal Drug, Dose, Volume, and Site of Administration

Drug Selection

There is little clinical evidence in the literature to help with the choice of drug. Almost all reports of intrathecal use have been with morphine. Meperidine, diamorphine, and β-endorphin have also been successfully instilled into the subarachnoid space (35,83,85). Morphine is the most popular extradural agent, but other narcotics are being increasingly employed. Fentanyl (110), hydromorphine (21), meperidine (46), diamorphine (56), methadone (21), alfentanil (27), pentazocine (61), buprenorphine (24), and β-endorphin have all been given with satisfactory results.

Morphine produces profound, prolonged analgesia of slow onset and is effective for single dose use where the onset time is not a factor as, for example, postoperatively where the agent can be administered either prior to the reversal of anesthesia or following reversal but before the onset of discomfort. It is also suitable for chronic pain conditions where bolus doses, given on a time-contingent basis, need only be administered once or twice daily. Delayed respiratory depression poses a significant potential problem when morphine is used. Lipophilic agents, such as meperidine and fentanyl, would be suitable for use in trauma, labor, and acute postoperative pain where the prompt establishment of analgesia is important.

There is conflicting evidence on the proposition that the addition of epinephrine 1:200,000 will prolong the action of epidural opioids, presumably by reducing the vascular absorption of the agent and intensifying all manifestations of spinal cord and brainstem uptake (18,21,96).

The choice of agent depends on the circumstances. For rapid onset, a lipophilic agent, such as fentanyl, should be selected. Morphine will have a slower onset time but a longer duration. Where appropriate, fentanyl could be given to establish analgesia and morphine used thereafter to maintain it.

Optimal Dose

Subarachnoid administration requires much lower doses than other systemic routes. These have been calculated to be between 1 and 100 μg of morphine (23), although larger quantities may be necessary to maintain a CSF reservoir. Intrathecal morphine is usually administered in a dose of 0.5 to 2 mg, with 1 mg being most popular. The amounts used have ranged between 0.03 mg (98) and 20 mg (92). It appears that effective prolonged analgesia and the virtual elimination of ventilatory depression can be obtained with lower doses of intrathecal morphine from 0.1 to 0.3 mg (69,98).

Bromage et al. (21) found that extradural morphine 2 mg was inadequate for analgesia in the early postoperative period and at least 5 mg was required. Three doses of extradural morphine (4, 6, and 8 mg) were compared in 24 patients after surgery (89). There was no difference in efficacy, but increasing the dose prolonged the duration of analgesia without increasing the side effects. On the other hand, a study of 29 postcaesarean-section patients who received saline or morphine 4 or 8 mg epidurally (25) demonstrated significant relief with the morphine compared to the saline controls. They noted dose-dependent side effects and concluded that 4 mg was reliable yet safer than 8 mg. Youngstrom et al. (116) also showed that morphine 4 mg could alleviate postcaesarean-section delivery pain. Morphine from 2 to 2.5 mg has, however, proved inferior for this purpose (37). In a preliminary report on the extradural administration of morphine 0, 2, 5, or 10 mg in 34 patients after femoropopliteal bypass surgery, 10 mg gave the best results (3).

Extradural fentanyl 12.5, 25, 50, 75, or 100 μg was administered to 22 patients following caesarean section (79). The minimum effective analgesic dose was 25 μg. Improved analgesia was noted with 50 μg, but no further benefit was apparent after increasing the dose.

Thus in the early postoperative period, following major body cavity surgery, the extradural narcotic dose may be similar to that required for other systemic routes (21,56). In these circumstances, morphine from 4 to 10 mg, meperidine from 50 to 100 mg, and fentanyl from 50 to 100 μg should suffice.

Lower doses have proved effective following body integument surgery and for cancer pain and nonmalignant chronic pain. Morphine from 2.5 to 5 mg (49) and meperidine from 20 to 60 mg (50) gave good results after orthopedic procedures to the lower limbs. Morphine from 2 to 4 mg has relieved intractable cancer pain for up to 24 hr (9), but the average daily dose is about 12 mg (4 mg every 8 hr) under these circumstances (38).

Assuming the site of action of the spinal opiate is in the spinal cord, doses should be given in absolute quantities and not by body weight.

Volume and Vehicle of Injection

The effects of using different volumes of opiate drug solutions in a standardized setting have not been investigated for either the intrathecal or extradural routes. The reported range of intrathecal use is 0.15 ml (94) to 10 ml (73) and 2 ml (70) to 20 ml (21) for the extradural route, with 1 ml and 10 ml, respectively, being the most popular volumes. The latter have been empirically derived and further studies must be done in order to identify the optimal volume. Dural permeability studies indicate that for dural transmission, the volume in which a given dose of drug is administered will, within reason, not be critical (78).

The vehicle usually employed for spinal injections is saline, but glucose solutions have been used for both the intrathecal (92) and extradural (70,75) routes. Hyperbaric glucose solutions in conjunction with appropriate positioning of the patient have been recommended for intrathecal use (92) to ensure localization of the opiate to the caudal regions of the spinal cord.

Spinal injections, especially intrathecal, should not be made with solutions containing preservatives (112).

Site of Injection

The injection site should be at or close to the desired level. With intrathecal narcotic administration, manipulation of dose, volume, baricity, and technique (e.g., barbotage) may compensate for injection at an inappropriate level because of the fluid connection with the thoracic CSF.

Extradural opiates are usually instilled in the lumbar region, frequently distant from the appropriate spinal segments. As with intrathecal use, adjustment of dose and volume may compensate to an uncertain extent for injection at a remote location. Conflicting evidence exists regarding whether or not the site of extradural injection is a constraint on the efficacy of the technique. Reports of the thoracic use of epidural morphine at low doses showed particular efficacy (35). Furthermore, it has been proposed that some of the negative findings in labor, where lumbar injection has been used, may be due to insertion of the agent at an unsuitable level. Conversely, other studies (30,80,95) comparing the lumbar and thoracic approaches for chest and upper abdominal pain have shown similar satisfactory analgesia, thereby indicating that the level of administration of extradural narcotics may not be critical for efficacy and casting doubt on the assertion that extradural narcotics act via an exclusive spinal action.

Onset and Duration of Analgesia

The onset and duration of analgesia are related to the dose, physico- chemical characteristics, and strength of receptor binding of the opiate. Thus, the clinical effects of various narcotics can be predicted to a large degree from their lipid solubility and specific receptor binding. Morphine is an agent with strong receptor binding and low lipid solubility which produces profound, prolonged analgesia of slow onset. The more lipophilic opiates, such as fentanyl and meperidine, have a rapid onset and an intense segmental effect of shorter duration than morphine.

Clinical Onset of Action

The latency and time to peak analgesia does not seem to be better for intrathecal use than other routes of administration (23). Clinical reports have varied widely with regard to the time of onset of analgesia following ex- tradural narcotic administration. There seems to be a general consensus that these agents have a latency of between 5 and 45 min, with most reports indicating some activity at 15 min. Peak analgesia may take from 30 to 60 min (23). An examination of the time of onset of extradural narcotic analgesia postoperatively showed the following order of drug onset times with ap- proximately equianalgesic doses: morphine 24 min, hydromorphone 13 min, methadone 12 min. Peak analgesia occurred as follows: morphine 37 min, hydromorphone 23 min, and methadone 17 min (21). Fentanyl (110), me- peridine (46), and diamorphine (56) often have some effect by 5 min, and after 15 min peak analgesia is usually present. These patterns are similar to those following intramuscular administration and could reflect absorption kinetics from the extradural site.

Clinical Duration of Analgesia

If the onset period and time to peak analgesia for spinal opiates are no better than for intramuscular use, there has to be some substantial advantage in the quality and duration of analgesia to warrant their use. The duration of the effects are proportional to the dose and dependent on the agent em- ployed. Major problems hamper interpretation of the available evidence on duration of action. The difficulties stem from differences in the dose of drug, level of injection, uncontrolled nature of the studies, and the types of procedures for which spinal opiates have been used. Clinical variability similar to that noted previously for time of onset has been reported.

In chronic pain there are consistent reports that small doses of extradural morphine (9,70), meperidine (35,46), and β-endorphin (82) provide prolonged analgesia. The drug time courses of a variety of extradural narcotics were assessed in patients suffering from cancer (112) and were as follows: meperidine 50 mg, 8 hr; fentanyl 100 μg, 14 hr; and morphine 5 mg, 22 hr. An even more prolonged effect is apparent with the intrathecal use of morphine (81,107), meperidine (35), or β-endorphin (83) in chronic pain.

For acute postoperative patients, the duration of analgesia from intrathecal opiates has extended from 14 hr to several days. Doses as high as 20 mg morphine do not appear to result in an increase in the duration of analgesia— 29 hr (92). The extradural use of opiates in acute postoperative pain has produced wide variations of duration between a few hours and several days. Morphine has a duration of between 8 hr and greater than 24 hr postoperatively as described for a range of doses (2–10 mg) following a variety of procedures (21,29,70). The duration of action of buprenorphine 60 μg appears to be about 12 hr (24). Diamorphine 5 mg (56) and pentazocine from 15 to 20 mg (61) last about 10 hr. Meperidine from 50 to 100 mg (35,47,101) and fentanyl from 50 to 100 μg (79,101,110) provide analgesia for about 6 hr.

Intrathecal morphine from 1 to 2 mg seems to provide analgesia for labor in excess of 8 hr (1,6,14,94), thereby often covering the entire period of labor. The duration of analgesia in labor from extradural narcotics is difficult to measure because the pain increases as labor progresses. Large doses of meperidine (100 mg) and fentanyl (80 μg) have provided from 1 to 2 hr of pain relief (54,59,86). As labor advances, the extradural opiate is less effective.

Adverse Side Effects

A variety of side effects, some irritating and others dangerous, are associated with spinal narcotic administration. Insertion of an opiate into either the extradural or spinal intrathecal space does not ensure that the agent will be confined to that limited region of the neuraxis. Spinal drugs may gain access to higher brain centers via absorption into the venous plexus in the extradural space (vertebral Batson's system) or by clearance into the blood through spinal tissues. Alternatively, there may be a bulk diffusion of the narcotic in the CSF to supraspinal centers. Therefore, the effects of the spinal injection may be complicated by an action at sites where opiate receptors may be associated with functions other than nociception. The factors governing this redistribution are discussed above.

A consequence of the intramuscular type of absorption from the extradural site is that of side effects similar to those seen following other routes of parenteral administration. These include nausea and vomiting, sedation, and early respiratory depression, which seem to be related to vascular uptake (23). There is no evidence that their incidence is different from systemic injection of the same dose (90). In the reports of early respiratory depression following extradural narcotics, other parenteral opiates had been given, thus complicating the interpretation. The use of spinal opiates in chronic pain raises the question of tolerance; this has been previously discussed above. Neurological sequelae associated with the spinal use of narcotics is a potential problem, although no cases have been reported at this time. A syndrome of side effects that includes pruritus, urinary retention, nausea and vomiting, and delayed respiratory depression has been reported following the administration of spinal narcotics. These are difficult to ascribe to parenteral absorption and may arise from pharmacodynamic variations in the CSF, neuraxis, and receptor site.

Delayed Respiratory Depression

Life-threatening late onset, unpredictable respiratory depression following spinal narcotics is rare but has proven to be the most significant untoward response. It is thought to be related to lipid/water solubility of the narcotic and to bulk flow of CSF within the subarachnoid and ventricular systems (17,112). The mechanism is suspected to be the diffusion and mixing of the opiate in the CSF so that it penetrates to the fourth ventricle and beyond. Late respiratory depression, unlike early depression, is not related to plasma levels but to rostral diffusion of the opiate. It may be intense, prolonged, and outlast a single dose of naloxone.

The Swedish Society of Anaesthetists conducted a retrospective nationwide survey of clinical experience with extradural and intrathecal opiates (47). Special interest was focused on the frequency and type of ventilatory depression. Extradural morphine had been given to approximately 6,000 to 9,000 patients, extradural meperidine to 220 to 450, and intrathecal morphine to 90 to 150 patients. Late respiratory depression was reported in 4 to 7% (6 patients) of patients treated with intrathecal morphine. Unfortunately, a paucity of series on patients given intrathecal morphine for postoperative pain has been recorded, thereby making an assessment of the incidence of delayed respiratory depression difficult. We must, therefore, rely on isolated clinical case reports. The characteristics of cases involving significant respiratory depression following intraspinal opiates are summarized in Tables 4 and 5.

A number of clinical reports of this phenomenon after subarachnoid morphine have been published (7,40,45,67), even with doses from only 0.8 to 1 mg (44) (see Table 4).

Respiratory depression following intrathecal narcotics may occur more frequently in association with the supine posture. After morphine 15 mg

intrathecally, respiratory arrest was reported 3 hr following transfer from a 40-deg upright incline to a supine position (67). The use of hyperbaric solutions and a head-up tilt of 30 to 40 deg appear to be necessary precautions to prevent respiratory depression following intrathecal morphine. In one series in which these measures were taken, no ventilatory difficulties occurred, even after doses of up to 20 mg intrathecal morphine (92).

All occurrences to date following intrathecal opiates have been observed in the postoperative period following general or spinal anesthesia. They have been associated with morphine which correlates with the pharmacology of the agent. Morphine, however, is the predominant drug used and it is at present not known if other agents would produce similar effects. In contrast, no life-threatening respiratory effects have been described after analgetically effective doses of spinal narcotics in ambulatory chronic pain patients and volunteers.

Naloxone provides reversal of the depressant effects of the spinal opiate, but repeated doses may be necessary in view of the short half-life (less than 30 min) of naloxone in brain (10). The analgetic effects and respiratory depression are reversed by naloxone. Small doses of naloxone, however, may relieve the respiratory depression and yet leave the analgesia intact. The basis of this observation relies on the presumption that the levels of opiate in the respiratory areas are much lower than in the spinal cord near the site of injection. Alternatively, the respiratory areas may be inhabited by a different opiate receptor population more sensitive to the effects of naloxone.

Delayed respiratory depression has also been described in connection with extradural narcotic administration (31). There have been isolated reports of unpredictable respiratory depression, some of which have been profound and delayed (see Table 5). Assessment of the late ventilatory effects after extradural narcotics has been complicated by the use of other parenteral opiates given either prior to or after the extradural dose. As with the intrathecal mode, all incidences having mortal significance have been observed in postoperative patients following general or spinal anesthesia, and no life-threatening respiratory depression has been reported in chronic pain patients or volunteers.

The overall incidence of clinically significant postoperative respiratory depression is difficult to assess. The Swedish survey (47) reported an incidence of from 0.25 to 0.40%. However, this figure is certainly an underestimate as the study was retrospective. Twenty-three instances of ventilatory depression requiring naloxone were reported after extradural morphine had been given to approximately 6,000 to 9,000 patients. The majority of cases occurred soon after administration of extradural morphine. Nine of the 22 patients who developed ventilatory depression within 1 hr after the last dose of extradural morphine received both extradural and systemic doses of opiates. Only 3 patients did not get narcotics additional to extradural morphine in the periods during or after operation. Only 2 of 22 patients experienced ventilatory depression later than 6 hr after the last dose of opiates (s.c., i.m., i.v., or extradural). Both were elderly (75 years) and high doses of morphine (in excess of 10 mg) had been given. The survey indicated that extradural administration of morphine is safe provided certain clinical factors are taken into consideration, specifically age, dose, concomitant use of systemic opiates, and impaired respiratory function. More than 6 hr after the last dose of opiate (s.c., i.m., i.v., or extradural), the risk of ventilatory depression was greatly reduced.

Large clinical series are being accumulated, confirming the safety of this technique. Inappropriate, unexpected, or delayed ventilatory impairment is not described with any regularity. In the clinical reports of delayed respiratory depression, extenuating circumstances, such as advanced age or concomitant parenteral narcotic administration, were frequently present (see Table 2). Alternatively, the depression has occurred too soon after injection to be explicable entirely by dural transfer and rostral CSF spread to the medullary region.

Investigations into the ventilatory effects of extradural narcotics show conflicting results. These substances do affect respiratory function even in cases where profound respiratory depression has not been observed (41). Some studies show the dose-related predictable behavior associated with the conventional routes of narcotic administration and show no evidence of specific, unpredictable, and/or delayed respiratory depression (34, 71,77,102). Others provide contradictory evidence of delayed and prolonged depression (63,74) and a biphasic pattern of ventilatory inhibition (60), but no instances of life-threatening severity have been reported. An identical biphasic pattern of ventilatory inhibition has been described following intravenous narcotic administration (8); therefore, it is not unique to the extradural route. Following intravenous opiate injection in the postoperative period, delayed, profound, and prolonged respiratory depression have been described postoperatively (2). I suspect that these rare episodes also occur following narcotic administration by alternative parenteral routes, and I am encountering the phenomenon of "differential scrutiny" whereby new techniques are evaluated and investigated with an intensity not previously encountered in the period when intramuscular and intravenous narcotics were initially utilized.

Opiates given epidurally were originally thought to redistribute by movement through the dura into the intrathecal space and then to higher centers. The observation that the depressant effects on respiration following extradural administration occur after a latency considerably shorter than that observed after intrathecal injection suggests it is unlikely that all the depression routinely occurs via absorption first into the intrathecal space. Epidural opiates must gain access to supraspinal centers via an additional route, probably the circulation. It seems likely that epidural venous plexus blood flow is important in controlling the redistribution of opiates from the epidural space.

The respiratory effects of extradural opioids are similar to parenteral opiates. No evidence exists for a respiratory effect that differs from other forms of parenteral narcotic therapy, except for intrathecal opiates. Reactions are explicable in terms of an overdose or intolerance, and similar behavior has been observed following alternate parenteral routes.

In contradistinction, intrathecal narcotics present a more sinister problem, and attempts should be made to limit their rostral spread by physical means, such as the use of hyperbaric solutions, steep head-up posture, and prevention of coughing and straining (92). Furthermore, it appears that the occurrence of delayed respiratory depression can be curtailed by limiting the dose of intrathecal morphine to 0.1 to 0.2 mg (98).

Pruritus

Spinal opiates may produce intense itching which can be very distressing. The sensation occurs particularly in parturient women (6,94) but also in chronic pain and postoperative patients. Its incidence varies from 0 to 80% and opinions vary as to whether the pruritus is dose related or not. Scratching behavior appears around or just after the development of analgesia and continues for its duration but may persist for days afterward. The sensation is not limited to segments of the spinal cord affected by the opiate; it may be generalized or local, affecting the trunk, legs, or face, especially the nose and palate.

The mechanism of itching is unknown. Though systemic opiates, particularly morphine, are known to release histamine, it remains uncertain if this mechanism is operative with spinal opiates as there are no cutaneous wheals or other stigmata that might suggest such a mechanism and the pruritus responds poorly to antihistamines (90). Experimental itch does not necessarily require histamine as a trigger, and the frequent affliction of the head, neck, and trunk suggest the phenomenon is related to a generalized modulation of cutaneous sensation rather than the effects of histamine. Furthermore, this pattern of involvement indicates the pruritus is not related to a sensation mediated by a direct segmental action of the spinal drug.

It has been suggested that the itching behavior may be associated with the presence of preservatives in the injectate (90). This has not been borne out in animal experiments or human clinical work where itching has been reported following intrathecal use where solutions have no additives. Although the itch may be abolished by naloxone, this should not be taken as conclusive evidence of a specific agonist/antagonist mechanism, as naloxone has also been shown to relieve cholestatic pruritus (97).

Urinary Retention

Failure to achieve spontaneous urination for periods sufficient to require catheterization has been observed following spinal opiates in postoperative

(90,94) and chronic pain patients (70). Its incidence has been variously reported as being from 0.3 to 90%. In the Swedish survey on adverse effects of spinal opiates (47), and incorporating from 6,000 to 9,000 cases, the stated frequency of patients requiring bladder catheterization varied from 0.3 to 25% with a median value of 10%. In a series of 1,200 patients who received epidural morphine 10 mg for postoperative pain, urinary retention was observed in 15% of cases (90). Problems with urination were noted in 90% (9 out of 10) of volunteers involved in an assessment of the nonrespiratory side effects of epidural morphine 10 mg (19). In another study urinary retention afflicted all 4 male volunteers given from 3 to 4 mg extradural morphine (102).

It is unlikely that the retention is related to a loss of sensation as the condition is extremely uncomfortable. In the postoperative period, 56 patients undergoing cholecystectomy or duodenal ulcer surgery received either intramuscular or extradural morphine from 5 to 10 mg and 4 mg, respectively (88). The incidence of urinary retention was about 35% in both groups (i.m. and extradural), and it is likely that the effect on the urinary bladder, if influenced by narcotics at all, is peripheral.

Preliminary studies indicate that spinal narcotics may promote oliguria by inducing ADH secretion (64).

Nausea and Vomiting

Nausea and vomiting have been reported in 9 of 12 parturients (75%) after 1 to 2 mg of intrathecal morphine (94). These were uncontrolled observations and nausea and vomiting are recognized concomitants of normal labor. Retching and emesis have been observed following intrathecal opiates in the primate (112) after variable intervals from 10 to 70 min, but the reported trials of intrathecal morphine in chronic pain and postoperative patients have not encountered this problem. The locus of action associated with nausea and vomiting is thought to lie in the vascularized area postrema lying superficially on the floor of the fourth ventricle as local application of chemicals or electrical stimulation of this system results in a powerful emetic response. Narcotic deposited intrathecally could migrate with the CSF circulation and reach this region.

In an attempt to diminish the frequent side effects seen with intrathecal morphine 1 mg for labor analgesia, the narcotic was followed after 1 hr by an infusion of intravenous naloxone (22). This significantly decreased the incidence of pruritus, urinary retention, and vomiting without affecting maternal analgesia or the progress of labor. Furthermore, respiratory depression was not observed in the 31 patients studied. Elective naloxone infusion is an interesting approach to the prophylaxis of adverse effects associated with intrathecal opiates, which, pending further evaluation, might prove a significant advance in the solution of this problem.

EXTRADURAL NARCOTICS—CONTROVERSIES AND UNCERTAINTIES

Two schools of thought exist regarding extradural narcotics—devotees and disbelievers. The former point out the theoretical advantages conferred by this form of therapy based on the proof that opiate receptors exist (5) and that the demonstration of the spinal action of opiates (113) provides a prospect of improved pain relief. The latter believe that a localized spinal action with prolonged analgesia and no central depressant effect is unlikely and that extradural opiates act through a combination of CNS effects involving spinal and supraspinal sites (23,56), as with other routes of administration with the probable exception of intrathecal opiates. Considering the pharmacokinetic data on blood and CSF opiate concentrations (16,35,46,49,50,54,80,99,108,116) as well as the prolonged clinical analgesia observed following extradural narcotic administration (26,56), it appears the answer lies somewhere in between.

Extradural Opiates—Comparison with Other Parenteral Routes

The extradural route will reproduce essentially intramuscular administration in addition to any regional component so that analgesia assessment of the extradural portion is impossible in the absence of an intramuscular control group. When the extradural and intramuscular routes are compared, they show similar behavior with respect to onset of action, time to optimal effect, degree of maximal analgesia, and clinically apparent systemic effects (56). The duration of analgesia is greater than would be expected from the same dose given intramuscularly.

Therefore the comparable clinical response, similar absorption profile, inadequate analgesia in the early postoperative period, failure in labor of low doses of extradural opiates, and efficacy despite injection at remote sites indicate that an exclusive spinal action with prolonged analgesia and no central depressant effect is unlikely. Furthermore, systemically administered narcotics display a spinal component of action via a receptor system functionally similar to that acted on by intrathecal narcotics (62).

The evidence available concerning the mode of action of extradural narcotics indicates a combination of CNS effects involving spinal and supraspinal sites, as with other routes of narcotic administration, except for intrathecal opiates. The importance of the direct effect on the spinal cord in relation to the total analgesic effect is not known. It is possible that the proportion varies inversely with the distance of deposition from the proposed site of action. Thus, by depositing the opioid closer to the ideal site of action, an accentuated spinal component may exist. This increased proportion of spinal binding may manifest clinically in a longer duration of effective analgesia.

Extradural Opioids—Specific Spinal Action: Yes or No?

The prime reason why extradural opiates should operate via a specific spinal effect is the proximity of injection to the proposed site of action. Since the presence of the dura represents an additional barrier between the locus of injection and the proposed site of action in the spinal cord, it should delay the opiate on its journey to the receptors in the dorsal horn. Consequently, one would expect the onset of analgesia of extradural opiates to be slower than that following intrathecal injection of narcotics. However, this is not the case and analgesia commences after a comparable period arising from differing mechanisms that coincidentally produce similar onset times. The start of analgesia following extradural opiate administration is probably determined by systemic uptake, which is reflected in an absorption profile analagous to that after intramuscular administration. Alternatively, the epidural drugs might initially gain access to the cord, not via diffusion through the dura but by absorption in the vasculature, which passes through the root sleeves and supplies the cord (112). Furthermore, the effect may be mediated by an action on the roots (42).

The dura mater forms a relatively thick barrier and displays low rates of diffusion. Polar, low molecular weight drugs, such as morphine, will have the most efficient dural transfer and a significant proportion of their effect could result from specific spinal binding. Lipophilic, high molecular weight narcotics, e.g., buprenorphine, probably have negligible transfer across the dura to the CSF and a predominantly supraspinal clinical effect is likely. Unlike local anesthetic agents, opiates have no proven regional action in the concentrations used, and until they traverse the dura and bind with their receptors in the dorsal horn, they are inactive.

The usual site of injection and the volume of the injectate used make it unlikely that high concentrations of narcotic will be available to bind at the spinal level(s) desired. The extradural space is extremely vascular and it is improbable that the opiate will preferentially transfer across the dura. Systemic absorption of the extradural bolus begins immediately and the plasma profile resembles the intramuscular route. As the drug is absorbed from the peridural site, the concentration gradient across the dura into the CSF must decrease. Therefore, the more rapidly that systemic absorption occurs, the less opiate will be transferred regionally into the neuraxis. Systemic absorption must make a contribution to the analgesia; the question is, how much?

CONCLUSION

It has been 5 years and many thousands of cases after the initial clinical use of spinal narcotics. There is little information on dose-response effects, best drug(s), and most effective dose and optimal volume of injectate. Furthermore, little is known about the factors determining the appearance of side effects. The available data has been gleaned from isolated, sporadic studies and observations. This situation has been created by the lack of properly controlled trials in large numbers of patients. Such studies are essential before the role of extradural and intrathecal narcotics in the management of pain can finally be defined.

Intrathecal opiates act within the spinal cord, independent of supraspinal control, to modify the transmission of information concerning noxious stimulation of peripheral receptors. The narcotics provide pure pain relief since their targets, the opiate receptors, are confined to the dorsal horn of the spinal cord. Analgesia is intense, prolonged, and free of sympathetic, motor, or nociceptive effects, which stands in remarkable contrast to the blockade achieved by subarachnoid local anesthetics. Systemic effects are absent and patients have both the ability and desire to ambulate at short postoperative intervals.

Unfortunately, unwanted side effects are not uncommon and delayed respiratory depression is potentially dangerous enough to warrant special nursing surveillance. The future appears gloomy from the viewpoint of routine, safe clinical application, for intrathecal opiates have failed to separate analgesia and respiratory depression as was initially anticipated when it was demonstrated that the deadlock between analgesia and systemically derived central depression could be broken by the subarachnoid application of narcotics.

The principles of management of patients receiving intrathecal opiates should involve the following:

1. For rapid onset and limited spread, use a lipid soluble agent. Lipid insoluble narcotics are more likely to cause delayed respiratory depression.

2. Use low doses, e.g., morphine from 0.1 to 0.2 mg.

3. Attempt to limit the rostral spread of the drug by physical means, such as steep head-up posture, use of hyperbaric solutions, and the avoidance of coughing and straining.

4. Ensure appropriate surveillance to detect and treat delayed respiratory depression.

Extradural opiates are safe in that unique respiratory effects are not a feature, and it appears they may be used with the same constraints as via the intramuscular route. They are effective provided the appropriate dose is administered. In a number of aspects they behave similarly to their intramuscular counterparts. The prolonged duration of action consistently observed following extradural use may be attributable to an increased proportion of spinal binding as a result of the proximity of injection to the proposed site of action. Alternatively, a sustained release effect from the adipose tissue in the extradural space may be operative.

It is possible that this route of administration is both utilized and withheld for the wrong reasons. Those who use it think it confers an exclusively spinal action; it is avoided because of the belief that it has specific depressant ventilatory effects. Neither premise has, at this juncture, been conclusively vindicated.

Extradural narcotics do not constitute the perfect form of analgesia that was initially proclaimed and they may merely be an exotic method of administering a deep systemic dose of opiate.

Future Trends in Spinal Opiate Analgesia

The Immediate Future

Superior analgesia in acute pain might be obtained by combining the intrathecal and systemic routes (intravenous) to provide optimal spinal/supraspinal synergy unattainable with extradural narcotics alone. In chronic pain the supraspinal component is less essential and the sole use of neuraxial narcotics is appropriate.

The Foreseeable Future

The local effect of intrathecal opiates could synergistically be augmented by the use of other drugs with actions involving alternative, specific synaptic systems capable of modulating spinal sensory processing. Such agents as clonidine, tricyclic antidepressants, baclofen, benzodiazepines, and substance P antagonists in various permutations may result in synergistic augmentation enabling subanalgesic doses to provide profound analgesia.

The ability of these alternate pharmacological systems to alter selectively the nociceptive threshold offers the opportunity of manipulating spinal function by the activation of intrinsic pharmacologically defined receptor systems through spinally administered agonists.

REFERENCES

1. Abboud, T. K., Shnider, S. M., Dailey, P. A., Raya, J., Khoo, S. S., Sarkis, S., De Sausa, B., Baysinger, C. L., and Miller, F. (1982): Hyperbaric intrathecal morphine for the relief of labor pain. *Anesthesiology*, 57:A384.
2. Adams, A. P., and Pybus, D. A. (1978): Delayed respiratory depression after the use of fentanyl during anaesthesia. *Br. Med. J.*, 1:278–279.
3. Allen, P. D., Walman, A. T., Cullen, D. J., Shesky, M., Patterson, K., and Covino, B. (1983): The effects of epidural morphine on postoperative analgesia. *Anesthesiology*, 57:A199.
4. Anonymous (1980): Editorial. Epidural opiates. *Lancet*, 1:962–963.
5. Atweh, S. F., and Kuhar, M. J. (1977): Autoradiographic localization of opiate receptors in rat brain. I. Spinal cord and lower medulla. *Brain Res.*, 124:53–67.
6. Baraka, A., Noueihid, R., and Hajj, S. (1981): Intrathecal injection of morphine for obstetric analgesia. *Anesthesiology*, 54:136–140.
7. Baskoff, J. D., Watson, R. L., and Muldoon, S. M. (1980): Respiratory arrest after intrathecal morphine. *Anesth. Rev.*, 7:12–15.

8. Becker, L. D., Paulson, B. A., Miller, R. D., Severinghaus, J. W., and Eger, E. I. (1976): Biphasic respiratory depression after fentanyl-droperidol or fentanyl alone used to supplement nitrous oxide anesthesia. *Anesthesiology*, 44:291–296.

9. Behar, M., Magora, F., Olshwang, D., and Davidson, J. T. (1979): Epidural morphine in treatment of pain. *Lancet*, 1:527–529.

10. Berkowitz, B. A., Ngai, S. H., Hempstead, J., and Spector, A. (1975): Disposition of naloxone: Use of a new radioimmunoassy. *J. Pharmacol. Exp. Ther.*, 195:499–504.

11. Besson, J. M., Wyon-Maillard, M. C., and Benoist, J. M. (1973): Effects of phenoperidine on lamina V cells in the cat dorsal horn. *J. Pharmacol. Exp. Ther.*, 187:239–245.

12. Binsted, R. J. (1983): Epidural morphine after caesarian section. *Anaesth. Intensive Care*, 11:130.

13. Boas, R. A. (1980): Hazards of epidural morphine. *Anaesth. Intensive Care*, 8:377–378.

14. Bonnardot, J. P., Maillet, M., Colau, J. C., Millot, F., and Deligne, P. (1982): Maternal and fetal concentration of morphine after intrathecal administration during labour. *Br. J. Anaesth.*, 54:487–489.

15. Booker, P. D., Wilkes, R. G., Bryson, T. H. L., and Beddard, J. (1980): Obstetric pain relief using epidural morphine. *Anaesthesia*, 35:377–379.

16. Boreus, L. O., Skoldefors, E., and Ehrnebo, M. (1983): Appearance of pethidine and norpethidine in cerebrospinal fluid of man following intramuscular injection of pethidine. *Acta Anaesthesiol. Scand.*, 27:222–225.

17. Bromage, P. R. (1981): The price of intraspinal narcotic analgesia: Basic constraints. *Anesth. Analg.*, 60:461–463.

18. Bromage, P. R., Camporesi, E. M., Durant, P. A., and Nielsen, C. H. (1983): Influence of epinephrine as an adjuvant to epidural morphine. *Anesthesiology*, 58:257–262.

19. Bromage, P. R., Camporesi, E. M., Durant, P. A. C., and Nielsen, C. H. (1982): Non-respiratory side-effects of epidural morphine. *Anesth. Analg.*, 61:490–495.

20. Bromage, P. R., Joyal, A. C., and Binney, J. C. (1963): Local anesthetic drugs: Penetration from the spinal extradural space into the neuraxis. *Science*, 140:392–397.

21. Bromage, P. R., Camporesi, E., and Chestnut, D. (1980): Epidural narcotics for postoperative analgesia. *Anesth. Analg.*, 59:473–480.

22. Brookshire, G. L., Shnider, S. M., Abboud, T. K., Kotelko, D. M., Nouiehed, R., Thigpen, J. W., Khoo, S. S., Raya, J. A., Foutz, S. E., and Brizgys, R. V. (1983): Effects of naloxone on the mother and neonate after intrathecal morphine for labor analgesia. *Anesthesiology*, 59:A417.

23. Bullingham, R. E. S., McQuay, H. J., and Moore, R. A. (1982): Extradural and intrathecal narcotics. In: *Recent Advances in Anaesthesia and Analgesia*, edited by R. S. Atkinson and C. Langton Hewer. pp. 141–156. Churchill Livingstone, New York.

24. Cahill, J., Murphy, D., O'Brien, D., Mulhall, J., and Fitzpatrick, G. (1983): Epidural buprenorphine for pain relief after major abdominal surgery. A controlled comparison with epidural morphine. *Anaesthesia*, 38:760–764.

25. Carmichael, F. J., Rolbin, S. J., and Hew, E. M. (1982): Epidural morphine for analgesia after caesarian section. *Can. Anaesth. Soc. J.*, 29:359–363.

26. Chambers, W. A., Sinclair, C. J., and Scott, D. B. (1981): Extradural morphine for pain after surgery. *Br. J. Anaesth.*, 53:921–925.

27. Chauvin, M., Salbaing, J., Perrin, D., Levron, J. C., and Viars, P. (1983): Comparison between intramuscular and epidural administration of alfentanil for pain relief and plasma kinetics. *Anesthesiology*, 59(3):A197.

28. Chauvin, M., Samii, K., Schermann, J. M., Sandouk, P., Bourdon, R., and Viars, P. (1981): Plasma concentration of morphine after IM extradural and intrathecal administration. *Br. J. Anaesth.*, 53:911–913.

29. Chayen, M. J., Rudick, V., and Borvine, A. (1980): Pain control with epidural injection of morphine. *Anesthesiology*, 53:338–339.

30. Christensen, P., Larsen, V. H., Iversen, A. D., and Andersen, P. K. (1983): Thoracic and lumbar epidural morphine after upper abdominal laparatomy. *Acta Anaesth. Scand.*, 27[Suppl.], 78:73.

31. Christensen, V. (1980): Respiratory depression after extradural morphine. *Br. J. Anaesth.*, 52:841.

32. Coombs, D. W., Saunders, R. L., Gaylor, R. S., Pageau, M. G., Leith, M. G., and Schaiberger, C. (1981): Continuous epidural analgesia via implanted morphine reservoir. *Lancet*, 2:425–426.

33. Coombs, D. W., Saunders, R. L., Gaylor, R. S., and Pageau, M. G. (1982): Epidural narcotic infusion reservoir; implantation technique and efficacy. *Anesthesiology*, 56:469–473.

34. Cooper, G. M., Goodman, N. W., Prys-Roberts, C., Jacobson, L., and Douglas, J. (1982): Ventilatory effects of extradural diamorphine. *Br. J. Anaesth.*, 54:239P.

35. Cousins, M. J., Mather, L. E., Glynn, C. J., Wilson, P. R., and Graham, J. R. (1979): Selective spinal analgesia. *Lancet*, 1:1141–1142.

36. Cox, B. M., Goldstein, A., and Li, C. H. (1976): Opioid activity of a peptide [BLTH(61–91)], derived from β-lipotropin. *Proc. Natl. Acad. Sci. USA*, 73:1821–1823.

37. Crawford, J. S. (1981): Experiences with epidural morphine in obstetrics. *Anaesthesia*, 36:207–209.

38. Crawford, M. E., Andersen, H. B., Augustenborg, G., Bay, J., Beck, O., Benveniste, D., Larsen, L. B., Carl, P., Djernes, M., Eriksen, J., Grell, A. M., Henriksen, H., Johansen, S. H., Jorgensen, H. O. K., Moller, I. W., Pedersen, J. E. P., and Ravlo, O. (1983): Pain treatment on outpatient basis utilizing extradural opiates; A Danish multicentre study comprising 105 patients. *Pain*, 16:41–47.

39. Crawford, R. D., Batra, M. S., and Fox, F. (1981): Epidural dose response for postoperative analgesia. *Anesthesiology*, 55:A150.

40. Davies, G. K., Tolhurst-Cleaver, C. L., and Tames, T. L. (1980): Respiratory depression after intrathecal narcotics. *Anaesthesia*, 35:1080–1083.

41. Doblar, D. D., Muldoon, S. M., Abbrecht, P. H., Baskoff, J., and Watson, R. L. (1981): Epidural morphine following epidural local anesthesia: Effect on ventilatory and airway occlusion pressure responses to CO_2. *Anesthesiology*, 55:423–428.

42. Fields, H. L., Emson, P. C., Leigh, B. K., Gilbert, R. F. T., and Iversen, L. L. (1980): Multiple opiate receptor sites on primary afferent fibers. *Nature*, 284:351–353.

43. Findler, G., Olshwang, D., and Hadani, M. (1982): Continuous epidural morphine treatment for intractable pain in terminal cancer patients. *Pain*, 14:311–315.

44. Gjessing, J., and Tomlin, P. J. (1981): Postoperative pain control with intrathecal morphine. *Anaesthesia*, 36:268–276.

45. Glynn, C. J., Mather, L. E., Cousins, M. J., Wilson, P. R., and Graham, J. R. (1979): Spinal narcotics and respiratory depression. *Lancet*, 1:356–357.

46. Glynn, C. J., Mather, L. E., Cousins, M. J., Graham, J. R., and Wilson, P. R. (1981): Peridural meperidine in humans: Analgetic response, pharmacokinetics and transmission into CSF. *Anesthesiology*, 55:520–526.

47. Gustafsson, L. L., Schildt, B., and Jacobsen, K. (1982): Adverse effects of extradural and intrathecal opiates: Report of a nationwide survey in Sweden. *Br. J. Anaesth.*, 54:479–486.

48. Gustafsson, L. L., Feychting, B., and Klingstedt, C. (1981): Late respiratory depression after concomitant use of morphine epidurally and parenterally. *Lancet*, 1:892–893.

49. Gustafsson, L. L., Friberg-Nielsen, S., Garle, M., Mohall, A., Rane, A., Schildt, B., and Symreng, T. (1982): Extradural and parenteral morphine: Kinetics and effects in postoperative pain. A controlled clinical study. *Br. J. Anaesth.*, 54:1167–1174.

50. Gustafsson, L. L., Garle, M., Johanisson, J., Rane, A., Stenport, J., and Walson, P. (1982): Regional epidural analgesia: Kinetics of pethidine. *Acta Anaesth. Scand. [Suppl.]*, 74:165–168.

51. Holland, A. C. J., Srikantha, S. K., and Tracey, J. A. (1981): Epidural morphine and postoperative pain relief. *Can. Anaesth. Soc. J.*, 28:453–458.

52. Hughes, J., Smith, T. W., Kosterlitz, H. W., Fothergill, L. A., Morgan, B. A., and Morris, H. R. (1975): Identification of two related pentapeptides from the brain with potent opiate agonist activity. *Nature*, 258:577–579.

53. Husemeyer, R. P., O'Conner, M. C., and Davenport, H. T. (1980): Failure of epidural morphine to relieve pain in labour. *Anaesthesia*, 35:161–163.

54. Husemeyer, R. P., Davenport, H. T., Cummings, A. J., and Rosankiewicz, J. R. (1981): Comparison of epidural and intramuscular pethidine for analgesia in labour. *Br. J. Obstet. Gynaecol.*, 88:711–717.

55. Husemeyer, R. P., Cummings, A. J., Rosankiewica, J. R., and Davenport, H. T. (1982): A study of pethidine kinetics and analgesia in women in labour following intravenous, intramuscular and epidural administration. *Br. J. Clin. Pharmacol.*, 13:171–176.

56. Jacobson, L., Phillips, P. D., Hull, C. J., and Conacher, I. D. (1983): Extradural versus intramuscular diamorphine: A controlled study of analgesic and adverse effects in the postoperative period. *Anaesthesia*, 38:10–18.

57. Johnston, J. R., and McCaughey, W. (1980): Epidural morphine. A method of management of multiple fractured ribs. *Anaesthesia*, 35:155–157.
58. Jurna, I., and Grossmann, W. (1976): The effect of the activity evoked in ventrolateral tract axons of the cat spinal cord. *Brain Res.*, 24:473–484.
59. Justins, D. M., Francis, D., Houlton, P. G., and Reynolds, F. (1982): A controlled trial of extradural fentanyl in labour. *Br. J. Anaesth.*, 54:409–414.
60. Kafer, E. R., Brown, J. T., Scott, D., Findlay, J. W. A., Butz, R. F., Teeple, E., and Ghia, J. N. (1982): Biphasic depression of the minute ventilation response to CO_2 following epidural morphine. *Anesthesiology*, 57:A482.
61. Kalia, P. K., Madan, R., Saksena, R., Batra, R. K., and Gode, G. R. (1983): Epidural pentazocine for postoperative pain relief. *Anesth. Analg.*, 62:949–950.
62. Kitahata, L. M., and Collins, J. G. (1981): Spinal action of narcotic analgesics. *Anesthesiology*, 54:153–163.
63. Knill, R. L., Clement, J. L., and Thompson, W. R. (1981): Epidural morphine causes delayed and prolonged ventilatory depression. *Can. Anaesth. Soc. J.*, 28:537–543.
64. Korinek, A. M., Languille, M., Bonnet, F., Lienhart, A., Thibonnier, M., Sassano, P., and Viars, P. (1983): Epidural morphine stimulates ADH secretion. *Anesthesiology*, 59(3):A202.
65. Lanz, E., Theiss, D., Reiss, W., and Sommer, U. (1982): Epidural morphine for postoperative analgesia. A double blind study. *Anesth. Analg.*, 61:236–240.
66. Lazorthes, Y., Gouarderes, C. H., Verdie, J. C., Monsarrat, B., Bastide, R., Campan, L., Alwan, A., and Cros, J. (1980): Analgesie par injection intrathecale de morphine. Etude pharmacocinetique et applicatior aux douleurs irreductibls. *Neurochirurgie*, 26:159–164.
67. Leslie, J., Camporesi, E., Urban, B., and Bromage, P. (1979): Selective epidural analgesia. *Lancet*, 1:151.
68. Liolios, A., and Hartmann Andersen, F. (1979): Selective spinal analgesia. *Lancet*, 2:357.
69. Lofstrom, J. B., Merits, H., and Bengtsson, M. (1983): Postoperative pain oblivation with morphine intrathecally in major hip surgery. *Acta Anaesth. Scand.*, 27[Suppl.], 78:73.
70. Magora, F., Olshwang, D., Eimerl, D., Shorr, J., Katzenelson, R., Cotev, S., and Davidson, J. T. (1980): Observations on extradural morphine analgesia in various pain conditions. *Br. J. Anaesth.*, 52:247–252.
71. Malins, A. F., Goodman, N. W., Cooper, G. M., Prys-Roberts, C., and Baird, R. N. (1984): Ventilatory effects of pre- and postoperative diamorphine. A comparison of extradural with intramuscular administration. *Anaesthesia*, 39:118–125.
72. Mather, L. E., and Meffin, P. J. (1978): Clinical pharmacokinetics of pethidine. *Clin. Pharmacokinet.*, 3:352–368.
73. Mathews, E. T., and Abrams, L. D. (1980): Intrathecal morphine in open heart surgery. *Lancet*, 1:543.
74. McCaughey, W., and Graham, J. L. (1982): The respiratory depression of epidural morphine. Time course and effect of posture. *Anaesthesia*, 37:990–995.
75. McClure, J. H., Chambers, W. A., Moore, E., and Scott, D. B. (1980): Epidural morphine for postoperative pain. *Lancet*, 1:975–976.
76. McDonald, A. M. (1980): Complication of epidural morphine. *Anaesth. Intensive Care*, 8:490–491.
77. Moller, I. W., Vester-Andersen, T., Steentoft, A., Hjortso, E., and Lunding, M. (1982): Respiratory depression and morphine concentration in serum after epidural and intramuscular administration of morphine. *Acta Anaesth. Scand.*, 26:421–424.
78. Moore, R. A., Bullingham, R. E. S., McQuay, H. J., Hand, C. W., Aspel, J. B., Allen, M. C., and Thomas, D. (1982): Dural permeability to narcotics: In vitro determination and application to extradural administration. *Br. J. Anaesth.*, 54:1117–1128.
79. Naulty, J. S., Johnson, M., Burger, G. A., Datta, S., Weiss, J. B., Morrison, J., and Ostheimer, G. W. (1983): Epidural fentanyl for post caesarean section delivery pain management. *Anesthesiology*, 59:A415.
80. Nordberg, G., Hedner, T., Mellstrand, T., and Dahlstrom, B. (1983): Pharmacokinetic aspects of epidural morphine analgesia. *Anesthesiology*, 58:545–551.
81. Onofrio, B. M., Yaksh, T. L., and Arnold, P. G. (1982): Continuous low dose, intrathecal morphine administration in the treatment of chronic pain of malignant origin. *Mayo Clin. Proc.*, 516–520.
82. Oyama, T., Fukushi, S., and Jin, T. (1982): Epidural Beta-endorphin in treatment of pain. *Can. Anaesth. Soc. J.*, 29:24–26.

83. Oyama, T., Jin, T., Yamaya, R., Ling, N., and Guillemin, R. (1980): Profound analgesic effects of Beta-endorphin in man. *Lancet*, 1:122.
84. Oyama, T., Matsuki, A., Taneichi, T., Ling, N., and Guillemin, R. (1980): β-endorphin in obstetric analgesia. *Am. J. Obstet. Gynecol.*, 137:613–616.
85. Paterson, G. M. C., McQuay, H. G., Bullingham, R. E. S., and Moore, R. A. (1984): Intradural morphine and diamorphine. Dose response studies. *Anaesthesia*, 39:113–117.
86. Perris, B. W. (1980): Epidural pethidine in labour: A study of dose requirements. *Anaesthesia*, 35:380–382.
87. Pert, C. B., and Synder, S. H. (1973): Opiate receptor: Demonstration in nervous tissue. *Science*, 179:1011–1014.
88. Petersen, T. K., Husted, S. E., Rybro, L., Schurizek, B. A., and Wernberg, M. (1982): Urinary retention during intramuscular and extradural morphine analgesia. *Br. J. Anaesth.*, 54:1175–1178.
89. Pybus, D. A., and Torda, T. A. (1982): Dose-effect relationships of extradural morphine. *Br. J. Anaesth.*, 54:1259–1262.
90. Reiz, S., and Westberg, M. (1980): Side-effects of epidural morphine. *Lancet*, 1:203–204.
91. Samii, K., Chauvin, M., and Viars, P. (1981): Postoperative spinal analgesia with morphine. *Br. J. Anaesth.*, 53:817–820.
92. Samii, K., Feret, J., Harasi, A., and Viars, P. (1979): Selective spinal analgesia. *Lancet*, 1:1142.
93. Scott, D. B., and McClure, J. H. (1979): Selective epidural analgesia. *Lancet*, 1:1410–1411.
94. Scott, P. V., Bowen, F. E., Cartwright, P., Mohan, R. A. O., Deeley, D. Wotherspoon, H. G., and Sumrein, I. M. A. (1980): Intrathecal morphine as sole analgesic during labour. *Br. Med. J.*, 2:351–353.
95. Shulman, M. S., Brebner, J., and Sandler, A. (1983): The effect of epidural morphine on postoperative pain relief and pulmonary function in thoracotomy patients. *Anesthesiology*, 59(3):A192.
96. Skjoldebrand, A., Garle, M., Gustafsson, L. L., Johansson, H., Lunell, N. O., and Rane, A. (1982): Extradural pethidine with and without adrenaline during labour: Wide variation in effect. *Br. J. Anaesth.*, 54:415–420.
97. Summerfield, J. A. (1980): Naloxone modulates the perception of itch in man. *Br. J. Clin. Pharmacol.*, 10:180–183.
98. Takasaki, M., and Asano, M. (1983): Intrathecal morphine combined with hyperbaric tetracaine. *Anaesthesia*, 38:76–77.
99. Tamsen, A., Sjostrom, S., Hartvig, P., Persson, P., Gabrielsson, J., and Paalzow, L. (1983): CSF and plasma kinetics of morphine and meperidine after epidural administration. *Anesthesiology*, 59(3):A196.
100. Torda, T. A., and Pybus, D. A. (1981): Clinical experience with epidural morphine. *Anaesth. Intensive Care*, 9:129–134.
101. Torda, T. A., and Pybus, D. A. (1982): Comparison of four narcotic analgesics for extradural analgesia. *Br. J. Anaesth.*, 54:291–294.
102. Torda, T. A., Pybus, D. A., Liberman, H., Clark, M., and Crawford, M. (1980): An experimental comparison of epidural and intramuscular morphine. *Br. J. Anaesth.*, 52:939–943.
103. Tseng, L. F., Loh, H. H., and Li, C. H., (1976): β-endorphin as a potent analgesic by intravenous injection. *Nature*, 263:239–240.
104. Tung, A., Maliniak, K., Tenicela, R., and Winter, P. M. (1980): Intrathecal morphine for intraoperative and postoperative analgesia. *JAMA*, 244:2637–2638.
105. Ventafridda, V., Figliuzzi, M., Tamburini, M., Gori, E., Parolaro, D., and Sala, M. (1979): Clinical observation on analgesia elicited by intrathecal morphine in cancer patients. In: *Advances in Pain Research and Therapy*, Vol. 3, edited by J. J. Bonica, J. C. Liebeskind, and D. G. Albe-Fessard, pp. 559–565. Raven Press, New York.
106. Wang, J. K. (1977): Analgesic effect of intrathecally administered morphine. *Reg. Anaesth.*, 2:3–8.
107. Wang, J. K., Nauss, L. A., and Thomas, J. E. (1979): Pain relief by intrathecally applied morphine in man. *Anesthesiology*, 50:149–151.
108. Weddel, S. J., and Ritter, R. R. (1981): Serum level following epidural administration of morphine and correlation with relief of postsurgical pain. *Anesthesiology*, 54:210–214.

109. Wolfe, M. J., and Nicholas, A. D. G. (1979): Selective epidural analgesia. *Lancet*, 2:150–151.
110. Wolfe, M. J., and Davies, G. K. (1980): Analgesic action of extradural fentanyl. *Br. J. Anaesth.*, 52:357–358.
111. Writer, W. D. R., James, F. M., and Wheeler, A. S. (1981): Double-blind comparison of morphine and bupivacaine for continuous epidural analgesia in labor. *Anesthesiology*, 54:215–219.
112. Yaksh, T. L. (1981): Spinal opiate analgesia: Characteristics and principles of action. *Pain*, 11:293–346.
113. Yaksh, T. L., and Rudy, T. A. (1976): Analgesia mediated by a direct spinal action of narcotics. *Science*, 192:1357–1358.
114. Yaksh, T. L., Jessel, T. M., Gamse, R., Mudge, A. W., and Leeman, S. E. (1980): Intrathecal morphine inhibits substance *P* release from mammalian spinal cord in vivo. *Nature*, 286:155–156.
115. Yaksh, T. L., Kohl, R. L., and Rudy, T. A. (1977): Induction of tolerance and withdrawal in rats receiving morphine in the spinal subarachnoid space. *Eur. J. Pharmacol.*, 42:275–284.
116. Youngstrom, P. C., Cowan, R. I., Sutheimer, C., Eastwood, D. W., and Yu, J. C. M. (1982): Pain relief and plasma concentrations from epidural and intramuscular morphine in post-cesarian patients. *Anesthesiology*, 57:404–409.
117. Zenz, M., Schappler-Scheele, B., Neuhaus, R., Piepenbrock, S., and Hilfrich, J. (1981): Long term peridural analgesia in cancer pain. *Lancet*, 1:91.

Advances in Pain Research
and Therapy, Vol. 7,
edited by C. Benedetti et al.
Raven Press, New York © 1984.

Calcitonin and Analgesia

*F. Fraioli, *A. Fabbri, *L. Gnessi, *C. Moretti, *C. Conti,
**G. Cruccu, **M. Inghilleri, **M. Manfredi, and †M. Felici

*Institute of Clinical Medicine V, and **Institute of Clinical Neurology V,
University of Rome; and †Hospital of St. Giuseppe, Marino, Rome, Italy

Calcitonin, discovered by Copp et al. in 1961 (24), until recently was considered the major Ca^{2+} regulating factor along with parathyroid hormone and vitamin D. However, the ubiquitous production of this substance (5,13,25,56), and the fact that complete removal of the thyroid gland does not affect circulating calcitonin levels (52), suggested that functions other than Ca^{2+} metabolism were linked to this hormone. In a recent editorial, Austin and Heath (2) describe calcitonin as a "hormone in search of a function" and, in fact, the exact role of calcitonin in human physiology is still controversial. It is generally accepted that calcitonin regulates plasma Ca^{2+} levels, probably through a mechanism related to gastrointestinal function. Calcitonin aids in absorption/binding of ingested Ca^{2+} and protects the skeleton (23,42). The hormone is thus efficacious in the treatment of Paget's disease of bone and in long-term treatment aimed at maintenance of skeletal mass (35,39).

Human calcitonin is a single-chain aminoacid polypeptide with a 3.5 K molecular weight (40). This calcitonin monomer results from the cleavage of a large precursor form (54). The peptide is species-specific and rat calcitonin is the molecule most closely resembling the human hormone, differing in only two aminoacids (43). The C parafollicular cells of the thyroid gland are the major source of calcitonin in humans (41,57). These cells originate from the embryonic neural crest (45) and migrate to their final position in the thyroid gland. However, calcitonin is produced in many tissues other than the thyroid gland (5,13,25,56); levels are not reduced and may be increased following thyroidectomy (52).

These facts prompt the suggestion that calcitonin is produced by all neural tissue. This would also be consistent with the concept of the APUD (amine precursor uptake and decarboxylation) system described by Pearse in 1968 (44). The presence of a human calcitonin-like molecule in the brain of protochordates and cyclostomes (31), of salmon calcitonin in the brain of lizard (29) and pigeon (30), and of calcitonin material in human brain extracts (5) suggests two considerations: that calcitonin has some functions in the central nervous system (CNS) of these species and that the bone-regulating function

of the substance may have evolved much later in vertebrate differentiation
(31).

Apart from this line of basic experimental studies, evidence has appeared
in the literature over the last few years suggesting that calcitonin acts on
the CNS. This evidence includes: (a) a neurotransmitter role (33,47); (b)
action on feeding (28) and other behavior (12); and (c) a central analgesic
effect (46,59). Regarding neurotransmission, calcitonin has been shown to
exert a clear influence on pituitary hormone secretion (8,11,33,36,47). In
particular, this peptide has been reported to exert an inhibitory effect on the
stimulated secretion of lutenizing hormone (36), growth hormone (8), thyroid-stimulating hormone (36), and on the basal and stress and thyrotropin-
releasing hormone-induced secretion of prolactin (PRL) (32,47). This inhibitory pattern appears to be mediated by a direct action on the CNS. As far
as the effects on feeding and other behavior are concerned, calcitonin has
been reported to inhibit feeding (28) and to have a clear sedative function
(12).

In the last few years, our research has been focused on the central analgesic effect. An analgesic effect of calcitonin was reported by Yamamoto
et al. (59), who presented pharmacologic data demonstrating that this peptide, on intraventricular injection, inhibited pain response in mice and the
potential evoked by electrical stimulation of the tooth pulp in rabbits. Earlier,
Pecile et al. (46) had shown that the analgesic effect of calcitonin is of a
morphine type but is more prolonged and does not induce dependence or
addiction. Significantly, this analgesic action is not reversed by the opiate
antagonists naloxone (7) and levallorphan (58). Nevertheless, these studies
refer mainly to the animal model. In humans, some clinical evidence has
indicated that calcitonin treatment in osteoarticular diseases has a pain-relieving effect that may occur concomitantly (35,39), or before the specific
action on bone (20).

On the basis of these findings, we carried out the three studies described
here to define the role of calcitonin in pain mechanisms in humans, using
three experimental models: (a) a case of congenital indifference to pain; (b)
subarachnoid injection of salmon calcitonin in patients with chronic pain;
and (c) subarachnoid injection of salmon calcitonin in subjects with experimentally induced pain.

A CASE OF CONGENITAL INDIFFERENCE TO PAIN

Over the past few years we studied a very rare case of an individual with
congenital indifference to pain. This very unusual condition is characterized
by the complete lack of pain in the absence of organic abnormalities in
nervous structures (4,22). We have already described the complete clinical
picture of this patient elsewhere (27,38). Briefly, high levels of opioid pep-

tides, detected by means of a radioreceptor assay technique, were found in the cerebrospinal fluid (CSF), suggesting that the presence of high amounts of pain-relieving substances might explain the pathogenesis of this syndrome.

Methods

Calcitonin levels were measured in peripheral plasma and CSF. Blood samples were collected by means of a syringe from a forearm vein and the plasma immediately frozen by means of an alcohol-dry ice mixture and stored at −70°C until assayed. Cerebrospinal fluid was obtained through an indwelling catheter introduced into the lumbar subarachnoid space with a lumbar puncture needle. The fluid was collected in tubes, immediately frozen, and stored at −70°C. Blood and CSF samples were collected using the same procedure 2 weeks later.

Immunoreactive calcitonin was measured by radioimmunoassay (RIA) in peripheral plasma and CSF. Before the assay, CSF (2 ml) was subjected to chromatography in a Sephadex G 50 column (a refrigerated 1 × 50-cm column), eluted in 0.05 M acetate buffer pH 5.6, and the assay was performed in the pooled fractions corresponding to the elution zone of the standard cold calcitonin. Radioimmunoassay reagents were purchased from Immunonuclear Company, Stillwater, Mi., and validated in our laboratory. The antibody used is specific for the amino acid sequence 17–32 in the calcitonin molecule and showed no significant cross-reaction with β-endorphin Met- and Leu-enkephalin, ACTH (1–39), and ACTH (1–24). Sensitivity of the method was 2.5 pg/tube. In our hands, inter- and intra-assay were 14 and 10%, respectively.

Results

The results of calcitonin assay are shown in Figure 1. Very high levels of immunoreactive calcitonin were found in CSF, whereas immunoreactive calcitonin in peripheral plasma remained within the normal range. Is this an artifact due to the methodology of the assay? Is this real calcitonin or a molecule cross-reacting in the radioimmunoassay system used with calcitonin? It is difficult to answer these questions at present, even if we used better validated radioimmunoassay techniques and separated the biological samples by gel-chromatography, assaying only the molecules eluting together with the standard calcitonin and thus in the range of its apparent molecular weight. It is interesting, however, that high-immunoreactive calcitonin molecules are present in the brain of a subject unable to feel pain.

TABLE 1. *Clinical details of patients*

Case no.	Age	Sex	Clinical details[a]
1	41	M	Ca. lung: bone metastases L1,L3. Severe low back pain.
2	49	F	Ca. rectum: right knee bone metastasis.
3	54	F	Ca. breast: multiple bone metastases. Severe shoulder pain.
4	63	M	Ca. tongue: cervical lymph gland metastases. Severe pain in the trigeminal area.
5	42	F	Ca. stomach: liver metastases.
6	58	M	Ca. prostate: L2,L3 metastases. Severe low back pain.
7	51	M	Myeloma. Multiple rib fractures. Severe chest pain.
8	57	M	Ca. thyroid: T2,T3 metastases. Severe back pain.

[a] Ca. = cancer.

SUBARACHNOID SALMON CALCITONIN INJECTION IN PATIENTS WITH CHRONIC PAIN

To our knowledge, this is the first report on the effect of calcitonin injected into the subarachnoid space. We chose the subarachnoid route in light of the results of experiments performed in animals (7,46,58), and to obtain rapid pain relief. In addition, peripheral salmon calcitonin injections cause only mild pain relief, which occurs in a mean time of 5.5 weeks after treatment (35).

Methods

This study consisted of 8 patients suffering from severe chronic pain (Table 1). The patients were informed of the nature and schedules of the experiment and all gave informed consent. The calcitonin was obtained through the courtesy of Armour Pharmaceutical, UK, and Armour Medicamenta, Italy batch E 19/Cl in aqueous solution free of additives and preservatives. To test for possible allergic reactions, the substance was injected intradermally 1 day before the experiment. Systemic medications including analgesics were withheld for at least 12 hr before the experiment. Pain was assessed by using the Visual Analog Scale of Scott and Huskisson (51) in which the patient's pain is assessed on a scale from 0 (no pain) to 10 (unbearable pain).

Amounts of 1.5 µg/kg body weight of calcitonin were injected in a single bolus through a lumbar puncture needle inserted at the L2–L3 interspace. To compare the effects of the subarachnoid injection of salmon calcitonin, the same patients were given alternatively at weekly intervals an injection of saline in the same volume as salmon calcitonin. Patients were not informed if saline or salmon calcitonin was being injected.

TABLE 2. *Pain behavior after subarachnoid injection of salmon calcitonin*[a]

Case no.	Pain score before sCT injection	Pain score after sCT injection (1.5 μg/kg body weight)						
		5 min	15 min	1 hr	6 hr	12 hr	24 hr	48 hr
1	10	0	0	0	0	0	0	0
2	10	10	1	1	1	1	1	1
3	9	7	6	4	4	4	4	4
4	10	0	0	0	0	0	0	0
5	10	0	0	0	0	0	0	0
6	10	4	0	0	0	0	0	0
7	10	5	0	0	0	0	0	0
8	10	0	0	0	0	0	0	0

[a] sCT = salmon calcitonin.

Results

The results are summarized in Table 2. As may be noted, before treatment all patients scored their pain as extremely severe, with 7 scoring pain intensity as 10, and 1 as 9. Within 3 to 5 min after injection of the salmon calcitonin, all patients showed considerable decrease of pain and the scores varied between 0 and 7. Fifteen minutes after injection, 7 patients reported complete relief of pain and 1 scored the pain as 6. For the ensuing 48 hr each patient reported an unchanged pain score. Between 48 and 60 hr, patients 3, 4, 6, and 8 scored their pain as 10; the remaining patients had persistent relief. On the morning of the sixth day, patients' assessment of pain returned to pretreatment scores. Thus it can be seen that pain relief lasted for at least 48 hr and for varying periods thereafter, depending on the patient. In contrast, following the saline injections, the patients experienced no pain relief and the pain score remained unchanged.

The only important side effects observed in any of the patients were nausea and vomiting about 1 hr after the salmon calcitonin injection (3 of 8 patients) and sustained diuresis lasting 24 hr after the injection (all patients). These effects of calcitonin following peripheral injection of the hormone had previously been described by other authors (3,35).

SUBARACHNOID SALMON CALCITONIN INJECTION IN EXPERIMENTALLY-INDUCED PAIN

Methods

Four male subjects with terminal cancer in pain-free phases with no systemic medications for at least 12 hr and no evidence of neurological and dental diseases volunteered to enter the study. Each patient was fully informed about the nature of the experiment and gave written consent, then was subjected to a painful stimulus: electrical stimulation of tooth pulp. Cortical evoked potentials were recorded. The techniques of stimulation and recording have been described elsewhere (1,6).

At the beginning of the session, subjects were asked to identify the weakest stimulus perceived (threshold) and the strongest bearable stimulus (tolerance level). Within this stimulation range, pulses of different intensities were delivered pseudorandomly until the supraliminal [(SL) a slight but clearly painful sensation] and submaximal (SM) levels were identified.

After the lumbar puncture needle was introduced into the subarachnoid space at L2–L3 level, the basal recording task was performed: 32-SL and 32-SM dental pulses were delivered pseudorandomly at 5 to 10/min, and the related evoked potentials were recorded and averaged. The 64 responses were always sufficient to provide a good signal-to-noise ratio and to permit precise measurement of the peak-to-peak amplitude of the major component, N 140-P 250 (Fig. 2). Fifteen, 30, 45, and 60 min after the injection of salmon calcitonin 0.4 μg/kg (the same preparation as that used in the previous experiment), the stimuli were repeated at the same levels as in the base-line session.

Results

Figure 3 shows the results dealing with the amplitude of the tooth pulp evoked potentials major component. An almost 50% decrease was observed at 60 min (from 30.88 ± 3.41 μV to 16.75 ± 3.43); the difference is statistically significant ($p < 0.01$). The very slow random rate of stimulation and delivery of pulses of differing intensity prevent, in our experience, any spontaneous time-related decays of sensation and amplitude of cortical responses. The late components of cortical evoked potentials are considered to be a sort of "pain potential" proportional to the perceived pain experience (17,19) and are used in the evaluation of analgesic procedures (18). Applying this concept, the decrease observed would be consistent with an objective pain-relieving action of calcitonin.

DISCUSSION

It is difficult, at the moment, to offer an explanation for the analgesic action of calcitonin. The dramatic pain relief following subarachnoid injection of salmon calcitonin, the significant reduction of the cortical evoked potentials after subarachnoid salmon calcitonin injection, and the presence of high levels of immunoreactive calcitonin in the CSF of a subject suffering from the inability to feel pain (i.e., congenital indifference to pain) are consistent with the possibility that calcitonin is involved in pain sensation in humans, as has already been shown in animals (46,59).

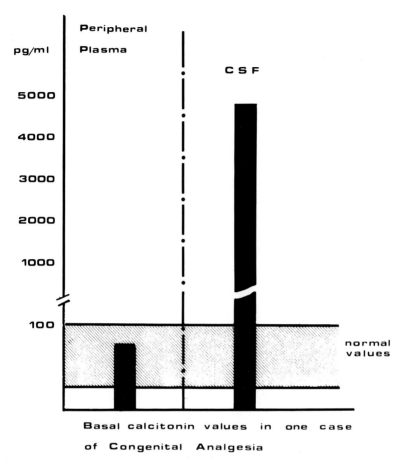

Fig. 1. Calcitonin radioimmunoassay values in the case of congenital indifference to pain indicated in the text. Cerebrospinal fluid (CSF) samples were gel-chromatographed before the assay (27).

The mechanism by which calcitonin acts is still unclear. Various hypotheses may be suggested: (a) calcitonin acts by increasing central opioid levels; (b) calcitonin exerts an agonist effect on opioid receptors; (c) calcitonin acts through the prostaglandin system; (d) calcitonin acts through variations in the central Ca^{2+} levels; and (e) calcitonin possesses its own receptors with an analgesic effect. Let us briefly consider these various hypotheses.

Does Calcitonin Act by Increasing Opioid Levels?

Our earlier findings (26) and those of others (55) exclude this possibility. The peripheral injection of salmon calcitonin does not lead to modification

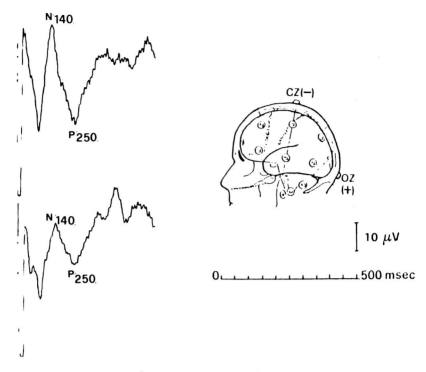

Fig. 2. Tooth pulp evoked potentials (TPEPs). **Right:** Recording electrodes disposition. **Left:** The TPEP obtained in basal conditions (**above**) and 60 min after sCT subarachnoid injection (**below**). Each potential is the average of 32 responses evoked by SL stimuli (0.9 mA, 1 msec). The decrease of amplitude of the N 140-P 250, component approaches 60%.

of endorphin levels. Furthermore, preliminary studies performed in the CSF of 2 of the present 8 patients with chronic intractable pain indicate also that when calcitonin is injected intrathecally it does not lead to an increase in endorphin levels but may even induce a decrease.

Does Calcitonin Act on Opioid Receptors?

One hypothesis advanced to explain the analgesic effect of calcitonin is that this peptide can bind the opiate receptor, evoking the analgesic action. Recent findings indicate that central opioid receptors are of at least two types, the so-called u and o receptors (15): u receptors have a high affinity for exogenous opiates (morphine and its antagonist naloxone), whereas o receptors show a high affinity for endogenous activity (mainly enkephalins). The possibility that calcitonin binds to u receptors is clearly excluded by the finding of Braga et al. (7), who report that naloxone does not reverse calcitonin analgesia. On the other hand, the binding of calcitonin to o receptors has been tested by us using a particular cell line, neuroblastoma

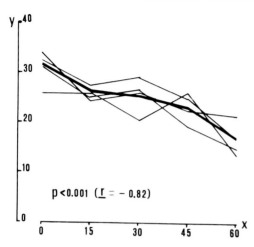

Fig. 3. Modulation of TPEPs after subarachnoid sCT injection. *x-axis:* Time (min) after sCT 0.4 ug/kg sub- arachnoid injection. *y-axis:* Peak- to-peak amplitude of the N 140-P 250 major component of the TPEPs. *Thin lines:* single subjects values. *Thick line:* average of the 4 subjects. The statistical signifi- cance of the decrease of TPEPs amplitude was evaluated by the Pearson's r coefficient of correla- tion for linear regression.

$p < 0.001$ ($r = -0.82$)

cells. Neuroblastoma is a tumor in which the receptor opioid activity of the cells is almost totally of the o type (16). Binding experiments using this model show that standard salmon calcitonin does not displace enkephalin binding at any concentration (Fig. 4). These data appear to refute the hypothesis that calcitonin action is mediated by opiate receptors.

Does Calcitonin Act Through the Prostaglandin System?

Studies have been performed on the possible involvement of the prosta- glandin system in calcitonin action. Ceserani et al. (14) have shown that calcitonin, like indomethacin, inhibits prostaglandin synthesis. This finding, however, has not been confirmed by others, who in fact report opposite effects (21,53). Moreover, our preliminary experiments in humans indicate that prostaglandin levels are not affected by subarachnoid injection of salmon calcitonin. Because of these discrepancies it is not possible to assign a def- inite role to the prostaglandin system in calcitonin analgesia.

Does Calcitonin Act Through Variations in Ca^{2+} Levels?

Ca^{2+} involvement has also been taken into consideration. It is common knowledge that calcitonin is a hypocalcemic substance (2) and a large number of reports indicate that administration of substances that cause a depletion of synaptosomal Ca^{2+} also provoke a narcotic effect (9,10,58). Furthermore, the intracerebroventricular injection of Ca ions antagonizes morphine an- algesia (49), and the injection of a Ca^{2+} chelator (e.g., EDTA, EGTA) by the same route potentiates the antinociceptive effect of morphine (50). As far as calcitonin is concerned, the finding that the analgesic effect of salmon calcitonin administered intracisternally in mice is inhibited by the simulta- neous injection of Ca^{2+} (49) is consistent with a Ca^{2+} explanation of salmon-

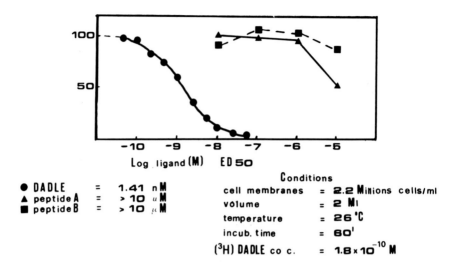

Fig. 4. ^{3}H-(Ala^2-D-Leu^5)-enkephalin (^{3}H-DADLE) binding on neuroblastoma-glioma cells. Peptide A refers to pure synthetic sCT, peptide B refers to pure porcine CT. Concentrations are indicated in the figure.

calcitonin-induced analgesia. Experiments are currently underway in our laboratory to establish if a similar occurrence also can be observed in humans.

Does Calcitonin Act on Its Own Receptors with an Analgesic Effect?

This hypothesis emerges since the analgesic effect of calcitonin cannot be completely explained on the basis of the above-mentioned hypotheses and if we take into consideration that the presence of calcitonin receptors in the CNS of rats has recently been reported (48). Although possessing a high affinity for salmon calcitonin, a molecule 50% different in amino acid composition from human calcitonin (2), these receptors show almost no affinity for human calcitonin. Does an endogenous ligand exist for salmon calcitonin receptors other than thyrocalcitonin?

The existence of an extrathyroidal calcitonin is well established (5,13,25,56). It is known that total thyroidectomy does not alter circulating levels of calcitonin (52,56) but may in some cases increase calcitonin tissue levels. Moreover, evidence has been obtained indicating that different forms of the hormone may circulate in human plasma (37). At this point it is tempting to postulate the existence of an endogenous ligand molecularly similar to salmon calcitonin but different from thyrocalcitonin, circulating in human CSF related to pain mechanisms. Moreover, the fact that CSF calcitonin in the patient with congenital indifference to pain, who shows high levels of this substance centrally, shows a different elution time from the human calcitonin standard also appears to be consistent with this hypothesis (Fig. 5).

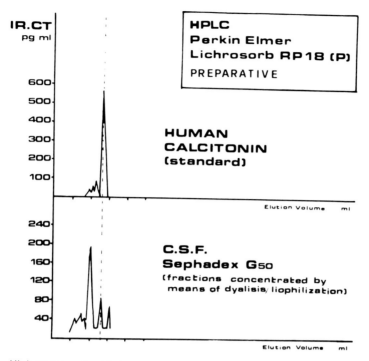

Fig. 5. High pressure liquid chromatography of CSF of the case of congenital indifference to pain described in the text. The HPLC was performed by means of reverse phase
and detected by means of RIA. Cerebrospinal fluid CT was compared in the same system
against human CT (Immunonuclear Corporation, Stillwater, Mi.).

Apart from any kind of speculation, the analgesic effect of salmon calcitonin
remains a most impressive finding. The administration of salmon calcitonin
seems to be at least as effective against pain as morphine (34) and it is
reasonable to believe that in humans, as in animals, it would not induce
dependence or addiction. Perhaps calcitonin "vestigial hormone" (2) may
offer new possibilities for the relief of human suffering.

REFERENCES

1. Accornero, N., Berardelli, A., Bini, G., Cruccu, G., and Manfredi, M. (1978): Potensiali
evocati corticali ottenuti mediante stimolazione della polpa dentaria. *Riv. Ital. EEG Neu-
rofisiol.,* 2:269–275.
2. Austin, L. A., and Heath, H. (1981): Calcitonin. *N. Eng. J. Med.,* 304:269–278.
3. Barnett, D. B., Edwards, I. R., and Smith, A. J. (1975): Antagonism by indomethacin of
diuretic response to calcitonin in man. *Br. Med. J.,* 3:686.
4. Baxter, D. W., and Olszewiski, J. (1960): Congenital universal insensitivity to pain. *Brain,*
83:381–393.
5. Becker, K. L., Snider, R. H., Moore, C. F., Monaghan, K. G., and Silva, O. L. (1979):
Calcitonin in extrathyroidal tissues of man. *Acta Endocrinol.* (Copenh.), 92:746–751.
6. Bini, G., Cruccu, G., and Manfredi, M. (1981): Acute experimental dental pain. A technique
for evaluating pain modulating procedures. *J. Neurosci. Meth.,* 3:301–309.

7. Braga, P., Ferri, S., Santagostino, A., Olgiati, V. R., and Pecile, A. (1978): Lack of opiate receptor involvement in centrally induced calcitonin analgesia. *Life Sci.*, 22:971–978.

8. Cantalamessa, L., Catania, A., Reschini, E., and Peracchi, M. (1978): Inhibitory effect of calcitonin on growth hormone and insulin secretion in man. *Metabolism*, 27:987–991.

9. Cardenas, H. L., and Ross, D. H. (1975): Morphine induced calcium depletion in discrete regions of rat brain. *J. Neurochem.*, 24:487–493.

10. Cardenas, H. L., and Ross, D. H. (1976): Calcium depletion of synaptosomes after morphine treatment. *Br. J. Pharmacol.*, 57:521–526.

11. Carman, J. S., and Wyatt, R. J. (1977): Reduction of serum prolactin after subcutaneous salmon calcitonin. *Lancet*, 1:1267–1268.

12. Carman, J. S., and Wyatt, R. J. (1979): Use of calcitonin in psychotic agitation or mania. *Arch. Gen. Psychiatry*, 36:72–78.

13. Catherwood, B. D., and Deftos, L. J. (1980): Presence by radioimmunoassay of a calcitonin-like substance in porcine pituitary glands. *Endocrinology*, 106:1886–1890.

14. Ceserani, R., Colombo, M., Olgiati, V. R., and Pecile, A. (1979): Calcitonin and prostaglandin system. *Life Sci.*, 25:1851–1856.

15. Chang, K. J., and Cuatrecasas, P. (1979): Multiple opiate receptors. *J. Biol. Chem.*, 254:2610–2618.

16. Chang, K. J., Hazum, E., and Cuatrecasas, P. (1980): Possible role of distinct morphine and enkephalin receptors in mediating actions of benzomorphan drugs (putative *k* and *o* agonists). *Proc. Natl. Acad. Sci. USA*, 77:4469–4473.

17. Chatrini, G. E., Canfield, R. C., Knauss, T. A., and Lettich, E. R. (1975): Cerebral responses to electrical tooth pulp stimulation in man. *Neurology*, 25:745–757.

18. Chen, A. C. N., and Chapman, C. R. (1980): Aspirin analgesia evaluated by event-related potentials in man: Possible central action in brain. *Exp. Brain Res.*, 39:359–364.

19. Chen, A. C. N., Chapman, C. R., and Harkins, S. W. (1979): Brain evoked potentials are functional correlates of induced pain in man. *Pain*, 6:365–374.

20. Chiarini, P., Matassi, L., and Fabrizi, G. (1978): Calcitonina e dolore somatico: Influenza dell'ormone sulla componente algogena della flogosi cutanea sperimentale da cantaridina. *Cl. Terap.*, 86:451–463.

21. Clopath, P., and Sizinger, H. (1980): Calcitonin increases porcine vascular prostacyclin formation. *Prostaglandins*, 19:1.

22. Comings, D. E., and Amromin, G. D. (1974): Autosomal dominant insensitivity to pain with hyperplastic myelinopathy and autosomal dominant indifference to pain. *Neurology*, 24:838–848.

23. Cooper, C. W. (1976): Recent advances with thyrocalcitonin. *Ann. Clin. Lab. Sci.*, 6:119–129.

24. Copp, D. H., Cockcroft, D. W., and Kuah, Y. (1961): Evidence for a new parathyroid hormone which lowers blood calcium. *Proc. Can. Federation Biol. Soc.*, 4:17.

25. Deftos, L. J., Burton, D., Bone, H. G., Catherwood, B. D., Parthemore, J. G., Moore, R. Y., Minick, S., and Guillemin, R. (1978): Immunoreactive calcitonin in the intermediate lobe of the pituitary gland. *Life Sci.*, 23:743–748.

26. Fabbri, A., Santoro, C., Moretti, C., Cappa, M., Fraioli, F., Di Julio, G. P., Galluzzi, T., and La Manna, V. (1981): The analgesic effect of calcitonin in man: Studies on the role of opioid peptides. *Clin. Pharmacol. Ther. Toxicol.*, 19:509–511.

27. Fraioli, F., Fabbri, A., Moretti, C., Santoro, C., and Isidori, A. (1981): Endogenous opioid peptides and neuroendocrine correlations in a case of congenital indifference to pain. *63rd Annual Meeting of the Endocrinology Society*. Cincinnati, Abstract 238.

28. Freed, W. J., Perlow, M. J. M., and Wyatt, R. J. (1979): Calcitonin: inhibitory effect on eating in rats. *Science*, 206:850–852.

29. Galan Galan, F., Rogers, R. M., Girgis, S. M., Arnett, T. R., Ravazzola, M., Orci, L., and MacIntyre, I. (1981): Immunochemical characterization and distribution of calcitonin in the lizard. *Acta Endocrinol. (Copenh.)*, 97:427–432.

30. Galan Galan, F., Rogers, R. M., Girgis, S. M., and MacIntyre, I. (1981): Immunoreactive calcitonin in the central nervous system of the pigeon. *Brain Res.*, 212:59–66.

31. Girgis, S. I., Galan Galan, F., Arnett, T. R., Rogers, R. M., Bone, Q., Ravazzola, M., and MacIntyre, I. (1980): Immunoreactive human calcitonin-like molecule in the nervous systems of protochordates and a cyclostome, Myxine. *J. Endocrinol*, 87:375–382.

32. Isaac, R., Merceron, R., Caillens, G., Raymond, J. P., and Ardaillou, R. (1980): Effects of calcitonin on basal and thyrotropin-releasing hormone-stimulated prolactin secretion in man. *J. Clin. Endocrinol. Metab.*, 50:1011–1015.

33. Iwasaki, Y., Chihara, K., Iwasaki, J., Abe, H., and Fujita, T. (1979): Effect of calcitonin on prolactin release in rats. *Life Sci.*, 25:1243–1248.
34. Jones, R. D. M., and Jones, J. G. (1980): intrathecal morphine: Naloxone reverses respiratory depression but not analgesia. *Br. Med. J.*, 281:645–646.
35. Kanis, J. A., Horn, D. B., Scott, R. D. M., and Strong, J. A. (1974): Treatment of Paget's disease of bone with synthetic salmon calcitonin. *Br. Med. J.*, 3:727.
36. Leicht, E., Birv, G., and Weinges, K. F. (1974): Inhibition of releasing hormone induced secretion of TSH and LH by calcitonin. *Horm. Metab. Res.*, 6:410.
37. Lumsden, J., Ham, J., and Ellison, M. L. (1980): Purification and partial characterization of high-molecular-weight forms of ectopic calcitonin from a human bronchial carcinoma cell line. *Biochem. J.*, 191:239–246.
38. Manfredi, M., Bini, G., Cruccu, G., Accornero, N., Berardelli, A., and Medolago, L. (1981): Congenital absence of pain. *Arch. Neurol.*, 38:507–511.
39. Martin, T. J. (1978): The therapeutic uses of calcitonin. *Scott. Med. J.*, 23:161–165.
40. McIntyre, I. (1978): The action and control of the calcium-regulating hormones. *J. Endocrinol. Invest.*, 1:277–284.
41. McMillan, P. J., Hooker, W. M., and Deftos, L. J. (1974): Distribution of calcitonin-containing cells in the human thyroid. *Am. J. Anat.*, 140:73–79.
42. Munson, P. L. (1976): Physiology and pharmacology of thyrocalcitonin. In: *Handbook of Physiology, Vol. 7*, edited by G. D. Aurbach, pp. 443–464. Waverly Press, Baltimore.
43. Otani, M., Noda, T., and Yamauchi, H. (1974): Isolation, chemical structure and biological properties of ultimobranchial calcitonins of the eel. In: *Proceedings of the 5th Parathyroid Conference*, edited by R. V. Talmage, M. Owen, and J. A. Parsons. pp. 111–115. Excerpta Medica, Amsterdam.
44. Pearse, A. G. E. (1969): The cytochemistry and ultrastructure of polypeptide hormone-producing cells of the APUD series. *J. Histochem. Cytochem.*, 17:303–313.
45. Pearse, A. G. E., Polak, J. M., and Van Noorden, S. (1972): The neural crest origin of the C-cells and their comparative cytochemistry and ultrastructure in the ultimobranchial gland. In: *Calcium, Parathyroid Hormone and Thyrocalcitonin*, edited by R. V. Talmage and P. L. Munson, pp. 29–40. Excerpta Medica, Amsterdam.
46. Pecile, A., Ferri, S., Braga, P. C., and Olgiati, V. R. (1975): Effects of intracerebroventricular calcitonin in the conscious rabbit. *Experientia*, 31:332–333.
47. Pecile, A., Olgiati, V. R., Luisetto, G., Guidobono, F., Netti, C., and Ziliotto, D. (1981): Calcitonin and pituitary secretion. In: *Proceedings of the International Symposium on Calcitonin*, edited by R. Decile, p. 183. Excerpta Medica, Amsterdam.
48. Rizzo, A. J., and Goltzman, D. D. (1981): Calcitonin receptors in the central nervous system of the rat. *Endocrinology*, 108:1672–1677.
49. Sattoh, M., Amano, H., Nakazawa, T., and Takagi, M. (1979): Inhibition by calcium of analgesia induced by intracisternal injection of porcine calcitonin in mice. *Res. Commun. Chem. Pathol. Pharmacol.*, 26:213.
50. Schmidt, W. K., and Leong Way, E. (1980): Hyperalgesic effects of divalent cations and antinociceptive effects of a calcium chelator in naive and morphine dependent mice. *J. Pharmacol. Exp. Ther.*, 212:22–27.
51. Scott, J., and Huskisson, E. C. (1976): Graphic representation of pain. *Pain*, 2:175–184.
52. Silva, O. L., Wisneski, L. A., Cyrus, J., Snider, R. H., Moore, C. F., and Becker, K. L. (1978): Calcitonin in thyroidectomized patients. *Am. J. Med. Sci.*, 275:159–164.
53. Sinzinger, H., Peskar, B. A., Clopath, P., Kovarik, J., Burghuber, O., Silberbauer, K., Leithner, C., and Woloszczuk, W. (1980): Calcitonin temporarily increases 6-oxo-prostaglandin $F_{1\alpha}$-levels in man. *Prostaglandins*, 20:611.
54. Steiner, D. F. (1976): Peptide hormone precursors: Biosynthesis, processing and significance. In: *Peptide Hormones*, edited by J. A. Parsons, pp. 49–65. University Park Press, Baltimore.
55. Tagliaro, F., Romanato, A., Plescia, M., and Luisetto, G. (1981): Immunoreactive calcitonin and β-endorphin in the plasma and CSF of normal subjects. In: *"RIA 81" 3rd International Symposium on Calciotropic Hormones*, edited by A. Alberini. Gardone Riviera 8–9 May, Abstract 93.
56. Watkins, W. B., Moore, R. Y., Burton, D., Bone, H. G., Catherwood, B. D., and Deftos, L. J. (1980): Distribution of immunoreactive calcitonin in the rat pituitary gland. *Endocrinology*, 106:1966–1970.

57. Wolfe, H. J., Voelkel, E. F., and Tashjian, A. H., Jr. (1974): Distribution of calcitonin-containing cells in the normal adult human thyroid gland: A correlation of morphology with peptide content. *J. Clin. Endocrinol. Metab.*, 38:688–705.
58. Yamamoto, H., Harris, R. A., Loh, H. H., and Way, E. L. (1978): Effects of acute and chronic morphine treatments on calcium localization and binding in brain. *J. Pharmacol. Exp. Ther.*, 205:255–264.
59. Yamamoto, M., Kumagai, F., Tachikawa, S., and Maeno H. (1979): Lack of effect of levallorphan on analgesia induced by intraventricular application of porcine calcitonin in mice. *Eur. J. Pharmacol.*, 55:211–213.

*Advances in Pain Research
and Therapy, Vol. 7,*
edited by C. Benedetti et al.
Raven Press, New York © 1984.

Recent Advances in Psychologic Pain Therapy

Richard A. Sternbach

Scripps Clinic and Research Foundation, La Jolla, California 92037

The deliberate use of psychologic techniques for the treatment of pain has a long past but a short history. Good doctors have always used such commonsensical psychologic methods as understanding, sympathy, encouragement, and practical advice on techniques for dealing with pain. Indeed, for many centuries, there were no other methods. Only comparatively recently have the somatic therapies of neurosurgery, nerve blocks, and analgesic drugs become available. Still more recently, in the middle of this century, the systematic application of psychologic methods to pain problems has emerged.

SOME HISTORICAL TRENDS

Perhaps the earliest deliberate use of a psychologic technique for pain control in recent times was the use of hypnosis. The review by Hilgard and Hilgard (3) of this phenomenon shows that hypnotic analgesia was used in a large series of surgical cases before the development of chemical anesthesia. Some attempt was made to explain this effect in terms of the science of the day, but no research was conducted except for the clinical application of the technique.

Freud incorporated his experience with hypnosis in hysteria into his psychoanalytic theory of neuroses. As Szasz (4) has noted, Freud did attempt to deal with the issue of pain. Szasz developed this into a more general psychoanalytic theory of pain. Whether somatic or psychologic in origin, pain was defined as the perception of a threat to the ego. If the threat were imagined or real (whether physical or mental), its perception would result in pain. If there were no perception of it, then there would be no pain, even if there were injury. The decision as to whether the pain was real or imaginary would depend on whether an observer found objective evidence of the threat. Such a decision is usually made by a physician looking for signs of a physical injury.

In the psychodynamic tradition, Engel (1) described the mechanisms of psychogenic pain in patients who repeatedly suffer painful disabilities. Such patients, he found, have excessive guilt feelings, and the experience of pain seems to serve as a punishment to relieve those feelings of guilt. Conversely, the patients appear to be intolerant of success in their lives. They repeatedly get themselves into situations or relationships in which they are hurt or defeated, and at these times their health is best. When their life situation improves, their pain returns.

This psychoanalytic approach tended to blur the differences between psychogenic and somatogenic pain. In contrast to hypnosis, which was a technique without a theory, the psychoanalytic approach to pain was a theory with no technique (except for the usual free association method). There was little to offer for the patient with, for example, causalgia or sciatica.

In the interim, behaviorism was developing in the United States as a theory to explain processes of learning, remembering, and changes in behavior. Initially founded on Pavlovian principles, it was enlarged by Skinnerian concepts of operant conditioning. Fordyce et al. (2) have applied these principles to the management of pain. They point out that behavior is governed by its consequences, and pain behavior is, likewise, enhanced or extinguished by the contingent consequence of positive or negative reinforcers. In practice, pain behaviors that are initially respondent to physical injury can be maintained by such reinforcers as, for example, bed rest, analgesics, avoidance of work, disability payments, and familial oversolicitousness. Treatment, then, consists in reversing the process, that is, failing to reinforce the pain behaviors and making the delivery of positive reinforcers contingent on the production of healthy behaviors.

SOME BASIC ASSUMPTIONS

It is obvious that any treatment of pain must be based on the implicit assumption that change is possible. Whether dealing with observable pain behaviors or subjective pain experiences, the psychologic therapies assume that these may be modified. This premise applies both to acute and to chronic pain. It also must be emphasized that the premise of modifiability applies as well to somatogenic pain as to psychogenic pain. One may infer that, if pain responses are modifiable, they must have been learned in the first instance; or, conversely, innate or nonlearned pain behaviors cannot be modified. But this inference is neither relevant nor supported by scientific evidence. All that is assumed, by the psychologic therapies, is that pain behavior can be changed.

However, the approach to this change is quite different among the therapies. There seem to be two basic schools of thought. The first, or centralist, school attempts to alter the subjective experience. This is most obvious in hypnosis, when the hypnotist suggests, for example, that the pain is another sensation, that its time course is different, or that it is in a different part of the body. When the patient perceives the pain differently, demeanor and bearing change, and the patient's voice and speech and other behaviors reflect the altered central state.

The psychodynamic therapies similarly focus on inner events. It is assumed, and case histories illustrate, that as inner conflicts or coping problems are resolved, with a relaxation of defenses, then psychogenic pain evaporates or the use of somatogenic pain as a defense mechanism becomes unnecessary. The resolution of such inner problems is reflected in changes in life-style, as invalidism or hypochondriasis associated with pain gives way to more adaptive and productive relationships.

Such orientations to pain treatment are clearly centralist in nature: alter the perception of the event and the behavior change will follow. In contrast, the peripheralist school emphasizes direct alteration of the outward behavior. This is most apparent in operant conditioning, in which pain behaviors such as downtime and drug use are targeted for modification. When the obvious pain behaviors are shaped to normal or healthy standards, the patient will become essentially indistinguishable from normals and simultaneously will experience less subjective pain.

The social modeling approaches to pain are, similarly, essentially peripheralist in nature. The emphasis is on the modifiability of pain behavior. Children acquire pain responses in a social setting, and these responses, both physiologic and behavioral, can be modified in social settings. This plasticity of pain responses is reflected in changed pain experiences and presumably is influenced by the role models to which the person is exposed.

The peripheralist philosophy is a strictly behaviorist one that was in large part influenced by the logical positivists. Only observable and measurable events are admitted as scientific data. Subjective experiences are private, not public, events and are inadmissible. Thus a phenomenon such as pain can be defined only in terms of objective and measurable behaviors, and pain reduction therefore must be a peripheral event. Whether or not a subjective experience of pain exists is both unprovable and irrelevant.

However, the behaviorists who do acknowledge the existence of subjective pain experiences actually predict that pain states will be felt as improved by patients whose pain behaviors are normalized. This follows from a principle known as "cognitive dissonance," which states that the perception of a disparity between a person's behavior and attitudes results in a tension state that produces a change in attitudes to conform to behavior. Thus a pain patient who is now active and productive and not using analgesics would find it hard to continue to think of himself as a disabled chronic pain patient and therefore would undergo a change in self-concept which included a significant reduction of pain.

It is interesting to observe that both the centralists and the peripheralists are monistic in their orientation, rather than dualistic, although in opposite directions. The centralists, at the very least, act as though pain is a mental event and outward behaviors are merely epiphenomena. The peripheralists, conversely, act as though behavior is all and mental events (if they exist) are mere epiphenomena of physical ones. Such differences, in both basic assumptions and applied methods, suggest that the centralist and peripheralist positions may be quite irreconcilable.

It is further interesting to note that these two different positions are merely the latest representatives of an ancient antagonism between two philosophies. The centralist position is in the tradition of emphasis on human spirituality and dignity, the primacy of thought and the search for truth, and (in terms of the Roman Church) the principle of salvation through faith. The peripheralist position is in the tradition of emphasis on practicality and social relationships, the primacy of performance and the search for standards, and (in ecclesiastical terms) the principle of salvation through works. Centralists emphasize insight and understanding; peripheralists emphasize training and performance. Centralists stress the uniqueness of human beings; peripheralists stress the human continuity with animals. Centralists derive hypotheses for understanding human behavior from studies of thinking and knowing; peripheralists derive hypotheses for changing human behavior from studies of animal training.

TOWARD A CONVERGENCE

Each of the two positions has seen a proliferation of derivative therapies applied to chronic pain. Gestalt therapy, transactional analysis, and autogenic training are some examples of variations on the centralist theme. Physical therapy and biofeedback are examples of peripheralist approaches.

Despite the many therapies available, program directors of pain clinics have been quite pragmatic and rather more interested in favorable outcome than in adherence to a philosophy. Accordingly both centralist and peripheralist therapies usually are represented in pain treatment programs. Most programs, for example, include group therapy as well as physical therapy, and relaxation training (either as biofeedback or as autogenics) as well as operant therapy.

Some attempt is being made now to combine the centralist and peripheralist approaches (which are basically antithetical) in a systematic way, in a system called "cognitive behavioral therapy." In this approach, an operant conditioning framework is used for the purpose of gradually extinguishing pain behaviors and substituting healthy behaviors. But, in addition, patients are deliberately taught mental strategies for dealing with pain. They are taught how to pace their activities to maximize satisfaction and minimize pain, how to relax, how to think differently about pain sensations (i.e., to interpret pain differently), and how to perceive themselves more in control of the pain than victims of it.

This cognitive behavioral approach, if properly applied by well-trained therapists, may enhance the probability of successful outcome in pain programs. It ensures that the benefits of both centralist and peripheralist techniques are applied to pain patients, and so maximizes their opportunity for improvement. It does make difficult the possibility of isolating the necessary and sufficient psychologic treatment for pain control, as several therapies are occurring at the same time. However, in terms of offering the most helpful practical treatment program to those with chronic pain, the cognitive behavioral therapy is a new and promising approach. After all, it is more important to help the patients than to prove a theory. Only future outcome studies will be able to compare this technique with others.

REFERENCES

1. Engel, G. C. (1959): "Psychogenic" pain and the pain-prone patient. *Am. J. Med.*, 26:899–918.
2. Fordyce, W. E., Fowler, R. S., Jr., Lehmann, J. F., and DeLateur, B. J. (1968): Some implications of learning in problems of chronic pain. *J. Chronic Dis.*, 21:179–190.
3. Hilgard, E. R., and Hilgard, J. R. (1975): *Hypnosis in the Relief of Pain*. William Kaufmann, Los Altos, Calif.
4. Szasz, T. S. (1957): *Pain and Pleasure: A Study of Bodily Feelings*. Basic Books, New York.

Advances in Pain Research
and Therapy, Vol. 7,
edited by C. Benedetti et al.
Raven Press, New York © 1984.

Evaluating Psychologic Interventions for Chronic Pain: Issues and Recent Developments

Judith A. Turner and Joan M. Romano

Pain Center, Department of Psychiatry and Behavioral Sciences, University of Washington, Seattle, Washington 98195

With the widespread acknowledgment that traditional medical techniques are all too often ineffective in relieving chronic pain (39,57,60) and that psychosocial variables seem in many cases to influence the persistence of chronic pain problems (19,55), there has been a growing application of psychologic treatments to these disorders. A rapid proliferation of pain clinics established to evaluate and treat chronic pain has occurred internationally (although particularly in the United States), and psychologists and psychologic interventions commonly are used in these settings.

In 1982, Turner and Chapman (60,61) reviewed the literature related to studies of various psychologic interventions for chronic pain. Such treatments were grouped according to the basic underlying concepts. Biofeedback and relaxation training were categorized as physiologic methods because they emphasize the control of physiologic factors believed to be involved in causing pain. Operant conditioning techniques, which aim to decrease learned pain behaviors by modifying the environmental consequences of the patient's actions, formed a second group. The third classification, cognitive-behavioral, included hypnosis and cognitive-behavioral therapies, which emphasize the role of cognitive factors in pain experience and behavior. (The reader is referred to the 1982 review for further details concerning underlying concepts and descriptions of these interventions.) The 1982 review (60,61) summarized and critically assessed studies evaluating relaxation training, biofeedback, operant conditioning techniques, hypnosis, and cognitive-behavioral therapies for chronic pain. A number of conclusions were drawn, and guidelines and directions for further research were suggested.

As the growth of research in this area is accelerating, it is now time to reevaluate the status of current knowledge and to appraise the major tasks that remain before proceeding further. This chapter will focus on selected treatment outcome studies that have been published since the 1982 review was prepared, emphasizing those that illustrate innovations in assessment and research design, as well as continuing methodologic issues. Suggestions for future research directions will be made. We will not review multidisciplinary multimodal treatment outcome studies in which the unique effects of psychologic interventions cannot be determined. This review also will be confined to studies using adult patients with nonmalignant chronic pain problems.

RELAXATION TRAINING

The use of relaxation techniques in the treatment of chronic pain is predicated on the assumption that high levels of muscle tension cause or exacerbate symptoms in a number of common pain syndromes (e.g., tension headache, low back pain, myofascial pain). Most commonly, relaxation training has used variations around the progressive muscle tensing and relaxing strategy first developed by Jacobson (32). However, autogenic training, which involves imagination of physiologic sensations of relaxation, also has been applied to chronic pain problems (4). As Turner and Chapman (60) noted, most investigations of relaxation training for chronic pain have been conducted with tension headache sufferers. Most of these studies found that relaxation produces significant reductions in headache frequency in a large proportion of patients and is generally as effective as electromyographic (EMG) biofeedback in the alleviation of headache symptoms.

As can be seen in Table 1, results of recent studies have not altered these conclusions and indicate that positive treatment effects generally are maintained at follow-up (14,44). One study (45) comparing EMG feedback and relaxation training at 1-year follow-up found that the continued practice of relaxation was the variable most highly associated with long-term success in controlling headache activity.

In a recent review of the headache treatment literature, Blanchard and Andrasik (8) reported that, across studies, the average percentage of improvement in tension headache patients treated by relaxation training has been 60%. They also concluded, given the number of studies done and consistency of results, that further direct comparison studies of relaxation training to no treatment or to EMG biofeedback alone have little utility.

A major focus of recent research has been on whether relaxation training can be enhanced by the addition of other strategies. For example, Philips and Hunter (44) compared progressive muscle relaxation training plus the use of imagery to relaxation alone in treating chronic tension headaches in a group of psychiatric patients. Headache activity was significantly decreased in both groups after treatment and at 6- to 8-week follow-up. There was no significant difference between conditions. Anderson et al. (4) compared autogenic relaxation training alone and "cognitive coping therapy" alone to a combination of these two approaches in 14 tension headache sufferers. Using a within-subjects design, these authors found that both treatments, alone or in combination, were highly effective in reducing self-monitored reports of headache activity. There seemed to be little additional benefit from the combined treatment, although in some cases further improvement occurred when coping skills and relaxation were used in conjunction. Turner (59) also compared progressive relaxation training with combined cognitive-behavioral therapy and relaxation training. This study is described in detail under the cognitive-behavioral section. In brief, both conditions, administered in an outpatient group format, were found to be effective in decreasing self-reported chronic back pain and associated problems, with some superiority of the combined condition over relaxation training alone in affecting certain measures.

The impact of other variables, such as treatment setting, on the efficacy of relaxation also has been examined. Home-based training using audiotapes was compared to traditional clinic-administered progressive muscle relaxation in a study of 35 patients with tension headache (58). If comparable effects could be obtained, the obvious advantages of decreased time and cost and increased convenience would argue for the implementation of home-based programs. The investigators found that both groups achieved significant and comparable degrees of improvement in headache activity (a composite measure reflecting frequency, duration, and intensity of headache). However, the clinic-based group showed a substantially lower rate of clinically significant improvement (only 23.5% of the group attained greater than 50% reduction in headache activity) than is ordinarily found in studies of clinic-administered relaxation, for reasons that were not clear. Thus further research comparing home- and clinic-based programs is needed before more definitive conclusions can be drawn as to the feasibility and efficacy of self-administered relaxation for this population.

A few recent reports of relaxation training for pain problems other than headache have appeared. Varni (64,65), in a series of systematic single-subject studies, has evaluated a package combining progressive relaxation, meditative breathing, and guided imagery in treating chronic arthritic pain secondary to hemophilia. Subjects showed substantial improvement in arthritic pain ratings and sleep, but not in episodes of bleeding or pain at times of bleeding. An interesting feature of these studies is the use of skin temperature measurement at a painful joint site as a means of independently assessing the efficacy of the treatment in producing physiologic changes. The guided imagery was constructed to help subjects imagine increased warmth and blood flow in painful arthritic joints, but no feedback was given to subjects during the treatment. All subjects showed increases in skin temperature at posttreatment testing, as well as decreased pain ratings. However, the use of multiple treatment techniques in combination prevents the assessment of the relative contributions of each.

TABLE 1. *Relaxation training: Experimental designs, populations, and treatment outcomes*

Author (ref.)	Population	N	Intervention(s)	Design	Control	Dependent measures	Follow-up	Results
Anderson et al. (4)	Tension headache	14	1. Autogenic relaxation 2. Cognitive coping skills 3. Combination of 1 and 2	Single subject	Multiple base line	Self-recorded headache frequency, intensity, duration	7 mo	All conditions generally equally effective in reducing headache activity
Cott et al. (14)			See under Biofeedback					
Philips and Hunter (44)	Tension headache (psychiatric patients)	16	1. Progressive muscle relaxation 2. Progressive muscle relaxation and imagery	Group outcome	None	Self-recorded headache frequency, duration, medication use; McGill Pain Questionnaire; Wakefield Depression Scale; pain complaint/ avoidance scale; EMG recordings; perceptions of treatment credibility and self-efficacy	6–8 wk	Both groups significantly improved in headache frequency, duration, McGill, pain complaint/ avoidance; no group differences; gains maintained at follow-up
Varni (64)	Arthritic pain secondary to hemophilia	3	Progressive muscle relaxation plus meditative	Single Subject	Multiple base line across subjects	Self-rated pain, mobility, sleep, medication use, bleeding	7–14 mo	All subjects substantially improved in pain, mobility,

Study	N	Condition	Treatment	Design	Measures	Follow-up	Results
			breathing and guided imagery		episodes; skin temperature recordings		sleep ratings, and increased skin temperature; gains maintained at follow-up
Varni (65)	2	Arthritic pain secondary to hemophilia	Progressive muscle relaxation plus meditative breathing and guided imagery	Single Subject Abbreviated multiple base line across subjects	Self-rated pain; skin temperature recordings	8 mo	Both subjects improved on pain ratings and increased skin temperature; gains maintained at follow-up
Turner (59)			See under Cognitive-Behavioral Therapies				
Teders et al. (58)	35	Tension headache	1. Home-based progressive muscle relaxation 2. Clinic-based progressive muscle relaxation	Group Outcome	Self-recorded headache frequency, intensity, duration; EMG recordings; MMPI, Beck Depression Inventory, State-Trait Anxiety, Buss-Durkee Hostility	None	Both groups significantly improved on headache activity with no difference between conditions

EMG = electromyograph; MMPI = Minnesota Multiphasic Personality Inventory.

BIOFEEDBACK

Biofeedback studies also have focused primarily on the treatment of chronic headache pain and have used several major treatment variants for different types of headache. Most common are (a) EMG feedback, which is aimed at decreasing levels of muscle tension, most often at frontal, temporal, or neck sites; (b) cephalic blood volume pulse (BVP) feedback, which targets reduction of blood flow in the cephalic temporal artery; and (c) thermal biofeedback, usually designed to increase skin temperature in fingers. Thermal and BVP procedures have been applied primarily to migraine headaches on the basis of the unproven assumption that this syndrome is associated with excessive cranial vasculature responsivity and that an increase in peripheral temperature and blood flow, or a decrease in cephalic blood flow, should decrease the cranial artery vasodilation believed to be associated with the headache. Electromyographic techniques have been applied primarily to tension (muscle contraction) headache, although some studies have examined the effects of EMG feedback on migraine as well as other problems, such as low back pain.

Turner and Chapman (60) concluded that the consensus of research at that time indicated a substantial treatment effect for biofeedback in the amelioration of migraine and tension headache. However, they also identified a number of areas of concern. First, biofeedback did not seem overall to be superior to relaxation training, a simpler and less expensive form of treatment. Second, the rationale and procedure of biofeedback could lead to overly simplistic notions of the nature of chronic pain conditions. Psychologic and behavioral factors contributing to the maintenance of pain can be overlooked if the focus of treatment remains strictly on the regulation of physiologic processes without embedding such training in the context of an overall management approach to stress, environmental reinforcers of pain behaviors, and other life problems.

Further, the reported efficacy of biofeedback for headache has not been demonstrated convincingly to be the result of the putative mechanisms on which it is based. Specifically, alterations in EMG levels of muscles in the head and neck, and in cerebral artery blood flow, generally have not been found to be strongly correlated with headache activity. Also, the biofeedback procedure often incorporates relaxation, thus confounding the effects of the two interventions. Turner and Chapman (60) and other reviewers (8) have questioned whether the effects of biofeedback are due to the acquisition of increased control over physiologic processes or rather are primarily the result of relaxation, or increased perceptions of self-efficacy, or other factors not assumed to be its "active ingredients."

Since the publication of that review, much has been done in the way of addressing a number of these issues. More progress has been made in researching the specific mechanisms and effects of biofeedback than with other psychologic interventions for pain. Some particularly interesting recent advances in research design and analysis will be highlighted toward the end of this section. To facilitate the organization of this complex area, studies of treatment outcome will be presented according to the type of pain problem addressed. Table 2 summarizes selected recent studies of biofeedback with each syndrome.

Tension Headache

A number of recent studies have examined the relation of EMG levels and procedural variations in training methods to treatment outcome in tension headache patients. Significant clinical improvement was noted in headache activity in several of these studies after biofeedback (15,26,51); however, studies that assessed EMG levels found no significant association between muscle tension levels and headache measures (15,24,26,43), consistent with the earlier results of Andrasik and Holroyd (5).

Variations in training techniques have been aimed at determining optimally effective procedures or elucidating the specific active components of biofeedback. For example, Hart and Cichanski (26) compared the effects of 15 sessions of frontalis muscle EMG feedback to an equivalent course of EMG feedback from neck muscles. They found significant decreases in headache activity for both, with significantly reduced medication consumption also reported for the latter condition. However, neither group showed a significant change in EMG levels and the correlations between these measures and headache activity were not significant.

Another study (15) used a very short course (three sessions) of EMG biofeedback in systematically analyzing the specific and nonspecific components of this intervention. Two feedback conditions (one with instructions to decrease muscle tension and the other to maintain tension levels) were compared to a condition in which patients were given relaxation and meditation with noncontingent feedback and to a headache-monitoring control group. Only the two feedback conditions produced significant reductions in headache activity, with the group instructed to lower tension also achieving significant reductions in EMG levels. Again, muscle tension measures and headache activity were unrelated. The meditation-relaxation group did not significantly improve, leading the author to conclude that the feedback information was crucial to the establishment of regulatory control over the neuromusculature, but that the method by which this control was established (increases or maintenance) was of less importance.

Gray et al. (24) compared the efficacy of biofeedback monitored from a site corresponding to the source of pain to that monitored from an unrelated site. A relaxation-only condition also was included. They found that EMG levels had not changed significantly at posttreatment testing, although within-session changes had been observed. Headache frequency was reduced significantly for the sample as a whole, primarily due to the response

TABLE 2. Biofeedback: Experimental designs, populations, and treatment outcomes

Author (ref.)	Population	N	Intervention(s)	Design	Control	Dependent measures	Follow-up	Results
Cram (15)	Tension headache	32	Compared: 1. EMG feedback to lower muscle tension level 2. EMG feedback to maintain muscle tension level 3. Meditation with non-contingent feedback 4. Headache monitoring	Group outcome	1. Meditation with non-contingent feedback 2. Headache monitoring	Self-recorded headache frequency, intensity; EMG recordings; State-Trait Anxiety, Manifest Anxiety Scales; MMPI	6 mo	Groups 1 and 2 significantly decreased headache activity. Group 2 maintained gains at follow-up; changes in EMG levels unrelated to headache measures
Gray et al. (24)	Tension headache	15	1. EMG feedback at site of pain 2. EMG feedback at a nonpainful site 3. Relaxation	Group outcome	Relaxation tapes	Self-recorded headache frequency, intensity, duration, and medication use; EMG recordings	1–6 mo	Relaxation group had significant decreases in headache frequency, intensity; no effects for BFB; at follow-up, no group differences, and gains maintained only for subjects with forehead as opposed to occipital pain.

Study	Headache type	N	Treatment	Outcome	Control	Measures	Follow-up	Results
Schlutter et al. (51)			See under Hypnosis					
Cott et al. (14)	Tension headache	8	1. EMG feedback and relaxation 2. Relaxation and noncontingent feedback	Group outcome	Relaxation and noncontingent feedback	Self-recorded headache location, intensity, duration and medication use	1 yr	Both groups were significantly improved at posttest in headache duration and severity; no group differences at posttest or at follow-up
Hart and Cichanski (26)	Tension headache	20	1. EMG feedback at frontal site 2. EMG feedback at neck site	Group outcome	None	Self-recorded headache frequency, duration, intensity, medication use; EMG recordings	6–12 mo	Both groups significantly decreased headache activity at posttest; only Group 2 significantly reduced medication use; EMG changes unrelated to headache measures

continued

TABLE 2. *Continued*

Author (ref.)	Population	N	Intervention(s)	Design	Control	Dependent measures	Follow-up	Results
Kremsdorf et al. (37)	Tension headache		See under Cognitive-Behavioral Therapies					
Philips and Hunter (43)	Tension headache (Psychiatric patients)	16	1. EMG feedback to lower muscle tension levels 2. EMG feedback to raise/maintain muscle tension levels	Group outcome	EMG feedback to raise/maintain tension levels	Self-recorded headache frequency, intensity, duration, and medication use; McGill Pain Questionnaire; EMG recordings; Wakefield Depression Scale; Pain Behavior Checklist	6–8 wk	No significant improvement in headache measures or McGill for either group; lower EMG levels in Group 1 posttreatment but no relationship between EMG and headache
Reinking and Hutchings (45)	Tension headache	18	Follow-up of study comparing: 1. Relaxation 2. EMG feedback 3. Relaxation and EMG feedback	Group outcome	None	Self-recorded headache activity and medication use; EMG recordings	12 mo	Overall treatment and group effects washed out; continued success related to home practice of relaxation
Holroyd and Andrasik (29)			See under Cognitive-Behavioral Therapies					

Study	Condition	N	Treatment	Outcome	Control	Measures	Follow-up	Results
Cohen et al. (13)	Migraine headache	42	1. Thermal BFB for forehead cooling 2. EMG feedback 3. Alpha EEG feedback 4. BVP feedback	Group outcome	None	Self-recorded headache frequency, intensity, duration, and disability; EMG, forehead temperature, heart rate, skin conduction, finger pulse amplitude recordings	8 mo	All groups showed significant and comparable reduction in headache frequency; other headache measures unchanged; deterioration for alpha training group noted at follow-up; physiological measures unrelated to outcome
Kewman and Roberts (35)	Migraine headache	34	1. Thermal BFB-hand warming 2. Thermal BFB-hand cooling 3. Headache recording	Group outcome	Headache recording only—no treatment	Self-recordings of headache frequency, duration, symptoms, impairment, and medications; finger temperature	6 wk	All three groups showed significant decreases in number of symptoms, impairment, and medication use; groups did not differ

continued

TABLE 2. *Continued*

Author (ref.)	Population	N	Intervention(s)	Design	Control	Dependent measures	Follow-up	Results
Elmore and Tursky (17)	Migraine headache	23	1. Thermal BFB-hand warming 2. Temporal BVP reduction	Group outcome	None	Self-recordings of headache frequency, duration, and psychophysically scaled ratings of pain intensity, reactivity and sensation, and medication use; finger and temporal pulse amplitude, hand temperature	None	BVP group superior to thermal in rating of pain sensation and reactivity and medication use; BVP group significantly improved on headache frequency and medication use and pain sensation; no significant improvement for thermal group
Gauthier et al. (22)	Migraine headache	24	1. Thermal BFB-hand warming 2. Thermal BFB-hand cooling 3. Thermal BFB-temple warming 4. Thermal BFB-temple cooling	Group outcome	None	Self-recordings of headache frequency, intensity, and duration, medication use, skin temperature at hand and temple; ratings of treatment credibility	6 mo	Significant reduction in number and duration of headaches and medication use; no differences among groups; gains generally maintained at follow-up

Study	Headache type	N	Treatment	Design		Measures		Results
Allen and Mills (2)	Migraine headache	8	BVP feedback	Single group outcome	None	BVP recordings at temporal artery and finger, pain estimates	None	Significant changes in BVP posttraining and during migraine attack; pain ratings significantly decreased by constriction but not dilation instructions
Blanchard et al. (11)	Tension, migraine, and combined headache	30	Progressive muscle relaxation, then EMG or thermal feedback	Group outcome	None	Self-recorded headache frequency, duration, intensity, and medication use; MMPI, Beck Depression Inventory, State-Trait Anxiety Inventory, EMG recordings	None	36% of tension and 44% of vascular headache nonresponders to relaxation improved significantly in headache activity after BFB

continued

TABLE 2. *Continued*

Author (ref.)	Population	N	Intervention(s)	Design	Control	Dependent measures	Follow-up	Results
Blanchard et al. (10)	Tension, migraine, and combined headache	91	Progressive muscle relaxation, then EMG or thermal feedback	Group outcome	None	Self-recorded headache frequency, duration, intensity, and medication use; MMPI, Beck Depression Inventory, State-Trait Anxiety Inventory, Rathus Assertiveness Schedule, Psychosomatic Symptom Checklist; Social Readjustment Rating Scale; EMG recordings	None	52% of tension and 22–30% of vascular patients rated "much improved" after relaxation training; BFB led to an additional 20% of tension and 25% of vascular groups "much improved," psychological tests significantly predicted outcome

Study	Condition	N	Treatment	Design	Measures	Control	Follow-up	Results
Nouwen and Solinger (42)	Chronic low back pain	25	1. EMG feedback 2. Waiting list—no treatment	Group outcome	Paraspinal EMG recordings; pain ratings	Waiting list control	3 mo	Significant decreases in EMG levels and pain ratings with feedback, but not in control condition; at follow-up, pain ratings but not EMG levels remained reduced
Dougherty (16)	Phantom limb pain	1	EMG feedback	Case report	Self-reported pain	None	5 wk	Decreased pain reported for 3 weeks following treatment; return of symptoms at 5-week follow-up
Achterberg et al. (1)	Rheumatoid arthritis	Study 1: 24	1. Relaxation plus thermal BFB-finger warming 2. Relaxation plus thermal BFB-finger cooling	Group outcome	ADL; Subjective Units of Discomfort; self-reported sleep, work, leisure time, pain hours; Profile of Mood States; walking time	None	None	Both groups reported significantly less discomfort, more sleep; no group differences

continued

TABLE 2. *Continued*

Author (ref.)	Population	N	Intervention(s)	Design	Control	Dependent measures	Follow-up	Results
		Study 2: 23	1. Thermal biofeedback 2. Physiotherapy	Group outcome	None	Same as above	None	Both groups significantly improved on walking time, ADLs; BFB more than physiotherapy in sleep and work time improvement
Wolf et al. (67)	Chronic low back pain	1	EMG feedback in static and dynamic activity	Single subject	Reversals to baseline condition	Paraspinal EMG recordings; McGill Pain Questionnaire	None	Clinically significant pain reduction during feedback phases; improvement in pattern of EMG activity during movement

EMG = electromyograph; BFB = biofeedback; BVP = blood volume pulse; EEG = electroencephalogram; MMPI = Minnesota Multiphasic Personality Inventory; ADL = activities of daily living.

of the relaxation group, which was the most improved. Intensity of headache was significantly lower in the relaxation group than in either of the biofeedback conditions at posttreatment testing. Of particular interest is the fact that EMG levels recorded from subjects as they were experiencing headaches during regular assessment sessions were not significantly different from nonheadache values. Although this study suffers from some limitations, such as the great diversity in the sample in pretest levels of headache symptomatology and questionable analysis of results, the findings that direct versus indirect feedback did not differ and that EMG levels did not covary with the reports of headache activity do not support the usual rationale for conducting biofeedback.

Philips and Hunter (43) assessed the efficacy of six sessions of EMG biofeedback for psychiatric patients with tension headache and elevated levels of muscle tension. Subjects were divided into two groups: those trained to decrease muscle tension and those instructed to maintain or raise EMG levels. They found that headache activity level as measured by self-monitoring diaries was not improved significantly by either treatment, nor were McGill Pain Questionnaire scores. A significant reduction in resting EMG level was found only in the group trained to decrease levels of muscle tension, but this was not associated with decreased pain or headache activity. The lack of clinical success in decreasing headache symptoms is at variance with most findings in this area (9) and possibly may have been associated with the fact that the subjects were psychiatric patients. A number were depressed, a factor found elsewhere to be associated with poor response to treatment (10).

Thus procedural variations in site of feedback and in instructions to subjects to lower or maintain tension levels seem to have little effect on outcome. The finding that decreased muscle tension does not seem to mediate improvement in headaches requires the generation and testing of alternate hypotheses for the effects of EMG feedback in relieving tension headaches. Areas to explore include enhancement of self-efficacy and awareness of antecedents to headache (8).

Migraine Headache

Previous reviewers (9,60) have concluded that a substantial proportion of migraine headache sufferers benefit to a significant degree from both thermal and BVP feedback training. However, as with EMG feedback, issues of comparative efficacy of different procedures and isolation of specific treatment mechanisms only recently have been addressed.

A persistent and puzzling finding in the literature is that changes in physiologic measures are unrelated to migraine headache activity (5,18). Recent studies of biofeedback training for migraine have continued to find positive treatment effects but little or no relation between physiologic recordings and outcome (13,17), just as physiologic factors have been observed to be unrelated to tension headache measures.

One interesting study (2) assessed the efficacy of bidirectional (increasing and decreasing) BVP training and examined the relation of patients' ability to demonstrate control over these responses to pain ratings while experiencing a migraine attack. Eight female migraine patients were trained to increase and decrease BVP as measured both from temporal artery and finger sites. Subjects then were assessed while experiencing a headache and were found to be able to produce significant increases and decreases in BVP under these conditions. Subjective pain ratings were significantly lower under instructions to decrease rather than increase BVP. In addition, the correlation between pain and actual BVP measurements were positive and highly significant. These results provide one of the few demonstrations that ability to influence selected physiologic processes during migraine headache is associated with changes in reported pain. The authors note that they selected subjects who described themselves as having no familiarity with biologic theories of migraine production and thus would not be biased in their reports of pain while increasing or decreasing BVP, but this possibility needs to be considered as an alternate explanation. These results also need to be replicated with a larger sample, and bidirectional BVP training compared to other treatments to assess further its effects on *in vivo* headache pain.

Attempts to determine the active ingredients of thermal biofeedback have compared hand warming training to hand cooling, a parallel task that presumably would control for the nonspecific effects of training. Several investigations (22,35) have found both hand warming and cooling biofeedback to decrease migraine headache activity and to be equally effective in doing so. Even when significant training effects in the targeted physiologic responses are obtained, these changes are virtually unrelated to headache activity (35). These results have been interpreted as providing support for the hypothesis that nonspecific factors are responsible for the efficacy of biofeedback (35). However, an interesting alternate hypothesis has been set forth by Gauthier et al. (22). Rather than attributing this lack of difference to the nonspecific "placebo" effects of biofeedback, they suggest that the hand warming and cooling conditions may both be "active" treatments that can increase patients' ability to gain control over and stabilize peripheral vasomotor activity, irrespective of the direction of targeted change. Thus it may be worthwhile to assess not only the magnitude of change in any direction from base line, but also the variability of responses to evaluate the relation of physiologic stabilization to headache activity.

Tension, Migraine, and Mixed Headache

Blanchard and colleagues (8–11) have conducted extensive research on the psychologic treatment of chronic headache, including tension, migraine, mixed (combined tension and migraine), and cluster types, the latter two representing underresearched populations. They have recently published a number of reports notable for their innovations and sophistication in methodology and statistical analysis. These will therefore be highlighted for the contributions they make toward resolving some issues previously raised.

Although controlled comparisons of biofeedback and relaxation have demonstrated fairly conclusively their comparable efficacy in decreasing headache activity, Blanchard et al. (9) argue that before concluding that the two interventions work in the same manner (e.g., by producing relaxation responses) or that there is little utility for biofeedback training, it is necessary to examine whether patients who fail to respond to relaxation might in fact demonstrate improvement when subsequently given biofeedback. Should this be the case, it may be argued that the treatments have different mechanisms of action or that, for some patients, the addition of feedback may be necessary to produce significant improvement.

Blanchard et al. (10,11) therefore conducted a series of studies in which headache subjects were treated first with relaxation training. Those who did not achieve at least a 60% reduction in headache activity were then treated with biofeedback. Tension headache patients were assigned to frontalis EMG feedback, and migraine and mixed headache patients were given skin temperature biofeedback. About 40% of those subjects who did not significantly improve after relaxation training did have a greater than 60% reduction in headaches compared to base line after treatment with biofeedback (11). To determine if continued response to the earlier relaxation training was responsible for these later improvements, data were reanalyzed excluding subjects who had shown a 10% or greater reduction in headache activity after relaxation. This smaller group of nonresponders exhibited a trend toward improvement after biofeedback, but this did not reach significance. The successful and unsuccessful responders to biofeedback of either type did not differ significantly in the degree to which either EMG level or hand temperature was altered. Response to EMG biofeedback, however, was related significantly to pretreatment depression and headache severity. Response to thermal biofeedback was related significantly to scores on the Hysteria scale of the Minnesota Multiphasic Personality Inventory (MMPI) (11).

In a larger scale study (10) using the same design, 91 patients (33 tension, 30 migraine, and 28 mixed) were evaluated with particular attention to delineating pretest variables predictive of response to each intervention. A significant reduction in headache activity was found for the sample as a whole after relaxation. Even so, only 52% of the tension headache sample and 26% of the vascular patients could be rated as much improved (more than 50% reduction in headache activity). Thus 59 patients entered either EMG or thermal biofeedback training according to headache type. Headache activity was decreased significantly in the tension and combined headache groups compared to postrelaxation levels and in all three groups when compared to base-line data. In addition, the proportion of patients rated as much improved after both treatments reached 73% of the tension group, 50% of the migraine group, and 54% of the mixed group. Finally, factors predicting treatment response were examined with multivariate statistical techniques. At least 72% of each headache group was classified correctly as to successful or unsuccessful outcome by a linear function of their pretest scores on selected psychologic measures.

The practical value of such prediction studies, of course, lies in their potential to facilitate selection of optimal interventions from information easily obtainable before treatment. These results can be regarded as only preliminary steps in this direction. More extensive work is needed, replicating these findings with a large sample size and cross-validating the predictive power of particular tests with different samples of patients. Also, these results do not address the prediction of long-term outcome, as no follow-up data were presented. These authors report that such data will in fact be collected.

This series of studies, although not designed to provide a definitive comparison of biofeedback and relaxation, did demonstrate that a substantial proportion of headache sufferers, especially those with vascular headaches, can benefit from biofeedback after a course of relaxation training. More importantly, these studies seem to point the field of headache research in a promising direction, not only toward determining efficacy of treatments, but also toward developing empirically based systems for assigning patients with particular types of pain and psychologic characteristics to optimal treatment choices.

Other Pain Syndromes

The paucity of controlled studies applying biofeedback to painful conditions other than headache noted by Turner and Chapman (60) persists. Although a few reports (1,16) have appeared, most have been uncontrolled and suffer from other methodologic shortcomings such as poor outcome measures or inappropriate statistical analysis of data. Therefore, additional research is needed in order to evaluate the utility of biofeedback training for these pain problems. This situation is puzzling given the widespread use of biofeedback in pain clinics and raises the suspicion that the lack of published reports reflects inability to achieve successful results.

Recently some innovative research in the use of EMG biofeedback for chronic low back pain patients has been reported by Wolf et al. (67). By gathering normative data on EMG levels in the paraspinal muscles during static and dynamic activity, they were able to document the existence of abnormal patterning of muscle activity during movement in chronic back pain patients. Preliminary results of a single case study using EMG feedback during movement training indicated that changes in EMG activity in the direction of normalization of these patterns was associated with reductions in McGill Pain Questionnaire scores. This method is interesting and worthy of further investigation.

OPERANT CONDITIONING

Developed by Fordyce, the operant conditioning approach and its theoretical rationale have been described in detail (19). Based on learning theory, this treatment focuses on decreasing learned (operant) pain behaviors and increasing behaviors inconsistent with the sick role. Toward this end, behaviors to be increased and decreased are defined, and reinforcers are identified and manipulated so that rewards are contingent on performance of desired behaviors; pain-behaviors are not rewarded (contingency management). Operant conditioning programs typically include a number of active components, including physical and occupational therapy, medication reduction, vocational counseling, biofeedback, and psychologic counseling, as well as training staff and family members to ignore pain-behaviors and reward well-behaviors (19).

Turner and Chapman (61) concluded that reports of inpatient operant conditioning programs suggest their effectiveness in increasing activity levels and decreasing medication use, and that there was some evidence of maintenance of such improvements at long-term follow-ups. However, Turner and Chapman (61) also noted that because these studies were uncontrolled, and interventions were multimodal, little could be concluded as to the contributions of contingency management versus those of other program components and nonspecific factors in modifying pain behaviors. A further problem was the careful selection of patients for such programs, resulting in limited generalizability of results.

Surprisingly few outcome studies of operant conditioning approaches have been published since the Turner and Chapman (61) review (Table 3). Positive results at 6 months to 3 years of follow-up were reported by one group (40). Forty patients who completed an inpatient pain management program of occupational and physical therapy, medication reduction, contingency management, and skills training in management of anxiety, depression, insomnia, and pain were mailed questionnaires; 32 responded. The percentage of patients using narcotics, nonnarcotic analgesics, and minor tranquilizers, although increased since discharge, was markedly less at follow-up compared to admission. Forty-eight percent rated their pain as decreased after the program. No patients had been employed or in training at admission, in contrast to 47% at follow-up. Such findings are certainly encouraging, but their significance is vitiated by the self-report nature and limited scope of assessment, lack of control condition, and lack of information concerning selection criteria for the program and rate of attrition.

In an article innovative in both research design and concept, Fordyce et al. (20) presented a single-subject study of a young man with abdominal pain,

TABLE 3. *Operant treatment programs: Experimental designs, populations, and treatment outcomes*

Author (ref.)	Population	N	Intervention(s)	Design	Control	Dependent measures	Follow-up	Results
Malec et al. (40)	Not specified ("benign organic pain")	32	Inpatient program with occupational and physical therapy, medication reduction, pain behavior reduction, and training in anxiety, depression, insomnia, and pain management	Group outcome	None	Questionnaire mailed at follow-up	6 mo–3 yr	Decreased use of medications; 48% reported pain decrease; 70% reported better mood; increased employment/training in 47%
Fordyce et al. (20)	Abdominal pain, dizziness	1	Systematic walking program, instructions to patient's mother to ignore "sick" behaviors and support walking, vocational counseling	Systematic single subject	None	Walking speed and distance, self-recorded activity and pain levels	21 mo	Improved ambulation, activity level, pain

Holzman et al. (30)	Low back pain	3	10 session outpatient program based on Fordyce (19)	Case studies	None	McGill Pain Questionnaire, State-Trait Anxiety Inventory, Beck Depression Inventory, Health Locus of Control, Locke-Wallace Marital Adjustment Scale, Pain Behavior Checklist	None	All showed some improvement; nature and extent of change variable
Sanders (49)	Low back pain	4	Base line, followed by 4 treatments given sequentially, and in different order for each subject: "functional pain-behavioral analysis training," relaxation training, assertion training, social reinforcement of activity	Multiple base line single subject	Multiple base line	Medication use, uptime, pain ratings	None	All treatments except functional pain-behavioral analysis led to improvement, and differentially affected dependent variables

dizziness, and gait disturbance. With the goal of nondistorted ambulation, a program was designed in which systematically increasing daily quotas of walking were assigned. The patient had the option of walking the assigned distance at a predetermined speed or walking twice the assigned distance at his own pace. A psychologist met regularly with the patient and his mother, who was instructed to ignore "immobilization behaviors" and encourage progress in ambulation. Vocational counseling also was given. The patient was able to ambulate freely at the end of treatment, and concurrent with progress in ambulation, there were decreases in self-recorded downtime at home and in reported pain severity. A 21-month follow-up revealed maintenance of treatment gains, with no further treatment required.

This study is commendable in its conceptual development, research design, and assessment of generalization and posttreatment maintenance of improvement. Although single-subject designs do have limitations, this study illustrates how they can be applied usefully to chronic pain treatment evaluations.

Although not strictly a treatment outcome study, another study is worthy of mention because of its innovative design. With the goal of assessing the effectiveness of single behavioral interventions in an inpatient pain treatment program, Sanders (49) assigned each of 4 low back pain patients who had already demonstrated improvement with treatment to a different base-line length. After base line, each subject received four different treatments in a different order. Each patient received five 1-hr sessions each of "functional pain-behavioral analysis training," progressive relaxation training, assertion training, and social reinforcement of increased activity level. Dependent measures were medication intake, uptime, and reported pain intensity. Sanders concluded that social reinforcement of increased activity primarily affected uptime, with slightly lesser effects on pain ratings and medication use and with a lesser effect on uptime. This use of a multiple base-line design is helpful in establishing that improvement is a function of treatment. As Sanders notes, replication on a larger group of patients is indicated.

In one of the few other studies of operant conditioning techniques, Holzman et al. (30) described three case studies of chronic low back pain outpatients seen for 10 sessions. Treatment was based on that described by Fordyce (19). All of the patients showed some improvement, but the nature and degree of change varied.

In summary, our conclusions are unchanged from those in the earlier review (61). Operant conditioning methods have been shown to be effective in increasing activity level and decreasing medication use, and perhaps also in leading to return to employment, but their impact on the individual's experience of pain is yet to be determined. Controlled investigations and component analyses of this complex intervention scheme are needed. Cost/benefit issues are also worthy of consideration, as operant programs typically involve lengthy and expensive inpatient hospitalizations. Research comparing inpatient versus outpatient treatments would be of great interest.

HYPNOSIS

It has been observed (61) that hypnosis has long been used for pain control. However, the actual mechanism by which hypnosis affects pain is still unclear. Cognitive processes such as mental relaxation, focusing of attention, and increased suggestibility seem to be major factors in hypnosis (28) and may be the active ingredients in producing hypnotic analgesia. Most studies on the relief of pain with hypnosis have been concerned with experimentally-induced pain. Although case reports of hypnotic treatment for clinical pain exist, they are less common, and there are almost no controlled studies of its application to chronic pain, leaving doubt as to its utility for this purpose.

Unfortunately, little progress has been made in this area since that review was prepared, although several reports have been published. Representative studies are described in Table 4. Friedman and Taub (21) reported the use of hypnosis and thermal imagery training with 23 female migraine patients. These authors pretested patients on a scale of hypnotic susceptibility; they administered standard trance induction to highly susceptible subjects and simulated trance induction to those who were found to be low on this measure. Both groups were instructed to use hand warming imagery and demonstrated significant decreases in reported headache frequency and intensity and medication use. These gains were maintained at a 6-month follow-up, with no differences between groups. Finger temperature was measured as an independent assessment of physiologic changes during treatment. Although some subjects produced increases in finger temperature while others produced no change or decreases, these changes were unrelated to the headache measures as well as to susceptibility. These results, although suggesting the utility of imagery in decreasing migraines, are difficult to interpret because no controls were used.

Hypnosis has been compared to EMG biofeedback with and without progressive relaxation in the treatment of tension headache (51). The hypnotic treatment produced significant decreases in pain intensity and duration equivalent to improvement seen in the other conditions. However, the extent to which trance induction was actually achieved in this group was not assessed. Also, a group receiving relaxation alone was not included, and thus the unique effects of hypnosis beyond relaxation remain unclear.

Howard et al. (31) report a case study in which a migraine subject received hypnosis, then "rational stage-directed hypnotherapy" (RSDH), after a base-line condition. In RSDH, patients are trained to substitute adaptive self-statements for maladaptive ones while in a hypnotic state. Although greater decreases in headache frequency were reported with RSDH than with hypnosis, definitive conclusions are prohibited because of a number of design shortcomings. Specifically, the base-line measurement period was quite short, and reversals or multiple base lines were not used; thus a direct relation between treatment techniques and headache activity could not be established.

TABLE 4. *Hypnosis: Experimental designs, populations, and treatment outcomes*

Author (ref.)	Population	N	Intervention(s)	Design	Control	Dependent measures	Follow-up	Results
Schlutter et al. (51)	Tension headache	48	1. Hypnosis 2. EMG feedback 3. EMG feedback plus relaxation	Group outcome	None	Self-recorded headache frequency, duration, intensity; psychophysical scaling of pain (tourniquet)	10–14 wk	All groups significantly improved in headache duration, intensity; no group differences; gains maintained at follow-up
Friedman and Taub (21)	Migraine headache	23	1. Hypnosis for high susceptible subjects 2. Simulated hypnosis for low susceptible subjects	Group outcome	None	Self-recorded headache frequency, intensity, medication use; finger temperature recordings	6 mo	Significant decreases in headache frequency, intensity and medication use over all subjects; no difference between groups
Howard et al. (31)	Migraine headache	1	1. Cognitive therapy plus hypnosis 2. Hypnosis alone 3. Base line	Case study	None	Self-recorded headache frequency; MMPI; Tennessee Self-Concept Scale	1 mo	Condition 1 resulted in greater improvement in headache frequency

EMG = electromyograph; MMPI = Minnesota Multiphasic Personality Inventory.

Given this continued paucity of well-designed studies and lack of convincing experimental evidence for the efficacy of hypnosis in alleviating chronic pain, we are forced to let stand the conclusion of Turner and Chapman (61) regarding doubt as to the merits of hypnosis for chronic pain problems. Systematic single-subject and controlled group outcome studies are needed to establish or refute the value of this technique for headache and other pain syndromes.

COGNITIVE-BEHAVIORAL THERAPIES

The concept of pain as a complex experience involving physical and psychologic responses is by now well accepted among interdisciplinary pain researchers (55). However, only recently have cognitive-behavioral approaches to chronic pain begun to be developed and systematically evaluated. The reader is referred to Turner and Chapman's review (60,61) for a definition and description of this treatment approach. This review indicated much promise for the application of cognitive-behavioral techniques to various chronic pain syndromes. Since then, there have appeared a number of studies evaluating cognitive-behavioral treatments and comparing them to other interventions (Table 5). Once again, most of these studies targeted headache pain.

Using a single-subject design, Anderson et al. (4) compared a "cognitive coping skills training" program to autogenic relaxation and to a combination of these two treatments with tension headache patients. All three conditions were effective in decreasing headache activity as assessed by single subject analyses. Little difference emerged between the two treatments at either posttreatment assessment or 7-month follow-up.

Similarly, Kremsdorf et al. (37) compared a stress coping procedure, EMG biofeedback, and a combination of both in two systematic case studies of tension headache patients. These authors found the presence of the coping procedure, alone or with biofeedback, to be the most influential factor in producing substantial reductions in headache activity. Commendably, these authors examined whether changes on EMG recordings occurred as a result of training. The biofeedback training did result in lower EMG levels; however, these changes were unrelated to decreases in headache activity.

A combined treatment package including "cognitive coping skills training," relaxation, and EMG biofeedback was evaluated by Bakal et al. (6) for a group of 45 tension and migraine headache sufferers. Significant improvement in the number of headache hours, the rated intensity of pain, and medication use were noted at posttreatment testing and maintained at a 6-month follow-up. The research design does not permit the identification of factors producing improvement nor the assessment of the degree of contribution of coping skills versus that of the other components. An attempt to identify predictors of outcome was generally unsuccessful; however, sub-

TABLE 5. *Cognitive-behavioral therapies: Experimental designs, populations, and treatment outcomes*

Author (ref.)	Population	N	Intervention(s)	Design	Control	Dependent measures	Follow-up	Results
Bakal et al. (6)	Tension and migraine headache	45	Coping skills plus EMG feedback plus relaxation	Group outcome	None	Self-recorded headache duration, intensity, frequency, symptoms, medication use	6 mo	Group improved significantly in duration, intensity and medication use; gains maintained at follow-up
Kremsdorf et al. (37)	Tension headache	2	1. Coping skills plus EMG BFB 2. EMG BFB 3. Coping skills plus EMG BFB	Single subject, with reversals	Subject as own control	Self-recorded headache intensity, frequency, duration; EMG recordings	None	Decreases in headache activity primarily occurred in coping condition
Anderson et al. (4)	See under Relaxtion Training							
Turner (59)	Chronic low back pain	36	1. Cognitive-behavioral therapy and relaxation 2. Relaxation only	Group outcome	Attention/ waiting list	SIP (self and other-rated); medication use; self-ratings of improvement;	1 mo and 1½–2 yr	Both Groups 1 & 2 were significantly improved at posttest on the SIP, Beck, and

Study	Condition	N	Treatment groups	Control	Outcome measures	Follow-up	Results
			3. Attention/ waiting list control		pain severity; Beck Depression Inventory; health care use; hours worked/week		pain ratings, and were significantly different from 3 but not from each other. Group 1 greater than Group 2 in self-rated tolerance of pain and activity at 1-mo follow-up; no group differences at 1½ to 2-yr follow-up
Holroyd and Andrasik (29)	Tension headache	19	Follow-up of comparison of: 1. Stress coping 2. EMG feedback	None	Group outcome; Self-recorded headache frequency, intensity, duration, headache symptoms, additional treatments used	2 yr	Group 1 maintained significant reduction in headache activity, significantly superior to Group 2

EMG = electromyograph; BFB = biofeedback; SIP = Sickness Impact Profile.

jects who reported continuous rather than intermittent headache pain were most likely to do poorly in this treatment.

One of the few controlled group outcome studies in the literature evaluated the comparative merits of cognitive-behavioral therapy, including relaxation training, relaxation training alone, and a waiting list–attention control group (59). Thirty-six patients with chronic low back pain were assigned randomly to one of these three conditions. Both progressive relaxation and cognitive-behavioral therapy patients were seen for 5 weekly sessions of group treatment. All subjects were assessed both before and after treatment, and at 1-month and 1-½- to 2-year follow-ups. Both the cognitive-behavioral and relaxation groups evidenced significant improvement at posttreatment testing compared to the waiting list controls on a measure of pain-related physical and psychosocial dysfunction rated both by patients and by a significant other, and on pain intensity ratings. Although the treatment groups did not differ from each other at posttreatment testing on these variables, the cognitive group did rate themselves as more improved in ability to tolerate pain and participate in normal activities. At 1-month follow-up, the cognitive therapy group reported significantly lower average pain and less use of somatic treatments for pain than did the relaxation group. By the final follow-up assessment, both treatment conditions had maintained significant improvement from their pretreatment assessment in average pain ratings and in the number of visits made to health care providers. Only the cognitive therapy group showed significant increases in the number of hours worked per week, which nearly doubled from before treatment to final follow-up.

This study provides clear evidence for the utility of psychologic treatments for chronic low back pain, with both relaxation and cognitive-behavioral therapy resulting in significant improvement on a number of measures. Some superiority of cognitive-behavioral treatment was found in the extent to which treatment gains were maintained and in patients' perceptions of ability to control pain and engage in daily activities. It should be kept in mind that this study relied heavily on self-report measures (although ratings also were completed by patients' spouses), and that all treatment groups were conducted by the author, thus potentially introducing a source of bias into the administration of treatment.

The results of these studies suggest several points. First, cognitive-behavioral techniques merit further refinement and standardization. Their efficacy and mechanisms of action need to be assessed with various chronic pain syndromes. Second, studies that compare the efficacy of cognitive-behavioral therapy with other interventions would be enhanced by long-term follow-ups to determine if there are differences in stability and generalization of treatment effects. Cognitive-behavioral therapies may have the potential for promoting maintenance of treatment gains by giving clients a wider range of skills for dealing with stress and pain. This issue was illustrated by a 2-year follow-up study (29) of tension headache patients who had received either cognitive-behavioral training in stress coping or EMG biofeedback.

The coping skills group had maintained significant reductions in headache activity from the pretest levels and had significantly fewer headaches and less overall headache activity than the biofeedback group. Also of interest is that the coping skills group reported significantly more improvement in other symptoms besides headache (increased control over dysphoric emotions and over other psychosomatic symptoms such as gastrointestinal distress).

METHODOLOGIC ISSUES: PROBLEMS AND SUGGESTIONS

In general, the methodologic problems that were identified in the Turner and Chapman (60,61) papers remain. We will summarize these briefly, note improvements that have been made, and highlight areas to be considered in future work.

Issues in Assessment

Knowledge about the absolute and comparative efficacy of various interventions is dependent on adequate pre- and posttreatment assessment. As noted previously (60,61), comprehensive assessment involves measuring multiple physical and psychosocial variables, ideally tapping self-report, observational, and physiologic sources of data. Published reports also should include information on pretreatment subject variables that may affect outcome and generalizability of results. These include pain location, frequency, severity, and chronicity; functional limitations; employment status; health care utilization; medication use; age; gender; previous treatments received; medical findings; education; and socioeconomic status.

A number of advances have been made very recently in assessment procedures and are summarized in a review by Keefe (33) and in the chapter by K. L. Syrjala and C. R. Chapman, *this volume.* These include the development by Keefe and Block (34) of a direct observation method for assessing pain behaviors (e.g., guarding, bracing, grimacing) in chronic low back pain patients. This assessment method seems to be reliable, to correlate with patients' verbal reports of pain intensity, and to be sensitive to treatment effects. Further, it was found to discriminate low back pain patients from pain-free, normal, and depressed subjects (34).

Some interesting preliminary work also has been done in the assessment of cognitive variables. Lefebvre (38) developed self-report measures to assess cognitive distortions in depressed low back pain patients. Rosenstiel and Keefe (47) described a questionnaire that assesses cognitive coping strategies (e.g., distraction, positive self-statements) used by pain patients, and found an association between certain coping strategies and functional impairment, pain, and depression in low back pain patients.

Attention also has been given to assessment of the patients' pain perception. A major advance was the development of the McGill Pain Questionnaire (41). This instrument attempted to assess multidimensional aspects of the pain experience and classified pain descriptors into sensory, affective, and evaluative categories. However, the questionnaire has limitations as a quantitative measure of pain (63). Tursky et al. (63) have emphasized the need to assess quantitatively multiple aspects of the pain experience. They argue that effects of treatments may be obscured when only simple pain intensity measures are used to evaluate results, and that measures of pain tolerance and psychologic reactions to pain are necessary. They have attempted to provide such a method of evaluating qualitative and quantitative aspects of the pain experience with the Pain Perception Profile (62,63). This four-part technique (a) measures sensation threshold and level of nociceptive stimulation judged to be uncomfortable, painful, and intolerable; (b) assesses the subject's magnitude estimates of nociceptive stimuli; (c) quantifies the subject's evaluation of pain descriptors; and (d) involves a pain diary using psychophysically scaled pain descriptors.

Heaton et al. (27) describe a structured interview, called the Psychosocial Pain Inventory, for evaluating psychologic and social factors in chronic pain. This evaluation system seems promising and was found in a small pilot study to predict success after treatment in patients with acute pain who were undergoing neurosurgical evaluation. However, more research in different settings is needed to establish its validity and utility.

A number of directions in the area of assessment are indicated. The Keefe and Block (34) method of assessing pain behaviors seems very promising, but must be replicated in other settings. Research is needed to explore the associations among these pain behaviors, other important aspects of the pain problem (e.g., presence of operant and respondent processes, patient's report of pain intensity), and patients' responses to various treatments. Similar rating methods for pain problems other than low back pain would be of interest.

The assessment of cognitive aspects of chronic pain is still very preliminary, and further development and refinement of instruments, with attention to reliability and relationship to objective measures, is needed. Potentially such tools could be of value in matching patients to treatments, in tailoring treatments to patients, and as process measures to elucidate the mechanisms of change associated with treatment. Similarly, considerable work is needed to refine measures of psychosocial variables that may influence response to treatment and that may be affected by treatment. The Psychosocial Pain Inventory (27) is one step in this direction. The Pain Perception Profile (63) holds promise as a measure of the patient's experience of pain. Evaluation of all or parts of this assessment system with various pain patient subgroups is warranted. It would be of interest to determine its relation to various observable pain-related behaviors and its utility in assessing responses to various treatments.

Although these new measures warrant more research, there is danger in continuing the trend of different research groups developing and using idiosyncratic instruments, and applying them to patient samples selected by varying criteria, with little standardization in assessment protocols across studies. Considerable refinement and standardization in the classification and assessment of other psychologic and behavioral disorders has been made in recent years. For example, in the field of depression, there are now widely accepted and used criteria for various diagnostic categories (Research Diagnostic Criteria, DSM-III) (3,54), commonly used self-report and clinician rating measures of symptom severity (Beck Depression Inventory, Hamilton Rating Scale for Depression) (7,25), and structured standard interview formats for gathering diagnostic information (Schedule for Affective Disorders and Schizophrenia, Diagnostic Interview Schedule) (46,53). These techniques facilitate the comparison and integration of results from different studies.

Likewise, standardized, commonly used methods are needed for diagnosing and evaluating chronic pain problems. The development of a diagnostic category with inclusion and exclusion criteria for "psychogenic pain disorder" in the American Psychiatric Association's diagnostic manual (DSM-III) (3) was an attempt to address the issue of diagnosis for at least a subset of the chronic pain population. However, limitations of this approach already have been noted and suggested revisions proposed (12,66). It is debatable whether chronic pain syndromes should be included in a manual of psychiatric disorders and whether other approaches to categorizing subgroups of pain patients might be preferable. Further dialogue among experts in different disciplines concerning these issues would seem useful. However, the development of criteria by which relatively homogeneous and well-defined samples of pain patients may be selected is important to continuing progress in chronic pain research. Currently, samples of subjects in treatment outcome studies differ in site and chronicity of pain, functional impairment, and psychosocial characteristics. The effect of such subject variability on response to different treatments is an unknown and confounding factor in evaluation research.

Similarly, validated standardized outcome measures are needed if meaningful conclusions across studies are to be drawn. One such instrument that has been widely used is the headache diary: a self-monitored daily account of headache frequency, intensity, and duration. The use of this measure has greatly facilitated the comparison of results across studies. The difficulty in establishing standard assessment protocols and patient classification systems is recognized; perhaps preliminary work could be done by a team of experts agreeing on guidelines for a standard assessment protocol to be used in treatment outcome studies.

Finally, attention to assessing reduction in financial cost associated with various pain problems as a result of treatment would be of value. Given the tremendous cost of pain problems to society, this factor is an important consideration in assessing the value of behavioral interventions. Amount of expenditure by individuals and by agencies for health care services, medications, disability compensation, and so on could be assessed. A model for such a study is an investigation by Schlesinger et al. (50) of Blue Cross/Blue Shield claims of federal employees with chronic disease. They found greater medical charges in the third year after diagnosis of the disease in those who had not received mental health treatment as compared to those who received over six mental health treatment sessions. Perhaps cooperative efforts between researchers and insurance providers could be made to determine effects of various psychologic treatments on frequency and cost of health care use.

Issues in Design of Outcome Research

As was evident in reviewing the recent outcome literature, problems persist in this area. These include lack of adequate detailed descriptions of treatments administered and lack of standardization of treatment within and across studies. Notable exceptions are studies by Blanchard and colleagues (8–11), who carefully detailed treatment and assessment procedures as well as experimental design. Such descriptions are needed especially in studies of operant programs, which may or may not include other active treatments such as physical therapy, occupational therapy, and marital sessions, and of cognitive-behavioral interventions, which may vary widely in nature across settings. There is also a continued lack of use of adequate control conditions, which are necessary to determine whether changes are due to active treatment ingredients or to nonspecific effects associated with receiving treatment. Similarly, checks on whether the treatment was actually delivered as intended, the extent to which the rationale for treatment was credible to patients, compliance with homework assignments, and adequate use of techniques taught are rare. Finally, the number of studies with long-term follow-ups is still small, although growing (29,36,45,59).

On the positive side, some commendable studies with significant improvements in research design have been published recently, particularly in the area of biofeedback. One such advance has been an effort by some researchers to assess process variables in treatment. For example, Philips and Hunter (43) measured perceived treatment credibility and self-control over headaches in a study of EMG biofeedback. Another notable research design feature was used by Allen and Mills (2). In an attempt to assess subjects' abilities to use techniques taught in treatment for pain control (in this case, self-regulation of BVP amplitude for migraine headaches), they asked subjects to come to the laboratory when they had prodromal signs and perform techniques that had been taught. Such a design allows assessment to be made in vivo of subjects' abilities to reduce pain as a result of treatment.

Some progress has been made toward identifying predictors of success after various treatments. Blanchard et al. (10), using multiple regression techniques, found that a number of indicators of psychologic disturbance predicted treatment response, and that the psychologic tests that were significantly associated with outcome were different for vascular versus tension headache patients. Obviously, these results need to be replicated in different patient samples.

Unfortunately, there have been fewer advances in research design with treatments other than biofeedback. Controlled evaluations and comparisons of other psychologic treatments for pain are still few in number. Turner's study (59) comparing group relaxation training and cognitive-behavioral therapy for back pain, although limited by the lack of a credible "pseudotherapy" control, was an improvement on earlier research by the inclusion of a waiting-list/attention control condition, in which patients were telephoned weekly by the therapist for the active treatments. Also, positive, long-term follow-ups of different treatments are appearing more often (20,40,59).

These advances in research methodology auger well for continued growth in knowledge about the effectiveness of psychologic interventions for chronic pain problems. Systematic programs of controlled research clearly are needed to continue this growth, particularly with interventions other than biofeedback and with nonheadache pain populations. We would like to emphasize several issues worth considering carefully in planning, conducting, and writing papers about such endeavors.

First, it would be helpful for researchers to specify the goals of treatment (e.g., decreased experienced pain, decreased pain behaviors, decreased health care use), as different therapies may be developed and applied for different purposes. Second, sample characteristics and criteria used in selecting subjects should be described; the implications for generalizability of results obtained are obvious. Third, treatment methods should be detailed clearly so that they can be replicated and compared with other studies. If two or more treatments are to be compared, they should be operationally distinguishable both in concept and in implementation. Checks on this and on subjects' reports of compliance with practice of treatments would be useful.

Fourth, in evaluating "unproven" treatments, credible control conditions should be included to equate for nonspecific treatment influences such as expectation of improvement. The difficulty of designing a condition that is equally credible to subjects yet lacks the hypothesized "active ingredients" of the treatment condition is recognized; some creativity in addressing this problem is needed. Subjects should, of course, be randomly assigned to treatment and control conditions, and their expectations for improving as a result of treatment should be assessed. It is also desirable that therapists have no vested interest in treatment outcomes.

It will be important to establish the clinical as well as statistical significance of results obtained; that is, what percentage of patients given a certain treatment show improvement as assessed by a predetermined standard? Sole focus on statistical comparison of group outcomes obscures individual differences in response to treatment. For example, there may be greater variability in outcome or a higher proportion of subjects showing improvement in one treatment than another, even though group means may be comparable. Examining such issues may form the basis for identifying which patients are likely to succeed in a particular treatment and for choosing one treatment over another in a clinical setting.

While treatments are being developed and refined, small controlled studies with defined subject samples are appropriate to address discrete questions about treatment efficacy. On the basis of findings from such studies, larger scale trials could be developed, possibly in the context of multicenter collaborative efforts. Further efforts also are needed to replicate and expand on earlier work identifying predictors of response to different treatments. A potentially fruitful area may be the analysis of which patients drop out or fail to respond to treatments, why this occurs, and whether such patients can benefit from other types of treatment.

Finally, long-term follow-up assessments are needed. Initial treatment effects and differential group outcomes may vary considerably from long-term results. Different factors may influence initial treatment-produced changes, their generalizability to the home environment, and their maintenance over time, with some treatments possibly having more or less impact at different stages. Other treatments received since the intervention under study should be determined at follow-up as well as the dependent variables assessed pre- and posttreatment.

Once certain treatments have been shown to be effective, there is a need for studies to determine the necessary and sufficient components of that treatment, how treatment effects can be maintained over time (e.g., by regular therapist telephone contact, alumni groups, booster sessions), and whether treatment effects can be enhanced by additional interventions. Also, researchers may wish to consider the comparative expenses associated with different treatments. Length of treatment, outpatient versus inpatient setting, level of training required for therapists, and necessary equipment are all related to the overall treatment cost. The issue of cost effectiveness will be particularly important in choosing which treatment to offer a patient if a number of approaches of comparable efficacy are available.

Issues in Meta-Analysis

As the volume of research on psychologic treatments for different types of chronic pain increases, researchers may consider drawing general conclusions about treatment efficacy by using meta-analytic techniques. Meta-analysis (23,48,52) is a relatively new and potentially quite useful technique for combining and analyzing results across studies of particular treatments. This methodology has been applied to studies of migraine and tension headaches by Blanchard et al. (9). Although, as they noted (9), meta-analysis has been criticized for obscuring study differences in sample characteristics, treatment and assessment procedures, and individual responses to treatment, this technique would still seem to be of help in making general conclusions regarding the efficacy of various psychologic interventions for different pain problems. It also can provide information about gaps in knowledge, suggesting directions for future research. Strube and Hartmann (56) also point out that meta-analysis can be used to study the relationship between different variables and study outcome. Thus plausible hypotheses can be constructed, then empirically tested in new research. It would be of interest to apply meta-analytic methods to outcome studies of chronic pain syndromes other than headache (e.g., low back pain). Obviously, however, the validity of conclusions from such analyses rests on the quality of assessment and treatment methodology in the individual studies included.

CONCLUSIONS

In conclusion, we would like to encourage researchers to move toward developing knowledge accumulated from systematic soundly designed investigations, rather than continue the proliferation of unrelated studies that are virtually impossible to integrate because of methodologic deficiencies and dissimilarities. This point is particularly applicable to common pain syndromes (e.g., low back, headache). However, there is also great need for research in special populations (e.g., child, geriatric, and cancer patients), where unique assessment and treatment strategies may need to be developed and applied. Thus, continuing challenges to the field are the refinement and systematic evaluation of existing assessment and treatment techniques, while developing innovative methods for addressing the diversity of chronic pain problems and populations.

ACKNOWLEDGMENT

During the writing of this article, J. M. Romano was supported by NIH #NSO7217.

REFERENCES

1. Achterberg, J., McGraw, P., and Lawlis, G. F. (1981): Rheumatoid arthritis: A study of relaxation and temperature biofeedback training as an adjunctive therapy. *Biofeedback Self Regul.*, 6:207–223.
2. Allen, R. A., and Mills, G. K. (1982): The effects of unilateral plethysmographic feedback of temporal artery activity during migraine head pain. *J. Psychosom. Res.*, 26:133–140.
3. American Psychiatric Association (1980): *Diagnostic and Statistical Manual of Mental Disorders (3rd ed.)*. Washington, D. C.
4. Anderson, N. B., Lawrence, P. S., and Olson, T. W. (1981): Within-subject analysis of autogenic training and cognitive coping training in the treatment of tension headache pain. *J. Behav. Ther. Exp. Psychiatry*, 12:219–223.

5. Andrasik, F., and Holroyd, K. A. (1980): A test of specific and non-specific effects in the biofeedback treatment of tension headache. *J. Consult. Clin. Psychol.*, 48:575–586.
6. Bakal, D. A., Demjen, S., and Kaganov, J. A. (1981): Cognitive behavioral treatment of chronic headache. *Headache*, 21:81–86.
7. Beck, A. T. (1967): *Depression: Clinical, Experimental, and Theoretical Aspects.* Hoeber, New York.
8. Blanchard, E. B., and Andrasik, F. (1982): Psychological assessment and treatment of headache: Recent developments and emerging issues. *J. Consult. Clin. Psychol.*, 50:859–879.
9. Blanchard, E. B., Andrasik, F., Ahles, T. A., and Teders, S. J. (1980): Migraine and tension headache: A meta-analytic review. *Behav. Ther.*, 11:613–631.
10. Blanchard, E. B., Andrasik, F., Neff, D. F., Arena, J. G., Ahles, T. A., Jurish, S. E., Pallmeyer, T. P., Saunders, N. L., Teders, S. J., Barron, K. D., and Rodichok, L. D. (1982): Biofeedback and relaxation training with three kinds of headache: Treatment effects and their prediction. *J. Consult. Clin. Psychol.*, 50:562–575.
11. Blanchard, E. B., Andrasik, F., Neff, D. F., Teders, S. J., Pallmeyer, T. P., Arena, J. G., Jurish, S. E., Saunders, N. L., Ahles, T. A., and Rodichok, L. D. (1982): Sequential comparisons of relaxation training and biofeedback in the treatment of three kinds of chronic headache or, the machines may be necessary some of the time. *Behav. Res. Ther.*, 20:469–481.
12. Blumer, D., and Heilbronn, M. (1982): Chronic pain as a variant of depressive disease: The pain-prone disorder. *J. Nerv. Ment. Dis.*, 170:381–406.
13. Cohen, M. J., McArthur, D. L., and Rickles, W. H. (1980): Comparison of four biofeedback treatments for migraine headache: Physiological and headache variables. *Psychosom. Med.*, 42:463–480.
14. Cott, A., Goldman, J. A., Pavloski, R. P., Kirschberg, G. J., and Fabich, M. (1981): The long-term therapeutic significance of the addition of electromyographic biofeedback to relaxation training in the treatment of tension headaches. *Behav. Ther.*, 12:556–559.
15. Cram, J. R. (1980): EMG biofeedback and the treatment of tension headaches: A systematic analysis of treatment components. *Behav. Ther.*, 11:699–710.
16. Dougherty, J. (1980): Relief of phantom limb pain after EMG biofeedback-assisted relaxation: A case report. *Behav. Res. Ther.*, 18:355–357.
17. Elmore, A. M., and Tursky, B. (1981): A comparison of two psychophysiological approaches to the treatment of migraine. *Headache*, 21:93–101.
18. Epstein, L. H., and Abel, G. G. (1977): An analysis of biofeedback training effects for tension headache patients. *Behav. Ther.*, 8:37–47.
19. Fordyce, W. E. (1976): *Behavioral Methods for Chronic Pain and Illness.* C. V. Mosby, St. Louis.
20. Fordyce, W. E., Shelton, J. L., and Dundore, D. E. (1982): The modification of avoidance learning pain behaviors. *J. Behav. Med.*, 5:405–414.
21. Friedman, H., and Taub, H. A. (1982): An evaluation of hypnotic susceptibility and peripheral temperature elevation in the treatment of migraine. *Am. J. Clin. Hypn.*, 24:172–182.
22. Gauthier, J., Bois, R., Allaire, D., and Drolet, M. (1981): Evaluation of skin temperature biofeedback training at two different sites for migraine. *J. Behav. Med.*, 4:407–419.
23. Glass, G. V. (1976): Primary, secondary, and meta-analysis research. *Educ. Res.*, 5:3–8.
24. Gray, C. L., Lyle, R. C., McGuire, R. J., and Peck, D. F. (1980): Electrode placement, EMG feedback, and relaxation for tension headaches. *Behav. Res. Ther.*, 18:19–23.
25. Hamilton, M. (1960): A rating scale for depression. *J. Neurol. Neurosurg. Psychiatry*, 23:56–62.
26. Hart, J. D., and Cichanski, K. A. (1981): A comparison of frontal EMG biofeedback and neck EMG biofeedback in the treatment of muscle-contraction headache. *Biofeedback Self Regul.*, 6:63–74.
27. Heaton, R. K., Getto, C. J., Lehman, R. A. W., Fordyce, W. E., Brauer, E., and Groban, S. E. (1982): A standardized evaluation of psychosocial factors in chronic pain. *Pain*, 12:165–174.
28. Hilgard, E. R., (1975): The alleviation of pain by hypnosis. *Pain*, 1:213–231.
29. Holroyd, K. A., and Andrasik, F. (1982): Do the effects of cognitive therapy endure? A two-year follow-up of tension headache sufferers treated with cognitive therapy or biofeedback. *Cogn. Ther. Res.*, 6:325–334.

30. Holzman, A. D., Kerns, R. D., Turk, D. C., and Ackerman, M. (1982): Evaluation of outpatient operant conditioning treatment for chronic pain patients. Paper presented at Association for Advancement of Behavior Therapy Annual Meeting. Los Angeles, Calif.
31. Howard, L., Reardon, J. P., and Tosi, D. (1982): Modifying migraine headache through rational stage directed hypnotherapy: A cognitive-experiential perspective. *Int. J. Clin. Exp. Hypn.*, 30:257–269.
32. Jacobson, E. (1932): *Progressive Relaxation.* University of Chicago Press, Chicago.
33. Keefe, F. J. (1982): Behavioral assessment and treatment of chronic pain: Current status and future directions. *J. Consult. Clin. Psychol.*, 50:896–911.
34. Keefe, F. J., and Block, A. R. (1982): Development of an observation method for assessing pain behavior in chronic low back pain patients. *Behav. Ther.*, 13:363–375.
35. Kewman, D., and Roberts, A. H. (1980): Skin temperature biofeedback and migraine headaches. *Biofeedback Self Regul.*, 5:327–345.
36. Khatami, M., and Rush, A. J. (1982): A one year follow-up of the multi-modal treatment for chronic pain. *Pain*, 14:45–52.
37. Kremsdorf, R. B., Kochanowicz, N. A., and Costell, S. (1981): Cognitive skills training versus EMG biofeedback in the treatment of tension headaches. *Biofeedback Self Regul.*, 6:93–102.
38. Lefebvre, M. F. (1981): Cognitive distortion and cognitive errors in depressed psychiatric and low back pain patients. *J. Consult. Clin. Psychol.*, 49:517–525.
39. Linton, S. J. (1982): A critical review of behavioural treatments for chronic benign pain other than headache. *Br. J. Clin. Psychol.*, 21:321–337.
40. Malec, J., Cayner, J. J., Harvey, R. F., and Timming, R. C. (1980): Pain management: Long-term follow-up of an inpatient program. *Arch. Phys. Med. Rehabil.*, 62:369–372.
41. Melzack, R. (1975): The McGill Pain Questionnaire: Major properties and scoring methods. *Pain*, 1:277–299.
42. Nouwen. A., and Solinger, J. W. (1979): The effectiveness of EMG biofeedback training in low back pain. *Biofeedback Self Regul.*, 4:103–111.
43. Philips, C., and Hunter, M. (1981): The treatment of tension headache. I. Muscular abnormality and biofeedback. *Behav. Res. Ther.*, 19:485–498.
44. Philips, C., and Hunter, M. (1981): The treatment of tension headache. II. EMG 'normality' and relaxation. *Behav. Res. Ther.*, 19:499–507.
45. Reinking, R. H., and Hutchings, D. (1981): Follow-up to: "Tension headaches: What form of therapy is most effective?" *Biofeedback Self Regul.*, 6:57–62.
46. Robins, L. N., Helzer, J. E., Croughan, J., and Ratcliff, K. S. (1981): National Institute of Mental Health Diagnostic Interview Schedule: Its history, characteristics, and validity. *Arch. Gen. Psychiatry*, 38:381–389.
47. Rosenstiel, A. K., and Keefe, F. J. (1980): Development of a questionnaire to assess cognitive coping strategies in chronic pain patients. Paper presented at Association for Advancement of Behavior Therapy Annual Meeting. New York, New York.
48. Rosenthal, R. (1983): Assessing the statistical and social importance of the effects of psychotherapy. *J. Consult. Clin. Psychol.*, 51:4–13.
49. Sanders, S. H. (1982): A component analysis of behavioral methods used in the treatment of chronic pain patients. Poster session presented at Association for Advancement of Behavior Therapy Annual Meeting. Los Angeles, Calif.
50. Schlesinger, H. J., Mumford, E., Glass, G. V., Patrick, C., and Sharfstein, S. (1983): Mental health treatment and medical care utilization in a fee-for-service system: Outpatient mental health treatment following the onset of a chronic disease. *Am. J. Public Health*, 73:422–429.
51. Schlutter, L. C., Golden, C. J., and Blume, H. G. (1980): A comparison of treatments for prefrontal muscle contraction headache. *Br. J. Med. Psychol.*, 53:47–52.
52. Smith, M. L., and Glass, G. V. (1977): Meta-analysis of psychotherapy outcome studies. *Am. Psychol.*, 32:752–760.
53. Spitzer, R. L., and Endicott, J. (1978): NIMH Clinical Research Branch Collaborative Program on the Psychobiology of Depression: *Schedule for Affective Disorders and Schizophrenia: Lifetime Version*, ed. 3. New York State Psychiatric Institute, Biometrics Research Division, New York.
54. Spitzer, R. L., Endicott, J., and Robins, E. (1978): Research diagnostic criteria: Rationale and reliability. *Arch. Gen. Psychiatry*, 35:773–782.
55. Sternbach, R. A. (1974): *Pain Patients: Traits and Treatment.* Academic Press, New York.

56. Strube, M. J., and Hartmann, D. P. (1983): Meta-analysis: Techniques, applications, and functions. *J. Consult. Clin. Psychol.*, 51:14–27.
57. Tan, S.-Y. (1982): Cognitive and cognitive-behavioral methods for pain control: A selective review. *Pain*, 12:201–228.
58. Teders, S. J., Blanchard, E. B., Andrasik, F., Jurish, S., Neff, D. F., and Arena, J. (1982): A controlled comparison of clinic-based and home-based relaxation training for the treatment of tension headache. Paper presented at Association for Advancement of Behavior Therapy Annual Meeting. Los Angeles, Calif.
59. Turner, J. A. (1982): Comparison of group progressive-relaxation training and cognitive-behavioral group therapy for chronic low back pain. *J. Consult. Clin. Psychol.*, 50:757–765.
60. Turner, J. A., and Chapman, C. R. (1982): Psychological interventions for chronic pain: A critical review. I. Relaxation training and biofeedback. *Pain*, 12:1–21.
61. Turner, J. A., and Chapman, C. R. (1982): Psychological interventions for chronic pain: A critical review. II. Operant conditioning, hypnosis, and cognitive-behavioral therapy. *Pain*, 12:23–46.
62. Tursky, B. (1976): Development of a pain perception profile. In: *Pain: New Perspectives in Therapy and Research*, edited by M. Weisenberg and B. Tursky. Plenum, New York.
63. Tursky, B., Jamner, L. D., and Friedman, R. (1982): The pain perception profile: A psychophysical approach to the assessment of pain report. *Behav. Ther.*, 13:376–394.
64. Varni, J. W. (1981): Self-regulation techniques in the management of chronic arthritic pain in hemophilia. *Behav. Ther.*, 12:185–194.
65. Varni, J. W. (1981): Behavioral medicine in hemophilia arthritic pain management: Two case studies. *Arch. Phys. Med. Rehabil.*, 62:183–187.
66. Williams, J. B. W., and Spitzer, R. L. (1982): Idiopathic pain disorder: A critique of pain-prone disorder and a proposal for a revision of the DSM-III category psychogenic pain disorder. *J. Nerv. Ment. Dis.*, 170:415–419.
67. Wolf, S. L., Nacht, M., and Kelly, J. L. (1982): EMG feedback training during dynamic movement for low back pain patients. *Behav. Ther.*, 13:395–406.

*Advances in Pain Research
and Therapy, Vol. 7,*
edited by C. Benedetti et al.
Raven Press, New York © 1984.

Recent Advances in Nerve Blocks and Related Procedures

Jose L. Madrid

*Department of Anesthesiology and Pain Clinic, City Hospital "1st October,"
Madrid, Spain*

Any peripheral nerve, cranial or spinal, can be reached with a needle and its function interrupted for hours with a local anesthetic or for months with a neurolytic agent. Thus nerve blocks with various local anesthetic agents can be used not only for surgical anesthesia, but in the management of a great variety of pain syndromes. The value of analgesic blocks for diagnostic, prognostic, prophylactic, and therapeutic purposes has been extensively documented (3).

The injection of neurolytic agents is a special form of symptomatic treatment aimed at modifying or blocking the painful impulses. As a rule, the main application of neurolytic injections is for those cancer patients whose physical state contraindicates neurosurgery or any type of palliative surgery. The success of a neurolytic block largely depends on how early it is performed. Partial neurolytic blocks do not, in most cases, last throughout the patient's lifetime even if the nerve pathways have been destroyed with maximum precision. In order to obtain long-term relief, the destruction of nervous input to any structure must be preganglionic, which can be accomplished by intrathecal injection of neurolytic drugs. In cases of pain of nonmalignant origin, however, neurolytic agents are contraindicated because of the inability to control them properly and the risk of producing motor root damage.

Failure to relieve pain may be due to technical errors, distortion of anatomy because of the pathologic process, or spread of the pain to zones and regions beyond the blocked dermatomas. The reinjection of intrathecal phenol usually is not as effective as the initial treatment because root sheathing and cerebrospinal fluid may preclude sensory root penetration (9).

In cases of pain of the upper extremity associated with apical lung carcinoma, the overall results with intra- and extradural injections of neurolytic drugs have been far from satisfactory due to the frequent occurrence of epidural tumor extension, which will explain the difficulty in performing an effective block. Batzdorf and Brechner (1) recommend that patients with Pancoast neoplasm should undergo myelography before therapeutic block is attempted. Therefore, it is my impression that because of the unreliability of neurolytic injections, we are using many fewer subarachnoid and extra-dural neurolytic blocks. On the other hand, blocks with local anesthetic, when properly carried out, constitute an effective therapy or adjunct to other therapies.

In this chapter I will briefly describe the use of nerve blocks and other therapies in four pain syndromes seen in our clinic frequently: (a) "the cervical syndrome" caused by osteoarthritis of the cervical spine; (b) pain due to peripheral vascular disease; (c) posttraumatic syndromes of the upper extremity; and (d) cancer pain. For more detailed description of the techniques, the reader is referred to the books by Bonica (3,4) and Mehta (9).

CERVICAL SYNDROME

We carried out a study on 77 patients with cervical syndrome. This term has become synonymous with symptoms and signs attributable to irritation of the cervical nerve roots within the region of the cervical intervertebral foramina. Impairment of movements of any part of the cervical spine can be responsible for pain, discomfort, and disability. Movement of the neck requires that the discs have sufficient integrity to permit distortion and recovery, the ligaments have adequate laxity to permit motion, and the posterior joints be sufficiently separated with capsular elasticity and smooth articular surfaces to allow movements in all directions necessary for normal neck movement.

The neck contains many sensitive tissues in a relatively small and compact area. Pain can result from irritation, injury, inflammation, or even infection of almost any of the contained tissues. The nerve roots within the spinal canal and in their course through the intervertebral foramina are obviously pain-sensitive tissues. Pain can also originate from ischemia of the muscle. Sustained contractions can accumulate catabolic products within the muscle while simultaneously constricting its intrinsic blood supply. These accumulated catabolic products of muscular contraction sensitize nociceptors and thus play an important role in the painful condition known as "cervical syndrome". The basic goals of treatment are to restore function, to correct or prevent deformities, and to relieve pain. Pain often causes loss of function in patients with cervical syndrome. The quality of their lives deteriorates, and many patients suffer economic hardships because of inability to work.

The rehabilitation department in our hospital attended 14,625 patients from July 1975 to May 1980; of those, 1,228 patients (8.40%) had cervicobrachial neuralgia with or without signs of cervicoarthritis. This is a good index of the importance and incidence of this syndrome.

A group of 77 patients (60 women; 17 men) 21 to 69 years old, irrespective of the pathogenesis of their root irritation, was assessed as to: (a) subjective painful symptomatology, (b) deformities, (c) objective painful symptomatology, (d) contractures, (e) joint motion, and (f) bone impairment.

Kinetic examinations revealed impairment in flexion movements in 57%. Extension movements were disturbed in 38% of the patients, and 30% had abnormal rotation movement of the neck. Pathologic radiographic changes were present in 82% of the cases.

In the management of these patients, we used three different approaches. In 30 patients the treatment consisted of kinesitherapy by means of massage, ultrasound, thermotherapy, and gradual cervical traction up to a total of 6 kg. Another group of 20 patients was treated with one cervical epidural injection per week for 3 consecutive weeks. With the patient seated and the neck flexed, the extradural cervical space was reached with a 6-cm 20-gauge, short-bevel needle inserted in the midline at the level of C4–C5, using Gutierrez's sign or "hanging-drop" method for identifying the epidural space. This site of injection was selected so as to place a high concentration of the drug near the involved nerve root(s). Once the epidural space was reached, the patient was placed in lateral decubitus position on the side of the pathology with a slight head-down tilt. Methylprednisolone acetate (60 mg in 5 cc normal saline) was injected slowly and the needle withdrawn; for the next 15 min the patient remained supine, then was allowed to ambulate.

The third group of 27 patients was treated with cervical extradural steriods in the same fashion as the second group, plus kinesitherapy right after the block was performed. The length of treatment in all three groups was 3 weeks.

All cervical epidural blocks but one were performed as a single-shot injection through a midline approach. In one case, technical difficulties due to intense interligament fibrosis prevented us from reaching the cervical epidural space through the midline and we had to use a lateral approach.

The results before and after the treatment regarding symptoms and physical examination are listed in Table 1. There is an evident decrease of the painful symptomatology with the three techniques, but the best results are those with a combined technique of epidural blocks plus kinesitherapy. This was especially the case for local pain and muscle contraction. It had been reported (6) that combined therapy of epidural steroid and manipulation should not be carried out at the same time in the treatment of sciatic pain because it may worsen the results. In our cases, however, it seems to be the contrary for cervicobrachial neuralgia.

The overall results at 2 months follow-up (Table 2) regarding pain relief show a significant improvement in the success rate in patients treated with epidural blocks plus kinesitherapy.

PAIN IN VASCULAR INSUFFICIENCY

The term *vascular insufficiency* includes a group of clinical entities in which there is reduction in the peripheral circulation. The obstruction to blood flow is the result of two components: organic occlusion and functional

TABLE 1. *Percentage of subjective and objective symptoms before and after treatment in patients with osteoarthritis of the cervical region*

Symptoms	Kinesitherapy (N = 30)		Epidural block (N = 20)		Kinesitherapy and epidural (N = 27)	
	Before	After	Before	After	Before	After
Local pain	83	32	83	39	85	16
Referred pain	68	32	78	39	92	41
Radicular pain	61	16	66	33	77	42
Vascular symptoms	45	22	44	22	70	16
Pain on spinous processes	75	39	72	45	69	33
Pain on transverse processes	81	32	78	39	61	25
Pain on supraclavicular fossa	74	32	77	39	62	25
Contractured muscles	81	29	66	39	84	17
Occipital pain	32	16	55	17	30	17

vasospasm, either or both of which may be present in varying degrees. The major complaint in patients with vascular insufficiency is pain and may be caused by chronic occlusive arterial disease, chronic venous insufficiency, trauma, or an inflammatory process. The common denominator of pain in the vascular tree is tissue ischemia. Besides pain, there are associated symptoms, such as muscle weakness, numbness, change in temperature, change in skin color, edema, trophic changes, and pulse abnormalities.

Despite the advances in vascular surgery, there are always a number of patients with occlusive vascular disease and ischemic problems of the lower extremity that for various reasons are not good candidates for reconstructive surgery. Because the vascular system is largely under control of the sympathetic nervous system and because vasoconstriction is the result of in-

TABLE 2. *Overall results in three groups of patients for pain relief at 2 months' follow-up[a]*

Procedure	N	Pain free	Less pain	No effect
Kinesitherapy	30	4	20	6
Epidural block	20	6	8	6
Epidural plus kinesitherapy	27	12	10	5
Total	77	22	38	17

[a] There is a significant improvement in the success rate in patients treated with kinesitherapy and epidural cervical blocks with steroids.

creased sympathetic activity, the use of local anesthetic blocks will cause interruption of sympathetic impulses in cases with vasoconstriction.

In our hospital we have many requests to treat patients with severe ischemic pain due to peripheral vascular diseases with nerve blocks not only as an analgesic therapy but also as an evaluation method for a possible surgical sympathectomy. In hospitalized patients, it is more convenient to use a continuous technique to provide lumbar sympathetic blocks, especially in patients with poor physical status. In this manner there is no need to subject patients to repeated needling. However, tachyphylaxis, a decline in effectiveness of a drug when it is given repeatedly, often is observed when a continuous nerve block is used over a long period of time. It is less likely to occur if a blocking agent is reinjected before the block is allowed to lapse. Tachyphylaxis may well prove to be the result of several unrelated clinical factors, such as perineural edema, microhemorrhage, or miniclots that may result from irritation by the catheter or from the anesthetic solution. Other plausible causes are hypernatremia due to the saline carrier of the anesthetic solution or acidosis from the anesthetic drugs by pH below 7.

A group of 10 patients was referred from the Department of Vascular Surgery to assess the potential therapeutic effect of an interruption of the sympathetic fibers. The indications for continuous sympathetic blocks were coldness of the foot and continuous rest pain. In addition, some patients had ulceration, gangrene, and cellulitis (Table 3); the duration of symptoms was 17 days to 3 months. In all of them, a preblock clinical assessment was carried out, including oscillometry, thermometry, cycloergometry, and infrared thermography. Continuous lumbar sympathetic blocks were performed with a modification of Wallace's technique (12). Under fluoroscopic control, a 16-gauge Teflon Abbocath catheter 12.7 cm in length was introduced until its tip was against the lateral surface of the second lumbar vertebral body. The catheter was secured with silk stitches at the skin exit for further intermittent injections.

Complete cooperation by the patient is essential for this procedure. The patient stays in bed and must be careful not to pull out the catheter. The rationale to use this technique instead of a lumbar sympathetic block by means of an epidural catheter was due to the fact that all patients had unilateral lesions, and we tried not to block both lumbar sympathetic chains in order to avoid an increased perfusion in regions not affected by disease (the steal phenomenon). If the perfusion pressure falls, the region distal to the obstruction will be the first to suffer (8).

Once the basal studies were completed, a volume of 12 ml of 0.25% plain bupivacaine was injected through the Abbocath catheter every 6 hr over 6 consecutive days. With this volume, we were able to obtain a complete sympathetic block as evidenced by the psychogalvanic reflex test. All patients had complete sympathetic interruption without motor involvement. After 6 days with an intermittent lumbar sympathetic block, the cycloergometric test was repeated under the same conditions as before the block.

TABLE 3. *Symptomatology of patients before management with continuous sympathetic blocks*

Case no.	Age	Gender	Diagnosis	Ulceration	Pain at rest	Claudication	Length of symptoms
1	53	M	Iliac occlusion	Yes	+	+ +	3 mo
2	72	F	Arteriosclerosis	Gangrene	+	+ +	1 mo
3	65	M	Thromboangiitis	Yes	+	+ + +	2 mo
4	58	M	Thromboangiitis	Yes	+ +	+ + +	1 mo
5	36	M	Popliteal thrombosis	Yes	+ +	+ + +	17 day
6	64	F	Ileofemoral occlusion	Yes	+	+ + +	19 day
7	59	M	Diabetic gangrene	Gangrene	+	+ + +	1 mo
8	61	M	Arteriosclerosis	Yes	+	+ + +	1 mo
9	57	F	Arteriosclerosis	Yes	+	+ + + +	2 mo
10	70	M	Arteriosclerosis	Yes	+ +	+ + + +	28 day

Pain: +, mild; + +, moderate; + + +, severe; + + + +, very severe.

TABLE 4. *Results of cycloergometry test after 6 days of continuous sympathetic blocks*

Case no.	Resistance (watt)	rpm	Appearance of pain after pedaling	
			Before block (sec)	After block
1	50	60	31	None at 3 min
2	50	60	17	2 min
3	50	60	60	None at 3 min
4	50	60	58	None at 3 min
5	50	60	72	None at 3 min
6	50	60	38	None at 3 min
7	50	60	55	None at 3 min
8	50	60	45	None at 3 min
9	50	60	22	70 sec
10	50	60	40	None at 3 min

All but 2 patients were able to pedal on the cycloergometer for 3 min without appearance of pain (Table 4). We discontinued the test after 3 min to prevent electrocardiographic alterations.

In an attempt to determine if this improvement was the result of a better perfusion of the ischemic limb, studies on temperature increase were carried out by infrared thermography. The study of alterations of the peripheral vascular system with infrared thermography is dynamic, atraumatic, easy to repeat, and good in studying the function of the peripheral circulation. It is a true heat photograph providing quantitative information regarding temperature of the surface under study. The results observed with infrared thermography showed a significant improvement of the ischemic areas revealed by an increase in temperature in the affected limbs. These results suggest that continuous lumbar sympathetic blocks in cases of intermittent claudication improve the leg nutritive muscle blood flow during exercise.

POSTTRAUMATIC PAIN SYNDROMES OF THE UPPER EXTREMITY

These are conditions that are often seen in everyday practice and constitute a serious problem. As these generally follow an apparently minor injury, they are often misdiagnosed and improperly treated. In these conditions, accidental or surgical trauma provokes local tissue changes and segmental and suprasegmental reflex responses, resulting in immediate pain, and altered circulatory dynamics and restricted function (3). In such posttraumatic pain syndromes, an irritative lesion is always present, which serves as a focus of noxious impulses producing a sympathetic hyperactivity and creating what Livingston (7) defines as a "vicious circle" between central and peripheral processes.

The role of diagnostic and therapeutic sympathetic blocks has been established as a specific treatment in these conditions and should not be delayed in order to obtain effective results. Bonica (5) points out that many patients with posttraumatic pain syndromes will be cured with the proper use of sympathetic nerve blocks, physical therapy, and exercise. It deserves emphasis that proper use of sympathetic block entails early diagnosis and prompt institution of the sympathetic interruption.

Posttraumatic pain syndromes are among the great variety of disorders included in so-called reflex sympathetic dystrophy. Two basic principles of therapy are, first, to recognize the syndrome, especially if there is evidence of traumatic injury; second, regardless of the pathogenesis, interruption of the appropriate sympathetic chain is nearly always curative of pain. The criteria to initiate treatment with sympathetic nerve blocks in a patient with pain and previous trauma are: (a) pain and tenderness in the extremity, (b) swelling of soft tissues, (c) vasomotor changes, and (d) diminished motor function. If not promptly treated, eventually there develops trophic skin changes and patchy osteoporosis.

In our hospital, we manage these cases as follows. A diagnostic stellate ganglion block is carried out with 10 ml of 1% lidocaine. Right after the block, sympathetic function tests are performed, including thermometry, oscillometry, digital plethysmography, psychogalvanic reflex, and sweating test with cobalt blue. If the sympathetic function tests are positive and there is pain reflief, we proceed to the next step. A continuous sympathetic nerve block of the upper extremity is carried out by inserting a catheter near the brachial plexus at axillary level and then producing brachial plexus block by the infraclavicular technique described by Raj et al. (10).

We use an 18-gauge 10-cm needle with a short bevel, directing its point laterally toward the brachial artery. Advance of the needle is monitored with a peripheral nerve stimulator. Once the muscular movements are lost after a test injection of 2 ml of 2% lidocaine, an epidural catheter is inserted through the 18-gauge needle and the tip of the catheter is confirmed to be placed on the brachial plexus by injection of a contrast medium. In many cases it was possible to observe diffusion of the contrast medium along the peripheral nerves of the brachial plexus, corroborating the correct placement of the catheter. Once the catheter was secured, a volume of 20 ml of 0.25% plain bupivacaine was injected every 6 hr for 6 consecutive days. Exercise and physical therapy, as part of the patient general rehabilitation program, was carried out during the length of the treatment with sympathetic blocks.

The rationale for using a continuous technique is based on a report by Vidal Lopez (11), who studied the effect on skin temperature with stellate ganglion block and an axillary perivascular brachial plexus technique performed simultaneously in a patient, by means of infrared thermography. He proved that, with a stellate ganglion block, the increase in temperature is very rapid, reaching its maximum effect at 10 min after the block. The increase in temperature in the extremity with an axillary perivascular block is slower beginning just over the ulnar nerve distribution. At 25 min, both hands have the same temperature. However, at 1 hr after the block, the hand where the stellate ganglion block was performed starts to cool, while the hand with the axillary block reaches its maximum increase in temperature.

According to these findings, it would be reasonable to use a continuous axillary block when a long period of treatment with sympathetic interruption is contemplated in order to sustain a more lasting beneficial effect. Although the continuous axillary block is more comfortable for the patient, we prefer the infraclavicular approach over the axillary technique because the former is easier to secure properly and is less likely to be displaced during exercises and movement of the extremity during rehabilitation. Moreover, the infraclavicular catheter is easier to keep clean.

CANCER PAIN

A significant percentage of patients with advanced malignant disease have intractable pain. In making a decision about cancer therapy, it is important to estimate the phase of the disease, the patient's longevity, the physical and mental condition of the patient, and the availability of the different methods of pain relief. Cancer pain problems deserve a careful appraisal and systematic plan for pain relief that will conserve the patient's resources and social usefulness as long as possible (3).

Peripheral nerve blocks, sympathetic blocks, and subarachnoid and extradural blocks are the main procedures in the treatment of pain of advanced cancer. Most patients can be managed and controlled with some different and refined techniques, such as percutaneous cervical cordotomy, thermocoagulation, cryoanalgesia, neuroadenolysis, or special neurosurgical procedures. All these techniques require hospitalization for several days and, depending on the medical demands and the availability of hospital beds in some areas, most of these procedures must be postponed.

Patients with intractable cancer pain who for some reason cannot be hospitalized may have the alternative of epidural morphine for pain control. Following the first reports by Yaksh and Rudy (14) and Wang (13), the use of subarachnoid and epidural morphine to treat chronic pain has become widespread. Numerous studies have demonstrated the efficacy of epidural morphine analgesia and the lack of sympathetic denervation, motor loss, or cerebral depression (2). This technique represents a very important addition to the methods used for the treatment of cancer pain (see L. Jacobson, *this volume*).

We have been using the technique of low-dose extradural morphine by means of an epidural catheter inserted in the cervical region for pain in the upper part of the body and in the lumbar epidural space for pain in the lower half of the body. However, we have observed that pain relief in any part of the body is achieved with this procedure independently of the injection level.

Once the selected space is chosen, a skin incision between two spinous processes is performed and the epidural space is reached with an 18-gauge

TABLE 5. *Complications and side effects in 118 patients treated with epidural morphine*

	Patients	
Side effects and complications	N	% of total
Constipation	24	20.3
Segmental itching	22	18.6
Urinary retention	10	8.4
Generalized itching	8	6.7
Pain during injection	6	5.0
Catheter obstruction	6	5.0
Local infection	3	2.5
Catheter extrusion	2	1.6
Paralysis lower extremity	1	0.8
Total	82	68.9

Hustead-type epidural needle. The catheter is inserted 8 cm lateral to the skin incision and passed subcutaneously so that its tip exits through the surgical incision. The catheter is threaded through the second needle (subcutaneous tunneling) and the proximal end of the catheter is placed in a small plastic bag and attached to the patient's skin with plastic tape.

A group of 118 patients was treated with this technique, all of whom had intractable cancer pain. The criteria for this form of treatment was, first, those cases where other therapeutic modalities had failed and the phase of disease was so far advanced that the estimated life expectancy was less than 4 months. Second, these patients were treated as outpatients in their own homes, so we asked for family acceptance and collaboration in the management of each case. Third, the catheter implant was carried out when a response to a single-shot epidural injection of 2 mg of morphine was able to provide analgesia lasting 18 or more hr.

The doses of epidural morphine in our cases were 2 mg of morphine in 5 ml of normal saline for injection in the cervical epidural space, and 2 mg of morphine in 10 ml normal saline for injection in the lumbar epidural space. In 42 patients, the epidural catheter was inserted in the cervical region at the C6–C7 level; the other 76 patients had an implanted epidural catheter in the lumbar region at L2–L3 level. The mean duration of the initial analgesia after the injection of 2 mg of morphine in the epidural space was 23 hr in the cervical group and 21 hr for the lumbar group. On the average, the epidural catheter was in place for 32 ± 4 days. The longest period of catheter implant was 5 months. The average number of injections after several days of treatment was once every 6 to 8 hr.

The most common side effects in our cases were constipation and segmental itching (Table 5). Pain during injection was observed in 6 patients after several days of intermittent injections; in two cases, injections of 40 mg of methylprednisolone solved the problem. The anti-inflammatory effect of the steroid would be of benefit to correct the edema and irritation caused by the catheter on the dura. In cases of catheter obstruction or catheter extrusion, a new catheter was inserted at a higher level. Most of the catheters underwent bacteriologic study; there were no reports of pathology.

One patient developed a paralysis of the right lower extremity after 15 days of treatment. He had a lumbar vertebra almost destroyed by metastases, and collapse of the bone structure could account for this complication. This patient died at home 5 days after the family reported this complication. Respiratory depression did not occur in this group of patients.

DISCUSSION

The injection of long-acting local anesthetic, neurolytics, and/or steroids into nerves or the spinal canal is a commonly used therapeutic technique in the management of chronic pain. Epidural-applied morphine is established as a method of alleviating pain, especially in cancer patients. However, this chapter deals with some nonmalignant chronic pain syndromes managed with techniques not frequently used but that have proved to be useful in association with other measures in the overall management of these conditions.

There are many reports on the mode of action of extradural injections with steroids. The ability to reduce inflammation around the nerve roots and to decrease formation of adhesions, minimizing nerve traction and subsequent pain production, will be of benefit for patients with radiculopathy. When the treatment is started early, not allowing the patients' disorder to become chronic, the analgesic response to the steroids and the association of a regime of manipulations gives better results. This justifies the combined technique of kinesitherapy and epidural injection of steroids.

Patients with extensive vascular involvement and rest pain and claudication must be treated by arterial surgery. If the surgical procedure cannot be performed because the lesions are too extensive or the patients are at high risk, a trial with continuous sympathetic blocks should be given to relieve both pain and claudication. Later, if the patient's general condition improves, vascular reconstruction or surgical or chemical sympathectomy can be reconsidered. The relief of pain by means of a sympathetic block reduces the painful impulses produced in the somatic afferent C fibers; this, in turn, reduces the activity in the internuncial neurons. Pain impulses may still pass to the spinothalamic tract via ordinary afferent fibers. This explains why sympathetic blockade does not always produce complete pain relief. Sympathetic blocks should be started early along with active motion. In order to provide a sustained sympathetic block, a continuous technique will enhance other conservative measures, will afford prolonged analgesia, and will allow major cooperation of the patient in the general management of these syndromes.

Treatment with epidural morphine in patients with severe cancer pain is an effective and relatively simple procedure to reduce and alleviate pain when carried out by physicians with experience in performing epidural blocks. The absence of changes in other sensory, motor, and sympathetic function indicates that this form of analgesia offers many advantages for relief of chronic malignant pain. This technique should not be regarded as a panacea. Depending on a number of different factors, such as lack of alternative techniques or unavailability of hospital beds, the apparent absence of serious complications, however, make it possible to have the patient at home surrounded by his family in a more pleasant environment. This plays a very important psychologic role in the patient's general condition. We are very satisfied to see that the families of patients with advanced cancer and intractable pain will prefer and willingly accept to have the patient at home rather than in the hospital.

REFERENCES

1. Batzdorf, U., and Brechner, V. L. (1979): Management of pain associated with the Pancoast syndrome. *Am. J. Surg., 137*:633–646.
2. Behar, M., Magora, F., Olshawang, D., and Davidson, J. T. (1979): Epidural morphine in the treatment of pain. *Lancet,* 1:527–529.
3. Bonica, J. J. (1953): *The Management of Pain.* Lea & Febiger, Philadelphia.
4. Bonica, J. J. (1959): *Clinical Application of Diagnostic and Therapeutic Nerve Blocks.* Charles C Thomas, Springfield, Ill.
5. Bonica, J. J. (1979): Causalgia and other reflex sympathetic dystrophies. In: *Advances in Pain Research and Therapy, Vol. 3,* edited by J. J. Bonica, J. C. Liebeskind, and D. Albe-Fessard, p. 141. Raven Press, New York.
6. Heyse-Moore, G. H. (1978): A rational approach to the use of epidural medication in the treatment of sciatic pain. *Acta Orthop. Scand., 49*:366–370.
7. Livingston, W. K. (1943): *Pain Mechanisms: A Physiologic Interpretation of Causalgia and Its Related States.* Macmillan, New York.
8. Lofstrom, B., and Zetterquist, S. (1969): Lumbar sympathetic blocks in the treatment of patients with obliterative arterial disease of the lower limb. *Int. Anesthesiol. Clin.,* 7:423.
9. Mehta, M. (1973): *Intractable Pain.* Saunders, London.
10. Raj, P. P., Montgomery, S. J., Nettles, D., and Jenkins, M. T. (1973): Infraclavicular brachial plexus block: A new approach. *Anesth. Analg., 52*:897–904.
11. Vidal Lopez, F. (1972): Progresos en anestesilogia, reanimacion y terapia del dolor. In: *Actas II Reunion International,* p. 24. Barcelona.
12. Wallace, G. (1955): A lateral approach for lumbar sympathetic nerve block. *Anesthesiology,* 16:254–260.
13. Wang, J. K. (1977): Analgesic effect of intrathecally administered morphine. *Reg. Anesth.,* 2:8.
14. Yaksh, T. L., and Rudy, T. A. (1976): Analgesia mediated by a direct spinal action of narcotics. *Science,* 192:1357.

*Advances in Pain Research
and Therapy, Vol. 7,*
edited by C. Benedetti et al.
Raven Press, New York © 1984.

Intercostal Nerve Block and Celiac Plexus Block for Pain Therapy

Daniel C. Moore

*Department of Anesthesiology, University of Washington, Seattle,
Washington 98195*

It has long been appreciated (3,4) and duly emphasized elsewhere in this volume that regional analgesia achieved with local anesthetics or neurolytic agents is a valuable diagnostic, prognostic, and therapeutic tool in managing patients with acute and/or chronic pain. Intercostal nerve block and celiac plexus block are among the most frequently used and most efficacious techniques for this purpose (3,14–16). This chapter contains concise discussions of the indications, techniques (including the anatomic bases and pharmacology), and complications of intercostal nerve block and celiac plexus block.

INTERCOSTAL NERVE BLOCK

Indications

Diagnosis

When thoracic or upper abdominal pain is present, intercostal nerve block is used to differentiate somatic from visceral pain. For example, intercostal nerve block will relieve pain arising in the thoracic wall caused by musculoskeletal or neurologic disorder but will not completely relieve thoracic visceral pain arising from such conditions as acute myocardial infarction and pulmonary embolus. Since nociceptive fibers from thoracic viscera pass to the spinal cord through the lower cervical and upper thoracic sympathetic chain, cervical thoracic sympathetic block extending from the middle cervical to the fifth thoracic ganglia, often referred to as stellate ganglion block, is effective in relieving these types of thoracic visceral pain. Likewise, upper abdominal pain arising from the abdominal wall will be relieved by intercostal nerve block; to abolish pain from the upper intraabdominal viscera, however, a celiac plexus block must be performed.

Therapeutics

For postoperative pain arising from incision of the thoracic and/or abdominal wall as well as pain from trauma to the thorax (fractured ribs), intercostal nerve block using 3 to 5 ml of bupivacaine (Marcaine®) per nerve in my opinion remains superior to other techniques, such as continuous segmental epidural block achieved with intermittent injection of local anesthetic. The complications that may accompany an intermittent epidural block are: (a) hypotension from extensive vasomotor blockade; (b) total spinal anesthesia from accidental subarachnoid injection of an epidural therapeutic dose; (c) migration of the tubing into a blood vessel with consequent systemic toxicity; and (d) loss of plastic tubing in the epidural space. These complications are not associated with intercostal block (15). Moreover, nausea, itching, apnea, and other complications of epidural narcotics do not occur with intercostal block and consequently the latter does not require the prolonged monitoring necessary with the former technique. Also, when metastatic cancer causes intractable somatic nerve pain limited to the thorax, as may occur with cancer of the breast, intercostal nerve block with absolute alcohol has resulted in complete pain relief for 3 months or longer.

Anatomic Considerations

Effective uncomplicated intercostal nerve block can be performed only by a physician who has a thorough understanding of the anatomy of the intercostal nerves and the ribs.

Intercostal Nerves

As described by Gray (10) and verified by me at autopsy by dissection of the intercostal nerves in eight corpses (17,24), the anterior rami of the second through the eleventh thoracic nerves lie in the costal grooves usually as far peripherally as 5 to 10 cm distal to the angles of the ribs (Fig. 1). At a distance of 5 to 8 cm anterior (peripheral) to the angle of the rib, the costal groove blends into the knife-like edge of the rib and then ceases to exist (Fig. 2). Even more important, before the termination of the costal groove, the main branches of the intercostal nerve have left the groove to pass between the internal intercostal muscles and the posterior intercostal membranes. Then they enter the substance of the internal intercostal muscles and run amidst their fibers as far as the costal cartilages.

The dura mater and the delicate arachnoid surrounding the anterior and posterior nerve roots pass to cover the formed spinal nerve and fuse with the epineurium at about the intervertebral foramen so that the pia mater is continuous with the epineurium of the nerve distal thereto (Fig. 3). Therefore, the perineural spaces of the intercostal nerves, particularly proximal

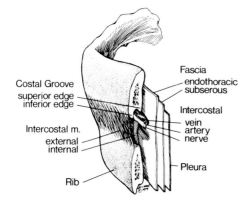

Costal Groove
superior edge
inferior edge

Fascia
endothoracic
subserous

Intercostal
vein
artery
nerve

Intercostal m.
external
internal

Pleura

Rib

FIG. 1. Cross-section at angle of rib. This relationship usually does not exist 5–8 cm lateral to the angle. m. = muscle.

FIG. 2. Anatomy of intercostal nerve (anterior division of thoracic spinal nerve) as it courses anteriorly, showing that its main branch does not lie under rib.

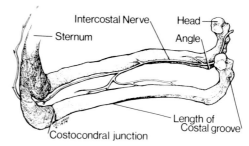

Intercostal Nerve   Head

Sternum   Angle

Length of
Costal groove

Costocondral junction

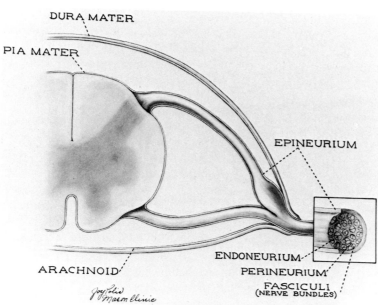

DURA MATER

PIA MATER

EPINEURIUM

ENDONEURIUM

PERINEURIUM

FASCICULI
(NERVE BUNDLES)

ARACHNOID

FIG. 3. Cross-section of spinal cord. Note that the epineurium of the nerve is a continuation of the pia mater. Therefore, fluid injected intraneurally may be trapped within the nerve. Although the interstices between the nerve bundles (fasciculi) are filled with connective tissue, they are called perineural spaces, and they are potential avenues for solutions injected intraneurally to undergo retrograde diffusion and reach the spinal cord.

to the angle of the rib, are potential canals by which fluids injected intra-neurally may spread centrally to the spinal cord, diffuse into the spinal fluid, and result in spinal anesthesia (12,13,25). Moreover, as is well known, the dermatomal distribution of each spinal nerve, including each intercostal nerve, overlaps so that, for example, the third intercostal nerve overlaps into the second and the fourth dermatomes. Therefore, to eliminate the pain of one dermatome, the intercostal nerve of that dermatome and the one above and the one below must be blocked. If the pain involves the midline structures such as the sternum, the intercostal nerves of both sides must be blocked in order to eliminate it.

Ribs

At the angle of the rib, that is, about 6 to 8 cm from the spinous process of the thoracic vertebra, the rib is the thickest and the costal groove is broadest and deepest but the groove does not extend beyond about 15 cm from the spinous process. The internal intercostal muscle attaches to the superior (internal) edge of the groove and the external intercostal muscles to its inferior (external) edge (Fig. 1). These muscles attach to the relatively narrow cephalad edge of the rib below. Between these muscles is a thin layer of fascia to which both muscles adhere (Fig. 1).

Covering the internal intercostal muscle is the endothoracic and subserous fasciae, as well as the pleura (Fig. 1). In a reasonably well-nourished patient, there is an accumulation of fat, which may be 2 to 3 mm or more, at the angle of the rib and between the subserous fascia and the pleura. This fat pad is seldom 2 to 3 mm thick at 15 cm or more distal to the spinous processes of the thoracic vertebrae. The fat pads and the width of the costal groove at the angle of the rib are added protection against a pneumothorax when the block is executed at this location.

Spread of the Injected Solution

When radiopaque solution, India ink, or blue liquid latex is injected into the costal grooves of ribs whose muscles and fasciae have not been disrupted by trauma, the anatomy causes these solutions to spread peripherally and centrally only in the groove of the injected rib (Fig. 4) (17,24). On the other hand, when injected into the intercostal muscles, the solutions pool in those muscles (Fig. 4) (24). However, if these barriers that limit spread are dis-rupted by trauma (e.g., fractured ribs, surgery, or removal of the thorax in cadavers), then the solution injected into the costal groove of one rib may spread to block more than one intercostal nerve (1,29). Finally, with com-puted tomography (CT), it is demonstrated that solutions injected into the costal grooves of the ribs do not spread to bathe the posterior branch of the

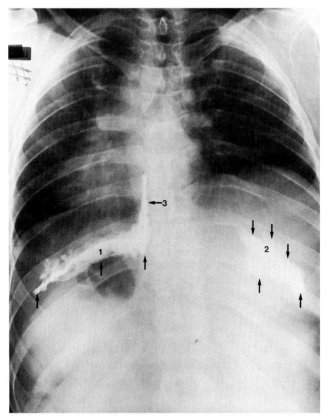

FIG. 4. (*1* and *3*) Spread of contrast medium solution along groove of human rib within 30 sec after injection of 5 ml [4 ml of 0.5% bupivacaine with 1 : 200,000 epinephrine and 1 ml of meglumine iothalamate USP 60 (Conray)] through needle correctly placed in groove 7.5 cm from spinous process of vertebra. (*2*) Spread from incorrectly placed needle into intercostal muscles. *Arrows* delineate extent of spread of contrast solution.

thoracic spinal nerves or the sympathetic ganglia, nor do they enter the epidural space (Fig. 5) (24).

Technical Considerations

Technique

If complications, particularly pneumothoraces, are to be kept to a minimum or avoided and the incidence of successful blocks kept high, the physician executing the block must know the previously described anatomy of the intercostal nerves and must meticulously adhere to the following steps in the technique of intercostal nerve block.

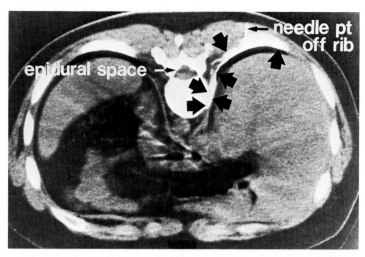

FIG. 5. Computed tomography scan of 5 ml of contrast solution [4 ml of 0.5% bupivacaine with 1 : 200,000 epinephrine and 1 ml of meglumine iothalamate USP 60 (Conray)] injected into costal groove of ninth rib 6.5 cm from spinous process of thoracic vertebra. *Arrows* delineate central and peripheral spread of the solution. The solution does not spread into the epidural space or anterior to the midpoint of the body of the vertebra to bathe the sympathetic ganglia.

The patient is placed in the prone position, with both arms hanging off the operating room table or cart, or in the lateral decubitus position (side), with the upper arm forward and cephalad. Both positions rotate the scapula upward and outward and away from the vertebral column, making palpation of the upper ribs easier. The prone position is preferred when a bilateral block is to be performed. The lateral position is selected when the block is unilateral and/or when the patient cannot lie on the abdomen. A line is drawn parallel to the spines of the vertebrae along the thoracic cage on the side to be blocked 6.5 to 7.5 cm (2½ to 3 inches) from the spines. The line should lie in the region of the angles of the ribs, just lateral to the sacrospinalis group of muscles. Then Xs are placed on this line at the lower border of the ribs to be blocked.

The Xs mark the optimal sites for injection of the local anesthetic solution because here: (a) the intercostal nerve lies in the rib's groove, and (b) the groove is the widest at this point, measuring 5 to 8 mm. The groove's depth at this point dictates that the length of the bevel of the needle's point should not exceed 3 mm. Furthermore, the use of radiopaque solutions in patients, as well as corpses, has demonstrated that 3 to 5 ml of solution injected into the rib's costal groove at this point is an adequate volume to block an intercostal nerve extensively (17,24).

The skin is aseptically prepared and draped. Skin wheals are raised at the determined points. When the physician anesthetist is right-handed, the full 10-ml syringe with the 3.8 cm short beveled, security-bead needle attached is held in the right hand while the index finger of the left hand palpates the inferior border of the rib. The left index finger pulls the skin which overlies the inferior border of the rib up and over the rib. The needle is introduced through the skin at the tip of the left index finger. The hub of the needle is inclined caudad so that the shaft forms an 80 degree angle with the skin. The needle is then slowly advanced until the point comes to rest on the lower edge of the rib. The left index finger releases the skin which had been pulled up and over the rib. Now the hub of the needle is held between the left thumb and index finger, and with the left middle (long) finger resting against the shaft of the needle, the needle's point is walked caudad off the rib. As the needle loses contact with the rib, the left hand resting on the back freezes the needle in place. The needle is then slowly advanced about 3 mm. Now, 3 to 5 ml of the anesthetic solution is deposited as the needle is constantly moved, that is, jiggled, first forward (inward) and then backward about 3 mm, guided by the left thumb and index finger. This technique is repeated on each of the intercostal nerves to be blocked and is known as "the shaking hand technique."

Drugs

For self-limiting somatic pain of the thorax and upper abdomen (e.g., fractured ribs, surgery), bupivacaine 0.25% or 0.5% with epinephrine (Adrenalin®) is the local anesthetic solution of choice. Special advantages of this drug are the long duration of action (9–18 hr when used for this block), absent tissue toxicity, and the low systemic toxicity (21). The optimal concentration of epinephrine is 1:200,000, i.e., 0.1 mg (0.1 ml of 1:1000 epinephrine) in 20 ml of the local anesthetic solution. The maximum amount of epinephrine added is 0.25 mg. Therefore, when 50 ml or less of the local anesthetic solution is required for the block, the optimal concentration of epinephrine is maintained. However, if more than 50 ml is required, then the concentration is less than optimal; for example, 0.25 ml of epinephrine in 80 ml of solution is a 1:320,000 concentration. Nonetheless, it is effective. Epinephrine is added because it slows absorption, and thereby: (a) prolongs the duration of the local anesthetic solution; (b) decreases its blood level, leaving more drug to diffuse to the nerves; and (c) consequently, intensifies the sensory and motor blockade. Equally important is epinephrine's positive inotropic effect on the heart, which offsets the depressant effects of the local anesthetic drug on the myocardium, should a systemic toxic reaction result (27).

For intractable cancer pain, 4 to 5 ml of absolute alcohol is injected into the costal groove. In the past, a maximum of 1.0 ml was injected, but numerous patients developed an intercostal neuritis, and the technique was abandoned (14). However, this has not occurred with the larger doses. One could theorize that, with the smaller dose, the nerve was only partially chemically destroyed and that, therefore, a causalgia-like pain resulted. With the larger amount, there is neurolysis of the entire nerve, and neuralgia does not occur. In attempts to relieve intractable pain of one rib, at least two intercostal nerves on that side need to be blocked, and if the sternum or middle of the abdomen is involved, the corresponding intercostal nerves on the other side may have to be injected.

Complications

Generalized Systemic Toxicity from the Local Anesthetics

During the 35-year-period 1947–1982, the author has not observed a severe systemic toxic reaction (e.g., unconsciousness, convulsion) during or after diagnostic or therapeutic percutaneous intercostal nerve block. However, when the statistics include the use of this technique for surgical operations for which the lower seventh intercostal nerves are usually blocked bilaterally, the incidence of systemic toxicity progressing to convulsions (all from absorption of the local anesthetic drug) was four in about 17,000 patients (0.024%). These convulsions occurred approximately 10 min after the injection of 70 to 80 ml of 0.5% bupivacaine (350–400 mg) with a final epinephrine concentration of 1:280,000 to 1:320,000. This is when the highest blood levels of the local anesthetic drug occur with intercostal nerve block. In one other like regional block procedure using 0.5% bupivacaine without epinephrine, asystole resulted without convulsions (27). These five reactions were treated with no untoward results (19). Therefore, from our experiences for these indications, the principal disadvantage of intercostal nerve block is the possibility of pneumothorax.

Pneumothorax

In the series of the author and his associates, pneumothorax consequent to intercostal nerve block occurred in only 14 of 17,000 patients (0.082%). The pneumothoraces did not result in major postoperative complications nor did they prolong hospitalization (7). Only one author has reported a high incidence of pneumothorax (19%) following intercostal nerve block (8). A number of anesthesiologists who have never done this block, or who have done it only occasionally, have stated that they do not use or teach the technique because the incidence of pneumothorax is too great. Obviously, our 0.082% incidence of pneumothorax and that of most others who have used this block in a significant number of patients, and thus have mastered the technique, do not support such statements (15). Also, to support my contention that pneumothorax occurs infrequently, routine preoperative anteroposterior roentgenograms were compared with ones taken on the second postoperative day in 200 consecutive surgical patients who received bilateral intercostal nerve blocks of the lower six or seven ribs as a step in the method of obtaining satisfactory anesthesia. In this study, one silent pneumothorax (no symptoms) with approximately a 25% collapse of the left lung occurred. No treatment was instituted and on the fifth postoperative day the chest X-ray showed that the lung had almost completely expanded (20). To conclude, our figures are impressive in view of the fact that 95% of the blocks were performed by resident physicians in all stages of anesthesiology training.

Cardiovascular Collapse

When the surgeon blocks the intercostal nerves before closure of the thoracotomy incision, it must be attempted intraneurally and as close as possible to the vertebral column (2,9,18,26,28,31). In the process, all or part of the local anesthetic solution may reach the subarachnoid space, perhaps through a long dural cuff, but more likely through the perineural spaces of the nerve (Fig. 3) (12,13,25). This can result in an unintentional spinal block with severe hypotension (2,9,18,26,28,31). When this has occurred, hypotension has been attributed to slowed metabolism of the local anesthetic drug and its depressing action on the cardiovascular system (9), or to deposit of the local anesthetic solution in the costal groove, with central spread bathing the sympathetic ganglia (9,31).

Our investigations, including CT of the spread of solutions injected into the costal groove of a rib at its angle (Fig. 5), do not confirm the theory of sympathetic blockade (17,24,28). Likewise, the theory of cardiovascular depression by the local anesthetic drug because of its reduced liver metabolism when intraneural injection of the intercostal nerves is done from within the thoracic cavity by the surgeon during an operation may be attributable to other than local anesthetic depression. It should be remembered that these patients receive general anesthesia, usually a halogenated hydrocarbon (e.g., halothane), which may contribute to cardiovascular depression. Percutaneous injection of the intercostal nerves in 17,000 patients, most for surgical procedures in which the bilateral intercostal nerve block was supplemented by general anesthesia consisting of nitrous oxide, oxygen, and very light concentration of halothane, have not produced hypotension (18,28).

To conclude, there are two ways to solve the problem of the intrathoracic approach resulting in cardiovascular collapse. First, no attempt should be made to inject the intercostal nerves intraneurally and centrad (mediad) to the angle of the rib. Second, the intercostal nerves can be blocked percutaneously before or after surgery. When performing percutaneous intercostal nerve blocks, my colleagues and I purposely avoid intraneural injections by jiggling the needle slightly as the 3 to 5 ml of solution is injected into the costal groove at the rib's angle; that is, the needle is moved a maximum of 3 mm forward and then backward (14).

CELIAC PLEXUS BLOCK

Indications

Diagnosis

The principal use of celiac plexus block is to differentiate upper abdominal musculoskeletal pain from that of the upper abdominal viscera (e.g., pancreas, gallbladder, liver, stomach) and to evaluate the effectiveness of chemical neurolysis in relieving intractable cancer pain of these organs. It may also be used to help in differential diagnosis of epigastric pain, which may be due to either disorders of the thoracic viscera or upper abdominal viscera. In the latter instance, celiac plexus block will relieve the pain but of course will not relieve pain of thoracic visceral origin.

Therapeutics

The principal use of celiac plexus block is to alleviate intractable pain from cancer of the pancreas for prolonged periods (3–12 months) using a neurolytic drug. However, it is also effective in abolishing pain from cancer of the other upper abdominal viscera. In over 600 such patients we have achieved immediate relief in 95% and long-term relief in 75 to 80% (16).

Celiac plexus block with either a local anesthetic drug or a neurolytic drug may not provide prolonged relief of pain due to acute or chronic pancreatitis. On the other hand, local anesthetic solutions containing steroids [80 mg of methylprednisolone (Depo-Medrol®) or triamcinoline (Aristocort®) in 50 ml of 0.5% bupivacaine with epinephrine 1:200,000 (0.25 mg in 50 ml)] have produced some promising results in treating acute pancreatitis with celiac plexus block, provided that one or more blocks are done early in the course of the disease.

Anatomic Considerations

Celiac Plexus and Ganglia

The celiac plexus consists of a number of prevertebral ganglia and a dense network of autonomic and sensory fibers that enmesh these ganglia (10). The autonomic fibers include sympathetic preganglionic fibers contributed by the greater splanchnic nerve that arises usually from T5 to T9 paravertebral sympathetic ganglia, the lesser splanchnic nerve that arises from T10 and T11 ganglia, and the lowest splanchnic nerve that arises from T12. The parasympathetic preganglionic fibers are contributed by both vagus nerves, particularly the right. The plexus gives off secondary plexuses to the diaphragm, liver, spleen, stomach, suprarenal gland, kidney, spermatic cord, abdominal aorta, and mesentery.

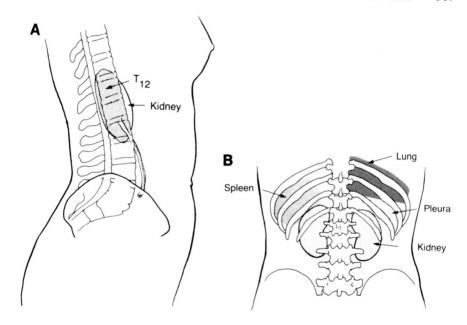

FIG. 6. **A:** Drawing showing position of kidneys lateral and opposite to vertebral column. **B:** Drawing of back of lumbar region, showing position of kidneys in relation to vertebrae, twelfth rib, pleura, lungs, and spleen.

The plexus is situated at the level of the upper part of the first lumbar vertebra and is composed of a right and left celiac ganglion and a dense network of nerve fibers connecting them. It surrounds the celiac artery and the base of the superior mesenteric artery. It lies in areolar tissue behind the peritoneum, the stomach, and the omental bursa, anterior to (below and in front of) the crura of the diaphragm and the commencement of the abdominal aorta, and between the suprarenal glands.

Kidneys

It is important to remember that the kidneys lie adjacent to the vertebral column and behind the peritoneum, surrounded by loose areolar tissue and a mass of fat. They are in the same compartment with the celiac plexus, the aorta, and the vena cava. Moreover, the medial surfaces of the upper and lower poles of the kidney lie about 5 and 7 cm, respectively, from the midline of the back (spinous processes of the vertebrae) with the right kidney 1 cm lower than the left (Fig. 6). The upper poles are at the level of the T12 vertebra and the lower poles at the upper border of the body of the L3 vertebra (Fig. 6). Finally, the twelfth ribs lie over the kidneys (Fig. 6). Obviously, therefore, if puncture of the kidneys is to be avoided, the needles must pass mediad to them in the 2 to 3 cm of tissue that normally lies between the kidneys and the lumbar vertebrae (11,16,22). In the patient with cancer, this distance may be markedly reduced on one or both sides by pressure from the tumor (22).

Diaphragm

The right crus of the diaphragm, broader and longer than the left, arises from the anterolateral surfaces of the bodies of the L1–L3 vertebrae and from their intervertebral discs. The left crus arises from the corresponding parts of the L1 and L2.

Technical Considerations

Technique

The celiac plexus may be blocked by one of three approaches: (1) the classic approach, which entails placing the needles and the solution cephalad to the diaphragm and blocking the greater, lesser, and lowest splanchnic nerves and the vagus nerves, all of which contribute to the plexus (Figs. 7 and 8) (11,14,16,22); (2) the transcrural approach, which results in blocking the celiac plexus and its ganglia caudad to the diaphragm (Fig. 9) (23,29); or (3) a combination of these (Fig. 10).

Since it was first described by Kappis (11) in 1919, the classic approach has been the most often used for diagnostic and therapeutic purposes without the aid of radiographic techniques (14). If the transcrural approach is to be used, CT is essential for accurate needle placement (21,29). Whether the transcrural approach has any advantage over the classic approach for the initial attempt to relieve the pain of cancer with a neurolytic drug is debatable (23).

Celiac plexus block is not difficult to master, and complications are minimal provided the technique of the block is meticulously followed (14). For any of the approaches, the patient is placed in the prone position with a pillow between the iliac crests and the rib cage so as to reduce the lumbar curve of the vertebral column to a minimum. Any other position increases significantly the likelihood of misplacing the needles.

The landmarks are the spinous process of the first lumbar vertebra and its cephalad edge under which the celiac plexus lies, and the lower borders of the twelfth ribs a maximum of 7.5 cm from the posterior midline of the body. These points are marked with Xs, and the Xs are connected by straight lines forming a flat triangle. The maximum of 7.5 cm from the midline to the ribs is critical because of the anatomical position of the kidneys (Fig. 6). If puncture of the kidneys is to be avoided, the needles must pass medial to them in the 2 to 3 cm of tissue that lies between the medial edges of the kidneys and the lumbar vertebrae. When the distance for inserting the needle

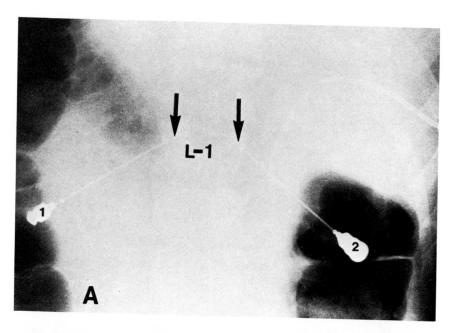

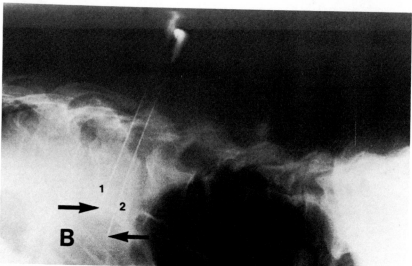

FIG. 7. A: Posteroanterior radiograph of needles depicted in most publications to be correctly and optimally placed for celiac plexus block anterior to and at cephalad lateral borders of body of L1 vertebra. These needles were placed by contacting the body of the L1 vertebra, walking the needles off the body of the vertebra, and then advancing them ventrally 1.5–2 cm. **B:** Lateral view shows needle on left and right anterior to body of vertebra. Although both needles are the same depth, the right one appears, from distortion, to be deeper than the left. Note that the needle on the right contains a removable metal cap so that it may be differentiated from the left on the lateral film.

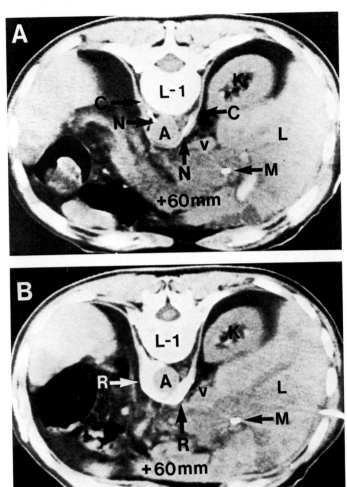

FIG. 8. A: Computed tomography scan at +60 mm (6 cm) cephalad from start of scanning (hubs of needles), with bevel of needle on left positioned unintentionally in wall of aorta and needle on right in correct position. **B:** Computed tomography scan at +60 mm, needle on left was withdrawn approximately 3 mm to free it from wall of aorta. Then 50 ml of 50% alcohol containing megulmine iothalamate was injected, i.e., 25 ml through each needle, and both needles were withdrawn. The solution spread cephalad to the diaphragm and surrounded the aorta. L-1 = first lumbar vertebra; A = aorta; v = vena cava; M = drainage tube in bile duct; C = crura of diaphragm; K = kidney; L = liver; N = points of needles; R = alcohol-iothalamate-local anesthetic drug solution.

is greater than 7.5 cm from the midline, the needle can pass through the kidney.

For the classic approach (needle's bevels placed cephalad to the diaphragm) a 20-gauge needle is placed through the Xs at the lower edge of the twelfth rib, at a 45 degree angle to the skin, on the left side. With the line

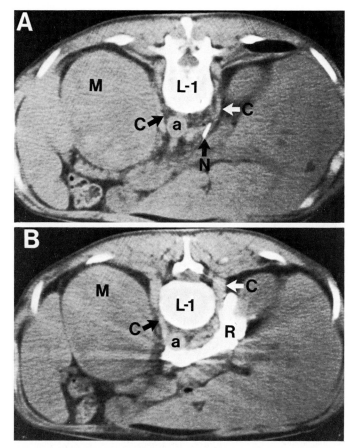

FIG. 9. When the transcrural approach is used, usually only one needle is placed on the right side at L1 because, even if CT is used, a needle inserted on the left side would in most instances pass through the aorta before puncturing the crus of the diaphragm, as can be ascertained from the CT scan. **A:** Needle's bevel anterior to crus of diaphragm. **B:** Spread from needle in A of 50 ml of 50% alcohol containing meglumine iothalamate. L-1 = body of first lumbar vertebra; C = crura of diaphragm; a = aorta; M = massive growth of lung metastasis in left adrenal gland; N = needle's bevel; R = spread of radiopaque solution in prevertebral space anterior to diaphragm.

of the side of the marked triangle as a guide, the needle is slowly advanced until its point contacts the lateral surface of the body of the first lumbar vertebra. The depth of the needle is noted. Then the needle is withdrawn 2.5 cm, and the angle between its shaft and the skin is increased by 10 degrees—that is, from 45 to 55 degrees—and then the needle is reinserted. This maneuver is repeated, increasing the angle slightly each time, until the needle is felt to slip off the body of the vertebra. Then it is inserted to a depth of 2 to 2.5 cm deeper than when the first contact with the lateral surface of the vertebra was made or until pulsations of the aorta are felt. If pulsations are felt, then the needle is withdrawn 3 to 4 mm so as to be certain it does

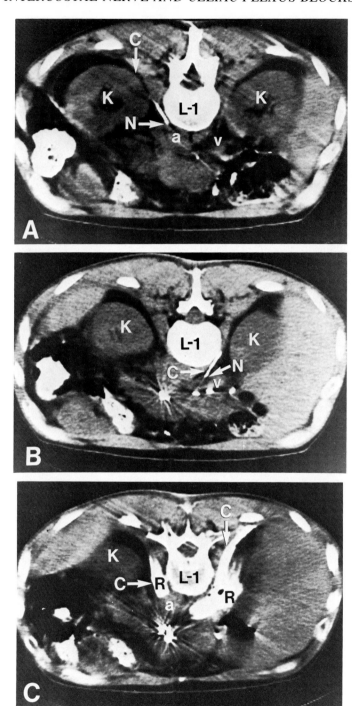

FIG. 10. Computed tomography scan of a combined approach in a patient whose previous block using classic approach gave only partial relief. **A:** Needle on left cephalad

not lie in the wall of the aorta. After placement of this needle, another 20-gauge needle is placed on the right side in an identical way and to the same or a slightly deeper depth as the needle on the left side.

For the transcrural approach (needle's bevel caudad to the diaphragm), all the steps of the classic approach are followed except one needle only is placed on the right side and advanced 4 to 5 cm or more anterior to the body of the vertebra so that its bevel traverses the right crus of the diaphragm.

For the combined approach, the needle on the left is placed as described for the classic approach and the needle on the right as for the transcrural approach.

When I perform a diagnostic and/or therapeutic block, I prefer to use a combination of the available radiographic techniques, i.e., posteroanterior and lateral radiographs for a diagnostic block with the local anesthetic drug (Fig. 7) and CT for a therapeutic block with alcohol (Fig. 8) (22). Doing so gives documentation of needle placement and, if the solution contains contrast medium, the extent of spread. Furthermore, using these radiographic aids constitute important educational tools when teaching residents. For the first attempt to relieve cancer pain, I select the classic approach for both the diagnostic and the therapeutic block. But if the transcrural approach is chosen, then only a single needle is placed on the right side (Fig. 9) because a needle placed on the left usually will pass through the aorta (Fig. 10A).

In the few instances where the cancer pain is not completely relieved within 24 to 48 hr using the classic approach, the block is repeated. Then the needle on the left side is placed behind the aorta (above the diaphragm) whereas that on the right is placed transcrurally (below it) (Fig. 10).

Advantages and Disadvantages of Radiography

The use of radiography has certain advantages and disadvantages other than cost, depending on the technique of blocking the plexus used.

Needles placed cephalad to the diaphragm (Classic Approach)

A posteroanterior radiograph can help avoid misplacement of the needles if: (a) there is a congenital absence of the twelfth rib, or if it is short and not palpable (this occurs in about 20% of patients); (b) the twelfth rib slopes markedly caudad; or (c) six lumbar vertebrae are present (Fig. 7A) (22). With CT, such variations cannot be demonstrated as rapidly. A lateral radiograph can assure that the needle does not traverse an intervertebral for-

---

to diaphragm. **B:** Needle on right caudad to diaphragm. **C:** Spread of solution after injection of 30 ml of 50% alcohol containing meglumine iothalamate through needle on left and 50 ml through needle on right. L-1 = first lumbar vertebra; K = kidneys; C = crus of diaphragm; N = needle's point; a = aorta; v = vena cava; R = spread of radiopaque solution.

amen and that the needle's point is positioned anterior to the body of the L1 vertebra (Fig. 7B) (22).

On the other hand, posteroanterior and lateral radiographs are of no value in establishing whether the needle has punctured an organ, the exact distance its point is located anterior to the L1 vertebra, or the exact spread of the injected solution (Fig. 8) (22). Fluoroscopy has the same advantages and drawbacks as radiography, but with it, to a limited extent, the spread of a radiopaque solution in relation to the pulsations of the aorta can be followed.

Computed tomography confirms the topographic anatomy of the kidney and further demonstrates that in order to avoid puncture of the kidneys in all patients, the site of insertion of the needles must be no more than 7 to 7.5 cm from the spinous process of the lumbar vertebra directly mediad to the lower edge of the twelfth rib (Figs. 8–10) (22). Even this distance may be too great in a patient with a large tumor; a needle has passed through the kidney when these distances were not exceeded (22).

Single needle placed caudad to the diaphragm (Transcrural Approach)

When this technique is used, CT is mandatory to be sure that the needle has traversed the diaphragm and lies caudad (Figs. 9 and 10).

One needle placed caudad to and one placed cephalad to the diaphragm (Combined Classic and Transcrural Approaches)

Again, with this technique, CT is mandatory to assure correct needle placement (Fig. 10).

Drugs

For the diagnostic block using the classic approach, 50 ml of 0.5% bupivacaine (250 mg with 1:200,000 epinephrine) is injected, i.e., 25 ml through each needle at the rate of 1.0 ml/sec. If only one needle is placed through the crus of the right diaphragm, the 50 ml is injected through it.

For the therapeutic block using these approaches, the 50 ml of solution contains: (a) 25 ml absolute alcohol; (b) 7 ml of meglumine iothalamate USP 60 (600 mg/ml), osmolarity = 1.5 mOsm/ml (Conray); and (c) 18 ml of 0.75% bupivacaine. This solution also is injected at the rate of 1 ml/sec (Figs. 8 and 9). However, when the initial block does not relieve the cancer pain and the block is repeated with one needle behind the aorta and the other transcrural (Fig. 10), 80 ml of solution is prepared. This solution contains: (a) 40 ml of absolute alcohol, (b) 8 ml of the meglumine iothalamate, and (c) 32 ml of 0.75% bupivacaine. Then 30 ml is injected through the needle behind the aorta and 50 ml through the other one (Fig. 10).

While CT assures correct needle placement, the addition of meglumine iothalamate allows determination of the actual extent of spread of the solution, which is particularly helpful if one or both blocks fail to relieve the patient's pain (Figs. 8B, 9B, and 10C). Contrary to other studies (23,29), it should be noted that when the transcrural approach is used, the solution does not spread around the aorta, as it does with the classic approach (cf. Figs. 9B and 10C with Fig. 8B).

Complications

If the needles are placed correctly as described (i.e., no more than 7.5 cm from the spinous process of the lumbar vertebra, immediately below the caudad edge of the twelfth rib and anterior to the body of the L1 vertebra, either cephalad to or caudad to the diaphragm and verified by conventional radiography and/or CT), the only complication that should occur is orthostatic hypotension for 24 hr. Therefore, fluids should be given intravenously during and after the block. Also, back pain lasting 24 to 36 hr may result from the alcohol. The intractable cancer pain usually disappears within 15 min, but occasionally it persists, even though markedly less intense, for 24 hr.

On the other hand, if the needles are incorrectly inserted through the skin more than 7.5 cm from the spinous process of a lumbar vertebra and if placement is not verified by posteroanterior radiographs or CT, the following complications may develop: (a) the kidney may be impaled, with subsequent hematuria, and if the pelvis of the kidney is also punctured, urine may extravasate into the tissues; (b) a lumbar somatic nerve may be blocked, with a motor and sensory deficit in the lower extremity; (c) the needle(s) may pass into the epidural or subarachnoid space, which, if not recognized, will result in epidural or spinal block; or (d) the lung(s) may be punctured and pneumothorax may result. Obviously, if these occur with a diagnostic block using a local anesthetic solution and if they are recognized and properly treated, permanent sequelae are unlikely to result. However, if a neurolytic therapeutic block is executed, the patient may be permanently paralyzed or lose the kidney. Both of these things have happened.

In conclusion, to avoid the complications of celiac plexus block, it is mandatory that the twelfth rib and the first lumbar vertebra be identified and that the distance from the midline to the point of needle insertion not exceed 7.5 cm.

ACKNOWLEDGMENT

Much of the work reported in this chapter was done in the Department of Anesthesiology, Virginia Mason Hospital, Seattle, Washington.

REFERENCES

1. Ballantine, R. I. W. (1980): Posterior intercostal nerve block (correspondence). *Br. J. Anaesth.*, 52:843.

2. Benumof, J. L., and Semenza, J. (1975): Total spinal anesthesia following intrathoracic intercostal nerve blocks. *Anesthesiology*, 43:124–125.
3. Bonica, J. J. (1953): *The Management of Pain*. Lea & Febiger, Philadelphia.
4. Bonica, J. J. (1974): Current role of nerve blocks in the diagnosis and therapy of pain. In: *International Symposium on Pain (Advances in Neurology, Vol. 4)*, edited by J. J. Bonica, pp. 445–453. Raven Press, New York.
5. Bonica, J. J., Akamatsu, T. J., Berges, P. U., Morikawa, K., and Kennedy, W. F., Jr. (1971): Circulatory effects of peridural block: II. Effects of epinephrine. *Anesthesiology*, 34:514–522.
6. Bonica, J. J., Kennedy, W. F., Jr., Akamatsu, T. J., and Gerbershagen, H. U. (1972): Circulatory effects of peridural block. III. Effects of acute blood loss. *Anesthesiology*, 36:219–227.
7. Bridenbaugh, P. O., Du Pen, S. L., Moore, D. C., Bridenbaugh, L. D., and Thompson, G. E. (1973): Postoperative nerve block anesthesia versus narcotic analgesia. *Anesth. Analg.*, 52:407–413.
8. Chivers, E. M. (1946): Pulmonary complications following regional analgesia for abdominal operations. *Br. J. Anaesth.*, 20:55–59.
9. Cottrell, W. M., Schick, L. M., Perkins, H. M., and Modell, J. H. (1978): Hemodynamic changes after intercostal nerve block with bupivacaine-epinephrine solution. *Anesth. Analg.*, 57:492–495.
10. Gray, H. (1980): In: *Anatomy of the Human Body, 36th ed.*, edited by P. L. Williams and R. Warwick, pp. 549, 1103–1106, 1131. Lea & Febiger, Philadelphia.
11. Kappis, M. (1919): Sensibilitat und lokale anasthesie im chirurgischen gebeit der bauchkokle mit besonderer berucksichtingung der splanchnicusanasthesie. *Beitr. Klin. Chir.*, 115:161–175.
12. Moore, D. C. (1953): Efocaine: Complications following its use. *West. J. Surg. Obstet. Gynecol.*, 61:635–638.
13. Moore, D. C. (1954): Complications following the use of Efocaine. *Surgery*, 35:109–114.
14. Moore, D. C. (1965): *Regional Block, 4th ed.*, pp. 148, 149–156, 156–158, 332–333. Charles C Thomas, Springfield, Ill.
15. Moore, D. C. (1975): Intercostal nerve block for postoperative somatic pain following surgery of the thorax and upper abdomen. *Br. J. Anaesth.*, 47:284–286.
16. Moore, D. C. (1979): Celiac (splanchnic) plexus block with alcohol for cancer pain for the upper intraabdominal viscera. In: *Advances in Pain Research and Therapy, Vol. 2*, edited by J. J. Bonica and V. Ventafridda, pp. 357–371. Raven Press, New York.
17. Moore, D. C. (1981): Intercostal nerve block: Spread of India ink injected to rib's costal groove. *Br. J. Anaesth.*, 53:325–329.
18. Moore, D. C. (1982): Anatomy of the intercostal nerve: Its importance during thoracic surgery. *Am. J. Surg.*, 144:371–373.
19. Moore, D. C. (1983): Systemic toxicity of local anesthetic drugs. In: *Seminars in Anesthesia, Regional Anesthesia, Vol. 2*, edited by R. L. Katz, pp. 62–74. Grune & Stratton, New York.
20. Moore, D. C., and Bridenbaugh, L. D. (1962): Pneumothorax: Its incidence following intercostal nerve block. *JAMA*, 182:1005–1008.
21. Moore, D. C., Bridenbaugh, L. D., Thompson, G. E., Balfour, R. I., and Horton, W. G. (1978): Bupivacaine: A review of 11,080 cases. *Anesth. Analg.*, 57:42–53.
22. Moore, D. C., Bush, W. H., and Burnett, L. L. (1981): Celiac plexus blocks: A roentgenographic, anatomic study of technique and spread of solution in patients and corpses. *Anesth. Analg.*, 60:369–379.
23. Moore, D. C., Bush, W. H., Burnett, L. L., and Singler, R. C. (1982): An improved technique for celiac plexus block may be more theoretical than real (correspondence). *Anesthesiology*, 57:347–349.
24. Moore, D. C., Bush, W. H., and Scurlock, J. E. (1980): Intercostal nerve block: A roentgenographic, anatomic study of technique and absorption in humans. *Anesth. Analg.*, 59:815–825.
25. Moore, D. C., Hain, R. F., Ward, A., and Bridenbaugh, L. D. (1954): Importance of the perineural spaces in nerve blocking. *JAMA*, 156:1050–1053.
26. Moore, D. C., and Reitan, J. A. (1978): Sudden total spinal block after intraoperative intercostal injections. *Anesth. Rev.*, 5:36–38.

27. Moore, D. C., and Scurlock, J. E. (1983): Possible role of epinephrine in prevention or correction of myocardial depression associated with bupivacaine. *Anesth. Analg.*, 62:450–453.

28. Moore, D. C., and Skretting, P. (1981): Hypotension after intercostal nerve block (correspondence). *Br. J. Anaesth.*, 53:1235–1236.

29. Nunn, J. F., and Slavin, G. (1980): Posterior intercostal nerve block for pain relief after cholecystectomy. *Br. J. Anaesthesiol.*, 52:253–260.

30. Singler, R. C. (1982): An improved technique for alcohol neurolysis of the celiac plexus. *Anesthesiology*, 56:137–141.

31. Skretting, P. (1981): Hypotension after intercostal nerve block during thoracotomy under general anesthesia. *Br. J. Anaesth.*, 53:527–529.

*Advances in Pain Research
and Therapy, Vol. 7,*
edited by C. Benedetti et al.
Raven Press, New York © 1984.

Contralateral Local Anesthesia in the Treatment of Phantom and Stump Pain

Dieter Gross

Niederraeder Landstrasse 58, D-6000 Frankfurt am Main 71, Federal Republic of Germany

This chapter includes information from an article that appeared in July 1982 (5). Therapeutic local anesthesia in the treatment of chronic pain due to injury of the peripheral nervous system has been used for many years (3). I have used this method since 1946 to manage a variety of pain syndromes that are manifested by disturbances of the vasomotor system, muscle tone, and local tissue health, and in this way disturb the functional symmetry (as measured plethysmographically) that exists between the two sides of the body (2). Acute disturbances lead to a hyperergic (plus) disturbance, whereas chronic ones produce hypoergic (minus) disturbance. Injection of a local anesthetic into a scar, chronic inflammatory site, trigger zone, or the sympathetic chain restores the functional symmetry; eliminates the associated dysesthesia, dyskinesia, dyscrasia and dysthymia; and promotes euesthesia, eukinesia, eucrasia and euthymia.

A beneficial result of local anesthetic injection suggests a correlation to the patterns of segmental or autonomic innervation (Fig. 1). During the past several years, I have used local anesthesia injected into sites of the contralateral limb in the treatment of phantom limb pain and stump pain (4,5). To date I have used this technique on 10 patients who had long histories of phantom limb pain and stump pain. In this chapter I will give details of one patient to illustrate the problems of diagnosis and therapy, summarize the management of three other patients, and mention the results obtained in the other six cases.

PATIENTS AND RESULTS

Case 1

In 1977 I saw a 63-year-old woman who had a long history of persistent pain in the stump and phantom limb that followed dysarticulation of the hip (Fig. 2). During the course of 2 years prior to the consultation, she had undergone three attempts at joint prosthesis, but she was left with a persistent abscess and fistula, necessitating dysarticulation. Promptly after the operation, she

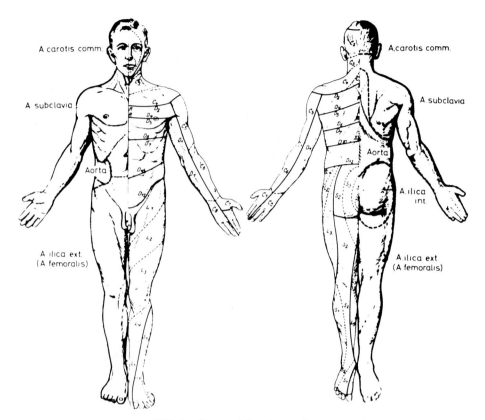

FIG. 1. Segmental and vascular zones.

began to have pain a few inches above her knee with radiation into her toes. The pain was of burning character and was associated with bouts of lancinating pain in the entire phantom. The pain awakened the patient at night and occurred frequently during the day, causing her to moan continuously. Analgesic and hypnotic medications were ineffective, as were local anesthesia injected into postcholecystectomy and postappendectomy scars.

Injection of the trigger areas in the opposite leg was then considered. The patient was asked to identify the region on her left leg that corresponded to the sites of her right phantom limb pain. These points were found to be hypersensitive to pressure in comparison to the surrounding areas. Within the hyperalgesic area, points that had a lower resistance to weak direct current (3 V) could be found. The hyperalgesic points on the left leg were identified and anesthetized with a fine needle with a total of 1.8 ml of 1% mepivacaine. This produced complete relief of pain for 1 hr, after which the pain recurred but of less intensity. Local anesthetic injection of the hyperalgesic points of the left leg on successive days produced similar results, and by the fourth day she complained only of a slight tingling sensation in the phantom limb. The treatment was continued, and by the end of 2 weeks the phantom pain disappeared completely. She remained pain-free for 6 months, when the phantom pain recurred in the toes and foot, prompting another series of contralateral anesthetic infiltration with similar results.

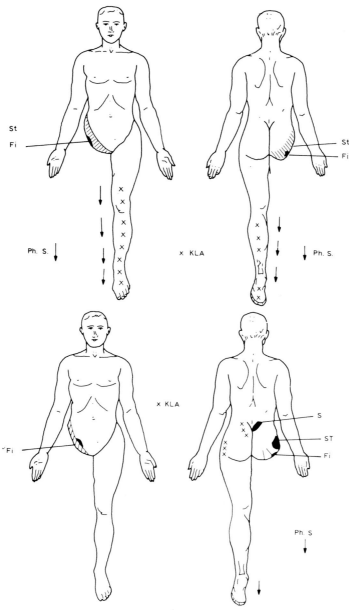

FIG. 2. *Case 1.* Sites of amputation pain and of contralateral therapeutic local anesthesia. The **upper** figure shows the site of phantom limb pain (Ph.S.), indicated by the arrow on the right side, and the site of injection of hyperalgesic points of the contralateral limb, while the **lower** figure shows the site of stump pain (St.) and the sites of the injection of the contralateral side to relieve it. Fi = fistula; S = sacroiliac joint; KLA = contralateral local anesthesia. (From Gross ref. 5, with permission.)

Two years later the patient reported almost no phantom pain, but she still complained of stump pain, especially above the right hip. This was increased by sitting. Systemic analgesics proved ineffective. Examination of the patient revealed hyperalgesic points above the right sacroiliac joint and the iliac crest, with corresponding contralateral hyperalgesia on the left side most readily elicited by pressure on the periosteum. Points of lower electrical skin resistance were noted, and at these sites the local anesthetic was injected down to the periosteum with a needle 8 cm long, using 1.8 ml of 1% mepivacaine. Promptly after the treatment there was complete pain relief, which lasted 6 hr. The hyperalgesic points above the right pelvis were again localized, and the corresponding points on the left were identified electrically. These were in the area of the sacroiliac joint, sacral nerve roots, ischium, and coccyx. Local anesthetic injected into these points on the left side produced complete pain relief and disappearance of the deeper hyperalgesic points. At a follow-up visit 1 year later, the patient was still pain-free.

This case has been described in detail because it demonstrates the possibility of using local anesthesia to treat phantom pain and stump pain. There are four salient points. First, local anesthesia has been helpful with persistent stump and phantom pain after a hip resection, accompanied by a wound fistula for years, which had resisted other pain therapy. Second, therapeutic local anesthesia of the stump itself and of other operation scars was ineffective. Third, on the periosteum of the normal leg, contralateral to the phantom, there were hyperalgesic points that could be detected by pressure with the finger. In these zones there were also points of lower skin resistance to direct current of 3 V. Small doses of a local anesthetic injected directly into these areas of the contralateral leg eliminated the patient's pain. Fourth, the surprising result was the long-term relief of the pain in phantom limb and stump on the side opposite to the injection sites.

Case 2

A 65-year-old man was referred because of pain on the outer side of his left thigh amputation stump, and phantom pain of the amputated left lower thigh (Fig. 3). Since the time of his injury in 1941, he had suffered from bouts of stump and phantom limb pain, which he described as "like being stabbed with a knife, especially when the weather changed and during the night." In addition to the intermittent phantom pain, there was also constant pain in the stump and phantom. The patient had hyperalgesia in the left buttock down to the stump. Examination of that region revealed an intense, sharp pain associated with a burning pain that came on with a slight latency. Stump and stump scar were painfully sensitive to pressure. Maximum pain was identified in the middle of the phantom tibia at the point of his original wound. The oscillometric examination of the upper thigh showed a clear reduction of amplitudes when contrasted with the left. The right oscillometric indices were astonishingly high, and the oscillometric quotient was 0.6 (5). Therapy, consisting of injection of the contralateral limb, was instituted with similar results. Follow-up for 4 years revealed that the phantom pain occurred sporadically about five times a year and became less and less, while the scar pain disappeared completely.

Case 3

A 60-year-old man was referred because of unbearable burning, lancinating pain in his phantom left big toe and heel (Fig. 4). The left foot and part of the lower thigh had been avulsed in 1943, and subsequently it was necessary to

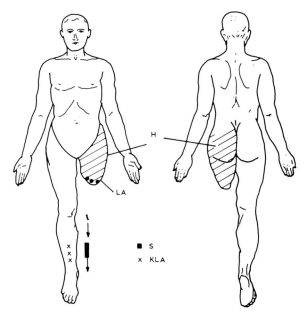

FIG. 3. *Case 2.* Phantom and stump pain. S = site of phantom and stump pain; H = hyperalgesia; LA = site of local anesthesia infiltration in the stump; KLA = site of contralateral local anesthesia injections. (From Gross, ref. 5, with permission.)

repeat the amputation on three occasions. The phantom pain in the toe began immediately after he was wounded. A left lumbar sympathectomy was performed in 1965 with significant improvement for a few years, but it did not eliminate completely the phantom pain that had plagued him night and day since 1978. Conventional analgesic therapy failed to give relief. Transcutaneous nerve stimulation for 3 months over the left peroneal nerve gave minimal relief. Contralateral local anesthetic was instituted in the same manner as previously described, and this produced complete relief of phantom pain for a 2-year period of follow-up.

Case 4

A 29-year-old man was run over by a bus in 1952. Bilateral below knee amputations were performed because of osteomyelitis of the right lower thigh and arterial insufficiency in the left lower thigh. The stumps were well healed with thick scarring, but a pressure ulcer of the left popliteal fossa failed to heal despite all forms of treatment. The patient experienced considerable pain when he bicycled with his prosthesis. This area, located above the medial popliteal nerve, was very sensitive to pressure. Contralateral local anesthesia was carried out as previously described. By the day after the injection, the pain had decreased considerably and, for the first time in 4 weeks, he also showed signs of healing. After a second injection on the right leg, pain in the region of the left-sided ulcer was markedly reduced. Five days later the ulcer was completely healed and the pain in the stomach had disappeared. At follow-up 6 months later, the pain relief in the stump and phantom limb persisted.

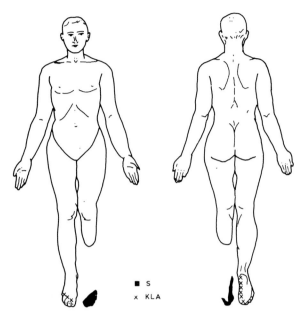

■ S
x KLA

FIG. 4. *Case 3.* Distribution of phantom limb pain indicated by the black missing foot. KLA = contralateral local anesthesia. (From Gross, ref 5, with permission.)

DISCUSSION

I have used this technique of contralateral anesthesia (CLA) in 6 other patients with similar results. The duration of pain in the 10 patients ranged from 2 to 39 years; the number of treatments required to relieve pain ranged from 2 to 34. The period of posttherapy observation ranged from 2 months to 4 years. Contralateral anesthesia provided immediate relief in all 10 patients, and long-lasting relief in 8. On the basis of this experience, I have developed the following technique of managing patients with phantom and stump pain with contralateral local anesthesia:

1. A comprehensive history of the patient is elicited, especially concerning the initial injury. This is followed by thorough neurologic, psychologic, medical, orthopedic, and radiologic examinations, often carried out in cooperation with other consultants.
2. The patient is asked to indicate the sites of his phantom limb pain and stump pain on the contralateral limb. Invariably, these "trigger" points are usually hypersensitive to pressure. They are marked on the skin.
3. The sensitivity of the skin of periosteum is then assessed by pressure exerted with a finger or with a probe.
4. Points within the hyperalgesic areas on the contralateral side, which have the characteristic of lower resistance of the skin against a weak DC electrical current (3 V), are identified, marked, and photographed.

5. At the point of lower skin resistance, the analgesic points are anesthetized, using the finest needle possible and injecting small volumes of local anesthetics (0.5–1.8 of 1% mepivacaine), with the injection carried down to the periosteum.
6. The next day the results of the contralateral local anesthesia are tested subjectively by the patient and objectively by testing the superficial hyperalgesia. Contralateral local anesthesia is repeated daily as required by the patient's progress.

Therapy of phantom pain by injection or stimulation of the contralateral intact limb has been tried with acupuncture by Bischko (*personal communication*) and Labrousse and Duron (7) and with transcutaneous nerve stimulation by Hiedl et al. (6), all of whom report some success. The mechanisms of these therapeutic approaches are not clear. Presumably, these procedures, like the contralateral local anesthesia, produce an inhibitory action at central nervous system sites where both limbs project (e.g., in medial structures of the thalamus or the brainstem reticular formation). Such inhibitory mechanisms have support from animal experiments. Neuronal hyperactivity in the thalamus of rats, which occurred after transection of dorsal roots, could be inhibited by electrical stimulation of the limb contralateral to the transected dorsal roots. Albe-Fessard and Lombard (1) have reported that electrical stimulation of the contralateral limb in these animals eliminated the behavioral signs of chronic pain during the period of stimulation.

I have used contralateral local anesthesia in the treatment of acute pain and other chronic pain syndromes with surprisingly good results. On the basis of my experience, I believe that the use of CLA deserves further trial in patients with phantom limb and stump pain as well as other acute and chronic pain syndromes.

SUMMARY

Phantom limb pain and stump pain were reduced or abolished by contralateral local anesthesia at hyperalgesic points on the opposite side in 10 patients with pain that had resisted other forms of therapy. The beneficial effects of CLA for these types of pain seem to be long term. The diagnostic and therapeutic techniques are described in the hope that others will use this method of managing patients with phantom limb and stump pain.

REFERENCES

1. Albe-Fessard, D. G., and Lombard, M. C. (1980): Animal models for chronic pain. In: *Pain and Society*, edited by H. W. Kosterlitz and L. Y. Terenius, pp. 299–310. Verlag Chemie, Weinheim.
2. Gross, M. (1976): Vergleichende Untersuchungen der Extremitatendurchblutung mit dem Doppler-Ultraschall-Verfahren, der Oscillographie, der Venenverschlussplethysmographie

und der Lichtplethysmographic an gesunden Versuchspersonen. Inaugural Dissertation. Med. Fakultat der Universitat Frankfurt.

3. Gross, D. (1979): *Therapeutische Lokalanasthesie. 2. Aufl.*, Hippokrates Verlag, Stuttgart.
4. Gross, D. (1981): Kontralaterale lokalanasthesia in der Therapise von Stumpf und Phantom-schmerz. In: *Phantomschmerz*, edited by J. Siegfried, A. Struppler and M. Zimmermann. Springer Verlag, Heidelberg.
5. Gross, D. (1982): Contralateral local anaesthesia in the treatment of phantom limb and stump pain. *Pain*, 13:313–320.
6. Hiedl, P., Struppler, A., and Gessler, M. (1979): TNS evoked long loop effects. *Appl. Neurophysiol.* 42:153–159.
7. Labrousse, J. L., and Duron, A. J. (1953): Traitement des algies des amputes par l'acupuncture. *Bull. Soc. Acupunct.*, 7.

Advances in Pain Research and Therapy, Vol. 7,
edited by C. Benedetti et al.
Raven Press, New York © 1984.

Lytic Saddle Block: Clinical Comparison of the Results, Using Phenol at 5, 10, and 15 Percent

S. Ischia, A. Luzzani, L. Pacini, and G. F. Maffezzoli

*Institute of Anesthesiology and Intensive Care, University of Padua,
37134 Verona, Italy*

Subarachnoid block is a useful technique for the treatment of perineal cancer pain. However, the frequent bilateral location of the pain, the involvement of the sphincters, often resulting from the block, and the duration of the antalgic effects are problems that have not been fully resolved.

Many authors have used Maher's (1) classic technique, which consists of injection of hyperbaric phenol in glycerin in the subarachnoid space at the L5–S1 level. The purpose of the present clinical research is to compare the results and complications obtained with the phenol concentrations normally advocated in the literature (5–7½%) against those obtained with higher concentrations of phenol (10–15%).

MATERIALS AND METHODS

We studied a group of 46 patients suffering from different neoplastic diseases: 28 patients had cancer of the rectum and sigmoid colon, 10 had cancer of the uterus, 5 had cancer of the vulva, 2 had cancer of the urinary bladder, and 1 had cancer of the prostate. The pain was exclusively located in the sacral spinal segments. All patients were treated with neurolytic subarachnoid block using 5% phenol (29 blocks in 20 patients), 10% phenol (16 blocks in 15 patients), and 15% phenol (11 blocks in 11 patients). The first block failed in 3 patients (5% phenol group) and was immediately repeated. A further 7 patients (6 belonging to the 5% phenol group, and 1 to the 10% phenol group) received a second block at varying time intervals after the first block.

Each patient was placed in a seated position, and a 20-gauge spinal needle was inserted at the L5–S1 level in the subarachnoid space. The bevel of the needle was carefully placed in the extreme posterior part of the subarachnoid space with the purpose of sparing the anterior nerve roots. Using an insulin syringe, we introduced the neurolytic solution very slowly in order to allow the phenol to slide caudad along the posterior aspect of the arachnoid sac and thus involve the posterior sacral roots. The quantity injected was standardized at 0.8 ml. Subsequently, the patient was seated with his spine tilted backwards at a 45 degree angle for a period of 3 hr. The degree of pain relief was evaluated 3 weeks after the block was performed, using the Scott-Huskisson (2) visual analog scale (below the 3 mark the results were considered positive; above the 3 mark results were considered negative).

RESULTS

In the first group, 7 of 20 patients (35%) treated with 5% phenol obtained positive results; 4 of 20 patients (20%) were already catheterized; and 2 of the remaining 16 patients (12%) developed postblock urinary retention. None of the patients suffered reduction of muscular strength in the lower extremities.

In the second group, 12 of 15 patients (80%) treated with 10% phenol obtained positive results; 4 of 15 patients (27%) were already catheterized; and 5 of the remaining 11 patients (45%) developed postblock urinary retention. One of the 15 patients (7%) presented moderate lower limb weakness of a transient nature (24 hr).

In the third group, 9 of 11 patients (82%) treated with 15% phenol obtained positive results; 5 of 11 patients (45%) were already catheterized; and 4 of the remaining 6 patients (67%) developed postblock urinary retention. One of the 11 patients (9%) had moderate lower limb weakness of a transient nature (48 hr).

It must be emphasized that in 14 patients from all 3 groups, other antalgic therapies, including percutaneous cervical cordotomy and pituitary neuroadenolysis, were given in addition to the subarachnoid blocks so as to control the pain arising from nonsacral dermatomes, or clearly lateralized incident pain.

CONCLUSIONS

In our experience as well as in that of others, the neurolytic subarachnoid block at L5–S1 level is a useful, efficacious, and very simple technique for controlling perineal pain of neoplastic origin. This is true whether the technique is used alone or in conjunction with other antalgic procedures.

As far as the concentrations used are concerned, it is fundamental to consider the clinical condition of the patient and the presence or absence of urinary catheter. The use of concentrations of 10% or above frequently causes sphincter complications. This price must be paid if one wants to obtain complete and lasting pain relief, which is often not obtained with the usual concentrations. Permanent motor complications of the lower limbs are avoidable if the correct procedure is followed.

REFERENCES

1. Maher, R. M. (1955): Relief of pain in incurable cancer. *Lancet,* 1:18–20.
2. Scott, J., and Huskisson, E. C. (1976): Graphic representation of pain. *Pain,* 2:175–184.

Advances in Pain Research and Therapy, Vol. 7,
edited by C. Benedetti et al.
Raven Press, New York © 1984.

Neurophysiological Foundations of Peripheral Electroanalgesia

Emilio Favale and Massimo Leandri

Department of Neurology, University of Genoa,
16132 Genoa, Italy

Despite the wide use of electrostimulation for pain relief, the underlying physiology of the procedure is still poorly understood (84). There is little doubt that electrostimulation activates neuronal mechanisms interfering with pain perception. This takes place either in the peripheral nervous system, accounting for a decrease in excitability of nociceptors, fatigue of peripheral nerve fibers, or both; or in the central nervous system through the activation of spinal, supraspinal inhibitory mechanisms, or both. In this chapter we will review the evidence pertaining to this issue.

PERIPHERAL MECHANISMS

In the past, nociceptors were usually considered mere physical transducers. It has been shown that, under particular conditions, their sensitivity can be either enhanced or reduced (92). This, however, does not seem to be the case when electrical stimulation is employed, unless autonomic fibers are concurrently activated. In fact, sympathetic efferents have been presumed to affect nociceptor sensitivity (128), the physiological basis of such a phenomenon being still largely unknown. In any case, the lack of effect of electrostimulation on the activity of sympathetic efferents, as demonstrated by microneurography (115), rules out their participation in electroanalgesia. Antidromic activation of peripheral fibers might modulate the microenvironment of nociceptors and, consequently, their excitability (95). However, this hypothesis has never been verified. Summing up, according to the data so far available, any possible role of nociceptors in the electrically-induced modulation of pain seems to be very unlikely.

Functional changes in peripheral nerve fibers involved in the transmission of pain impulses have been repeatedly investigated during electrostimulation procedures by means of both neurographic (20) and microneurographic (58) methods. The validity of the latter technique has been questioned somewhat, subjective ratings being held more reliable in the estimation of stimulus intensity than the discharge rates of individual C fibers (47). Two peripheral stimulation techniques are currently being used: transcutaneous electrical stimulation (TES) and electroacupuncture (EAP) (4,7,14,37,51,62,87). In both cases, square wave pulses are given. Constant current and constant voltage stimulators have been used, but the latter is preferred for safety reasons. Recently, short trains of stimuli (EAP-like stimulation) instead of single pulses have been employed (33,34,107,108) thus allowing the use of considerably lower intensities of stimulation. Apart from the type of electrode and stimulus waveform used, the EAP-like technique seems to be very similar to the "brief, intense, transcutaneous somatic stimulation" recently proposed by Melzack (82). The TES uses high frequency-low intensity stimuli (50–100 Hz; 1–2 sensory threshold [St]) delivered through surface electrodes; EAP uses low frequency-high intensity stimuli (1–2 Hz; 6–8 St) given through needle electrodes. The type of electrode used does not seem crucial, many authors using either surface or needle electrodes in both cases (4). In contrast, electrode positioning with respect to the site of pain seems to be of the utmost importance.

Functional changes in peripheral fibers, accounting for the relief of pain, may depend either on the intensity or the frequency of stimulation. In fact, TES can be surmised to activate the low-threshold peripheral fibers predominantly (if not exclusively), whereas EAP should activate both low- and (at least in part) high-threshold peripheral fibers. In other words, TES is selective, whereas EAP is relatively broad (42) or to the limit of the subject's tolerance. Incidentally, clinical pain temporarily made worse by particularly intense electrical stimulation (14). Unlike the choice of intensity, that of frequency of stimulation was not motivated by any neurophysiological strategy and was largely arbitrary and empirical at best (87). Nevertheless, the frequency of stimulation also could have important neurophysiological implications. Repetitive stimulation could fatigue pain-mediating afferents in the course of both TES and EAP. Since the intensity of stimulation used in TES, although not painful, also activates A delta fibers (58), a peripheral electrogenic blockade of this contingent (7) due to the high frequency of stimulation used should be considered. Stimulation frequencies comparable to those used in EAP may provoke fatigue of the C fibers (114), provided they have been truly activated (4,58). However, it has been claimed that the current intensity required to activate C fibers cannot be tolerated by the subjects (26). It should be pointed out that activation of C fibers is not necessarily related to painful stimuli (113). Whichever the case, activation of a significant number of unmyelinated fibers by the electrical stimulations currently used is highly unlikely, at least in the conscious subject.

The reduction in amplitude of the A delta component of the neurogram, previously attributed to fatigue of the corresponding fiber group (20), would actually be due to the increased jitter of individual spikes, resulting in an artifactual amplitude decrement in surface-recorded neurograms (58), particularly at higher stimulation rates. Briefly, the data so far available indicate that analgesia by electrostimulation is unlikely to be due specifically to fatigue of the pain-mediating peripheral fibers, as demonstrated by examination of the different sensory modalities in the course of stimulation (56).

It has been noted that electrostimulation can be effective even when the position of electrodes is not anatomically related to the site of pain. Obviously, in such cases, the analgesic effect cannot be attributed to fatigue of the peripheral fibers involved in the transmission of impulses from the painful area (50). Nevertheless, the hypothesis of peripheral fatigue, apparently discounted by this latter finding, cannot be completely ruled out in view of the following. Peripheral nerve stimulation can be effective when the stimulus is proximal to the site of pain, in agreement with the concept of "peripheral block" (60) much in vogue among physiotherapists, but loses all effectiveness when distal to it (71). Similarly, the sensory threshold of a given cutaneous area increases when the stimulation is proximal to it (20,94), but remains unchanged during distal stimulation (94). Paradoxically, TES at clinically effective intensity and frequency improves sensation in the painful limb (86), but is almost ineffective in the normal limb (19,57). This may support the hypothesis that electrical analgesia is brought about by a peripheral blockade of the activity of some but not all of the small fibers, thus accounting both for a reduction in clinical pain and improvement of sensory perception (19,57,89). This outcome implies a contribution by a central (spinal) gating mechanism as well (19,57).

Although there is no experimental support for the hypothesis of diminished receptor sensitivity induced by electrical stimulation, the hypothesis of peripheral fatigue still holds a certain value when the stimulus is delivered to an area anatomically related to the site of pain.

SPINAL MECHANISMS

Spinal mechanisms are described by the gate theory of pain (83), the introduction of which has renewed interest in electrical stimulation of the nervous system for analgesic purposes. In fact, from the gate hypothesis stemmed the pioneer observations of Wall and Sweet (118) and Shealy et al. (105) regarding the possibility of temporarily abolishing pain using electrical stimulation applied either peripherally (118) or to the dorsal columns (105). The latter effect has been attributed to the antidromic activation of the collaterals of large diameter fibers ending in the posterior horns. Such observations further strengthen the theoretical postulate that the beneficial effects of TES are due to selective stimulation of large peripheral fibers. In particular, the negative feedback mechanism triggered by high levels of activity in the A fibers would close the spinal gate, preventing the small diameter fibers from transmitting pain impulses to the posterior horn cells (83).

The experimental basis for the theory can be summarized as follows. At the level of the posterior horns there exist at least two types of neurons responsive to nociceptive stimuli (49,55): (a) the so-called convergent or type 2 neurons, activated either by noxious or nonnoxious stimuli; and (b) the so-called nonconvergent or type 3 neurons, activated exclusively by nociceptive stimuli. In both populations (49,55), the activity evoked by nociceptive stimuli can be inhibited by stimulation of large peripheral fibers coming from the pertinent receptive field (54). A similar effect occurs in the spinothalamic neurons (41).

It may be of interest to mention that, in accordance with clinical observations by Wall and Sweet (118) and Shealy et al. (105), inhibition of nociceptive responses of the posterior horn cells can be obtained by stimulating both the peripheral nerves (49,55) and the dorsal columns of the spinal cord (49). Briefly, in both cases a phenomenon of segmental interaction between nociceptive and nonnociceptive afferents would take place. Such a mechanism could involve pre- or postsynaptic inhibition or both (54). Recent reports are consistent with the idea that A afferents interact presynaptically with C fibers to reduce their synaptic effectiveness (40). The length of time impulse transmission is depressed parallels the extracellular potassium elevation in the spinal cord (116). The duration of this interaction exceeds only slightly that of the conditioning stimulus, and would be independent of descending influences (10). In fact, the same findings can be obtained even in the spinal animal (66,125). Also, trigeminal nociceptive neurons can be inhibited by local (segmental) afferent influences from A alpha/beta fibers innervating orofacial tissues (104,127).

The existence of a segmental interaction between nociceptive and nonnociceptive afferents has been demonstrated using the changes in amplitude of the nociceptive polysynaptic reflex (120). It is well known that nociceptive reflexes and pain sensation share common mechanisms at the level of the posterior horns (78,120). In particular, it was shown that at the level of the posterior horns, neurons exist, the axons of which, directed contralaterally to the anterolateral quadrant of the spinal cord, give rise to collaterals projecting ipsilaterally to the anterior horns of the spinal cord (75). This explains why both pharmacological analgesia (78) and electroanalgesia (15) are accompanied by a depression of nociceptive reflexes, even though recently the relationship between nociceptive reflexes and pain sensation in humans (120) has been the object of controversy (17,18,122).

Finally, the concept of a spinal gating mechanism is supported, at least in part, by changes in somatic sensation occurring during transcutaneous electrical stimulation in clinical pain states (19,57); this effect could not be reproduced in normal subjects (88).

Two practical considerations derive from these facts. First, stimuli used for analgesic electrostimulation should activate primarily, if not exclusively, the large-diameter peripheral fibers. Second, the stimulating electrodes should be located over an area or a nerve trunk anatomically related to the site of pain. In other words, the stimulation should be selective and segmental. Actually, selective stimulation of the peripheral nerve is not a simple matter (53). Each class of nerve fibers has its own strength-duration curve; relatively short pulses will stimulate large fibers before exciting small ones. A pulse duration short enough to allow a maximal large fiber stimulation while keeping A delta fiber excitation as low as possible should be chosen. Unfortunately, published data comparing, within a given range of pulse durations, different thresholds for afferent and efferent excitability are not available (53).

It has been suggested that the range lying between 2 and 50 μsec be explored (53). It should be pointed out, however, that the possible usefulness of this range was extrapolated from strength-duration curves obtained with a particular wave-form (haversine waves), and with the anode placed proximal to the cathode in relation to the recording electrode (68). A selective blockade of the peripheral nerve known to be effective in animals (16) proved difficult to apply and quite unselective in humans (119). The best recommendation is to use the minimal pulse-width effective with any given stimulator (53). The effective choice of stimulus intensity seems to be one that gives the patient a definite tingling or vibratory feeling over the painful area (53); if the patient does not feel the right sensation in the right place, either the stimulator is inadequate or the electrode placement incorrect. The tingling sensation induced by electrical stimulation is thought to be brought about by a discharge of large-diameter myelinated fibers (26,53).

Recently, use of high intensity electrical stimuli (4,9,36,58,59,62,73,82) delivered through electrodes not necessarily located over areas or nerve trunks related to the site of pain (67,70) has gained acceptance in some circles, despite Long's contention (71) that no published data currently available substantiate the choice. Even the reaction to experimental pain in human subjects has been reduced by TES only at very high intensities of stimulation (20,88,124); moderate intensities failed to modify the pain threshold (88,124). It has been observed that cutaneous electrical stimulation can be effective in raising the pain threshold even in contralateral limbs (102). In other words, a massive extrasegmental stimulation could be used instead of a selective segmental one. This philosophy underlies the usage of EAP (4), EAP-like stimulation (33), and of the "brief, intense, transcutaneous somatic stimulation" proposed by Melzack (82), which has been outlined above. Several lines of evidence indicate that the analgesic effects of electrical stimuli of high intensity involve supraspinal mechanisms, especially when applied to an area anatomically unrelated to the site of pain.

SUPRASPINAL MECHANISMS

The use of remote, high-intensity electrical stimuli for analgesic purposes is conceptually related to the so-called hyperstimulation analgesia (81). Intense somatic stimulation causes pain and, at the same time, activates a mechanism that inhibits noxious signals from other sources, such as those related to pathological pain (59). This empiric concept has found ample experimental support. In 1969 Wagman and Price (117) observed that the nociceptive responses of posterior horns could be inhibited by extrasegmental painful stimuli. Inhibiting influences from the entire cutaneous surface impinging on the neurons of the spinal trigeminal nucleus activated by tooth pulp stimulation have been reported (111). Finally, Le Bars et al. (65,66) demonstrated the activity evoked by nociceptive stimuli in convergent posterior-horn neurons can be inhibited by a painful stimulus applied to a completely unrelated area of the body. We can conclude that local, painful stimuli can produce a diffuse inhibition of nociceptive spinal, as well as trigeminal (28), responses. Such inhibition could be pre- or postsynaptic in origin, or both (65). Quite recently, the occurrence of a diffuse inhibition following noxious stimulation of remote areas of the body surface has been confirmed but, at variance with the above description, its effects were not limited to convergent neurons (45).

Le Bars et al. (65) considered this phenomenon the outcome of a control mechanism they called "diffuse noxious inhibitory control" (DNIC). This differs from the "gate control" in three ways. First, inhibition is provoked by nociceptive stimuli, i.e., by the activation of small diameter peripheral fibers. On the other hand, activation of large diameter fibers does not show inhibitory effects other than those occurring at the segmental level (65). Second, the inhibition is both segmental and extrasegmental; in fact, it can be obtained by stimulating areas other than anatomically related ones (65). Third, the inhibition is supraspinal in origin; this is clearly demonstrated by the fact that DNIC is no longer obtained in the spinal preparation (66). Evidence suggests that DNIC is exerted through supraspinal structures containing 5-HT neurons, such as the nucleus raphe magnus (NRM) (65,98). It has been proposed that DNIC and NRM-mediated inhibition share common mechanisms (29). On the other hand, it is unusual for a neuron to be inhibited both by peripheral stimulation of low-threshold afferents and by NRM stimulation (27). Fourth, endogenous opiates are involved in DNIC (64). In particular, DNIC has been considered the expression of a possible enkephalinergic neuronal mechanism of analgesia based on the counter-irritation principle (i.e., pain relief by painful or unpleasant stimuli).

These aspects suggested that DNIC could be the mechanism responsible for EAP analgesia. Electroacupuncture analgesia also requires the use of painful stimuli that can be applied to body areas different from the painful one. Both EAP and DNIC analgesia are thought to be supraspinal in origin (4,13,14,31,51,62,63,66,78,106,109). Both DNIC (64) and EAP (22,25,79,107,108) analgesia are antagonized by naloxone. However, the analogy between DNIC and EAP is only partial since the onset of the neuronal inhibition provoked by DNIC is almost immediate (65), whereas EAP analgesia takes place gradually (4,5,23,51). This could depend, at least in part, on different experimental conditions.

There is an extraordinary similarity between EAP analgesia and the analgesia produced by stimulation of the periaqueductal gray substance (PAG) (4,13,38,74,77,78,112), the latter being obviously much stronger than the former. In both cases, the analgesia is gradual in onset and diffuse, although mainly segmental. Moreover, both types of analgesia are antagonized by naloxone (1,3,22,25,52,79,107,108). However, the naloxone reversal of PAG analgesia was not confirmed by other investigators (43,93,126). In particular, the effects of naloxone on analgesia (1,3,43,52,93,126), as well as on the inhibition of dorsal horn neurons (21,32) following PAG stimulation, are still controversial (64). It has been proposed that PAG stimulation inhibits ascending activity evoked by noxious stimuli by mechanisms not necessarily influenced by endogenous opiates (61).

In EAP analgesia, both gradual induction and naloxone's antagonist effect indicate a neurochemical mechanism (in which the main link could be a "neuromodulator" rather than a classic neurotransmitter) that would inhibit transmission of the nociceptive impulses at the level of the posterior horns of the spinal cord (39,46,69,80,90,123), as well as the level of the nucleus of the descending trigeminal root (10,99,103). A simple segmental mechanism could hardly explain its gradual onset, its diffuse character (even if prevalently segmental), and its slow regression (5,7). The mainly segmental effect of PAG stimulation could be due to the somatotopic organization of this structure (78), whereby the resulting analgesic effects are stronger in the corresponding peripheral region (14). Electroacupuncture analgesia also is mostly segmental (8,23). This could be accounted for by the addition to the diffuse suprasegmental effects of the local effects of spinal origin related to simultaneous stimulation of the large-diameter peripheral fibers. The occurrence of an EAP-induced diffuse (i.e., extrasegmental) increase of the pain threshold is not unanimously accepted, being usually attributed to psychological factors.

The supraspinal structures responsible for EAP analgesia are located in the brainstem (31,106). The analgesic effect disappears in the spinal preparation, whereas it persists in the decerebrate animal. Furthermore, it was demonstrated that the related descending influences travel in the posterior lateral column of the spinal cord close to the posterior horn (106), and more precisely in the dorsolateral funiculus (DLF). The latter takes origin, at least in part, from the NRM (10), which is thought to receive the excitatory influence of PAG (10,12,96). The PAG neurons do not appear to connect directly with the spinal nerve cells that transmit the incoming pain signals nor to inhibit them (74). See, however, Carstens et al. (21). Rather, neurons in the NRM may serve as a relay station between the higher brain centers and the spinal nerve cells (10,74). In fact, the electrical stimulation of this nucleus gives rise to potent analgesic effects in animals (91,97), and its electrolytic destruction (63), as well as the section of DLF (106), can abolish EAP analgesia. The latter could be due to an inhibition of the posterior horn cells (39,46,69,80,90,123), particularly those of the spinothalamic tract (11,123) and of the nucleus of the descending trigeminal root (63) following excitation of NRM. The analysis of the response properties of individual NRM neurons has shown they are most effectively activated by noxious stimuli (10). The same holds true for the nucleus reticularis gigantocellularis (48); therefore, its possible functional contribution to electrically-induced analgesia should be considered. The mechanism by which the NRM inhibits dorsal horn neurons is not entirely clear (10). At any rate, a postsynaptic inhibition of primate spinothalamic neurons by NRM stimulation has been recently demonstrated (44).

Analgesia by stimulation of the NRM can be inhibited by both p-clorophenylalanine (p-CPA) (2) and naloxone (91), possibly because the serotoninergic output of NRM is conveyed to the posterior horn cells through enkephalinergic interneurons (10). The reduction of the inhibitory effect of NRM stimulation could even originate at the level of NRM itself, since this nucleus contains neurons rich in enkephalin. On the other hand, in the experiments by Duggan and Griersmith (32), the NRM-mediated inhibition was unaffected by intravenous naloxone (the animals, however, were under general anesthesia). Moreover, the administration of p-CPA does not seem to affect EAP analgesia (25). It is apparent, therefore, that the recent implication of serotoninergic and enkephalinergic pathways in NRM modulation of dorsal horn neurons (98) and, possibly, in EAP analgesia, still awaits validation by further experimental data.

For other details on the supraspinal mechanisms responsible for pain suppression, the reader is referred to the most recent reviews on the subject (38,76,128).

CONCLUSIONS

The bulk of present evidence indicates that the analgesia produced by stimulation of the large fibers depends on segmental mechanisms rather than on the activation of a descending system. On the other hand, the latter is more effectively activated by noxious volleys transmitted by small-diameter fibers than by innocuous inputs relayed by large-diameter fibers. It follows that the two types of pain suppression should be considered quite different from one another. These concepts can be applied respectively to the TES and to EAP-induced analgesia, taking into account their respective features. The relationships between the changes induced by TES and EAP are still largely undefined, as suggested by the following data:

1. It is generally maintained that TES analgesia is localized at variance with EAP analgesia, which is diffuse, although mainly localized (4). However, according to Chapman et al. (23), acupunctural stimulation has almost a pure intrasegmental sensory effect with no significant response bias, whereas the nonsegmental changes previously reported by Andersson et al. (5) were largely psychological in origin. On the

other hand, in a subsequent unpublished study, Chapman demonstrated that TES, when applied to the same sites used for acupunctural stimulation, yielded approximately the same analgesic response as the latter technique. Finally, it has been recently reported that, besides changes in pain threshold within the territory of the stimulated nerve, TES can induce marked changes elsewhere throughout the body as well (129).

2. The fast modifications of pain threshold considered typical of TES (7) can hardly be reconciled with recent neurophysiological evidence showing that high-frequency stimulation of large-diameter fibers, when sufficiently prolonged, induces a gradual inhibition of the posterior horn cells (30). The recovery of neuronal activity after cessation of the high frequency stimulus occurs in a progressive manner as well (30). Indeed, according to the current clinical views about electrically-induced analgesia, these changes would be more consistent with the effects of a low- rather than a high-frequency stimulation (4).

3. It is commonly held that TES differs from EAP for its refractoriness to naloxone (4,25,37,72,95,107,108,112). This has been challenged by various authors (100,125) who support a recent concept of Woolf (124) that only experimental models who are morphine sensitive are affected by TES. Furthermore, Salar et al. (101), in contrast with Terenius (112), have shown that TES increases the concentration of endorphins in the cerebrospinal fluid.

4. On the other hand, although there is little doubt that acupuncture stimulation can alter pain sensation, it has been recently denied that such a phenomenon could be reversed by naloxone, one or more mechanisms other than those mediated by endorphins being thus involved in acupuncture analgesia (24).

5. The partial abolition of TES analgesia brought about by the administration of p-CPA (25) suggests the effect of TES is, in some measure, supraspinal in origin, possibly related to the raphe-spinal projections (25). In fact, at variance with the intact preparation, in the spinal animal, the antinociceptive effect produced by TES was unaltered by a pretreatment with p-CPA (85). Moreover, it seems noteworthy that stimulation of the ventral PAG, at variance with that of its dorsal part, produces an analgesic pattern very similar to that induced by TES (110). This suggests that the current opinion that TES analgesia, unlike that produced by EAP, is completely spinal in origin, should be reexamined (see also 95). In fact, several lines of evidence (pharmacologic, surgical, and biochemical) seem to lead to the conclusion that the analgesia induced by high-frequency electrical stimulation is mediated by the raphe-dorsal longitudinal fascicle serotoninergic system.

6. The therapeutic indications are no longer as strict as in the past. Classically, TES was employed in chronic pain (4,6,7,25) and EAP in acute pain (4,6,7,25). It now seems beyond question that TES and EAP can be usefully employed in both conditions (33–35,108).

In brief, apart from a particular experimental approach in which the effects of EAP turn out to be clearly different from those of TES (121), the most recent findings support the hypothesis that similar mechanisms may operate in both electrostimulation procedures (124). Obviously it cannot be excluded that any given pain condition may selectively respond to either EAP or TES. According to Eriksson et al. (34), both stimulation methods should be tried whenever a patient is not relieved by one of them.

REFERENCES

1. Adams, J. E. (1976): Naloxone reversal of analgesia produced by brain stimulation in the human. *Pain*, 2:161–166.
2. Akil, H., and Mayer, D. J. (1972): Antagonism of stimulation-produced analgesia by pCPA, a serotonin synthesis inhibitor. *Brain Res.*, 44:692–697.
3. Akil, H., Mayer, D. J., and Liebeskind, J. A. (1976): Antagonsim of stimulation-produced analgesia by naloxone, a narcotic antagonist. *Science*, 191:961–962.
4. Andersson, S. A. (1979): Pain control by sensory stimulation. In: *Advances in Pain Research and Therapy, Vol. 3,* edited by J. J. Bonica. J. C. Liebeskind, and D. G. Albe-Fessard, pp. 569–585. Raven Press, New York.
5. Andersson, S. A., Ericson, T., Holmgren, E., and Lindquist, G. (1977): Analgesic effects of peripheral conditioning stimulation. I. General pain threshold effect on human teeth and a correlation to psychological factors. *Acupuncture Electro-Therapeut. Res. Int. J.,* 2:307–322.
6. Andersson, S. A., Hansson, G., Holmgren, E., and Renberg, O. (1976): Evaluation of the pain suppressive effect of different frequencies of peripheral electrical stimulation in chronic pain conditions. *Acta Orthop. Scand.*, 47:149–157.
7. Andersson, S. A., and Holmgren, E. (1978): Analgesic effects of peripheral conditioning stimulation. III. Effect of high frequency stimulation: Segmental mechanisms interacting with pain. *Acupuncture Electro-Therapeut. Res. Int. J.*, 3:23–36.
8. Andersson, S. A., Holmgren, E., and Roos, A. (1977): Analgesic effects of peripheral conditioning stimulation. II. Importance of certain stimulation parameters. *Acupuncture Electro-Therapeut. Res. Int. J.*, 2:237–246.
9. Augustinsson, L. E., Bohlin, P., Bundsen, P., Carlsson, C. A., Forssman, L., Sjoberg, P., and Tyreman, N. O. (1977): Pain relief during delivery by transcutaneous electrical nerve stimulation. *Pain*, 4:59–65.
10. Basbaum, A. I., and Fields, H. L. (1978): Endogenous pain control mechanisms: Review and hypothesis. *Ann. Neurol.*, 4:451–462.
11. Beall, J. E., Martin, R. F., Applebaum, A. E., and Willis, W. D. (1976): Inhibition of primate spinothalamic tract neurons by stimulation in the region of the nucleus raphe magnus. *Brain Res.*, 114:328–333.
12. Behbehani, M. M., and Fields, H. L. (1979): Evidence that an excitatory connection between the periaqueductal gray and nucleus raphe magnus mediates stimulation produced analgesia. *Brain Res.*, 170:85–93.
13. Bishop, B. (1980): Pain: Its physiology and rationale for management. Part III. Consequences of current concepts of pain mechanisms related to pain management. *Phys. Ther.*, 60:24–37.
14. Boureau, F., and Willer, J. C. (1979): *La Douleur. Exploration, Traitement par Neurostimulation et Electro-Acupuncture.* Masson, Paris.
15. Boureau, F., Willer, J. C., and Dehn, H. (1977): L'action de l'acupuncture sur la douleur. Bases physiologiques. *Nouv. Presse Med.*, 6:1871–1874.
16. Brindley, G. S., and Craggs, M. D. (1980): A technique for anodally blocking large nerve fibres through chronically implanted electrodes. *J. Neurol. Neurosurg. Psychiatry*, 43:1083–1090.
17. Bromm, B., and Treede, R. D. (1980): Withdrawal reflex, skin resistance reaction and pain ratings due to electrical stimuli in man. *Pain*, 9:339–354.

18. Bromm, B., and Treede, R. D. (1981): Nociceptive reflexes and pain sensation in man. *Pain*, 10:408–410.
19. Callaghan, M., Sternbach, R. A., Nyquist, J. K., and Timmerans, G. (1978): Changes in somatic sensitivity during transcutaneous electrical analgesia. *Pain*, 5:115–127.
20. Campbell, J. N., and Taub, A. (1973): Local analgesia from percutaneous electrical stimulation: A peripheral mechanism. *Arch. Neurol.*, 28:347–350.
21. Carstens, E., Yokota, T., and Zimmermann, M. (1979): Inhibition of spinal neuronal responses to noxious skin heating by stimulation of mesencephalic periaquaductal gray in the cat. *J. Neurophysiol.*, 42:558–568.
22. Chapman, C. R., and Benedetti, C. (1977): Analgesia following transcutaneous electrical stimulation and its partial reversal by a narcotic antagonist. *Life Sci.*, 21:1645–1648.
23. Chapman, C. R., Chen, A. C., and Bonica, J. J. (1977): Effects of intrasegmental electrical acupuncture on dental pain: Evaluation by threshold estimation and sensory decision theory. *Pain*, 3:213–227.
24. Chapman, C. R., Colpitts, Y. M., Benedetti, C., Kitaeff, R., and Gehrig, J. D. (1980): Evoked potential assessment of acupunctural analgesia: Attempted reversal with naloxone. *Pain*, 9:183–197.
25. Cheng, R. S. S., and Pomeranz, B. (1979): Electroacupuncture analgesia could be mediated by at least two pain-relieving mechanisms: Endorphin and nonendorphin systems. *Life Sci.*, 25:1957–1962.
26. Collins, W. F., Nulsen, F. E., and Randt, C. T. (1960): Relation of peripheral nerve fibre size and sensation in man. *Arch. Neurol.*, 3:381–385.
27. Dickenson, A. H., Hellon, R. F., and Woolf, C. J. (1981): Tooth pulp input to the spinal trigeminal nucleus: A comparison of inhibitions following segmental and raphe magnus stimulation. *Brain Res.*, 214:73–87.
28. Dickenson, A. H., Le Bars, D., and Besson, J. M. (1980): Diffuse noxious inhibitory controls (DNIC). Effects on trigeminal nucleus caudalis neurones in the rat. *Brain Res.*, 200:293–305.
29. Dickenson, A. H., Rivot, J. P., Chaouch, A., Besson, J. M., and Le Bars, D. (1981): Diffuse noxious inhibitory controls (DNIC) in the rat with or without p-CPA pretreatment. *Brain Res.*, 216:313–321.
30. Dickhaus, H., Pauser, G., and Zimmermann, M. (1978): Hemmung im Ruckenmark, ein neurophysiologischer Wirkungsmechanismum bei der Hypalgesie durch Stimulationsakupunktur. *Wien. Klin. Wochenschr.*, 90:59–64.
31. Du, H. J., and Chao, Y. F. (1976): Localization of central structures involved in descending inhibitory effect of acupuncture on viscero-somatic reflex discharges. *Sci. Sin.*, 19:137–148.
32. Duggan, A. W., and Griersmith, B. T. (1979): Inhibition of the spinal transmission of nociceptive information by supraspinal stimulation in the cat. *Pain*, 6:149–161.
33. Eriksson, M., and Sjolund, B. (1976): Acupuncturelike electroanalgesia in TNS-resistant chronic pain. In: *Sensory Functions of the Skin*, edited by Y. Zotterman, pp. 575–581. Pergamon Press, Oxford.
34. Eriksson, M. B. E., Sjolund, B. H., and Nielzen, S. (1979): Long term results of peripheral conditioning stimulation as an analgesic measure in chronic pain. *Pain*, 6:335–347.
35. Ersek, R. A. (Ed.) (1981): *Pain Control with Transcutaneous Electrical Neuro Stimulation (TENS)*, Warren H. Green, Inc., St. Louis.
36. Favale, E., and Leandri, M. (1979): Stimolazione elettrica del sistema nervoso periferico nella terapia del dolore cronico. *Atti del XXI Congresso della Societa Italiana di Neurologia*, pp. 111–128. Catania.
37. Fields, H. L. (1981): Pain II: New approaches to management. *Ann. Neurol.*, 9:101–106.
38. Fields, H. L., and Basbaum, A. I. (1978): Brainstem control of spinal pain transmission neurons. *Annu. Rev. Physiol.*, 40:193–221.
39. Fields, H. L., Basbaum, A. I., Clanton, C. H., and Anderson, S. E. (1977): Nucleus raphe magnus inhibition of spinal cord dorsal horn neurons. *Brain Res.*, 126:441–453.
40. Fitzgerald, M., and Woolf, C. J. (1981): Effects of cutaneous nerve and intraspinal conditioning on C-fibre afferent terminal excitability in decerebrate spinal rats. *J. Physiol. (Lond.)*, 318:25–39.
41. Foreman, R. D., Beall, J. E., Applebaum, A. E., Coulter, J. D., and Willis, W. D. (1976): Inhibition of primate spinothalamic tract neurons by electrical stimulation of dorsal column

of peripheral nerve. In: *Advances in Pain Research and Therapy, Vol. 1*, edited by J. J. Bonica and D. G. Albe-Fessard, pp. 405–410. Raven Press, New York.

42. Fu, T. C., Halenda, S. P., and Dewey, W. L. (1980): The effect of hypophysectomy on acupuncture analgesia in the mouse. *Brain Res.*, 202:33–39.
43. Gebhart, G. F., and Toleikis, J. R. (1978): An evaluation of stimulation-produced analgesia in the cat. *Exp. Neurol.*, 62:570–579.
44. Giesler, G. J., Jr., Gerhart, K. D., Yezierski, R. P., Wilcox, T. K., and Willis, W. D. (1981): Postsynaptic inhibition of primate spinothalamic neurons by stimulation in nucleus raphe magnus. *Brain Res.*, 204:184–188.
45. Gray, B. G., and Dostrovsky, J. O. (1981): Inhibition of cat dorsal horn neurons by noxious cutaneous stimulation of anatomically remote areas of the body surface. (Abstract) *Pain* (Suppl. 1):S183.
46. Guilbaud, G., Oliveras, J. L., Giesler, G., and Besson, J. M. (1977): Effects induced by stimulation of the centralis inferior nucleus of the raphe on dorsal horn interneurons in cat's spinal cord. *Brain Res.*, 126:355–360.
47. Gybels, J., Handwerker, H. O., and Van Hees, J. (1979): A comparison between the discharges of human nociceptive nerve fibres and the subject's ratings of his sensations. *J. Physiol. (Lond.)*, 292:193–206.
48. Haber, L. H., Martin, R. F., Chung, J. M., and Willis, W. D. (1980): Inhibition and excitation of primate spinothalamic tract neurons by stimulation in region of nucleus reticularis gigantocellularis. *J. Neurophysiol.*, 43:1578–1593.
49. Handwerker, H. O., Iggo, A., and Zimmermann, M. (1975): Segmental and supraspinal actions on dorsal horn neurons responding to noxious and nonnoxious skin stimuli. *Pain*, 1:147–165.
50. Hiedl, P., Struppler, A., and Gessler, M. (1979): Local analgesia by percutaneous electrical stimulation of sensory nerves. *Pain*, 7:129–134.
51. Hole, K., and Berge, O. G. (1981): Regulation of pain sensitivity in the central nervous system. *Cephalalgia*, 1:51–59.
52. Hosobuchi, Y., Adams, J. E., and Linchitz, R. (1977): Pain relief by electrical stimulation of the central gray matter in humans and its reversal by naloxone. *Science*, 197:183–186.
53. Howson, D. C. (1978): Peripheral neural excitability. Implications for transcutaneous electrical nerve stimulation. *Phys. Ther.*, 58:1467–1473.
54. Iggo, A. (1976): Peripheral and spinal "pain" mechanisms and their modulation. In: *Advances in Pain Research and Therapy, Vol. 1*, edited by J. J. Bonica and D. G. Albe-Fessard, pp. 381–394. Raven Press, New York.
55. Iggo, A., Ogawa, H., and Cervero, F. (1976): Inhibition of nociceptor-driven dorsal horn neurons in the cat. In: *Advances in Pain Research and Therapy, Vol. 1*, edited by J. J. Bonica and D. G. Albe-Fessard, pp. 99–104. Raven Press, New York.
56. Ignelzi, R. J., and Nyquist, J. K. (1979): Excitability changes in peripheral nerve fibers after repetitive electrical stimulation. Implications in pain modulation. *J. Neurosurg.*, 51:824–833.
57. Ignelzi, R. J., Sternbach, R. A., and Callaghan, M. (1976): Somatosensory changes during transcutaneous electrical analgesia. In: *Advances in Pain Research and Therapy, Vol. 1*, edited by J. J. Bonica and D. G. Albe-Fessard, pp. 421–425. Raven Press, New York.
58. Janko, M., and Trontelj, J. V. (1980): Transcutaneous electrical nerve stimulation: A microneurographic and perceptual study. *Pain*, 9:219–230.
59. Jeans, M. E. (1979): Relief of chronic pain by brief, intense transcutaneous electrical stimulation: A double-blind study. In: *Advances in Pain Research and Therapy, Vol. 3*, edited by J. J. Bonica, J. C. Liebeskind, and D. G. Albe-Fessard, pp. 601–606. Raven Press, New York.
60. Jenkner, F. L. (1977): *Peripheral Nerve Block. Pharmacologic: By Local Anesthesia. Electric: By Transdermal Stimulation*. Springer-Verlag, Wien.
61. Jurna, I. (1980): Effect of stimulation in the periaqueductal grey matter on activity in ascending axons of the rat spinal cord: Selective inhibition of activity evoked by afferent A delta and C fibre stimulation and failure of naloxone to reduce inhibition. *Brain Res.*, 196:33–42.
62. Kaada, B. (1976): Neurophysiology and acupuncture: A review. In: *Advances in Pain Research and Therapy, Vol. 1*, edited by J. J. Bonica and D. G. Albe-Fessard, pp. 733–741. Raven Press, New York.

63. Kaada, B., Jorum, E., Sagvolden, T., and Ansethmoen, T. E. (1979): Analgesia induced by trigeminal nerve stimulation (electro-acupuncture) abolished by nuclei raphe lesions in rats. *Acupuncture Electro-Therapeut. Res. Int. J.*, 4:221–234.
64. Le Bars, D., Chitour, D., Kraus, E., Dickenson, A. H., and Besson, J. M. (1981): Effect of naloxone upon diffuse noxious inhibitory controls (DNIC) in the rat. *Brain Res.*, 204:387–402.
65. Le Bars, D., Dickenson, A. H., and Besson, J. M. (1979): Diffuse noxious inhibitory controls (DNIC). I. Effects on dorsal horn convergent neurones in the rat. *Pain*, 6:283–304.
66. Le Bars, D., Dickenson, A. H., and Besson, J. M. (1979): Diffuse noxious inhibitory controls (DNIC). II. Lack of effect on non-convergent neurones, supraspinal involvement and theoretical implications. *Pain*, 6:305–327.
67. Leandri, M., and Favale, E. (1981): Punti e tecniche di stimolazione nel trattamento del dolore cronico. In: *Le Cefalee. Farmacologia e Agopuntura*, edited by A. Agnoli and F. Negro, pp. 117–122. Verduci Editore, Roma.
68. Li, C. L., and Bak, A. (1976): Excitability characteristics of the A- and C-fibers in a peripheral nerve. *Exp. Neurol.*, 50:67–79.
69. Liebeskind, J. C., Guilbaud, G., Besson, J. M., and Oliveras, J. L. (1973): Analgesia from electrical stimulation of the periaqueductal gray matter in the cat: Behavioral observations and inhibitory effects on spinal cord interneurons. *Brain Res.*, 50:441–446.
70. Linzer, M., and Long, D. M. (1976): Transcutaneous neural stimulation for relief of pain. *IEEE Trans. Biomed. Eng.*, 23:341–345.
71. Long, D. M. (1979): Current status of neuroaugmentation procedures for chronic pain. In: *Mechanisms of Pain and Analgesic Compounds*, edited by R. F. Beers, Jr. and E. G. Bassett, pp. 51–69. Raven Press, New York.
72. Long, D. M., Campbell, J., and Freeman, T. (1981): Failure of naloxone to effect chronic pain or stimulation induced pain relief in man. (Abstract.) *Pain* (Suppl. 1):S111.
73. Mao, W., Ghia, J. N., Scott, D. S., Duncan, G. H., and Gregg, J. M. (1980): High versus low intensity acupuncture analgesia for treatment of chronic pain: Effects on platelet serotonin. *Pain*, 8:331–342.
74. Marx, J. L. (1977): Analgesia: How the body inhibits pain perception. *Science*, 195:471–473.
75. Matsushito, M. (1969): Some aspects of the interneuronal connections in cat's spinal gray matter. *J. Comp. Neurol.*, 136:57–80.
76. Mayer, D. J. (1979): Endogenous analgesia systems: Neural and behavioral mechanisms. In: *Advances in Pain Research and Therapy, Vol. 3*, edited by J. J. Bonica, J. C. Liebeskind, and D. G. Albe-Fessard, pp. 385–410. Raven Press, New York.
77. Mayer, D. J., and Liebeskind, J. C. (1974): Pain reduction by focal electrical stimulation of the brain: An anatomical and behavioral analysis. *Brain Res.*, 68:73–93.
78. Mayer, D. J., and Price, D. D. (1976): Central nervous system mechanisms of analgesia. *Pain*, 2:379–404.
79. Mayer, D. J., Price, D. D., and Rafii, A. (1977): Antagonism of acupuncture analgesia in man by the narcotic antagonist naloxone. *Brain Res.*, 121:368–372.
80. Mayer, D. J., Wolfle, T. L., Akil, H., Carder, B., and Liebeskind, J. C. (1971): Analgesia from electrical stimulation in the brainstem of the rat. *Science*, 174:1351–1354.
81. Melzack, R. (1973): *The Puzzle of Pain*. Basic Books, New York.
82. Melzack, R. (1975): Prolonged relief of pain by brief, intense transcutaneous somatic stimulation. *Pain*, 1:357–373.
83. Melzack, R., and Wall, P. D. (1965): Pain mechanisms: A new theory. *Science*, 150:971–979.
84. Meyerson, B. A. (1981): Electrostimulation procedures. Their effects, presumed rationale and mechanisms. (Abstract.) *Pain* (Suppl. 1):S159.
85. Mitchell, D., and Woolf, C. F. (1979): Descending tryptaminergic pathways and the antinociceptive effect produced by peripheral electrical stimulation in the rat. *J. Physiol. (Lond.)*, 293:59–60.
86. Nathan, P. W. (1960): Improvement in cutaneous sensibility associated with relief of pain. *J. Neurol. Neurosurg. Psychiatry*, 23:202–206.
87. Nathan, P. W. (1978): Acupuncture analgesia. *Trends Neuro.*, 1:21–23.
88. Nathan, P. W., and Rudge, P. (1974): Testing the gate-control theory of pain in man. *J. Neurol. Neurosurg. Psychiatry*, 37:1366–1372.

89. Nyquist, J. K., and Eriksson, M. B. E. (1981): Effects of pain treatment procedures on thermal sensibility in chronic pain patients. (Abstract.) *Pain* (Suppl. 1):S91.

90. Oliveras, J. L., Besson, J. M., Guilbaud, G., and Liebeskind, J. C. (1974): Behavioral and electrophysiological evidence of pain inhibition from midbrain stimulation in the cat. *Exp. Brain Res.*, 20:32–44.

91. Oliveras, J. L., Redjemi, F., Guilbaud, G., and Besson, J. M. (1975): Analgesia induced by electrical stimulation of the inferior centralis nucleus of the raphe in the cat. *Pain*, 1:39–45.

92. Perl, E. R. (1976): Sensitization of nociceptors and its relation to sensation. In: *Advances in Pain Research and Therapy, Vol. 1*, edited by J. J. Bonica and D. G. Albe-Fessard, pp. 17–28. Raven Press, New York.

93. Pert, A., and Walter, M. (1976): Comparison between naloxone reversal of morphine and electrical stimulation induced analgesia in the rat mesencephalon. *Life Sci.*, 19:1023–1032.

94. Pertovaara, A., and Hamalainen, H. (1981): Threshold elevations found during high-frequency TENS due to peripheral mechanisms. (Abstract.) *Pain* (Suppl. 1):S182.

95. Pertovaara, A., and Kemppainen, P. (1981): The influence of naloxone on dental pain threshold elevation produced by peripheral conditioning stimulation at high frequency. *Brain Res.*, 215:426–429.

96. Pomeroy, S. L., and Behbehani, M. M. (1979): Physiologic evidence for a projection from periaquaductal gray to nucleus raphe magnus in the rat. *Brain Res.*, 176:143–147.

97. Proudfit, H. K., and Anderson, E. G. (1975): Morphine analgesia: Blockade by raphe magnus lesions. *Brain Res.*, 98:612–618.

98. Rivot, J. P., Chaouch, A., and Besson, J. M. (1980): Nucleus raphe magnus modulation of response of rat dorsal horn neurons to unmyelinated fiber inputs: Partial involvement of serotonergic pathways. *J. Neurophysiol.*, 44:1039–1057.

99. Ruda, M. A., Hayes, R. L., Price, D. D., Hu, J. W., and Dubner, R. (1976): Inhibition of nociceptive reflexes in the primate by electrical stimulation or narcotic microinjection at medial mesencephalic and diencephalic sites: Behavioral and electrophysiological analyses. *Proc. Soc. Neurosci.*, 2:952.

100. Salar, G., Iob, I., and Mingrino, S. (1980): Cortical evoked responses and transcutaneous electrotherapy. *Neurology (Minneap.)*, 30:663–665.

101. Salar, G., Iob, I., Mingrino, S., Bosio, A., and Trabucchi, M. (1981): Effect of transcutaneous electrotherapy on CSF beta-endorphin content in patients without pain problems. *Pain*, 10:169–172.

102. Satran, R., and Goldstein, M. N. (1973): Pain perception: Modification of threshold of intolerance and cortical potentials by cutaneous stimulation. *Science*, 180:1201–1202.

103. Sessle, B. J., Dubner, R., Greenwood, L. F., and Lucier, G. E. (1975): Descending influences of periaqueductal gray matter and somatosensory cerebral cortex on neurones in trigeminal brainstem nuclei. *Can. J. Physiol. Pharmacol.*, 54:66–69.

104. Sessle, B. J., and Greenwood, L. F. (1976): Inputs to trigeminal brainstem neurones from facial, oral, tooth pulp and pharyngolaryngeal tissues. I. Responses to innocuous and noxious stimuli. *Brain Res.*, 117:211–226.

105. Shealy, C. N., Mortimer, J. T., and Reswick, H. P. (1967): Electrical inhibition of pain by stimulation of the dorsal columns. *Anaesth. Analg. (Lond.)*, 46:489–491.

106. Shen, E., Tsai, T. T., and Lan, C. (1975): Supraspinal participation in the inhibitory effect of acupuncture on viscero-somatic reflex discharges. *Chin. Med. J. (Engl.)*, 1:431–440.

107. Sjolund, B. H., and Eriksson, M. B. E. (1979): Endorphins and analgesia produced by peripheral conditioning stimulation. In: *Advances in Pain Research and Therapy, Vol. 3*, edited by J. J. Bonica, J. C. Liebeskind, and D. G. Albe-Fessard, pp. 587–592. Raven Press, New York.

108. Sjolund, B. H., and Eriksson, M. B. E. (1979): The influence of naloxone on analgesia produced by peripheral conditioning stimulation. *Brain Res.*, 173:295–301.

109. Takeda, K., Taniguchi, N., Kuriyama, H., and Matsushita, A. (1979): Experimental study on the mechanism of acupuncture anesthesia. In: *Advances in Pain Research and Therapy, Vol. 3*, edited by J. J. Bonica, J. C. Liebeskind, and D. G. Albe-Fessard, pp. 623–628. Raven Press, New York.

110. Takeshige, C., Luo, C. P., Sato, T., and Oka, K. (1981): The different role of dorsal PAG-SPA and ventral PAG-SPA associated with ascending and descending pathways in acupuncture and morphine analgesia. (Abstract.) *Pain* (Suppl. 1):S281.

111. Tamari, J. W., and Jabbur, S. J. (1976): Modulation of tooth pulp input into the spinal trigeminal nucleus by electrical stimulation of remote cutaneous areas in the cat. In: *Advances in Pain Research and Therapy, Vol. 1*, edited by J. J. Bonica and D. G. Albe-Fessard, pp. 191–194. Raven Press, New York.

112. Terenius, L. (1979): Endorphins in chronic pain. In: *Advances in Pain Reserach and Therapy, Vol. 3*, edited by J. J. Bonica. J. C. Liebeskind, and D. G. Albe-Fessard, pp. 459–471. Raven Press, New York.

113. Torebjork, H. E., and Hallin, R. G. (1973): Perceptual changes accompanying controlled preferential blocking of A and C fibre responses in intact human skin nerves. *Exp. Brain Res.*, 16:321–332.

114. Torebjork, H. E., and Hallin, R. G. (1974): Responses in human A and C fibres to repeated electrical intradermal stimulation. *J. Neurol. Neurosurg. Psychiatry*, 37:653–664.

115. Torebjork, H. E., and Hallin, R. G. (1979): Microneurographic studies of peripheral pain mechanisms in man. In: *Advances in Pain Research and Therapy, Vol. 3*, edited by J. J. Bonica, J. C. Liebeskind, and D. G. Albe-Fessard, pp. 121–131. Raven Press, New York.

116. Vyklicky, L., and Sykova, E. (1981): May increased extracellular potassium be responsible for analgesic effects of electroacupuncture? (Abstract.) *Pain*, (Suppl. 1):S282.

117. Wagman, I. H., and Price, D. D. (1969): Responses of dorsal horn cells of *M. mulatta* to cutaneous and sural nerve A and C fiber stimulation. *J. Neurophysiol.*, 32:803–817.

118. Wall, P. D., and Sweet, W. H. (1967): Temporary abolition of pain in man. *Science*, 155:108–109.

119. Whitwam, J. G., and Kidd, C. (1975): The use of direct current to cause selective block of large fibres in peripheral nerves. *Br. J. Anaesth.*, 47:1123–1133.

120. Willer, J. C. (1977): Comparative study of perceived pain and nociceptive flexion reflex in man. *Pain*, 3:69–80.

121. Willer, J. C., Boureau, F., and Luu, M. (1981): Differential effects of electroacupuncture (EA) and transcutaneous nerve stimulation (TNS) on the nociceptive component (R2) of the blink reflex in man. (Abstract.) *Pain* (Suppl. 1):S280.

122. Willer, J. C., Dehen, H., Boureau, F., Cambier, J., and Albe-Fessard, D. (1981): Nociceptive reflexes and pain sensation in man. *Pain*, 10:405–407.

123. Willis, W. D., Haber, L. H., and Martin, R. F. (1977): Inhibition of spinothalamic tract cells and interneurons by brainstem stimulation in the monkey. *J. Neurophysiol.*, 40:968–981.

124. Woolf, C. J. (1979): Transcutaneous electrical nerve stimulation and the reaction to experimental pain in human subjects. *Pain*, 7:115–127.

125. Woolf, C. J., Mitchell, D., and Barrett, G. D. (1980): Antinociceptive effect of peripheral segmental electrical stimulation in the rat. *Pain*, 8:237–252.

126. Yaksh, T. L., Yeung, J. C., and Rudy, T. A. (1976): An inability to antagonize with naloxone the elevated nociceptive thresholds resulting from electrical stimulation of the mesencephalic central gray matter. *Life Sci.*, 18:1193–1198.

127. Young, R. F. (1978): Response properties of neurons in trigeminal nucleus caudalis to noxious and innocuous stimuli under chloralose anaesthesia. *Exp. Neurol.*, 58:521–534.

128. Zimmermann, M. (1979): Peripheral and central nervous mechanisms of nociception, pain and pain therapy: Facts and hypotheses. In: *Advances in Pain Research and Therapy, Vol. 3*, edited by J. J. Bonica, J. C. Liebeskind, and D. G. Albe-Fessard, pp. 3–32. Raven Press, New York.

129. Zoppi, M., Francini, F., Maresca, M., and Procacci, P. (1981): Changes of cutaneous sensory threshold induced by non-painful transcutaneous electrical nerve stimulation in normal subjects and in subjects with chronic pain. *J. Neurol. Neurosurg. Psychiatry*, 44:708–717.

Advances in Pain Research
and Therapy, Vol. 7,
edited by C. Benedetti et al.
Raven Press, New York © 1984.

Multidisciplinary Approach to Managing Pain

Terence M. Murphy and Steen Anderson

Clinical Pain Service, University of Washington, Seattle, Washington 98195

The causes of various chronic pain syndromes are not well understood. Although successful diagnostic and therapeutic methods have been developed for some specific causes of pain such as cancer and reflex sympathetic dystrophy, no adequate explanation for the symptomatology is available for some of the most common chronic pain problems such as low back pain and headache. Therefore, many patients with chronic pain do not receive effective treatment. In such patients, many different therapies have been used empirically, ranging from treatment directed at removing damaged tissue, to attempts to change the patient's behavior without addressing therapeutic efforts to any specific somatic site. These diverse therapeutic efforts reflect: (a) insufficient knowledge of the basic mechanisms of various pain syndromes; and (b) inadequate application of knowledge and therapeutic modalities currently available.

These difficulties were recognized by Bonica (1) early in his experience in treating patients with intractable pain in a large military hospital during World War II. As a result of this experience, he realized there were fundamental differences between acute and chronic pain. With more and more experience, he began to appreciate the multidimensional characteristics of chronic pain, and the fact that causes ranged from chronic tissue damage in a viscus or in somatic structures through injury of the peripheral and/or central nervous system or both, to psychologic and behavioral disorders, with many patients presenting a very puzzling picture. It became obvious that solution of complex pain problems required vast knowledge and clinical experience, more than one individual could possess. This led to the concept that such complex problems could be more effectively managed by a team of specialists representing different disciplines, each of whom contributed to development of the most appropriate therapeutic strategy. After the war, Bonica put this concept into practice in a private community hospital. In 1961 he started a facility at the University of Washington. During the early 1950s, similar facilities for pain diagnosis and therapy were organized by Alexander and by Livingston and his associate Haugen.

For two decades, Bonica traveled extensively and expended considerable time and effort to arouse interest in the concept, but it was not until the late

1960s and early 1970s that this type of facility began to be developed in other medical centers. During the past decade, multidisciplinary facilities, typically called pain clinics or pain centers, have been developed.

These facilities take many different forms and there is, as yet, no universally consistent strategy for diagnosis and treatment. For the most part, pain clinic staff acknowledge the causal complexity of chronic pain and enlist individuals with expertise in different fields to help in the diagnosis and management of these problems (2). The "ideal" pain clinic should possess facilities to evaluate patients for medical, psychological, social, and environmental causes and effects of chronic pain. The pain clinic should have procedures for integrating this information expeditiously and formulating a diagnostic opinion. Moreover, the clinic should be able to implement a management strategy that includes not only conventional medical therapies, but also psychologic and psychiatric therapies, and efforts to change responses of such individuals as the patient's immediate relatives, and employers. This approach is used at the University of Washington Pain Center and most pain clinics use similar methods. Thus the procedures outlined below can be considered representative of multidisciplinary pain management.

ADMISSION AND DIAGNOSIS

Procedure for Admission

Initially when a patient is referred to a pain diagnostic facility, the referring physician is asked to send a comprehensive summary of all diagnostic and therapeutic procedures to date, with emphasis on the patient's primary health problem; surgical, medical, and psychiatric therapies used; and the results of these treatments, along with any radiographs. The summary is carefully reviewed by an attending physician and, often with the help of colleagues, he or she decides whether the patient will be admitted to the program. The information not only helps in screening patients, but also avoids excessive delay for the out-of-town patients who otherwise must wait while the records are being collected.

Once the decision is made to accept the patient, the referring physician and patient are notified of the appointment date. The pain clinic promptly sends the patient: (a) a pain center brochure that explains the procedures of admission and the comprehensive evaluation, and emphasizes the need for the spouse or another relative to accompany the patient to the first appointment; and (b) "diary" forms for recording, at hourly intervals during the day, the frequency and intensity of pain, the amount of medication taken, and the amount of time the patient is lying down, walking, standing, and engaging in various activities. The completed diary gives an overview of how the patient behaves and functions over time in his or her domestic environment. The cover letter reemphasizes the importance of having the spouse or a relative accompany the patient for the interview at the initial visit. The reason for interviewing the spouse or family member is to obtain information concerning the patient's pain complaint and behavior (without his or her personal biases) to supplement that given by the patient, and also to confirm the data contained in the "diary."

Initial Visit

The initial visit is for the purpose of carrying out a screening evaluation. A conventional medical history is elicited and a physical examination is carried out. This is intended to complement and confirm the referral information and to seek a medical explanation for the patient's continued pain. The patient also undergoes a psychosocial evaluation and the spouse or other close relative is interviewed by the clinical psychologist. Once these interviews have been completed, the physicians, psychologists, and social workers who participated in the screening process discuss the patient's problem, develop a diagnosis, and then outline what they think is the best therapeutic strategy for it. This information is given to the patient and the referring physician, who decide whether the therapy will be carried out in the pain center facility or by the referring physician.

When the preliminary evaluation indicates the patient has an exceedingly complex pain problem that is being generated not only by tissue damage, but also by psychologic, behavioral, and environmental factors, a comprehensive multidisciplinary inpatient evaluation or treatment program or both is needed. A recommendation to this effect is made at this early stage for consideration by the patient and the referring physician. If this is agreed on, the patient is admitted to the pain ward for a more comprehensive psychosocial evaluation, further medical evaluation, and consultation with other specialists.

Psychologic and Psychosocial Evaluation

The psychologic and psychosocial evaluation is done by a clinical psychologist or psychiatrist very early in the process, at which stage the patients and relatives will frequently accept such evaluation as a necessary part of the process. On the other hand, if psychological intervention is suggested at a later stage—after the patient has undergone medical evaluation and a trial of conventional medical therapies such as pills, injections, or stimulators has failed—patients and their families are usually reluctant to undergo such evaluation, and some flatly refuse it. Many patients conceive that a psychologic evaluation after trial of medical therapies is a veiled suggestion that the pain is "unreal," "in their heads," or "imaginary." Other patients with refractory pain problems exhibit the phenomena of denial (10); at this stage, a suggestion of further psychologic, psychiatric, or behavioral assessment is strongly resented because it is interpreted that the pain facility staff considers the pain to be caused by "psychologic" factors. Thus it is vitally important to carry out the evaluation by the clinical psychologist and psychiatrist early.

A complete psychologic and sociologic evaluation is essential because chronic pain in many patients is an expression of a complex array of physical, psychologic, behavioral, and affective reactions provoked by operant mechanisms. Information is obtained not only about the developmental history but also the present interaction of the patient with his or her work and family environment. Clinical interviews by psychologists and social workers include assessment of the effects of pain on the lives of patients and their families. The use of psychologic tests, such as the Minnesota Multiphasic Personality Inventory (MMPI), and the illness behavior questionnaire affords the pain team vital information regarding specific functional aspects of the chronic pain experience. The interview covers intake of drugs, alcohol, and tobacco; the amount of physical activity during each day; the impact of pain on sexual relations, social activities, and family attitudes and responses; and what life stresses occurred at the time of the onset of pain and since then. This account of daily life helps determine the presence of depression, anxiety, personality disorders, or behavioral factors and to what extent these may contribute to the pain complaint.

Intellectual function, particularly in older patients, is an important consideration. Both simple and sophisticated tests of intellectual function are available. Intellectual and other mental deficits in older patients are increasingly recognized as generators of pain complaints, which serve to protect them from social or occupational circumstances in which cortical defects would become embarrassingly apparent. Psychologic and psychosocial evaluation is critical to an accurate diagnosis and helps indicate whether behavioral therapy or counseling or both should be included in the pain management plan. It deserves strong emphasis that a diagnosis of psychologic, behavioral, and environmental factors as predominant causes of the pain cannot be made merely on the lack of physical findings, but should be made from positive evidence derived from the psychosocial evaluation.

Medical Evaluation

The medical evaluation includes a complete history and physical examination that invariably includes neurologic, orthopedic, and/or other special examinations, as well as selected radiographic and laboratory studies and when indicated, electromyography.

The history-taking interview emphasizes the patient's previous health, and detailed accounts of previous experiences with medical or surgical care. Excessive and inappropriate medication ingestion is characteristic of a subgroup of chronic pain patients and may well be a contributing factor to their ongoing pain. Special attention is therefore given to eliciting a medication history and a list of current prescriptions. The interviewer tries to obtain precise information about circumstances contributing to the pain, its location, distribution, quality, intensity, and duration at three time periods: when it first began, since it started, and at the present time. Information is elicited about what factors aggravate and relieve the pain, along with specific details about associated phenomena such as muscle spasm, muscle weakness, paresthesia, autonomic dysfunction, and local tenderness. As with most other problems, a family history is elicited.

The physical evaluation begins with careful examination of the painful region to determine the presence or absence of tenderness, hyperesthesia, and other abnormal findings. This is followed by a general physical examination. Although patients referred to pain clinics frequently have undergone many complete physical examinations in regard to their pain problem, it is important to search thoroughly for evidence of pathophysiology responsible for chronic pain, such as reflex, sympathetic dystrophy, or sensory deficits and other neurologic signs of peripheral nerve damage and/or denervation dysesthesia as occurs following nerve damage caused by injuries, surgery, or infection. In patients with evidence of neurologic or musculoskeletal problems, it is desirable to obtain consultations from appropriate colleagues to confirm the findings.

In many patients with chronic pain, other diagnostic procedures are indicated. Clinical laboratory tests and complete radiographic examinations are often essential. In some patients, the skillful application of diagnostic nerve blocks may provide additional information. In those with muscle dysfunction suspected to be caused by neurologic disorders, electromyography is an essential part of the examination. Some pain clinics are using thermography as another valuable diagnostic procedure.

Decision Making: The Pain Conference

Patients for whom the diagnosis or therapy or both are uncertain are discussed at the conferences of the pain group. Those who have evaluated the patient as well as those who may be able to contribute valuable information attend. The patient's managing physician and house officer summarize the history and physical findings and then ask the consultants who have seen the patient to make additional comments. Members of the pain group who have not seen the patient are given an opportunity to ask questions and make comments. In many facilities, the patient and spouse or family member are usually present during part of the conference. The discussion continues in a coordinated, to-the-point manner, until a consensus is reached about the diagnosis and therapeutic strategy. After the conference, the decision made by the group is conveyed to the patient and spouse and subsequently to the referring physician, who also receives a comprehensive summary of the findings and recommendations.

MULTIDISCIPLINARY TREATMENT STRATEGIES

A comprehensive pain clinic offers both multidisciplinary diagnostic capability and comprehensive treatment alternatives—from advanced medical, surgical, psychologic, and psychiatric modalities to innovative social readjustment and behavior modification strategies. Most comprehensive pain clinics will use most, if not all, of the treatment modalities summarized below.

Medications

Review of Current Medications and Detoxification

Systemic analgesics, both nonnarcotic and narcotic as well as sedatives and related drugs, are much used and abused in the treatment of chronic pain. As emphasized by Halpern (*this volume*), all these drugs are used frequently and often inappropriately because they are economical and simple to administer. The nonnarcotic anti-inflammatory drugs, which usually do not produce dependency and tolerance, are highly effective in a variety of chronic pain syndromes caused by peripheral mechanisms.

The use of narcotic analgesics is rarely a good long-term solution to nonmalignant chronic pain. It deserves emphasis that many patients with chronic pain present at pain clinics with dependency on narcotics. These drugs tend to confuse the patient and aggravate pain behavior. In such patients, it is essential to initiate a "detoxification" program early in the treatment. Indeed, it may be necessary to do so during the evaluation program to come to a final diagnosis. Detoxification requires hospital admission and includes the following steps. (a) The problem is discussed with the patient and family and the procedure of detoxification is explained thoroughly. Consent is obtained from the patient, and all drugs in the patient's possession are taken away. (b) During a 48-hr period, the patient is allowed to request and take whatever drugs he or she has been taking, as much and as often as usual. These dosage data are recorded by the nurse. (c) By means of equivalency tables, a comparable amount of long-acting narcotic, such as methadone, or long-acting sedative hypnotic, such as phenobarbital or both, are substituted, dissolved in a masking vehicle and administered by mouth. (d) The drug is given at regular intervals (time contingency basis), rather than as needed, to ensure a steady blood level of the ingredients. (e) A period of stabilization ensures control of the patient's symptoms. Then as other treatment strategies are introduced, the amount of each ingredient is gradually reduced until the patient can do without the medication or with minimum medication. This "weaning" process can take place expeditiously over a week or so, or it may be necessary to continue it for several weeks or even months.

For patients with chronic pain due to advanced or terminal cancer, narcotics properly administered play a predominant role in pain management. This is discussed in detail by T. Ferrer-Brechner and V. Ventafridda (*this volume*).

Neuraxial Narcotics

An innovative use for narcotic analgesics for acute and chronic pain control has been to administer these directly into the epidural or subarachnoid space or both. They appear to produce their selective analgesic effects in the area of the dorsal horn of the spinal cord, either by direct subarachnoid application or diffusion from epidural deposits. There is a burgeoning literature attesting to the analgesic efficacy of this new form of analgesic administration (see L. Jacobson, *this volume*). The problem at the moment is the delivery system. Implantable pumps have been attached to indwelling epidural catheters, although these are exceedingly expensive devices, particularly for individuals with a very short life expectancy. In regard to neuraxial narcotics for patients with long life expectancies, a surprising but gratifying factor has emerged: it is possible to leave conventional epidural catheters in place to deliver this treatment over prolonged periods of time (3), and this technique has been used satisfactorily in the patient's home. This approach can often be successful if the clinic has skilled regional anesthesiologists and staff, such as visiting nurses or physicians prepared to do housecalls, who can monitor the catheters after the patient goes home. Most centers using epidural catheters for analgesic delivery minimize the risk of respiratory depression by closely observing the patient in the hospital 48 hr before commencing long-term therapy continuing either in the hospital or at home.

Antidepressants

Tricyclic antidepressants and similar drugs were initially introduced in attempts to control the chronic pain of postherpetic neuralgia by combining these with other centrally active drugs (14). However, patients and physicians noted that benefits seemed to accrue from the antidepressants themselves. Although chronic pain patients frequently resemble depressed individuals, the degree of depression is often less than that met with in conventional psychiatry. Pain patients often benefit from smaller doses of antidepressants than those needed for conventional therapy in psychiatric patients. Since the pharmacology and clinical application of tricyclic antidepressants are discussed by S. Butler (*this volume*), nothing more will be said here except to emphasize that smaller doses than usual seem to control chronic pain syndromes.

Anticonvulsants

Some of the chronic pain problems that occur with denervation in spinal cord injury, trigeminal neuralgia, postherpetic neuralgia, and so on, are believed to be due to abnormal afferent activity along the damaged afferent nerve paths. Anticonvulsant drugs—phenytoin (Dilantin®) and carbamazepine (Tegretol®)—have been used successfully in such patients (6). In those patients whose pain is associated with some evidence of damage to the peripheral nervous system, these drugs are worth a trial. Phenytoin is well tolerated in doses of 100 mg three times a day, although it is rarely successful in the more refractory types of chronic denervation pain.

Carbamazepine, 250 to 1,000 mg/day, is often more effective but is associated with the side effects of disorientation, unsteadiness of gait, nausea, and hemopoietic depression. Therefore, it should be started in very low doses and gradually increased until it produces a therapeutic effect. If side effects occur, it should be reduced to previously tolerated levels for a few days before attempting to increase the dosage again. By using such strategies, it is often possible to arrive at a dose that is effective and tolerable. Carbamazepine tends to be more useful for the episodic spasmodic chronic pain problem such as trigeminal neuralgia, and is less effective for the relentless denervation dysesthesias such as postherpetic neuralgia, which is perhaps better treated with such drugs as fluphenazine, 1 to 2 mg four times per day. Although these particular drugs are often effective in the denervation dysesthesias, the response to these agents is not uniformly good. Such problems as postherpetic neuralgia often continue to be refractory to therapeutic efforts at this time.

Treatment of Chronic Pain Due to Peripheral Mechanisms

Myofascial Pain Syndromes

Chronic pain due to peripheral mechanisms is often associated with degenerative diseases, but patients with these problems are rarely referred to pain clinics. They usually receive care from general practitioners, rheumatologists, physiatrists, and orthopedists. However, patients with chronic myofascial pain syndromes are frequently seen in pain clinics (15). The etiology, possible mechanisms, and various patterns of pain, as well as treatment of these disorders, are discussed in detail by A. E. Sola (*this volume*).

Reflex Sympathetic Dystrophies

The subgroup of patients with reflex sympathetic dystrophies are characterized by excessive activity of the sympathetic efferent nervous system. They usually respond well to nerve blocks of the stellate ganglion for upper extremity pain, or the lumbar sympathetic chain for lower extremity pain (1). In fact, the diagnosis of reflex sympathetic dystrophy is often made on the basis of positive response to these blocks. This type of pain develops not infrequently following accidental or surgical injury to a limb, or following various disease states, but unfortunately it is frequently not recognized until irreversible trophic changes have occurred. Consequently, only a small percentage of patients with this chronic pain problem are seen in multidisciplinary clinics. This and other aspects of the problem are discussed by R. Rizzi et al. (*this volume*).

Neurolytic Nerve Blocks

Prolonged or permanent destruction of nerves is rarely if ever indicated in nonmalignant chronic pain problems. These measures are reserved for the control of pain of advanced or terminal cancer. Such procedures as neurolytic celiac plexus block for cancers of the pancreas and other abdominal viscera, neurolytic destruction of the segmental nerves to the thorax for carcinoma of the breast, and neurodestructive cranial nerve blocks such as glossopharyngeal nerve block for carcinoma of the pharynx, can be very effective in reducing and even eliminating the nociceptive component of the pain complaint of patients with terminal cancer. This technology has the potential for significant paralytic sequelae in both sensory and motor function. It should, therefore, be undertaken only by those individuals experienced in its use, and certainly not before several diagnostic blocks indicate that such an irrevocable course is necessary. This modality is discussed in more detail by J. L. Madrid and D. C. Moore (*this volume*).

Stimulation-Produced Analgesia

Nerve stimulation to relieve pain has been in use from ancient times, beginning with cupping and acupuncture. In these methods, an alternative stimulus to the pain is supplied to the painful area or a related part. The "gate" theory of Melzack and Wall (8) has provided a plausible neurophysiologic explanation as to how these procedures work and stimulated a renewed interest in providing such therapies through acupuncture and the more modern application of transcutaneous nerve stimulation. (For a review of their neurophysiologic basis, see E. Favale and M. Leandri, *this volume*.)

Transcutaneous electrical stimulators are now available in a wide variety of models—mainly battery-powered units delivering an electric current via flat rubber electrodes to the painful part. This form of therapy appears to work best in myofascial syndromes, peripheral neuropathies, stump pains, and phantom limb pains (7). Stimulators are less effective but nevertheless are much used for low back and neck pain. In contrast to many of the other potential therapies for this refractory type of pain, transcutaneous stimulation (along with biofeedback) has the advantage that there is virtually no morbidity attached to its use. It has been proved to be more effective than placebo in chronic back and neck pain, but it does not solve these problems. Although the stimulator units are expensive, they are economically competitive with the other forms of therapy used by this group of patients.

Attempts to deliver the electrical stimulation at more central sites in and around the neuraxis have met with varied success. Most informed opinion nowadays regards electrical stimulation of the central nervous system itself as still experimental, although percutaneous introduction of such electrodes, either to the dorsal columns or to more central brain sites with radiologic and stereotactic control, can conceivably be done without the morbidity of open operative procedures. This approach also permits removal of the electrodes if relief is not obtained, again without major surgical trespass. The place of electrical stimulation of the central nervous system in pain management awaits full delineation (11).

Psychological Methods Used in Pain Clinics

Nonspecific psychologic support is an integral part of maintenance for patients with chronic pain as is the more recently introduced biofeedback technology. Despite uncertainty regarding psychologic and biologic mechanisms of biofeedback, it does, like transcutaneous stimulation, appear to be valuable in the management of chronic refractory pain (5). In somatically focused patients, it reinforces the other components of the multidisciplinary treatment strategy. For those patients with a muscle tension pain, an electromyographic-mode biofeedback machine is used with which the patient practices and, it is hoped, becomes proficient in relaxing the groups of muscles involved. For a comprehensive review of various psychologic interventions, see J. A. Turner and J. M. Romano (*this volume*).

Behavior Modification Therapy

Most pain clinics include some variation of behavior modification as pioneered by Fordyce (4), where "well-behavior" is substituted for the "chronic pain-behavior" characteristic of many patients referred to pain clinics. Most patients suitable for this modality have reduced their physical activity, apparently in response to their pain complaint. The highly structured exercise component of the behavior modification strategy increases physical activity (well-behavior) to replace inactivity (pain-behavior) in the patient's life-style.

In addition to a gradually increasing exercise, programs to reduce dependence on medications and regain productivity complete the behavior modification strategy. Pain cocktail regimens as described previously wean patients from dependence on medication. Subsequently, the patient is introduced into "job stations," which are often located in supportive hospital facilities such as the laundry room and mailroom, where the patient attempts to relearn job skills. In patients with chronic pain due to operant mechanisms, this process can take anywhere from 3 to 12 weeks. On resuming life at home, the patient frequently experiences a relapse. The patient and spouse are reassured that if this occurs, ongoing contact is available to help them regain and maintain the capabilities acquired during the inpatient behavior modification program. This general theme forms the core of most programs offered by pain clinics.

Neurosurgical Ablative Techniques

With improved knowledge of neuroanatomical pathways conducting pain sensation, it is possible to interrupt these pathways neurosurgically. Although these methods are often effective in relieving pain for finite periods of time, the pain usually returns eventually, or a denervation dysesthetic pain develops in a few months (16). Neurosurgical ablation is often very effective in relieving severe cancer pain caused by peripheral and peripheral-central mechanisms, as discussed by C. A. Pagni (*this volume*). It is much less suitable for chronic nonmalignant pain when the patient's life expectancy greatly exceeds the expected period of relief, about a year at most. The exception to this rule is the use of neurosurgical ablation for trigeminal and glossopharyngeal neuralgia, discussed in detail by C. A. Pagni (*this volume*). The various neurosurgical techniques used for cancer pain are also considered by Pagni. The use of neuroadenolysis, a procedure conceived and practiced by Moricca, is discussed in detail by A. B. Levin, and G. Gianasi, *this volume*.

RESULTS

The results of the efforts of multidisciplinary pain clinics are most difficult to evaluate because the clinics vary so much. It is also exceedingly difficult to obtain follow-up data on a group of patients who are characteristically refractory to medical treatment. If the results are not to their satisfaction, they move on to other medical attendants. Many authors, however, have made valiant attempts to assess the efficacy of such treatment centers.

Since the vast majority of pain clinics have considered behavioral factors important in the generation of chronic pain complaints, and therefore have used behavioral techniques as a significant part of their therapeutic efforts, it is understandable that most of the objective gains observed in these clients have been in the behavioral aspects of pain rather than in the pain symptomatology.

Thus pain clinics seem to be quite effective at modifying the secondary behavior changes that result from the pain. Pain clinics are very effective at reducing the amount of medication patients take for their pain, and most reviews attest to the fact that graduates of pain programs are much less likely to undergo further surgical therapy for their pain complaints. Although the rate of return to normal activity and gainful employment is less than spectacular, by and large it is improved for patients treated in pain clinics compared with control groups in the limited studies that have been conducted in this regard (12). It certainly seems that the number of invasive procedures performed for reduction of pain is greatly reduced once a patient has been through a pain management program.

Sadly, however, the actual pain complaint is probably the factor least influenced by most pain management programs. The typical graduate of such a program demonstrates a reduction in pain but frequently only a modest one. In one of the more detailed follow-up studies that demonstrated some significant functional and behavioral gains at 18-months follow-up (9), it is interesting that the pain levels were virtually unchanged from the initial presenting complaint. Most program evaluations, however, still depend on the patient's subjective report by such methods as mailed questionnaires, which are notoriously unreliable. Seres and Newman (13), however, followed up 100 graduates of a pain program via follow-up visits at 3 months after discharge and determined that 80% were not seeking other medical care at that time. Approximately one-third of these patients were contacted again at 18 months (9) and apparently 30% of this group were back at work. Despite this almost spectacular modification of behavior, the patients' pain complaints remained more or less unchanged.

Current pain treatment facilities that attempt to correct the secondary behavior changes produced by chronic pain seem to be effective at doing that. They reduce inactivity by restoring physical function; they seem to reduce dependency on medications. They seem to deter patients from seeking further medical care. Most of the graduates of these clinics still persist with a pain complaint, despite immense efforts spent addressing this primary concern. We are at this time little nearer to a solution to the chronic pain complaint problem itself.

SUMMARY

Pain clinics, management programs, and pain centers seem to be effective (but not spectacularly so) in reversing many of the undesirable behaviors associated with chronic pain, particularly with regard to health care utilization, medications, and ineffective surgery. At this time, the pain treatment center approach is probably most effective at dealing with refractory nonmalignant pain problems for those patients who by definition tend to be failures of the conventional medical system.

REFERENCES

1. Bonica, J. J. (1953): *Management of Pain*, Lea & Febiger, Philadelphia.
2. Bonica, J. J., Benedetti, C., and Murphy, T. M. (1983): Function of pain clinics and pain centers, In: *Relief of Intractable Pain, Vol. 3*, edited by M. Swerdlow. Elsevier Science Publishers, Amsterdam.
3. Crawford, M. E., and Senn, H. B., (1983): Pain treatment on an outpatient basis utilizing extradural opiates. A Danish multicenter study comprising 105 patients. *Pain*, 16:41–47.
4. Fordyce, W. F. (1976): *Behavioral Methods for Chronic Pain and Illness*. C. V. Mosby, St. Louis.
5. Jessup, B. A., Neufeld, R. W. J., and Merskey, H. (1979): Biofeedback therapy for headaches and other pain. *Pain*, 7:225–270.
6. Loeser, J. D. (1978): What to do about tic douloureux. *JAMA*, 239:1153–1155.
7. Long, D. M., and Hagfors, N. (1975): Electrical stimulation in the nervous system: The current status of electrical stimulation in the nervous system for relief of pain. *Pain*, 1:109–174.
8. Melzack, R., and Wall, P. D. (1965): Pain mechanisms: A new theory. *Science*, 150:971–979.
9. Newman, R. I., Seres, J. L., Yospe, L. P., and Garlington, B. (1978): Multidisciplinary treatment of chronic pain. Long-term follow-up of low back patients. *Pain*, 4:293.
10. Pilowsky, I., and Spence, N. D. (1976): Illness behavior syndromes associated with intractable pain. *Pain*, 2:61–71.
11. Richardson, D. E., and Akil, H. (1977): Pain reduction by electrical brain stimulation in man. *J. Neurosurg.*, 47:178–183.
12. Roberts, A. H., and Rheinhardt, L. (1980): The behavioral management of chronic pain. Long-term follow-up with comparison groups. *Pain*, 8:151–162.
13. Seres, J. L., and Newman, R. I. (1976): Results of treatment of chronic low back pain at the Portland Pain Center. *J. Neurosurg.*, 45:32–36.
14. Taub, A., and Collins, W. F. (1974): Observations on the treatment of denervation dysesthesia with psychotropic drugs: Post-herpetic neuralgia, anesthesia dolorosa, peripheral neuropathy. *Adv. Neurol.*, 4:309–315.
15. Travell, J. G., and Simons, D. G. (1983): *Myofascial Pain and Dysfunction: The Trigger Point Manual*. Williams & Wilkins, Baltimore.
16. White, J. C., and Sweet, W. H. (1979): Anterolateral chordotomy: Open vs. closed, comparison of end results. In: *Advances in Pain Research and Therapy, Vol. 3*, edited by J. J. Bonica, J. C. Liebeskind, and D. Albe-Fessard. Raven Press, New York.

*Advances in Pain Research
and Therapy, Vol. 7,*
edited by C. Benedetti et al.
Raven Press, New York © 1984.

Pathophysiology and Therapy of Postoperative Pain: A Review

*Costantino Benedetti, *John J. Bonica, and
**Gualtiero Bellucci

**University of Washington, Department of Anesthesiology, Seattle, Washington
98195; and **Chair of Anesthesiology, Policlinico, 53100 Siena, Italy*

Effective control of postoperative pain is one of the most important pressing issues in the field of surgery and one that has a significant impact on our health care system. This importance stems from three facts: (a) Of hundreds of millions of people worldwide who will undergo operations this year, most will experience postoperative pain of varying intensity. (b) In too many patients the pain will be treated inadequately, causing them needless suffering, and many will develop complications as an indirect consequence of the pain. (c) There are analgesic modalities that, if properly applied, can prevent or at least minimize the needless suffering and complications. In this chapter the following aspects of the subject will be considered: (a) the incidence, intensity (severity), and duration of postoperative pain and the factors that influence it; (b) the mechanisms, pathophysiology, and complications of postoperative pain; (c) the current status of therapy and reasons for existing deficiencies; and (d) prophylaxis and treatment of postoperative pain. This is an update and expansion of previous reports (10,12,13).

MAGNITUDE OF POSTOPERATIVE PAIN

The incidence, intensity, and duration of pain experienced by patients after various operations are not precisely known. This is simply because well-designed studies of the time-intensity profile of pain following specific operations have not been done under controlled conditions that would permit evaluation of the various factors that affect postoperative pain. Indeed, comprehensive epidemiologic studies have been done on virtually every aspect of any surgical and medical problem; however, there are no data on the incidence of postoperative pain across the entire surgical population. We can get an insight, albeit a crude one, by summarizing the data in published reports (2,10,26,39,46,55,59,66,67,69,81,82,96,98,102) where the number of doses and the total amount of narcotics, and the interval between doses, were used as criteria, and in clinical articles that correlated the amount of

TABLE 1. *Incidence, intensity and duration of postoperative pain following various operations*

Site and type of operation	Steady wound pain		Pain on movement/ reflex spasm		Duration in days of moderate/severe pain
	Moderate	Severe	Moderate	Severe	Mean (range)
Intrathoracic					
Sternotomy	25–35	60–70	25–35	65–75	4 (2–7)
Thoracotomy	25–35	45–65	30–40	60–70	3 (2–6)
Upper intraabdominal					
Gastrectomy	20–30	50–75	25–35	65–75	3 (2–6)
Cholecystectomy and others	25–35	45–65	30–40	60–70	2 (1–5)
Lower intraabdominal					
Hysterectomy and colectomy	30–40	35–55	40–50	50–60	2 (1–4)
Simple appendectomy	35–45	20–30	70–80	20–30	1 (0.5–3)
Renal					
Nephrectomy, pyelolithotomy	10–15	70–85	30–40	60–70	5 (3–7)
Laminectomy	15–20	70–80	30–40	60–70	4 (2–7)
Major joint			(reflex spasm)		
Hip (replacement/ reconstruction)	20–30	60–70	20–30	70–80	3 (2–6)
Knee (patellectomy replacement)	25–30	55–65	30–40	60–70	3 (2–6)
Shoulder or elbow reconstruction or replacement	25–35	45–60	30–40	60–70	3 (2–6)
Simple nailing of joint	40–50	15–30	—	—	3 (2–6)
Other limb operations					
Major hand or foot	15–20	65–70	40–50	50–60	3 (2–6)
Open reduction graft/amputation	20–30	55–70	—	—	2 (1–4)
Closed reduction	40–50	15–30	—	—	1 (0.5–3)
Vascular	35–40	20–35	—	—	1.5 (1–3)
Bladder and prostate	15–20	65–75	—	—	1 (0.5–4)
Perineal					
Anorectal	25–30	50–60	—	—	2 (1–5)
Vaginal	35–40	15–20	—	—	1 (0.5–3)
Scrotal	35–45	15–35	—	—	1 (0.5–3)
Maxillofacial surgery	25–35	35–55	—	—	2 (1–6)
Skin					
Major graft	30–40	40–55	—	—	2.5 (1–5)
Minor graft	40–50	—	—	—	0.5 (0.5–2)
Head and neck	35–45	5–15	—	—	1 (0.5–3)
Abdominal wall					
(Ventral hernia)	35–45	15–25	40–50	25–35	1.5 (1–3)

TABLE 1. (*Continued*)

Site and type of operation	Incidence and intensity (severity)				Duration in days of moderate/severe pain Mean (range)
	Steady wound pain		Pain on movement/ reflex spasm		
	Moderate	Severe	Moderate	Severe	
Thoracic wall					
Radical mastectomy	40–50	10–30	50–60	20–35	1.5 (1–3)
Minor mastectomy (excision lipoma, etc.)	40–45	5–15	—	—	0.5 (0–1)

pain with personality factors (21,37,56,110). All of these data suggest that the incidence, intensity, and duration of postoperative pain vary considerably from patient to patient, from operation to operation, from one hospital to another, and, indeed, from one country to another.

Thus, this suggests that the most important factors that influence the occurrence, intensity, quality, and duration of postoperative pain include (a) the site, nature, and duration of the operation; the type of incision; and the amount of intraoperative trauma; (b) the physiologic and psychologic makeup of the patient, (c) the preoperative psychologic, physical, and pharmacologic preparation of the patient by each member of the surgical team; (d) the presence of serious complications related to the operation; (e) the anesthetic management before, during, and after the operation; and most, importantly, (f) the quality of postoperative care.

The Operation

Extensive clinical observations and published reports (2,10, 26,31,39,55,59,61,66,67,81–83,96,98,102,109) indicate that postoperative pain occurs more often and is more severe following intrathoracic, intraabdominal, and renal surgery; extensive surgery of the spine, major joints, and large bones in the hand and foot; and other major surgical procedures. Table 1 was compiled from published and unpublished data and contains the ranges and approximate average figures for the incidence and duration of pain that occurs after the more commonly done operations. For the sake of clarity, data on "no pain" or "mild pain" are omitted. Until more precise data become available, *these must be considered rough estimates*.

It is noted that after intrathoracic, intraabdominal, and, to a lesser extent, renal operations, movements that place tension on the incision, such as deep breathing, coughing, or extensive body movements, increase the intensity of the pain. The type of incision is also important: For cholecystectomy, a subcostal incision is followed by less pain than a midline one; a transverse abdominal incision also damages fewer intercostal nerves and causes less pain (1,10). Moreover, after replacement or reconstruction of the hip, many patients experience bouts of moderate to excruciating pain caused by severe reflex spasm of the quadriceps and other thigh muscles—pain that occurs at frequent intervals and that is superimposed on the incisional pain. Bouts of severe pain caused by reflex muscle spasm and/or movement also occur after other major joint surgery and/or rectal surgery and certain other operations as noted in the table.

In contrast, superficial operations of the head and neck, limbs, chest wall, and abdominal wall are usually followed by severe pain in 5 to 15% of the patients, moderate pain in 30 to 50%; more than 50% have minimal or no pain and require no narcotic analgesics. Exceptions to this are extensive major skin grafts for burns or other plastic operations and radical mastectomy, which have a slightly higher incidence of severe pain.

The Patient

The incidence and severity of postoperative pain is also influenced by the physical, psychological, emotional, motivational, and personality characteristics of the patient; by social, cultural, and interpersonal factors; and the patient's previous experience with pain (10,19–21,27,56,110). The degree of preoperative and postoperative anxiety, apprehension, and fear is important. Anxiety may be influenced by such preoperative life-changing and disturbing events as emotional, economic, or family problems.

Chapman and associates (20,21) and others (56,73,101,110) noted that preoperative and postoperative anxiety changed dramatically over the course of the postoperative period, particularly in patients inadequately prepared psychologically. Prior to the operation, many, if not most, patients who are inadequately informed and otherwise unprepared develop anxiety, apprehension, and fear about the impending anesthesia and operation, which they carry over into the postoperative period. Also preoperatively, patients may experience the fear of death, of losing consciousness, of being physically helpless, and of losing inhibitions that may cause them to perform irresponsible acts or behavior. Preoperatively, most patients also have fear of, and develop anxiety about, the possible resultant complications of anesthesia and/or surgery, as well as about the possibility of severe pain (10,19–21,58,90).

It has been impressively shown that admission to the hospital produces anxiety and stress that correlate highly with the incidence and intensity of postoperative pain (19,56,110). Volicer (110) has shown that patients scoring high in "hospital stress" preoperatively had more pain and lower physical status ("more morbidity") postoperatively and less improvement after discharge than patients having a low stress score. In this study, some of the factors used to measure hospital stress were unfamiliar surroundings, separation from spouse and family, isolation from other people, lack of information, and previous experience with inadequate pain medication.

Chapman (20) has pointed out that the postoperative patient's state of anxiety is composed of, or caused by, three basic determinants: fear or fright, uncertainty, and helplessness. Fright is a reaction to the onslaught of pain as soon as the effects of anesthesia disappear. The pain and suffering seem to be worse than expected, and the patient feels frantic and threatened, especially if this is the first such experience. Uncertainty, the second component, has a serious impact on anxiety, especially in those who are uninformed of what to expect after the operation. The patient experiences unexpected discomforts and feelings aggravated by the unfamiliar machines, infusion bottles, and other paraphernalia that usually surround the postoperative patient. The confusion created by these imperceptions feeds the anxiety, and the patient remains hypervigilant and anxious, which in turn decreases the pain threshold and increases the patient's perception of pain. Thus a vicious circle is created. This is further enhanced by helplessness, the third component of anxiety. The patient is placed in a fixed position, and, because movement aggravates the pain, he or she feels unable to cope except perhaps to ask the nurse for medication.

Surgical and Anesthetic Management

Other factors that influence postoperative pain are the necessary surgical and anesthetic management including preoperative preparation of the patient, the operative and anesthetic techniques, and postoperative care. The skill of the surgeon and extent of the operative procedure determine the amount of surgical trauma, which, in turn, partly determines the amount of postoperative pain and complications. Similarly the quality of preanesthetic, intraanesthetic, and postanesthetic care influences the incidence and intensity of postoperative pain both indirectly and directly. Traumatic tracheal intubation and generalized muscle pain consequent to succinylcholine-induced muscle spasm directly contribute to the patient's postoperative discomfort. Inadequate muscle relaxation and other problems that prolong the operation will contribute indirectly by increasing the amount and duration of surgical trauma.

NATURE AND PATHOPHYSIOLOGY OF POSTOPERATIVE PAIN

In order to prevent and effectively treat postoperative pain, it is essential for every member of the surgical team to have knowledge of the neurophysiology, biochemistry, psychology, and modulation of acute pain in general and the pathophysiology of postoperative pain in particular. Since other chapters in this volume provide a summary of the basic aspects of pain in general, only those aspects relevant to postoperative pain are included here.

Mechanisms

Surgical operations, like accidental injuries or disease, produce local tissue damage and a barrage of noxious stimuli that are transduced by nociceptors into impulses which are transmitted to the neuraxis by A-delta, and C fibers. Consequent to cellular damage, there is liberation of endogenous substances such as K^+, H^+, lactic acid, serotonin, bradykinin, and prostaglandins, which stimulate and sensitize nociceptors (119). As is well known, nociceptive impulses from the body below the head are transmitted via fibers that synapse with interneurons or second-order neurons in the dorsal horn of the spinal cord; impulses from the head are transmitted via fibers in cranial nerves V, VII, IX, and X that synapse with neurons in the trigeminal sensory nucleus caudalis, the homolog of the spinal dorsal horn.

On reaching the dorsal horn or the nucleus caudalis, nociceptive impulses are subjected to modulating influences coming from the periphery, from local small interneurons, and from supraspinal descending control systems, which together with other factors, determine their further transmission. Some of the nociceptive impulses pass to the anterior and anterolateral horns of the same and adjacent segments of the spinal cord to stimulate somatomotor and sympathetic preganglionic neurons, respectively, and thus promoting segmental, autonomic (nocifensor) reflex responses. Other nociceptive impulses from the periphery stimulate dorsal horn neurons, the axons of which make up ascending afferent systems in the spinal cord and higher parts of the neuraxis, thereby transmitting nociceptive information to various parts of the brainstem and brain, where they provoke suprasegmental and cortical responses, respectively.

Segmental Reflex Responses

Segmental (spinal) reflexes may and often do enhance nociception and produce alteration of ventilation, circulation, and gastrointestinal and urinary function. Thus stimulation of the somatomotor cells results in an increase in skeletal muscle tension. This decreases chest wall compliance and initiates positive feedback loops that generate nociceptive impulses from the muscles (119). Stimulation of sympathetic preganglionic neurons in the anterolateral horn of the spinal cord causes an increase in heart rate and stroke volume and, consequently, in cardiac work and myocardial oxygen consumption. Moreover sympathetic hyperactivity causes segmental vasoconstriction, decreases gastrointestinal tone which may progress to ileus, and decreases urinary bladder function resulting in urinary retention.

Suprasegmental Reflex Responses

Suprasegmental reflex responses result from nociceptive-induced stimulation of the respiratory and other medullary centers, of autonomic centers in the hypothalamus, and of some limbic structures (10,12,62,114,119). These responses include alteration in ventilation (usually increased in the awake individual) and an increase in neural sympathetic tone. The latter causes increases in heart rate and stroke volume, generalized vasoconstriction, and consequent increase in total peripheral resistance and liberation of catecholamines by the adrenal medulla. These, in turn, produce a further increase in cardiac output and blood pressure, and, as a result, an increase in the cardiac workload as well as in general metabolism and oxygen consumption. Moreover, the increased sympathetic tone aggravates the segmentally induced inhibition of gastrointestinal and urinary function.

Finally, and most importantly, suprasegmental reflex responses include a marked increase in the secretion of neuroendocrines characteristic of the stress response (10,62,114). The endocrine stress response to trauma (including surgery) consists of increased secretion of catabolically acting hormones, such as catecholamines, cortisol, ACTH, ADH, glucagon, and aldosterone, and a concomitant decrease in the secretion of the anabolically acting hormones, such as insulin and testosterone. These endocrine changes in turn cause a number of metabolic effects, including increases in blood glucose, plasma cyclic AMP, free fatty acids, ketone bodies, and blood lactate, as well as an increase in general metabolism and oxygen consumption. These endocrine and metabolic changes result in substrate mobilization from storage to central organs and the traumatized tissues. Ultimately, a catabolic state with negative nitrogen balance will exist. The degree and duration of these endocrine and biochemical changes are related to the degree and duration of tissue damage, and many of the biochemical changes last for days (8).

Cortical Responses

Cortical responses occur in the awake individual and are provoked by nociceptive impulses that reach the highest parts of the brain. There they activate very complex systems concerned with integration and perception, or recognition, of the sensation of pain. Simultaneously, cognitive, analytical, judgmental, and memory processes interpret the type, quality, and meaning of the pain within the framework of the individual's learning, personality, culture, ethnic background, experience, motivation, interpersonal influences, and psychologic condition at the time the pain is perceived. These highly complex interactions of sensory, motivational, and cognitive processes that produce pain sensation act on the autonomic and somatic motor systems and initiate psychodynamic reactions of anxiety, apprehension, and fear. These, in turn, collectively produce the complex physiologic, psychologic, and behavioral responses that characterize the multidimensional pain experience. It deserves emphasis that anxiety, especially when severe, greatly enhances the hypothalamic response. Indeed, cortisol and catecholamine secretion in response to anxiety may exceed the hypothalamic response provoked directly by nociceptive impulses (51). Moreover, anxiety and emotional stress may cause cortically-induced increased blood viscosity (95) and clotting (33), fibrinolysis (79), and platelet aggregation (118).

Influence of Anesthesia

During an operation performed with modern, general, balanced anesthesia, the cortical responses are obviated by the anesthetic, while muscle relaxants used as part of the anesthesia prevent reflex muscle spasm. However, unless excessive concentrations of inhalation agents or anesthetic doses of narcotics (e.g., 2 mg i.v./kg body-weight) are used, the sympathetic, neuroendocrine, and biochemical responses provoked by the injury-induced nociceptive input are reduced only slightly or not at all (10,62). This lack of depression or elimination of reflex responses during general anesthesia is often reflected by increases in cardiac output and blood pressure or even by cardiac arrhythmia provoked by intense noxious stimulation, such as sternotomy, intense traction on the hilum of the lung, or an abdominal viscus or trauma to the periosteum. It is also reflected by all of the aforementioned biochemical changes characteristic of the stress response.

During the operation, general anesthesia often is associated with hypoxemia that extends into the postoperative period for a variable time (71,72). General anesthesia lasting more than 30 min for nonabdominal operations is followed by postoperative hypoxemia that persists for about 3 hr and then returns to normal within the first postoperative day (71). If general anesthesia is given for surgery involving the upper abdomen, hypoxemia usually does not resolve within the first day but worsens during the ensuing several days (72). In contrast, in surgery carried out with regional anesthesia that covers *all* of the operative site, the nociceptive input is blocked before it reaches the neuraxis and thus prevents the various segmental, suprasegmental, and neuroendocrine/biochemical responses (10,62). After an intraabdominal operation performed with effective regional anesthesia, hypoxemia does not occur until the block wears off and the postoperative pain develops; at that point the Pao_2 decreases, thus indicating the important role pain plays in postoperative hypoxemia (15).

Responses in the Postoperative Period

In the postoperative period when the effects of surgical anesthesia disappear, the patient's injury persists and pain-producing (algesic) substances continue to be liberated. These substances greatly reduce the threshold of nociceptors so that tenderness ensues and innocuous stimuli, such as touch, produce pain. Moreover, damaged nerves become sensitive and may add to the afferent barrage (112). These pathophysiologic changes are greatly enhanced by sympathetic hyperactivity and consequent liberation of norepinephrine, which sensitizes nociceptors and damages nerves (112).

In operations involving the chest or thoracic viscera, the total pain experience is produced by input from three sites of injury—the skin, the deep somatic structures, and the involved viscus or viscera (10,12):

The cutaneous component that results from both liberation of algesic substances and damaged nerves is characterized by a sharp stimulating quality, is well localized, and often is accompanied by a burning sensation.

The deep somatic component also results from both liberation of algesic substances and the consequent lowering of nociceptive threshold as well as the damaged nerves in fascia, muscle, pleura, or peritoneum. It produces a diffuse, aching discomfort that is felt locally and/or in an area of reference.

The visceral component of pain results from the pathophysiology inherent in the surgical disorder and from tension and contraction of the smooth muscles of the viscera. The pain is characterized by a dull, aching, diffuse quality and is felt locally and/or in an area of reference in the abdominal wall or chest.

Major joint operations entail massive nociceptive input from the richly innervated joint tissues that produce continuous deep somatic pain and severe reflex spasm of muscles supplied by the same and adjacent spinal cord segments that supply the site of surgery (10). Similarly, operations on the thoracic spine and on the maxillofacial region, as well as other operations entailing noxious stimulation of cutaneous and deep somatic "pain-sensitive" structures, including periosteum, produce similar responses.

Pathophysiology and Complications

A number of postoperative dysfunctions are related directly or indirectly to postoperative pain. The most important of these are pulmonary, circulatory, gastrointestinal, and urinary dysfunction; impairment of muscle metabolism and function; thromboembolic processes; and undesirable psychologic and emotional reactions which may be transient or prolonged.

Pulmonary Dysfunction

Pulmonary dysfunction is the most common and most important postoperative complication that occurs, especially after thoracic or intraabdominal surgery. A combination of factors, including reflex muscle spasm and involuntary splinting of the thoracic and abdominal muscles, produces ventilation/perfusion abnormalities. This is further aggravated by ileus with consequent abdominal distension that impairs excursion of the diaphragm and by tight abdominal binders or dressings. Fear of producing or aggravating pain may cause a patient to suppress the urge to breathe deeply or to cough (10,38,39). Bronchiolar spasm may result from activation of cutaneovisceral reflexes (9). Moreover, it has been demonstrated that stimulation of the central end of cut intercostal nerves causes reflex (involuntary) inhibition of respiration (57). The pain-induced medullary stimulation produces hyperventilation (60,83), but this is offset by a decrease in vital capacity (VC) and functional residual capacity (FRC), which produces hypoxemia.

The results of recent studies, summarized by Craig (28), emphasize the importance of the site of operation and the consequent severity of pain, segmental reflex responses, injury to muscles and other tissues, and possible other pathophysiologic factors in producing pulmonary dysfunction. Patients who have undergone intrathoracic or intraabdominal surgery with general anesthesia show a restrictive pattern of ventilation postoperatively with severely reduced inspiratory capacity (IC) and VC, plus a smaller, but more important, reduction in FRC. These alterations in pulmonary function are greatest after upper intraabdominal surgery; VC is reduced to about 40% of the preoperative value within 1 to 4 hr after the operation, remains at this level for 12 to 24 hr, slowly increases from 60 to 70% of the preoperative value at 7 days, and returns to the preoperative level during the ensuing week or so. Immediately after surgery, FRC is near the preoperative level, but by 24 hr postoperatively it is decreased to about 70% of the preoperative level and remains depressed for several days. It then gradually returns to normal by day 10.

Reduction of total lung capacity, and therefore FRC due to abdominal or thoracic pain, produces a higher than atmospheric pleural pressure in gravity-dependent areas of the lung, resulting in negative transpulmonary pressure and causing the small airways to narrow or close. The outcome is a low ventilation/perfusion relationship which impairs gas exchange and leads to hypoxemia. Moreover, failure of an airway to reopen will, in time, lead to total collapse of the lung unit served by that airway, producing the clinical syndrome of atelectasis. If a rapidly absorbed gas, such as nitrous oxide or oxygen, is trapped behind a closed airway, atelectasis will occur more rapidly. These pathophysiologic processes are likely to occur more rapidly and to a greater degree in patients who are elderly, obese, or heavy smokers (28). In patients with preexisting pulmonary disease, these are superimposed on their pulmonary dysfunction. Moreover, certain types of midline abdominal incisions cause greater dysfunction than others (e.g., subcostal) (1,10).

Pulmonary dysfunction caused by postoperative pain also occurs with operations in other parts of the body, although not to the same degree. Modig (77) studied a group of elderly patients who had undergone total hip replacement to evaluate pentazocine and epidural block for the relief of postoperative pain. Those patients managed with pentazocine had a decrease of

Pao_2 from a preoperative level of 82 to a range of 68 to 70 mm Hg on the first and second postoperative days and to 67 mm Hg on the third day. That the hypoxemia was probably due to pain and nociceptively induced reflex responses is suggested by the fact that patients managed with epidural analgesia were completely pain-free and their Pao_2 values remained essentially the same as the preoperative values for the entire 3 days. Patients managed with pentazocine had lower tidal volume and higher respiratory frequency that those of the epidural group, a condition that probably led to a less uniform ventilation with more alveolar closure than in the epidural group. Moreover radiographic studies revealed marked elevation of the diaphragm due to abdominal distension, a condition not seen in the epidural group. The decrease in Pao_2 was due mainly to ventilation/perfusion disturbance that persisted in the third postoperative day despite routine physical therapy. These findings emphasize that postoperative hypoxemia can and does occur after major surgery of the extremities, especially in elderly patients, and is probably due to inadequate pain relief and the aforementioned reflex responses.

It has long been appreciated that unless vigorous prophylactic and therapeutic measures are carried out, pulmonary dysfunction may progress to pneumonitis and increased morbidity. The reported incidence of postoperative pulmonary complications varies from about 5 to 25% or more (10,15,34,44,63,80,83,84,91,105,113), depending on the criteria used and the type of operation. In young adults in otherwise good physical condition, superficial or extremity surgery is not associated with any ongoing abnormality of lung volumes (28). However, urgent operations for gastrointestinal bleeding carry up to a 60% rate of pulmonary complications (113). Moreover, in elderly patients or those at risk from one of the aforementioned factors, atelectasis and hypoxemia, and even pneumonitis, may develop (28). If fever, cough, increased production of sputum, or leukocytosis are used as indices of pulmonary complications, the incidence across all postoperative patients is said to vary between 5 and 10% (63,84,113). After thoracic and upper abdominal operations, atelectasis and pneumonitis are said to occur in approximately 20 to 30% of patients (7,10,22,29,44,80,84); however, in one study where radiographs and blood gas studies were used as criteria for atelectasis, the incidence was 60% (83).

Circulatory and Metabolic Dysfunctions

Postoperative pain and the segmental and suprasegmental reflex responses produced by the continued nociceptive input cause increased cardiac output, blood pressure, metabolism, and oxygen consumption (10–12). That these are due to postoperative pain is suggested by the results of studies in which narcotics and epidural analgesia were evaluated as mentioned in the next section.

Gastrointestinal Complications

Ileus with accompanying nausea and, in some cases, vomiting is also the direct result of postoperative nociceptive impulses arising in the viscera and somatic structures. Studies have demonstrated the presence of powerful cutaneovisceral and visceral-visceral reflexes resulting in sympathetic hyperactivity and consequent reflex inhibition of gastrointestinal function (9,10,64). These complications are due to reflex responses, not only those initiated in thoracic and abdominal viscera but also in extremities and other parts of the body, as was impressively demonstrated by Modig (77). Following total hip arthroplasty, patients who were managed with epidural analgesia had good bowel sounds and frequent flatus. This was in contrast to patients who were managed with pentazocine; they were sedated and drowsy, had nausea and absence of bowel sounds, and a marked elevation of the diaphragm due to abdominal distension. The latter probably resulted from the pain-induced reflex inhibition and, perhaps, the effects of the narcotic. Moreover, persistent nociceptive input in the postoperative period may have caused reflex inhibition of the urinary tract with consequent urethral and bladder hypomotility and difficulty with urination (10,12).

Impairment of Muscle Metabolism and Muscle Function

These are pain-induced complications of major surgery in the hip, knee, and other major joints. In a study at the Karolinska Hospital (Stockholm) of patients who underwent knee surgery (E. Erickson, *personal communication*), persistent postoperative pain and consequent limitation of motion was noted to produce marked impairment of normal muscle metabolism, cause muscle atrophy, and significantly prolong return of normal muscle function. The pain and reflex vasoconstriction, and possibly other reflex responses, were probably the cause, since the patients managed with epidural analgesia had complete pain relief, much less limitation of motion, and, consequently, less muscle atrophy with much quicker return to normal function.

Thrombus Formation of the Lower Limbs

This complication occurs with greater frequency in postoperative patients whose pain is inadequately relieved and who reduce their physical activity for fear of aggravating the pain (10). The development of thrombi is likely to be further increased by pain-induced anxiety, which as previously mentioned, causes cortically mediated increased blood viscosity and clotting, fibrinolysis, and platelet aggregation. The potential danger of thromboembolic phenomena needs no elaboration.

Psychological/Emotional Effects

In some patients, severe postoperative pain if unrelieved may produce serious long-term emotional disturbances which may impair the patient's mental health (19). In many patients, inadequate relief of postoperative pain causes undue fear and anxiety in the event that these patients require subsequent surgery.

CURRENT STATUS OF POSTOPERATIVE PAIN THERAPY

The experience of the second author (J. J. B.) with a number of major operations he has been subjected to, his interviews of thousands of postoperative patients, and numerous reports in the literature (24,32,35,42,68,70,75,76,108) lead us to the deep conviction that in all too many patients, postoperative pain has been and continues to be improperly managed. A study carried out by Marks and Sachar (70) of Montefiore Hospital (New York) revealed that in three-quarters of the patients with acute and chronic pain, the pain remained unrelieved following administration of narcotic analgesics. A review of the patient's chart revealed that house officers prescribed narcotics (usually meperidine) in amounts that were approximately 50 to 65% of what had been established as effective doses of this narcotic for severe pain. (Two-thirds of the patients were prescribed 50 mg meperidine every 4 hr p.r.n.) Moreover, nurses administered approximately 40 to 50% of the inadequate amounts prescribed. Consequently, patients with severe pain were given an average of 90 mg meperidine per day.

In their review article on postoperative pain, Utting and Smith (108) cite more than a dozen reviews, editorials, and letters dealing with postoperative pain published during the past decade; nearly all stressed the inadequacy of treatment. They cited the case of C. MacInnes, the late well-known English novelist and journalist who, after a major operation, described the treatment of his postoperative pain as the "great defect in English public hospital treatment, which to my mind . . . is a cruel and callous disgrace" (68). This subjective account of inadequate postoperative pain relief stimulated an editorial in *The Lancet* on "tight-fisted analgesia" in which the attitude of the medical profession toward postoperative pain was castigated (35). Utting and Smith also cited the report of a professor of obstetrics in which he stated that his pain after open heart surgery "defies description"; this provoked another, similar editorial comment (32). The inadequacy of postoperative pain relief at night was the object of another devastating account by a medical man (42). One of the present authors (J. J. B.) had similar experiences following 3 of 11 hip operations and 4 ear plastic procedures which produced severe, sometimes excruciating pain that was inadequately relieved because of insufficient amounts of narcotics given. (This was in contrast to the other 8 hip operations, a cholecystectomy, and several other procedures managed with regional analgesia that did provide effective pain relief.)

Cohen (24) studied the adequacy of relief of postoperative pain in 109 patients in five central Illinois hospitals. The patients were interviewed and their charts reviewed on the third postoperative day. After all patient interviews were completed, 121 nurses on the same units responded to a questionnaire that evaluated their knowledge of the pharmacology of drugs, attitude about pain, and skills in pain relief. The results of the patient interviews indicated that 75% of the patients given narcotics for pain continued to experience moderate or marked pain and distress after narcotic therapy. Moreover, 70% of the patients stated that pain interfered with their sleep, and in 40% it was disturbed to a marked degree. When asked if they experienced the return of pain before receiving the next dose of analgesia, 88% indicated they did; of these, 38% stated the pain had returned more than 1 hr before their next dose and 45% stated the pain caused them to "cry out."

Mather and Mackie (75) surveyed 170 children recovering from surgery in two major teaching hospitals in Adelaide, Australia. The survey revealed that analgesic medication was not ordered for 16% of the patients and was not administered to 31%. In 25% of the patients where narcotic or nonnarcotic analgesic medication was ordered, only the nonnarcotic drug was given. Consequently, only 25% of the patients were pain-free on the day of surgery with 13% reporting severe pain. On the first postoperative day, 17% still reported severe pain.

Reasons for Deficiencies

For nearly three decades, Bonica has repeatedly studied the reasons for inadequate management of pain in general and postoperative pain in particular (10–13). The reasons have remained the same and can be grouped into two major categories: (a) voids in knowledge about basic mechanisms and other aspects of postoperative pain because of insufficient research and (b) inadequate application of the knowledge and therapeutic modalities currently available. Since these reasons have been discussed in detail elsewhere (11), only two comments relevant to postoperative pain are made here.

Despite its clinical importance, no well-designed studies of the time-intensity profile of pain following each operation have been done. Until recently, no studies had been done on such basic mechanisms as the biochemical and neurophysiologic substrates of pain caused by damaged nerves, and the inflammatory response to injury. Equally important, very few comprehensive psychologic studies have been done to evaluate the influence of personality, ethnic background, and the personal interactions of the patient, the house staff, and other members of the surgical team on anxiety and its influence on postoperative pain.

Inadequate or improper application of knowledge and therapies currently available is certainly the most important factor resulting in inadequate postoperative pain relief. We *do have* sufficient information and a variety of narcotic drugs and other modalities that, if properly applied, would provide effective relief for most patients with postoperative pain. This deficiency has resulted from a lack of organized instruction of medical and nursing students and of surgeons in training (11,12,24,70,75), inadequate sources of relevant information on postoperative pain in surgical textbooks and journals, and a lack of appreciation by surgical teams of the various factors that influence the intensity and duration of postoperative pain.

Several studies have provided impressive evidence that a lack of knowledge of clinical pharmacology of narcotics by surgical house officers and nurses contributes to the inadequate management of postoperative pain. As part of their study, Marks and Sachar (70) sent a questionnaire to 102 physicians and surgeons-in-training in two major hospitals in New York. This part of the study revealed that because of inadequate knowledge of the pharmacology of narcotics, most of the house staff physicians and surgeons underestimated the effective dose range of these drugs, overestimated the duration of their action, and had an exaggerated opinion of the danger of addiction. Cohen (24) found similar deficiencies among the 121 nurses who responded to the questionnaire. The data revealed that nurses were overly concerned about the possibility of addiction, their choices of analgesic medications seemed irrational, and their knowledge of the drugs was inadequate. From their survey, Mather and Mackie (75) also concluded there is a critical need to improve postoperative pain management in children, and this must be based on improved education of medical and nursing staff, as well as improved communication between staff, parents, and patients.

There is also evidence that many house officers and nurses do not know or appreciate the importance of preoperative evaluation and preparation of each individual patient. Moreover, there is insufficient appreciation of the value of psychologic approaches, including the provision of psychosocial support in the form of information, the manifestation of a sympathetic attitude, and other positive interpersonal factors that enhance the patient's coping skills and decrease or eliminate fear, anxiety, and other psychologic factors known to increase postoperative pain.

Inadequate interest or concern about the problem of postoperative pain is further attested by the fact that very little, if any, information about pain management is found in the surgical literature, voluminous as it is. A review of the seven most important textbooks on the principles and practice of surgery in the United States revealed that only one (13) contains a chapter devoted to postoperative pain; the other six (25,36,45,86,92,97) devote only 19 pages, out of a total of 8,252, to the *symptomatic* therapy of postoperative pain. Moreover, in reviewing numerous surgical journals, it is difficult to find an article on the subject. From these data, the only conclusion that can be drawn is that pain has not been considered important by surgical scientists, educators, and clinicians. They have been satisfied to leave the matter to their house officers who apparently, as previously mentioned, are uninformed about this important aspect of surgical practice.

MANAGEMENT OF POSTOPERATIVE PAIN

Prophylactic Measures

The incidence, severity, and duration of pain and suffering during the postoperative period can be decreased by proper preoperative and postoperative psychologic care (11,13,19,20,56). One of the most obvious and effective methods of decreasing its magnitude is to directly manipulate anxiety, the cardinal psychologic component of postoperative pain. One thing surgeons, anesthesiologists, and nurses can affect is the cognitive-judgmental aspect of patients' suffering with the goal of reducing uncertainty and the consequent anxiety. Several investigators have shown that if the patient is given adequate information before the operation, encouraged to ask questions, and given a careful explanation of what will happen and when it will happen, then uncertainty will be eliminated or significantly reduced and the patient will have less pain and suffering. For example, Egbert et al. (37) provided one group of surgical patients with a combined cognitive-behavioral intervention consisting of information about the surgical procedure and the expected sensation *plus* instructions regarding physical relaxation, deep-breathing exercise, and body maneuvers designed to decrease discomfort during the postoperative period; this group was then compared to another group receiving only procedural information. The combined group required smaller amounts of narcotics after surgery and was discharged earlier than the control group. A number of other studies (40,65,94,115) have demonstrated that behavioral coping strategy in combination with some form of preparatory information is effective in increasing patients' abilities to cope with surgical stress.

The assurance by members of the surgical team that modern science has much to offer to prevent pain during the operation and to decrease the degree of discomfort and suffering after the operation can help the patient overcome any feeling of helplessness. This will help the patient become aware that he or she can control disagreeable sensations by strategic shifts of attention, by autosuggestion, and by using other coping skills, all of which will tend to reduce anxiety and pain (19–21,39,56). Such psychologic manipulations may possibly stimulate the endogenous antinociception system with consequent liberation of enkephalin and other endorphins to impair transmission of nociceptive information, thus contributing significantly to the patient's welfare.

During the preoperative period the anesthesiologist can contribute significantly to the efforts of the other members of the surgical team in decreasing preoperative anxiety by an ample preanesthetic visit and providing effective psychologic and pharmacologic preparation of the patient (27,90). All should be done to fully inform the patient about the anesthetic to be used with the intent of dispelling any fears about the procedure and by inspiring confidence and developing rapport. If regional analgesia is used for the operation, it is best to use a long-acting agent or a continuous technique to prolong the analgesia for at least the time the patient is in the recovery room. This, combined with minimal sedation, can provide excellent analgesia plus an awake, calm, and cooperative patient. When the block regresses, pain usually can then be controlled with a reinjection of local anesthetic or, if regional anesthesia is discontinued, the residual analgesic action permits prescribing reduced doses of systemic analgesics. Balanced general anesthesia also may provide residual analgesia that reduces the requirements of systemic narcotics postoperatively. This is particularly true with certain volatile anesthetics and, of course, with narcotic analgesia used for the operation and continued during the first postoperative day, as is often done for patients who have undergone cardiac surgery.

Optimal surgical care also helps decrease the severity of the pain. Skillful and gentle handling of tissues, carrying out the operation with dispatch, and observance of other surgical principles by the surgeon and assistants will minimize trauma. Proper postoperative care to help decrease the magnitude of postoperative pain involves continuing psychologic support, proper care of wounds, early ambulation, and good nursing care.

ACTIVE TREATMENT

Postoperative pain may be partially or completely relieved by one or more of the following methods: (a) systemic analgesics and adjuvant drugs; (b) regional analgesia achieved with local anesthetics; (c) regional analgesia achieved with intraspinal narcotics; (d) electrical analgesia achieved by transcutaneous electrical stimulation, electroacupuncture, or spinal cord stimulation; and (e) psychologic analgesia in the form of hypnosis or suggestion.

Systemic Analgesics and Adjuvant Drugs

Narcotics

Morphine and other narcotic analgesics remain the most commonly used, standard method of treating postoperative pain. The immense popularity and widespread use of these drugs are due to the fact that they are readily available, easy to use, and inexpensive, and when properly administered, they provide good (though not complete) relief of pain. As previously mentioned, all too often these drugs are improperly used; consequently, many patients do not derive good pain relief. The most common error is routine administration without regard to the intensity of the pain and associated phenomena; the emotional makeup, physical status, and age of the patient; and the various other factors previously mentioned. This, in turn, is due to the traditional practice of ordering narcotics p.r.n. without first evaluating the efficacy of the initial dose. Many physicians and nurses do not fully appreciate the great variability in the pharmacokinetics, analgesic efficacy, and side effects of different narcotics in different individuals.

Intramuscular administration

Recent pharmacokinetic studies have shown that after intramuscular administration there is great variability in the time of onset, degree, and duration of analgesia. For example, Austin et al. (3) studied the pharmacokinetics and analgesic efficacy of 100 mg meperidine administered intramuscularly at the end of surgery and every 4 hr thereafter, and found that the interpatient peak meperidine concentration (PMC) varied fivefold and the intrapatient PMC varied twofold. The time to reach PMC ranged from 15 to 106 min with a mean $\pm$ SD of 45 $\pm$ 17 min. With the first injection, the PMC varied from 0.24 to 1.21 μg/ml with a mean $\pm$ SD of 0.44 $\pm$ 0.14 μg/ml; it lasted from 45 to 60 min and then decayed to 0.25 μg/ml. With the second injection the mean PMC was 0.58 $\pm$ 15 μg/ml and then decayed to a mean of 0.44 μg/ml. With subsequent injections, the mean $\pm$ SD PMC was 0.75 $\pm$ 0.20 μg/ml and then decayed to a mean of 0.40 to 0.45 μg/ml at 24, 28, and 32 hr. These data indicate there was systemic accumulation of meperidine as the blood concentration gradually increased in the first two dosing intervals, and it appeared to reach a steady state. Pain control was very poor during the first 4-hr dosing interval (none of the patients derived effective relief), but improved somewhat during the second dosing period and even more with subsequent doses. However, even with the later doses, effective (almost complete) relief was achieved in about 45 min, lasted from 75 to 90 min, and then pain increased steadily to severe levels by the fourth hour. In another study (4) they estimated the minimum effective analgesic concentration (MEAC) of meperidine to be a mean of 0.5 μg/ml, and the drug remained above the MEAC for only 35% of the 4-hr dosing interval (approximately 85 min). In view of these data, it is no wonder that patients derived only transient effective analgesia even after they had reached a steady state. These and other data emphasize the critical need to both instruct the patient to request analgesia as soon as the pain returns and monitor the patient carefully during the first three dosing intervals to assess accurately the efficacy and duration of analgesia and any adverse side effects.

Evaluation of the efficacy of narcotics is the responsibility primarily of the surgical staff but also requires joint efforts by the nurses and patient. The dose then can be revised, if necessary, and given at regular intervals that are from 15 to 20 min shorter than the duration of analgesia or given as needed provided the patient is willing to ask for an analgesic and the nurse or other personnel is available to promptly administer it. This will help produce a more even and sustained analgesia and will avoid the repeated peaks of pain feared by most patients.

Intravenous administration

In order to eliminate variability in the peak plasma concentration and the time to reach this peak, narcotics can be given intravenously (10,13,50,103). In addition to eliminating the variability of absorption, the intravenous route has important advantages (50):

1. There is rapid onset of action that produces prompt relief of pain and decreases the incidence of anxiety and other emotional effects of severe pain.
2. The early occurrence of the peak effects facilitates the titration of the drug to meet the needs of the individual patient.
3. The rapid decline of the blood concentration limits the time in which undesirable effects are likely to occur.

To obtain these advantages it is necessary to observe the patient for 15 to 20 min after the first injection and assess the pain relief and any undesirable effects. To achieve effective analgesia and at the same time minimize the incidence of undesirable side effects, small doses (e.g., 2 to 3 mg morphine or 20 to 30 mg meperidine diluted in 3 to 5 ml of saline) are given *slowly*. Initially it will be necessary to give 2 or 3 doses at intervals of 15 to 20 minutes to achieve good analgesia, but the intervals can be increased to 45 to 60 min to maintain a steady rate. Roe (88) reported that with small intravenous doses, patients consumed significantly less narcotic to obtain a more even analgesia than with intramuscular injections. Of course, this method requires more time and effort on the part of the nursing and surgical house staff and may not be practical in certain hospitals.

Continuous infusion

Continuous infusion of narcotics requires careful monitoring of the patient and adjusting the rate of infusion as needed to achieve good pain relief. On the basis of available pharmacokinetic data (3,50,74,103,104), the intravenous infusion containing the narcotic is started at rates of 0.1 mg/min (6 mg/hr) of morphine or 1 mg/min (60 mg/hr) meperidine or equianalgesic doses of other narcotics for the first hour; the infusion rate is then decreased to half these amounts during the second and third hour, and thereafter to maintenance doses of 2 to 3 mg of morphine or 20 to 30 mg meperidine per hour for the rest of the period. Obviously the patient must be monitored closely during the first several hours and frequently thereafter in order to increase or decrease the rate as necessary. Since this infusion rate may require from 2 to 3 hr to reach minimum analgesic concentration (103), it may be desirable to administer 5 mg morphine or 50 mg meperidine in a slow intravenous bolus at the beginning of the infusion and repeating it in about 30 min (50). These bolus injections permit achieving MEAC promptly, and this is likely to last for approximately 120 to 150 min, at which time the intravenous infusion would achieve MEAC (103).

Patient-administered narcotic analgesia

Another option is to use a system that permits "on-demand" analgesia known as PACAT, or patient-controlled analgesic therapy. The practicality of this method has been demonstrated by a number of clinicians including Tamsen (104), in his thesis on the subject in which he reviews the literature. Tamsen demonstrated that intravenous self-administration of preset doses of each analgesic can be accomplished by means of a press-button-activated, programmable drug injector that permits infusion of wide ranges of drug doses and rates of injection. The injector is programmed to allow a maximum of 1 dose per 15 min. The patient must be informed thoroughly about the procedure and instructed on how to manipulate the apparatus. Near the end of the surgery, patients should receive a bolus of morphine or one or more boluses of meperidine; as soon as postoperative pain is felt, the patient is allowed to begin self-administration of 20 or 30 mg of meperidine or 2 or 3 mg of morphine, or equianalgesic doses of other narcotics, every 15 min or longer as soon as pain returns.

Tamsen noted that individual analgesic consumption remained virtually constant throughout the PACAT period. Most patients established and maintained a pseudo-steady-state plasma concentration by triggering new doses as the plasma concentration dropped to a critical level of MEAC. They found the mean plasma analgesic concentration for meperidine similar to that reported by Mather et al. (3,4,74,103). The hourly consumption of the analgesic was as follows (in milligrams): meperidine 26 ± 10, morphine 2.6 ± 1.2, and ketobemidone 2.3 ± 0.8, which represent the 4-hourly totals similar to the recommended 4-hourly doses for these drugs given intramuscularly, except that these patients derived almost continuous pain relief.

Like Mather, Tamsen found a substantial interpatient variation in doses consumed and in the mean plasma concentration achieved. Interestingly, they found that individual meperidine levels in plasma and cerebrospinal fluid were inversely related to each individual's level of endorphins. Moreover, substance P decreased in individuals with a CSF meperidine concentration greater than 200 μg/ml. These results suggest that endorphins may play an important role in the modulation of acute postoperative pain and in regulating the demand for narcotic analgesic after surgical trauma. Tamsen concluded that PACAT is an effective way of providing postoperative pain relief.

Conclusions

Whatever the route of administration, a cardinal rule is to give the patient sufficient amounts of narcotics to provide effective and sustained pain relief with minimal side effects. Even though narcotics do produce respiratory depression, this is not clinically significant. In a study of patients who had undergone upper abdominal thoracic operation, Keats and Kirgis (60) gave intravenous meperidine in increments of 10 to 15 mg repeated at 15-min intervals until significant pain relief was achieved. Following effective analgesia the Pa_{CO_2} increased a mean of 2 mm Hg, and the Pa_{O_2} increased almost 8 mm Hg. Thus, although narcotics given to patients in pain depress respiration slightly, they decrease the ventilation/perfusion abnormality. Equally important is that the pain relief permits patients to breathe more deeply and cough somewhat better when they are so instructed by the surgical/nursing staff. Patients who are elderly, debilitated, or hypovolemic will require significantly less drug. Special care also should be exercised in administering narcotics to patients with chronic lung disease, head injury, or advanced liver disease (43), or to those who have been on monoamine-oxidase-inhibiting drugs.

Addiction among medically treated patients rarely if ever occurs. In a study of nearly 40,000 hospitalized medical patients monitored for narcotic addiction, Porter and Jick (85) of the Boston Collaborative Drug Surveillance Program found that among the nearly 12,000 patients who had received narcotics, there were only four documented cases of addiction, and only one of these had major addiction. These and other data (5) suggest that medical use of narcotics is rarely associated with development of addiction and should not cause physicians and nurses to avoid prescribing and/or administering effective doses of narcotics. Moreover, physical dependence rarely, if ever, occurs in patients given narcotics for several days.

Adjuvants

An alternative method is to combine morphine (or another narcotic) given in smaller doses with hydroxyzine or dextroamphetamine. It has been shown that hydroxyzine potentiates the analgesic efficacy of narcotics and, at the same time, relieves anxiety and decreases the incidence of nausea and vomiting (6,52,93). For example, Hupert (52) showed that 5 mg of morphine combined with 100 mg of hydroxyzine produced a degree of analgesia equivalent to that produced by 10 mg of morphine.

The ability of amphetamines to potentiate the analgesic action of narcotics was first demonstrated nearly four decades ago and, subsequently, Bonica (10) advocated their use in the management of acute and chronic pain. More recently Forrest et al. (41) showed that 5 and 10 mg of dextroamphetamine increased narcotic analgesia 1.5- and twofold, respectively. For example, 10 mg dextroamphetamine combined with 6 mg morphine produced relief of postoperative pain similar in degree to that achieved with 12 mg morphine alone. Evidence suggests the analgesia induced by amphetamine is due to an increased secretion of serotonin and, presumably, to enhancement of the function of the bulbospinal descending inhibitory system (54). In addition to potentiating analgesia, amphetamines counteract narcotic-induced central nervous system depression, appear to decrease anxiety and improve mood, and enhance a feeling of well-being.

Weak Analgesics

Mild to moderate postoperative pain can be relieved effectively with 325 to 650 mg of aspirin combined with 64 mg of codeine. Obviously since this combination is taken by mouth, it can only be used in patients who have no gastrointestinal dysfunction.

Regional Analgesia with Local Anesthetics

Regional analgesia achieved with local anesthetics properly administered is one of the most effective methods of relieving postoperative pain. Regional analgesia not only provides complete or near complete relief of pain but interrupts the afferent limb of segmental and suprasegmental reflex responses and the consequent endocrine and biochemical changes (12,13,62). By completely or almost completely relieving pain and the associated skeletal muscle spasm, it permits better pulmonary ventilation than is possible with narcotics. Moreover, since regional analgesic blocks, unlike systemic narcotics, afford complete relief of pain without depressing respiration and the cough reflex, the patient can cough effectively and cleanse the tracheobronchial tree. Because better ventilation, greater activity in bed, and earlier ambulation are made possible by the high degree of analgesia, the decrease in VC, FRC, and consequent pulmonary shunting and hypoxemia is less, and hospitalization is shorter than obtained with narcotic analgesia (17,23,28,39,48,49,69,77,83,100). However, since decreases in VC, FRC, and peak expiratory flow rates (PEFR) following upper abdominal and thoracic surgery are the result not only of pain and reflex muscle spasm but also of the operation-induced impairment of chest wall and diaphragmatic function, regional analgesia does not completely eliminate these changes (28).

For optimal results, regional anesthetic techniques must be carried out with skill and the patient must be managed properly during and after execution of the block. Although this method is more complicated to administer than narcotics and requires more time and effort, in skilled hands these are relatively minor disadvantages and not sufficient to preclude its use. The disadvantage of the need to repeat the injection can be minimized by using bupivacaine (Marcaine®) as the local anesthetic of choice.

Regional analgesia can be achieved by injecting the local anesthetic into the spinal canal via a catheter to produce continuous segmental epidural block, by injecting nerves at their exit from the intervertebral foramina (paravertebral block), or by injecting the intercostal spaces or near peripheral nerves.

Continuous Segmental Epidural Block

Continuous segmental epidural block is, from both the patient's and anesthesiologist's points of view, one of the best and most satisfactory methods for providing postoperative analgesia. Many investigators (17,18,23, 39,48,62,69,77,83,87,100) have shown that patients managed with continuous epidural analgesia develop significantly less pulmonary shunting and hypoxemia during the postoperative period than patients managed with narcotic analgesics. Moreover, in patients with epidural analgesia, it causes VC, FRC, and Pao_2 to be restored to higher levels than after narcotics. For example, Maneyuki et al. (69) noted that following upper abdominal surgery in patients managed with meperidine in intravenous increments of 10 mg until almost complete analgesia developed, the Pao_2 was decreased significantly; whereas, in the group managed with continuous epidural analgesia, it increased slightly. They showed that differences between decreased physiologic shunt in the epidural group and increased shunt in the meperidine group were statistically significant. A reduction of the 7 to 8% oxygen consumption was observed in both groups during analgesia without significant changes in metabolic factors. Somewhat similar results were reported by Hollmen and Sukkonen (48) who compared the effects of narcotic analgesia with that of epidural analgesia in 20 patients who had undergone cholecystectomy and biliary surgery.

Bromage (17) cites his own data and those of others to show that epidural analgesia is more effective in relieving postoperative pain after upper or lower intraabdominal or intrathoracic surgery than narcotics. This superiority is demonstrated by the differences in the percentage of restoration of pulmonary function as measured by VC toward preoperative levels which Bromage calls the respiratory restoration factor (RRF). With epidural analgesia, RRF was 50 to 70% in the early postoperative period compared with 16 to 35% with narcotics. He also reported that PEFR, after being reduced from a preoperative level of about 300 liters/min to about 90 liters/min after upper abdominal surgery, was restored to approximately 150 to 200 liters/min by effective epidural analgesia. On the other hand, systemic analgesia caused an appreciably smaller improvement. Bromage (17), Wahba et al. (111), and others have shown that the reduction in FRC is less with epidural analgesia than it is with narcotics. Bromage emphasizes the importance of encouraging the patient to breathe deeply, cough, and ambulate early in order to obtain the maximum benefits from epidural analgesia.

Renck (87) compared morphine with lumbar epidural analgesia for postoperative pain in patients who had prostatectomy and found oxygen uptake increased after surgery in both groups, but the increment was less in the epidural group. This suggests the latter group tended to have a hyperkinetic circulation; that is, cardiac output increased proportionately more than oxygen uptake, which gave a more favorable situation of oxygen transport compared to the group given morphine, which had a hypokinetic circulation.

The findings of Modig (77) in patients who underwent total hip replacement have already been mentioned. It is important to note that patients managed with epidural analgesia were completely pain-free and able to move their lower limbs actively, which together with increased blood flow due to sympathetic block likely reduced thromboembolic disease. Moreover, patients in the epidural group had greater tidal volumes and lower respiratory frequency which led to a more uniform ventilation with lesser alveolar closure than was seen in patients in the narcotic group who had rapid and shallow breathing patterns, factors responsible for hypoxemia in this group. The beneficial effects of epidural analgesia on gastrointestinal function have also been mentioned.

Pflug et al. (83) compared continuous epidural analgesia with morphine analgesia in 24 patients who had undergone upper abdominal surgery and 16 patients who had major hip surgery. They found patients managed with regional analgesia had a more benign postoperative course as manifested by earlier walking and ambulation and earlier return of appetite. In the upper abdominal patients, they found lesser decreases of VC and PEFR with epidural analgesia than with morphine. Finally, and importantly, they found a much shorter convalescent period among patients managed with epidural analgesia as compared with those managed with morphine (4.8 ± 0.2 vs 7.8 ± 0.6 days for the combined group). The difference was even more impressive for those patients who had hip surgery: their mean convalescence was 4.2 days shorter with epidural analgesia than with morphine (4.7 ± 0.3 vs 8.9 ± 1 days). This was attributed to complete relief without the sedative effect of morphine that allowed earlier ambulation and more physical therapy.

In addition to the greater efficacy of epidural and other regional techniques in providing pain relief, these procedures minimize or eliminate the endocrine and metabolic responses to the surgical stress that continues in the postoperative period. Kehlet (62) cites a number of studies that have shown continuous epidural analgesia prevents or minimizes most of the endocrine and metabolic responses. In this way it minimizes the stress-induced catabolic state, the increased demands on various body organs, and a negative nitrogen balance, all of which contribute to increased postoperative morbidity. These beneficial effects on minimizing the responses and decreasing morbidity can be obtained only if the regional blockade includes *all* the surgically damaged tissue and consequently interrupts all the nociceptive input.

Continuous segmental epidural analgesia has the following advantages over other regional techniques. It entails the insertion of one needle and a catheter that can be placed at any level and produces analgesia that can extend from two to ten spinal segments depending on the need. The blockade can be achieved with intermittent injections or continuously with an infusion pump (83,99). It may be used effectively for postoperative pain in any part of the body below the neck (10,13,17). Epidural block eliminates pain arising in somatic structures and viscera, and interrupts efferent sympathetic pathways and thus eliminates the sympathetically induced inhibition of gastrointestinal and genitourinary function caused by the pain and associated reflexes. Continuous segmental epidural block can be initiated before the operation, used for surgical anesthesia, and extended for 1 to 3 postoperative days. The continuous technique affords maximum flexibility in controlling the extent, duration, and intensity of analgesia. If the surgical incision does not extend below T12, segmental analgesia does not interfere with ambulation.

The most important disadvantage of this procedure is that it produces a vasomotor block with varying degrees of hypotension, especially if the analgesia is extensive or the patient is hypovolemic. This problem can be minimized by infusing fluids prior to the block or otherwise making certain the patient is normovolemic, and by limiting the analgesia to those segments involved in the surgical incision. An additional prophylactic measure is to have the patient use elastic stockings and an abdominal binder to minimize the amount of blood pooled in the lower limbs and pelvis, especially when the patient ambulates. As previously mentioned, the use of these procedures after hip and knee surgery has been found to markedly decrease the impairment of muscle metabolism and muscle function that is caused to a significant degree by persistent pain and by limitation of motion during the postoperative period.

Intercostal Block

Intercostal block is a simple and effective technique that can be used to relieve severe postoperative pain in the chest and abdomen. It is particularly effective after cholecystectomy, gastrectomy, mastectomy, thoracotomy, or superficial operations on the chest wall or abdomen. As with epidural block, this procedure not only relieves pain but reduces or eliminates muscle spasm and other reflex phenomena. Since the block does not include visceral afferent fibers, it relieves neither the visceral component of the pain nor the other noxious impulses that arise in the operated viscus. Nevertheless, even in these cases it produces greater relief of pain and muscle spasm than can be had with narcotics or with means other than epidural blockade.

Many investigators have shown the superiority of intercostal block over narcotic analgesia for the relief of pain after upper intraabdominal and intrathoracic operations (16,38,39,78,106). The regional block not only produced more effective pain relief but better pulmonary function. For example, Engberg (38) found that with unilateral intercostal block following cholecystectomy, achieved through a subcostal oblique incision, peak expiratory flow (PEF), forced vital capacity (FVC), and forced expiratory volume in 1 second (FEV$_1$), which were reduced to 40 to 48% of preoperative values in the control group, were significantly improved after two or more intercostal blocks. Moreover, the Pao$_2$ decreased much less with intercostal block than with narcotic analgesia. This improvement in lung function was sustained during the second postoperative day.

Important advantages of intercostal block over segmental epidural block are (a) little or no risk of hypotension and (b) production of analgesia two to four times the duration achieved with the same drug injected into the epidural space. The latter effect is obviously due to a large amount of drug being deposited right near each of the nerves in the intercostal spaces. Moore (78) reported the duration of analgesia achieved with 4 ml of 0.25% bupivacaine with 1:200,000 epinephrine injected into each intercostal space to produce intercostal block that lasted from 10 to 12 hr. This length makes it practical to induce bilateral intercostal block analgesia in the morning and have the patient ambulate, cough, and be as active as possible during the analgesic state for the rest of the day. If necessary, the block can be repeated in the evening, or at least repeated each morning.

Disadvantages of intercostal block when compared with epidural block are the following:

1. The need to make multiple injections once or twice a day
2. Noninvolvement of the visceral afferent (pain) fibers
3. Risk of pneumothorax.

The discomfort of multiple injections can be minimized by skillfully using sharp needles and performing the first injection while the patient is still anesthetized. For subsequent injections, the discomfort can be prevented by giving the patient an intravenous bolus of from 75 to 100 mg of thiopental, which produces amnesia for the time needed to carry out the procedure, after which the patient awakens and is alert. Usually visceral pain is not severe, but if it is, the block needs to be supplemented with narcotics that can be used in smaller doses than would be needed if the block were not effective. Although the incidence of pneumothorax has been reported to be as high as 19%, this must be attributed to lack of anatomic knowledge, skill, and experience. That its incidence can be kept to a very acceptable minimum is attested by the data of Moore (78), who has used this technique in over 12,000 patients in whom over 110,000 individual nerves were blocked and reported an incidence of pneumothorax of less than 0.1%, as well as the data of others, who have reported incidences of from 0.3 to 0.8% (see ref. 78 for references).

Other Regional Techniques

Continuous caudal analgesia for the relief of postoperative pain has the same advantages of segmental epidural block except it does involve the lumbar and sacral segments; thus, it interferes with bladder and rectal function and may cause significant weakness of the lower limbs. Analgesia with this technique should be limited to the sacral and lower lumbar segments for the management of pain in the anorectal and perineal regions and lower limbs.

Block of one or more of the other nerves of the limbs or trunk, or even the face, may be used in special circumstances when postoperative pain is excruciating and cannot be relieved with large doses of narcotics. Wiklund and Holmdahl (as reported in ref. 49) compared splanchnic celiac plexus block with narcotic analgesia for pain in the immediate postcholecystectomy period. The group given splanchnic block had improved postoperative bowel function with ability to ingest fluids on the day of operation and had normal Pao_2; whereas, in the group given narcotics there was a significant decrease in Pao_2.

Epidural and Intrathecal Narcotics

Following the reports by Yaksh (116) of an animal model that permitted the injection of small doses of morphine and other narcotics into the subarachnoid space resulting in elevation of the pain threshold without affecting nonnoxious reflexes or somatic or autonomic responses, subarachnoid and later epidural injections of narcotics have been used to relieve acute and chronic pain in humans (18). (See also L. Jacobsen, *this volume*.) Most of the reports have impressively demonstrated the efficacy of this method in producing postoperative analgesia, but a number of cases with delayed respiratory depression have been recorded (30,116,117). The obvious advantage of the technique over epidural analgesia with local anesthetics is that it provides pain relief without affecting somatic motor and sympathetic functions (18). Like regional analgesia, intrathecal narcotics minimize the reflex responses and thus tend to stabilize the patient's hemodynamics.

For subarachnoid injection, the dose of narcotics should be limited to 0.5 to 1 mg morphine or 10 to 30 mg meperidine, or equianalgesic doses of other drugs diluted to 1 ml. With morphine, analgesia will develop in 15 to 30 min and will last from 18 to 24 hr; with meperidine, it will occur in 5 to 10 min and will last from 15 to 20 hr. For epidural injection, a dose of 5 to 10 mg of morphine or 50 to 100 mg of meperidine diluted in 5 to 10 ml of saline produces analgesia that lasts from 15 to 20 hr. Because meperidine is more lipophilic than morphine, it traverses the dura and penetrates the spinal cord to attach to the opiate receptors faster than does morphine.

The complications of this technique include pruritus in 15 to 20% of patients, urinary retention in 15 to 20%, nausea in 15 to 25%, and delayed respiratory depression in a small but very significant number. This suggests that (a) the patient should be monitored closely for approximately 18 to 20 hr after the injection of the drug and (b) the pharmacokinetics and optimal dose of various narcotics for epidural and subarachnoid injections need to be studied further before the method is used routinely.

Electrical Stimulation

Another form of postoperative pain control is the use of transcutaneous electrical nerve stimulation (TENS) near the site of the incision. Sterile stimulating electrodes are attached in strips to the margin of the wound before the bandage is applied and high-frequency, low-intensity stimulation is initiated before the patient awakens from the anesthetic (107).

With this procedure, partial to complete pain relief is said to be experienced by 60 to 75% of the patients. A number of studies have shown that the use of TENS significantly reduces narcotic requirements by postoperative patients (2,26,46,53,89,96,102,107,109). Some reports have shown that in addition to relieving pain, TENS has a pulmonary function sparing effect. Ali and associates (2) reported that postoperative VC in treated patients was approximately 60% of preoperative values compared to approximately 40% in the control group, and FRC was approximately 80% with TENS in 60% of the control group. Moreover, postoperative Pa_{O_2} was unchanged from preoperative values. Hymes et al. (53) reported that in addition to producing an 80% reduction in the intensity of postoperative pain, TENS given continuously or intermittently for 4 or 5 days after surgery, produced a significant decrease in the incidence of postoperative atelectasis and ileus and a reduction of $1\frac{1}{2}$ days in the average length of stay in the postoperative intensive care unit. Cooperman et al. (26) also noted that three-quarters of the patients who had undergone upper abdominal surgery and were managed with TENS derived good to excellent pain relief, but found no difference between this group and the group of patients given meperidine with regard to the incidence of postoperative atelectasis or pneumonia and duration of postoperative ileus on the length of stay in the postoperative intensive care unit. Rosenberg et al. (89) also noted that patients who had undergone cholecystectomy showed a threefold reduction in narcotic requirements as compared to a control group, but found no influence on respiratory function as measured by arterial blood gas tensions, maximum expiratory flow rate, FEV_1, and VC, and no difference in the incidence of postoperative atelectasis or the duration of ileus.

Stabile and Mallory (102) used TENS for postoperative pain relief in a prospective randomized study of patients undergoing total hip replacement or total knee replacement. Patients managed with TENS required significantly less postoperative narcotics than did patients who were managed with narcotics alone. Harvie (46) used TENS after surgery in 34 patients who had total knee replacement, synovectomies, menisectomies, knee arthrotomies, patella plasties, or open reduction of fractures of the knee joint. Stimulation was applied as soon as the patient was fully recovered from the anesthesia; the patient controlled the unit for a period of from 4 to 7 days, and quadriceps and range of motion exercise was instituted. Decrease in the use of narcotics associated with TENS ranged from 75 to 100% and 5 patients required no narcotics. Moreover, the use of TENS was associated with improvements in straight leg raising and range of motion exercises, and there was a decrease in the length of hospital stay. Schuster and Infante (96) noted that patients with postoperative pain who were managed with TENS for 72 hr following low back operations required 4.65 ± 3.66 doses of narcotics compared with 10.92 ± 6.17 doses in the control group.

The results obtained to date, summarized by Tyler et al. (107), suggest that TENS is often effective in relieving postoperative pain and reducing narcotic requirements. TENS appears to be most effective in relieving pain caused by trauma to muscles, bones, and peripheral nerves. Patients with well-localized visceral pain and those who are anxious or depressed are less likely to benefit from TENS. Notwithstanding the discrepant results regarding pulmonary function, it appears that TENS is useful in relieving postoperative pain. Although requiring special instrumentation, the technique is attractive because of its simplicity and because it has no adverse side affects. In view of these considerations, this method should be given further trial.

The percutaneous insertion of epidural electrodes that would permit stimulation of the dorsal column has been suggested and is currently being used on an experimental basis. From preliminary studies it appears this technique causes segmental analgesia. However only a small number of patients have been treated and even if the preliminary data seem encouraging, it is too early to draw meaningful conclusions.

Psychologic Methods

The value of cognitive-behavioral therapies in reducing postoperative anxiety, stress, and pain has already been mentioned. Finer (39), like Egbert et al. (37), demonstrated that encouragement given to patients before and after cholecystectomy resulted in significantly greater increases toward normal in regard to VC, FEV_1, and peak expiratory flow rate (PEFR) in 1 min during the second to fourth postoperative days than without encouragement. The use of hypnosis to control postoperative pain has not been extensively applied and reported in the literature. Some reports are available, however, about the application of this technique for surgical anesthesia with concurrent use of posthypnotic suggestion to alleviate postoperative pain (14,19). Hilgard and Hilgard (47) stress the need to devote more attention to the postoperative period. They suggest that instead of relying only on posthypnotic suggestion, fresh hypnotic reassurance be added to obtain better control of postoperative pain. Finer (39) reported increases toward normal of VC, FEV, and PEFR.

The method used most often to evaluate the analgesic effect of hypnosis postoperatively is a comparison of use of narcotics in two similar groups of patients, one receiving hypnosis or suggestion, and the other the usual post-surgical care. The few studies on this subject are concordant in reporting a decrease of narcotic intake by hypnotically prepared patients, but the percentage of reduction varies (14,47).

SUMMARY

Postoperative pain is an important clinical problem that deserves greater attention by members of the surgical team. There is a need to do careful epidemiologic studies and investigate other aspects of the problem. More importantly, there is a critical need for specific educational programs for medical, nursing, and dental students and for surgeons-in-training that will enhance their capabilities to carry out more effective prophylaxis and treatment of postoperative pain.

Prophylactic measures include psychologic evaluation and preparation of the patient during the preoperative period to decrease the degree of postoperative fear and anxiety, optimal anesthesia and skillful surgery to minimize the degree of trauma, and postoperative enhancement of the patient's coping skills. Effective therapy requires evaluation of the patient and the pain to determine the optimal method of pain relief. Narcotics remain the mainstay of therapy, and if properly prescribed and administered, they provide effective relief. This requires close monitoring of the patient before and after the administration of at least the first 2 or 3 doses of narcotics and during the rest of the time the patient has pain.

The wider use of regional analgesia of a local anesthetic should be encouraged because it is a more effective method of relieving pain, but it does require special skill and precautionary measures to avoid serious side effects and complications. Finally, the newer techniques of epidural or subarachnoid injection of narcotics and transcutaneous nerve stimulation have the promise of being very useful and should be given extensive clinical trials to ascertain their efficacy and side effects.

REFERENCES

1. Ali, J., and Khan, T. A. (1979): The comparative effects of muscle transection and median upper abdominal incisions on postoperative pulmonary function. *Surg. Gynecol. Obstet.*, 148:863–866.
2. Ali, J., Yaffe, C., and Senette, C. (1981): The effect of transcutaneous electric nerve stimulation on postoperative pain and pulmonary function. *Surgery*, 89:507–512.
3. Austin, K. L., Stapleton, J. V., and Mather, L. E. (1980): Relationship of meperidine concentration and analgesic response. *Anesthesiology*, 53:460–466.
4. Austin, K. L., Stapleton, J. V., and Mather, L. E. (1980): Multiple intramuscular injections: A major source of irritability in analgesic response to meperidine. *Pain*, 8:47–62.
5. Ball, J. C., and Chambers, C. D. (1970): *The Epidemiology of Opiate Addiction in the United States*. Charles C Thomas, Springfield, Ill.
6. Beaver, W. T. (1976): Comparison of morphine, hydroxyzine, and morphine plus hydroxyzine in postoperative pain. *Hosp. Pract.* (Special Report), January, p. 23.

7. Beecher, H. K. (1933): Effect of laparotomy on lung volume. Demonstration of a new type of pulmonary collapse. *J. Clin. Invest.*, 12:651.
8. Bessman, F. P., and Renner, V. J. (1982): The biphasic hormonal nature of stress. In: *Pathophysiology of Shock, Anoxia and Ischemia*, edited by R. A. Cowley and B. F. Trump, pp. 60–65. Williams & Wilkins, Baltimore.
9. Bing, H. I. (1936): Viscerocutaneous and cuteanovisceral thoracic reflexes. *Acta Med. Scand.*, 89:57–68.
10. Bonica, J. J. (1953): *The Management of Pain*, pp. 1240–1261. Lea & Febiger, Philadelphia.
11. Bonica, J. J. (1980): Pain research and therapy: Past and current status and future needs. In: *Pain, Discomfort and Humanitarian Care*, edited by L. K. Y. Ng and J. J. Bonica, pp. 1–48. Elsevier/North-Holland, Amsterdam.
12. Bonica, J. J. (1983): Current status of postoperative pain therapy. In: *Current Topics in Pain Research and Therapy*, edited by T. Yokota and R. Dubner, pp. 169–189. Excerpta Medica, Tokyo.
13. Bonica, J. J., and Benedetti, C. (1980): Postoperative pain. In: *Surgical Care: A Physiologic Approach to Clinical Management*, edited by R. E. Condon and J. J. DeCosse, pp. 394–415. Lea & Febiger, Philadelphia.
14. Bonilla, K. B., Quigley, W. F., and Bowers, W. F. (1961): Experience with hypnosis on a surgical service. *Milit. Med.*, 126:364–370.
15. Boutros, A. R., and Weisel, M. (1971): Comparison of effects of three anesthetic techniques on patients with severe pulmonary obstructive disease. *Can. Anaesth. Soc. J.*, 18:286–292.
16. Bridenbaugh, P. O., DuPen, S. L., Moore, D. C., Bridenbaugh, L. D., and Thompson, G. E. (1973): Postoperative intercostal nerve block analgesia versus narcotic analgesia. *Anesth. Analg.*, 52:81–85.
17. Bromage, P. R. (1978): *Epidural Analgesia*. Saunders, Philadelphia.
18. Bromage, P. R., Camporesi, E., and Chestnut, D. (1980): Epidural narcotic for postoperative analgesia. *Anesth. Analg.*, 59:473–480.
19. Cantor, A. J., and Fox, E. A. N. (eds.) (1956): *Psychosomatic Aspects of Surgery*. Grune & Stratton, New York.
20. Chapman, C. R. (1978): Psychologic aspects of pain. *Hosp. Pract.* (Special Report), January, pp. 15–19.
21. Chapman, C. R., and Cox, G. B. (1977): Anxiety, pain and depression surrounding elective surgery: A multivariate comparison of abdominal surgery patients with kidney donors and recipients. *J. Psychosom. Res.*, 21:7–15.
22. Churchill, E. D., and McNeil, D. (1927): The reduction in vital capacity following operation. *Surg. Gynecol. Obstet.*, 44:483–487.
23. Cleland, J. G. P. (1949): Continuous peridural and caudal analgesia in surgery and early ambulation. *Northwest Med.*, 48:26–34.
24. Cohen, F. L. (1980): Postsurgical pain relief: Patients' status and nurses' medication choices. *Pain*, 9:265–274.
25. Cole, W. H., and Zollinger, R. M. (1970): *Textbook of Surgery*, 9th ed. Appleton-Century-Crofts (Meredity Corp.), New York.
26. Cooperman, A., Hall, B., Mikalacki, K., Hardy, R., and Sadar, E. (1977): Use of transcutaneous electrical stimulation in the control of postoperative pain. *Am. J. Surg.*, 133:185–187.
27. Corman, H. H., Hornick, E. J., Kritchman, M., and Terestman, N. (1958): Emotional reactions of surgical patients to hospitalization, anesthesia, and surgery. *Am. J. Surg.*, 96:646–659.
28. Craig, D. B. (1981): Postoperative recovery of pulmonary function. *Anesth. Analg.*, 60:46–52.
29. Cutler, E. D., and Hoerr, S. O. (1944): Postoperative pulmonary complications. *Proceeding of the Interstate Postgraduate Medical Association, Cleveland*, pp. 232–237.
30. Davies, G. K., Tolhurst-Cleaver, C. L., and James, T. L. (1980): Central nervous system depression from intrathecal morphine. *Anesthesiology*, 52:280.
31. Denton, J. E., and Beecher, H. K. (1949): New analgesics. I: Methods in the clinical evaluation of new analgesics. *JAMA*, 141:1051–1057.
32. Donald, I. (1976): At the receiving end. *Scott. Med. J.*, 21:49–57.

33. Dreyfuss, F. (1956): Coagulation time of the blood, level of blood eosinophiles and thrombocytes under emotional stress. *J. Psychosom. Res.*, 1:252–257.
34. Dripps, R. D., and Deming, M. V. N. (1946): Postoperative atelectasis and pneumonia. *Ann. Surg.*, 124:94–110.
35. Editorial (1976): Tight-fisted analgesia. *Lancet*, 1:1338.
36. Edmonson, A. S., and Grenshaw, A. H. (1980): *Campbell's Operative Orthopaedics, 6th ed.* Mosby, St. Louis.
37. Egbert, L. D., Battit, G. E., Welch, C. E., and Bartlett, M. K. (1964): Reduction of postoperative pain by encouragement and instruction of patients. A study of doctor-patient rapport. *N. Engl. J. Med.*, 270:825–827.
38. Engberg, G. (1975): Single-dose intercostal nerve block with etidocaine for pain relief after upper abdominal surgery. *Acta. Anaesthesiol. Scand. [Suppl.]*, 60:43–49.
39. Finer, B. (1970): Studies of the variability in expiratory efforts before and after cholecystectomy: with special reference to certain psychological and pharmacological aspects. *Acta. Anaesthesiol. Scand. [Suppl.]*, 38:7–68.
40. Fortin, F., and Kirouac, S. (1976): A randomized controlled trial of preoperative patient education. *Int. J. Nurs. Stud.*, 13:11–24.
41. Forrest, W. H., Jr., Brown, B. W., Brown, C. R., Defalque, R., Gold, M., Gordon, H. E., James, K. E., Katz, J., Mahler, D. L., Schroff, P., and Teutsch, G. (1977): Dextroamphetamines with morphine for the treatment of postoperative pain. *N. Engl. J. Med.*, 296:712–715.
42. Freed, D. L. J. (1975): Inadequate analgesia at night. *Lancet*, 1:519.
43. Gildea, J. (1968): The relief of postoperative pain. *Med. Clin. North Am.* 52:81–90.
44. Hamilton, W. K. (1965): Postoperative respiratory complications. In: *Respiratory Therapy, Clinical Anesthesia*, edited by P. Safar, pp. 259–281. Davis, Philadelphia.
45. Hardy, J. D. (editor) (1977): *Rhoads' Textbook of Surgery: Principles and Practices*, 5th ed. Harper & Row, New York.
46. Harvie, K. W. (1979): A major advance in the control of postoperative knee pain. *Orthopedics*, 2:26–27.
47. Hilgard, E. R., and Hilgard, J. R. (1975): *Hypnosis in the Relief of Pain.* William Kaufmann, Los Altos, Calif.
48. Hollmen, A., and Sukkonen (1972): The effects of postoperative epidural analgesia versus centrally-acting opiate on physiological shunt after upper abdominal operation. *Acta Anaesthesiol. Scand.*, 16:147–154.
49. Holmdahl, M. G., and Modig, J. (1975): Patient management: The role of regional block versus parenteral analgesics on the treatment of postoperative pain. *Br. J. Anaesth.*, 47:264–270.
50. Hug, C. C., Jr. (1980): Improving analgesic therapy. *Anesthesiology*, 53:441–443.
51. Hume, D. M. (1969): The endocrine and metabolic response to injury. In: *Principles of Surgery*, edited by S. E. Schwartz. McGraw-Hill, New York.
52. Hupert, C. (1978): Treatment of postoperative pain—analgesic potentiation. *Hosp. Pract.* (Special Report) 13:27–31.
53. Hymes, A., Raab, D., Yonehiro, E., Nelson, G., and Printy, A. (1974): Acute pain control by electrostimulation: a preliminary report. *Adv. Neurol.*, 4:761–767.
54. Innes, I. R. (1963): Action of desamphetamine on 5-hydroxytryptamine receptors. *Br. J. Pharmacol. Chemother.*, 21:427–435.
55. Jaggard, R. S., Zager, L. L., and Wilkins, D. S. (1950): Clinical evaluation of analgesic drugs: A comparison of Nu-2206 and morphine sulphate administered to postoperative patients. *Arch. Surg.*, 61:1073–1082.
56. Janis, I. L. (1958): *Psychologic Stress. Psychoanalytic and Behavioral Studies in Surgical Patients.* Wiley, New York.
57. Kahn, A. J. (1940): Studies on intercostal nerve physiology. *Proc. Soc. Exp. Biol. Med.*, 44:514–517.
58. Kaufman, W. (1956): The physician's role in the preparation of a patient for surgery. In: *Psychosomatic Aspects of Surgery*, edited by A. J. Ganter and A. N. Fox, pp. 1–10. Grune & Stratton, New York.
59. Keats, A. S. (1956): Postoperative pain, research and treatment. *J. Chronic Dis.*, 4:72–83.
60. Keats, A. S., and Kirgis, K. Z. (1968): Respiratory depression associated with relief of pain by narcotics. *Anesthesiology*, 29:1006–1013.

61. Keats, A. S., Beecher, H. K., and Mosteller, F. C. (1950): Measurement of pathological pain in distinction to experimental pain. *J. Appl. Physiol.*, 1:35–44.
62. Kehlet, H. (1978): Influence of epidural analgesia on the endocrine-metabolic response to surgery. *Acta Anaesthesiol. Scand.*, 70:39–42.
63. King, D. S. (1933): Postoperative pulmonary complications. I. A statistical study based on 10 years' personal observation. *Surg. Gynecol. Obstet.*, 56:43–50.
64. Kuntz, A. (1953): *The Autonomic Nervous System*, 4th ed. pp. 488–490. Lea & Febiger, Philadelphia.
65. Lindeman, C. A., and Van Aernam, B. (1971): Nursing intervention with the presurgical patient: The effects of structured and unstructured teaching. *Nurs. Res.*, 20:319–332.
66. Loan, W. B., and Dundee, J. W. (1967): The clinical assessment of pain. *Practitioner*, 198:759–768.
67. Loan, W. B., and Morrison, J. D. (1967): The incidence and severity of postoperative pain. *Br. J. Anaesth.*, 39:695–698.
68. MacInnes, C. (1976): Cancer ward. *New Society*, 36:232–234.
69. Maneyuki, M., Ueda, Y., Urabe, N. Takeshita, H., and Inamoto, A. (1968): Postoperative pain relief and respiratory function in man: Comparison between intermittent intravenous injections of meperidine and continuous lumbar epidural analgesia. *Anesthesiology*, 29:304–313.
70. Marks, R. M., and Sachar, E. F. (1973): Undertreatment of medical inpatients with narcotic analgesics. *Ann. Intern. Med.*, 78:173–181.
71. Marshall, B. E., and Millar, R. A. (1965): Some factors influencing postoperative hypoxaemia. *Anaesthesia*, 20:408–428.
72. Marshall, B. E., and Wyche, M. Q. (1972): Hypoxaemia during and after anesthesia. *Anesthesiology*, 37:178–209.
73. Martinez-Urrutia, A. (1975): Anxiety and pain in surgical patients. *J. Consult. Clin. Psychol.*, 43:437–442.
74. Mather, L. E., Lindop, M. J., Tucker, G. T., and Pflug, A. E. (1975): Pethidine revisited: Plasma concentration and effects after intramuscular injection. *Br. J. Anaesth.*, 47:1269–1275.
75. Mather, L., and Mackie, J. (1983): The incidence of postoperative pain in children. *Pain*, 15:271–282.
76. McCaffrey, M. (1976): Undertreatment of acute pain with narcotics. *Am. J. Nurs.* 76:1586–1591.
77. Modig, J. (1976): Respiration and circulation after total hip replacement surgery. *Acta Anaesthesiol. Scand.*, 20:225–236.
78. Moore, D. C. (1975): Intercostal nerve block for postoperative somatic pain following surgery of thorax and upper abdomen. *Br. J. Anaesth.*, 47:284–286.
79. Ogston, D., McDonald, G. A., and Fullerton, H. W. (1962): The influence of anxiety in tests of blood coagular ability and fibrinolytic activity. *Lancet*, 2:521–523.
80. Palmer, K. N. V., and Sellick, B. A. (1953): The prevention of postoperative pulmonary atelectasis. *Lancet*, 1:164–168.
81. Papper, E., Brodie, B. B., and Rovenstine, E. A. (1952): Postoperative pain: its use in the comparative evaluation of new analgesics. *Surgery*, 32:107–110.
82. Parkhouse, J., Lambrechts, W., and Simpson, B. R. J. (1961): The incidence of postoperative pain. *Br. J. Anaesth.*, 33:345–352.
83. Pflug, A. E., Murphy, T. M., Butler, S. H., and Tucker, G. T. (1974): The effects of postoperative peridural analgesia on pulmonary therapy and pulmonary complications. *Anesthesiology*, 41:8–17.
84. Pooler, H. E. (1949): Relief of postoperative pain and its influence on vital capacity. *Br. Med. J.*, 2:1200–1203.
85. Porter, J., and Jick, H. (1980): Addiction rare in patients treated with narcotics. *N. Engl. J. Med.*, 302:123.
86. Randall, H. T., Hardy, J. D., and Moore, F. D. (1967): *Manual of Preoperative and Postoperative Care*. (American College of Surgeons) Saunders, Philadelphia.
87. Renck, H. (1969): The elderly patient after anesthesia and surgery: with special reference to certain respiratory, circulatory, metabolic, and muscular function. *Acta Anaesthesiol. Scand. [Suppl.]*, 34:1–13.
88. Roe, B. B. (1963): Are postoperative narcotics necessary? *Arch. Surg.*, 87:912–915.

Advances in Pain Research
and Therapy, Vol. 7,
edited by C. Benedetti et al.
Raven Press, New York © 1984.

Apomorphine-Induced Headache

F. Sicuteri, M. Fanciullacci, U. Pietrini, and F. Cangi

*Institute of Internal Medicine and Clinical Pharmacology, University of Florence,
50134 Florence, Italy*

The preeminent pharmacologic pattern exhibited by sufferers of idiopathic headache (IH) is the hyperresponsiveness to specific drugs (in a few cases to an impressive extent). When speculating on such drug susceptibility, two hypotheses can be considered: (a) susceptibility concerns the functions that are impaired during migraine; and (b) all drugs capable of unmasking IH susceptibility are strong dopamine (DA) agonists. The disturbances caused by IH—such as vomiting, impaired thermoregulation and blood pressure control, hallucinations, mood changes, and nociception—are directly or indirectly correlated with the dopaminergic system. In view of this correlation, DA was suggested as a "second protagonist" some years ago (5HT being considered the first) in the mechanism of the clinical manifestations of IH (19,24).

Hypersensitivity to DA agonists is concerned mainly, although not exclusively, with the most impaired functions in patients; in fact, sufferers of hyperemetic, hyperpyretic, or collapsing migraine react to the same dopaminomimetic, with vomiting, fever, and vascular collapse. If DA susceptibility is one of the IH mechanisms, or the sole mechanism, a dopaminomimetic agent should provoke natural-like symptoms. The reactions to a dopaminomimetic, therefore, could be predicted for both quantity and quality on the basis of the spontaneous clinical manifestations of the patient undergoing tests. Moreover, a reduction of the basic DA susceptibility of IH sufferers is expected from a chronic treatment with dopaminomimetic drugs, in agreement with the classic concept of receptor subsensitivity after persistent increased concentrations of the specific ligand (DA or dopaminomimetic). The chronic treatment with conventional ergot derivatives such as methysergide and lisuride, considered as strong dopaminomimetics (6,11,12), therefore could correct DA supersensitivity through a process of DA-receptor desensitization, which improves the clinical picture.

Recently migraine has been considered as a sort of "quasi self (endorphin) abstinence syndrome" (21). This hypothesis was postulated on the chemical and clinical evidence. *Chemically*, endogenous opioids are lower in cerebrospinal fluid (CSF) during migraine attack (22), as well as in plasma (2). Even in plasma of chronic (daily) IH sufferers, beta-endorphin concentrations seem to be persistently lowered (8). *Clinically*, migraine crisis is unique in its physiognomy because it has no analogus patterns except for the acute syndrome of sudden withdrawal (or from naloxone administration) in opiate addicts (20).

The triadal syndrome (vegetative, affective, nociceptive) during the acute opiate abstinence is almost indistinguishable from a migraine attack. Further, pharmacologic evidence is compatible with the withdrawal simulation of migraine and other IH to opiate abstinence: the increased reactivity in humans *in vivo* of the smooth muscle (iris and hand dorsal vein) to monoamines (9,23). In addition, there is evidence that correlates the dopaminergic system with morphine analgesia, tolerance, and abstinence (7,13,16,18,28).

Dopamine was emphasized particularly as a transmitter (together with 5HT and endorphins) of the antinociceptive system (1,3). In view of the chemical evidence (in CSF and in plasma) of an endogenous opioid system deficiency, one could postulate that the susceptibility of IH sufferers to dopaminomimetics is due to a deficient modulation of the terminal ending of DA neurons (resulting in an incontinent and, consequently, "empty" neuron). Such a concept was formulated many years ago by our group, and since then we have collected other observations. The aim of this chapter is that of a critical synthesis of past and recent (unpublished) results.

The rationale of the present research is based on the hypothesis that most clinical phenomena (including pain) exhibited by IH sufferers are due to an impairment of some sections of the dopaminergic central system as a consequence of endorphinergic deficiency. In fact, close interaction between endorphinergic and dopaminergic systems generally is acknowledged (14,17,27).

METHODS AND CLINICAL MATERIAL

Drugs

Considering their safe use in humans, a pure dopaminomimetic apomorphine (APH) and two impure dopaminomimetics, lisuride and bromocriptine, were used. Apomorphine was administered sublingually in doses of 100 μg and intravenously in amounts of 0.5 mg in 100 ml of saline solution for rapid infusion; lisuride in 25 μg doses was injected intravenously as a bolus; and 2.5 mg of bromocriptine was administered orally. The drug tests were evaluated on a random and single-blind basis versus placebo. Apomorphine tests were repeated at weekly intervals by administering saline, domperidone (10 mg i.m.), or haloperidol (0.5 mg i.m.) on random and single-blind basis 15 min before APH.

Clinical Materials

According to the clinical feature, subjects were grouped into mixed headache and migraine headache patients. The mixed headache group (so-called

TABLE 1. *Questionnaire for apomorphine-induced symptoms*

Yawning	Rhinorrhea
Sedation	Hypersalivation
Sleepiness	Sweating
Tiredness	Nausea
Light-headed feeling	Vomiting
Sadness	Perceptive body distortion
Lacrimation	Headache

vascular plus muscular headache) consisted of 18 sufferers from migraine attacks (4 to 8 per month) with an interattack period occupied by a less intense, daily headache. There were 11 female and 7 male patients 24 to 59 years of age. Migraine patients consisted of 10 female and 5 male patients 15 to 52 years of age. They were affected by typical migraine attacks (2 to 8 per month), with headache-free intervals.

Clinical Parameters

Considering the APH-induced behavioral effects in humans (5), a questionnaire was submitted to the subjects. This questionnaire is a list of expected symptomatology, mainly concerning the vegetative, vigilance, psychic, and nociceptive changes (Table 1). The subjects had to report what symptoms, and their time-course, were elicited by the drug, as listed in the questionnaire; they were questioned about the possible onset of nonlisted, unexpected effects. Subjects also were asked to report whether the described symptoms were distinguishable from those complained of during spontaneous headache attacks. When the phenomena were distinguishable, the patients described the difference in quality, intensity, and time-course of the phenomena. Particular attention was given to the most common symptoms experienced by patients during their own attacks, such as yawning, lacrimation, nasal obstruction, cold-warm sensation, sleepiness, irritability, sadness, photophonoosmophobia, and pulsating or not pulsating headache.

Dopamine does not mimic migraine attacks because it does not cross the blood-brain barrier (BBB). Therefore, if APH and other dopaminomimetics mimic migraine by interacting with DA receptors located in the central nervous system, these drugs must penetrate into the BBB in order to induce migraine phenomena. To verify this assumption, antidopamine agents capable (haloperidol) or incapable (domperidone) of crossing the BBB were administered before APH and lisuride, and their ability to prevent dopaminomimetic-induced symptoms was established.

RESULTS

According to the present and past investigations concerning the involvement of the dopaminergic system in headache mechanisms, the following findings are noteworthy:

1. DA, incapable of crossing the BBB when injected as a bolus or by venous infusion, did not provoke or exacerbate a headache. When infused in larger doses, DA slightly increased the headache, but not the usual non-pain phenomena of the attack.
2. Placebo did not produce subjective or objective changes in any headache patients.
3. In sufferers from serious mixed headache, dopaminomimetics administered in the interattack period reproduced the symptoms of the spontaneous attack in almost 90% of patients in regard to quality, quantity, and chronologic sequence. The similarity of symptoms concerns not only pain (distribution, throbbing, associated paresthesias) but also nonpain phenomena, such as somnolence, yawning, lacrimation, cold-warm sensation, nausea and vomiting, and hyperesthesias. All the subjects noted that the symptoms induced by dopaminomimetics were indistinguishable from the spontaneous ones.
4. In migraine patients, dopaminomimetics elicited the attack in 30% of the cases. Most negative cases were characterized by a few attacks (2 to 3 per month). Haloperidol, the antagonist of DA receptors, prevented all the symptoms induced by dopaminomimetics in all patients, whereas domperidone prevented the nonpain phenomena but not the headache.
5. As previously mentioned (4,10), bromocriptine also induces headache in IH patients with a hypotensive reaction, which can be severe in some patients.

DISCUSSION

It has been postulated that the dopaminergic system is involved in the mechanism of IH, not only at the peripheral level (vascular or muscular) but also at the central (noci-antinociceptive system) level (19). The following observations indirectly support this assumption: (a) The migraine attack cannot be precipitated by DA, which is not able to cross the BBB. (b) An attack whose physiognomy is indistinguishable from the spontaneous one is evoked by the pure agonist APH of DA receptors, capable of crossing the BBB. (c) The domperidone DA antagonist, which does not cross (or only partially crosses) the BBB, does not prevent APH-precipitated crises. (d) The haloperidol DA antagonist, which crosses the BBB, is capable of preventing APH headache. (e) Even impure but powerful DA agonists, lisuride and bromocriptine, both of which cross the BBB, precipitate the headache attack as APH. Patients are unable to recognize APH attacks from those provoked by lisuride and bromocriptine. Also, the attacks precipitated by these "impure" DA agonists are prevented by haloperidol but not by domperidone.

Three important additional observations have to be made on the interpretation of dopaminomimetic headache:

1. *Latency:* Despite venous or sublingual administration of the drugs, the onset of clinical phenomena arises after a latency of 1 to 2 hr. This latency

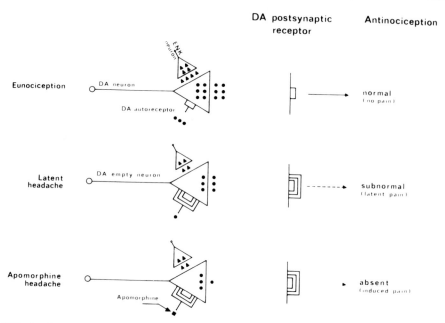

FIG. 1. Speculative mechanism of DA "empty-neuron" and apomorphine-induced headache. A poor enkephalinergic modulation causes a chronic deficiency and then total exhaustion of DA neuron. Apomorphine, acting on presynaptic supersensitive DA receptors, inhibits DA (intended as a pain-suppressing neurotransmitter) release and induces or aggravates headache.

suggests that the evoked phenomena do not result from a direct, immediate action but rather from an indirect or mediated action. For example, these agonists could activate presynaptic DA receptors, located on DA neurons, which inhibit the release of DA (Fig. 1).

2. *Identity of symptomatology:* Different headache-precipitating agents such as nitroglycerine, histamine, bradykinin, and reserpine mainly provoke painful phenomena, distinguishable from the naturally occurring symptoms. Patients noted that pain and nonpain manifestations induced by dopaminomimetic agents are identical and indistinguishable from spontaneous ones. Dopaminomimetic agents produce also the nonpain phenomena of yawning, vomiting, collapse, and perceptive distortions, which emerge spontaneously during the natural attack.

3. *Tachyphylaxis:* If the same dose of apomorphine or other dopaminomimetic drugs are administered daily, the drug gradually becomes incapable of evoking migraine-like phenomena (including pain) within a few days. This type of DA desensitization could be the basic role in the therapeutic mechanism of those classic antimigrainous ergot derivatives, methysergide and lisuride, with dopaminomimetic activity.

These results and considerations further emphasize the participation of the dopaminergic system in the mechanism of pain and other symptoms of

IH. It is generally accepted that DA is involved directly or indirectly in causing impairment of functions such as thermoregulation, emesis, blood pressure, sexual excitation, vigilance, sleep, and sensory perception during migraine attacks. However, there are different opinions concerning the role of DA in noci-antinociceptive systems. Results from investigations on decerebrate cats suggest that the DA mechanism plays a role in the inhibition produced by the brainstem on nociceptive-activated cells in the spinal cord, thus indicating that a dopaminergic link has access to the descending inhibitory system on transmission of "pain impulses" (3). The investigations on the effect of 6-hydroxydopamine on the antinociceptive action of morphine also conclude with the assumption that dopaminergic neurons mediate morphine analgesia in rats (25).

The pharmacologic depletion of DA decreases the analgesia elicited by the stimulation of periaqueductal gray matter; the DA precursor (L-Dopa) and APH increase this analgesia, thus suggesting that DA, like 5HT, facilitates the analgesia inhibited by noradrenaline (1). Apparently opposite results indicate that direct or indirect dopaminergic receptor stimulants (APH, L-Dopa) enhance the reactivity of mice to a nociceptive stimulus and antagonize morphine analgesia (16,26,28).

Our conclusions from present and past investigations (24) seem to confirm that the dopaminergic system is deeply involved in the mechanism of those diseases provisionally classified as "idiopathic head pains." The fact that no one headache-provoking agent, such as histamine, bradykinin, or reserpine, is capable of reproducing all nonpain phenomena (e.g., somnolence, yawning, nasal obstruction) and pain phenomena is thought-provoking. Even the constant tolerance to DA receptor stimulation could be correlated to the dopaminomimetic activity of the classic antimigrainous ergot derivatives and to the mechanism of the so-called prophylactic treatment of migraine.

Finally, the fact that the closest pharmacologic and biochemical interactions of opioids are with dopaminergic (17) and noradrenergic (15) systems is of great interest. These correlations are evident even in morphine-dependent humans (23) and animals (14). Moreover, APH-induced headache is an intriguing and promising new tool for a better understanding of headache mechanisms.

SUMMARY

In most sufferers from migraine and other correlated headaches, the pure (apomorphine) and impure (lisuride, bromocriptine) dopaminomimetic agents, administered in small doses (amounts that do not elicit definite reactions in subjects exempt from spontaneous headaches), elicit painful and nonpainful manifestations, indistinguishable from those of the spontaneous attacks. Between sublingual or venous administration of apomorphine and the onset of the clinical manifestations, a latency of 1 to 2 hr constantly occurs; such a latency suggests that an indirect neuronal (prereceptoral) mechanism is triggered rather than a direct (postreceptoral) one. Another constant aspect of the dopamine-evoked headache is the tachyphylaxis that develops after a few days of daily administration of apomorphine. This is compatible with an indirect (neuronal) mechanism and also could be an explanation for the therapeutic mechanism of ergot derivatives (all dopaminomimetics) in migraine and other analogue headaches, which might correct a condition of DA receptor supersensitivity. The superreactivity of headache sufferers to the dopaminomimetic agents is also compatible with an involvement of the endogenous opioids, even in view of the intimate relation between the endorphinergic and dopaminergic systems.

ACKNOWLEDGMENT

This work was supported by a grant from the National Research Council (Finalized group "Chimica Fine e Secondaria"), Rome, Italy.

REFERENCES

1. Akil, H., and Liebeskind, J. C. (1975): Monoaminergic mechanisms of stimulation produced analgesia. *Brain Res.*, 94:279–296.
2. Baldi, E., Salmon, S., Spillantini, M. G., Cappelli, G., Brocchi, A., and Sicuteri, F. (1982): Intermittent hypoendorphinaemia in migraine attack. *Cephalalgia*, 2:77–81.
3. Barnes, C., Fung, S. J., and Adams, W. L. (1979): Inhibitory effects of substantia nigra on impulse transmission from nociceptors. *Pain*, 6:207–215.
4. Boccuni, M., Fanciullacci, M., Michelacci, S., and Sicuteri, F. (1981): Impairment of postural reflex in migraine: Possible role of dopamine receptors. In: *Apomorphine and Other Dopaminomimetics. Vol. 2, Clinical Pharmacology*, edited by G. U. Corsini and G. L. Gessa, pp. 267–273. Raven Press, New York.
5. Corsini, G. U., Piccardi, M. P., Bocchetta, A., Bernardi, F., and Del Zompo, M. (1980): Behavioural effects of apomorphine in man: Dopamine receptor implications. In: *Apomorphine and Other Dopaminomimetics. Vol. 2, Clinical Pharmacology*, edited by G. U. Corsini and G. L. Gessa, pp. 13–24. Raven Press, New York.
6. Da Prada, M., Bonetti, E. P., and Keller, H. H. (1977): Induction of mounting behaviour in female and male rats by lisuride. *Neurosci. Lett.*, 6:349–353.
7. Eidelberg, E., and Erspamer, R. (1974): Dopaminergic mechanisms of opiate actions in brain. *J. Pharmacol. Exp. Ther.*, 192:50–57.
8. Facchinetti, F., Nappi, G., Savoldi, F., and Genazzani, A. R. (1981): Primary headaches: Reduces circulating beta-endorphin and beta-lipotropin level with impaired reactivity to acupuncture. *Cephalalgia*, 1:196–201.
9. Fanciullacci, M., Del Bianco, P. L., and Sicuteri, F. (1978): Iris and vein adrenoceptors in migraine and central panalgesia. In: *Recent Advances in the Pharmacology of Andrenoceptors*, edited by E. Szabad, C. M. Bradshaw, and P. Bevan, pp. 295–303. Elsevier/North-Holland, Amsterdam.
10. Fanciullacci, M., Michelacci, S., Curradi, C., and Sicuteri, F. (1980): Hyperresponsiveness of migraine patients to the hypotensive action of bromocriptine. *Headache*, 20:99–102.
11. Horowski, R. (1978): Differences in the dopaminergic effects of ergot derivates bromocriptine, lisuride and d-LSD as compared with apomorphine. *Eur. J. Pharmacol.*, 51:157–166.
12. Johnson, A. M., Vigouret, J. M., and Loew, D. M. (1973): Central dopaminergic action of ergotoxine alkaloids and some derivatives. *Experientia*, 29:763.
13. Kuschinsky, K. (1981): Psychic dependence on opioids: By dopaminergic mechanisms in the striatum? *TIPS*, 287–289.

14. Lal, H. (1976): Narcotic dependence, narcotic action and dopamine receptors. Mini review, *Life Sci.*, 17:483–496.
15. Llorens, C., Martres, M. P., Baudry, M., and Schwartz, J. C. (1978): Hypersensitivity to noradrenaline in cortex after chronic morphine: Relevance to tolerance and dependence. *Nature*, 274:603–605.
16. McGilliard, K. L., and Takemori, A. E. (1979): The effect of dopaminergic modifiers on morphine-induced analgesia and respiratory depression. *Eur. J. Pharmacol.*, 54:61–68.
17. Pollard, H., Llorens-Cortes, C., and Schwartz, J. C. (1977): Enkephalin receptors on dopaminergic neurones in rat striatum. *Nature*, 268:745–747.
18. Schulz, R., and Herz, A. (1977): Naloxone-precipitated withdrawal reveals sensitization to neurotransmitters in morphine tolerant/dependent rats. *Naunyn Schmiedebergs Arch. Pharmacol.*, 299:95–99.
19. Sicuteri, F. (1977): DA: The second putative protagonist in headache. *Headache*, 17:129–131.
20. Sicuteri, F. (1979): Headache as the most common disease of the antinociceptive system: Analogies with morphine abstinence. In: *Advances in Pain Research and Therapy. Vol. 3*, edited by J. J. Bonica, J. C. Liebeskind, and G. Albe-Fessard, pp. 359–365. Raven Press, New York.
21. Sicuteri, F. (1979): Phenomenal similarities of migraine and morphine abstinence. *Headache*, 19:232–233.
22. Sicuteri, F., Anselmi, B., Curradi, C., Michelacci, S., and Sassi, A. (1978): Morphine like-factors in CSF of headache patients. In: *Advances in Biochemical Psychopharmacology. Vol. 18*, edited by E. Costa and M. Trabucchi, pp. 363–366. Raven Press, New York.
23. Sicuteri, F., Del Bianco, P. L., and Anselmi, B. (1979): Morphine abstinence and serotonin supersensitivity in man: Analogies with the mechanism of migraine? *Psychopharmacology (Berlin)*, 65:205–209.
24. Sicuteri, F., Fanciullacci, M., and Del Bene, E. (1977): Dopamine system and idiopathic headache. In: *Headache: New Vistas*, edited by F. Sicuteri, pp. 239–250. Biomedical Press, Florence, Italy.
25. Slater, P., and Blundell, C. (1978): The effect of 6-hydroxydopamine on the antinociceptive action of morphine. *Eur. J. Pharmacol.*, 48:237–247.
26. Tulunay, F. C., Sparber, S. B., and Takemori, A. E. (1975): The effect of dopaminergic stimulation and blockade on the nociceptive and antinociceptive responses of mice. *Eur. J. Pharmacol.*, 33:65–70.
27. Van Loon, G. R., and Kim, C. (1978): Beta-endorphin-induced increase in striatal dopamine turnover. *Life Sci.*, 23:961–970.
28. Vander Wende, C., and Sporlein, M. T. (1973): Role of dopaminergic receptors in morphine analgesia and tolerance. *Res. Commun. Chem. Pathol. Pharmacol.*, 5:35–43.

*Advances in Pain Research
and Therapy, Vol. 7,*
edited by C. Benedetti et al.
Raven Press, New York © 1984.

Headache Therapy

Giovanni Nattero

*Headache Center, Institute of Internal Medicine, Turin University,
10126 Turin, Italy*

Headache therapy is such a complicated subject that it would be very difficult to cover in only one chapter. In fact, the therapy for headache and some forms of craniofacial pain includes pharmacological agents, psychotherapy, biofeedback, varied surgical techniques, as well as the use of homeopathic treatment, acupuncture, and physiotherapy.

The still incomplete knowledge of the pathogenetic mechanism of some forms of idiopathic headache, as well as the frequent association of many pathogenetic components in generating the headache in the same patient, justifies any therapeutic attempt, either surgical or physiotherapeutic, provided that it brings a lasting relief to a suffering commonly termed "the pain that does not kill but does not let you live."

The main aspect of headache therapy considered here concerns the so-called idiopathic headaches, whose treatment is at present mainly pharmacological. Biofeedback is a procedure quite recently adopted and now widely employed. In the past, when medical therapies failed to yield appreciable results, various surgical techniques were attempted. Today, surgical techniques (and also acupuncture), are still employed, but these techniques are still to be organically collected and checked with reference to idiopathic headaches.

The current study is based on the medical therapy of idiopathic headaches, referring only to the literature of Appenzeller (1), Barolin (2), Diamond and Dalessio (3), Heyck (4), Lance (5), Nattero (6–9), Sicuteri (10), Vinken and Bruyn (11), and Wolff (12).

This task does not seem any easier when we realize that there have been more than 400 therapies in use for migraine alone in the last decade.

ACUTE THERAPY

It is widely known that, among the ergot alkaloids currently used in therapy, ergotamine tartrate appears to be helpful in the acute migraine attack if administered when the prodromal vasoconstriction intracranial stage is followed by the extracranial (and probably also intracranial) stage of vasodilatation and edema. The table published by Wolff (12), shows that under the action of this potent agent (injected either intramuscularly or intravenously) the pain reduces proportionately, according to the reduction of the pulse amplitude, registered on the superficial temporal artery.

However, several reports in the literature warn that, with incorrect use or overdosage, ergotamine tartrate may cause harmful side effects on the cardiovascular system, including hypertension, angina pectoris, and vascular, peripheral changes.

Some cases of ergot addiction (although a migraine sufferer never becomes a morphine addict) showed EKG alterations due to coronary disease and sphygmographic reduction of the index on the four limbs. While all these changes regressed rapidly after a few days of abstinence from the drug, the arteriography showed a consistent stenosis in the arterial area of the hand.

A compound of indomethacin, caffeine, and prochlorperazine does not cause these undesirable side effects. Under the action of this agent, in the rapid extinction stage of the migraine crisis, the sphygmic, dynamographic, and rheographic values (consistently higher homolaterally to the pain-affected side of the head) underwent an evident reduction. By contrast, an increase in the contralateral sphygmic parameters was observed, resulting in a renewed hemodynamic balance at the cephalic level. Contraindication to the use of this remedy, as well as to that of ergotamine compounds, is the presence of gastric ulcer, cerebrovascular insufficiency, or hypertension.

Pirazolic derivatives, phenacetin (at present sub-judice), aspirin, metochlopramide, and paracetamol, administered alone or with barbiturates, are widely employed in less severe headache of various origins. Results have varied and are difficult to evaluate.

PROPHYLAXIS AND CHRONIC THERAPY

Before starting a patient on a long-term therapy, the physician should identify every possible cause of headache. Once again, it must be emphasized that muscle contraction headache does not only include depression and conversion forms, but also headaches that might involve skeletal musculature and be referred to the most varied causes.

By means of a brief questionnaire and a short test, eventual temporomandibular joint dysfunction and dental malocclusion, often associated with bruxism and causing headache, can be diagnosed. The assessment consists of asking the patient whether he or she is in the habit of grinding the teeth and clenching the jaws; whether there is any neck and shoulder pain other than headache; and whether there is any impairment in dental sensitiveness or at the temporo-mandibular joint level. The examiner then verifies the position of the condyles in the temporo-mandibular cavity by palpating the temporo-mandibular joint, as well as by measuring the aperture of the "bite." Longitudinal studies show that elimination of the etiology of this dental problem frequently relieves or eliminates these headaches.

Furthermore, studies at Turin University Headache Center showed that a pathogenetic correlation does exist between some headaches and ocular disorders. After a thorough investigation—refraction and visus examination, examination of the intrinsic and extrinsic motility, state of binocular vision, campimetry, perimetry, tonometry, and ophthalmoscopy—it could be concluded that the "migrainous status" is the headache less affected by vision impairment. On the contrary, classic and common migraine may be considerably relieved by correcting eventual refractive errors. In the case of headache associated with an increase in intraocular pressure, a marked decrease in pain was observed as soon as this hypertension was reduced.

Other ocular disorders whose correction results in alleviation of migraine pain include astigmatism, sometimes accompanied by myopia, and hypermetropia. Common migraine seems to be much more benefited by the ophthalmic treatment than classic migraine.

To illustrate the most recent progress in headache prophylaxis and therapy, Table 1 provides a general outline of the most effective and potent agents in headache treatment. The various idiopathic headaches were listed in the following order: "tic douloureux," cluster headache, migrainous variants, migraine, mixed headaches, tension headache, and headache associated with depression.

Tic douloureux is greatly improved by the use of carbamazepine and diphenylhydantoin, which are the most commonly used remedies for their well-known anticonvulsant action. However, the results vary from patient to patient and from one administration cycle to another.

For cluster headache, the histamine desensitization is still very much debated, especially by American authors. Corticosteroids are also employed for their antiphlogistic action. Lithium is mainly known as a modifier of the electric conductivity in the CNS. As to their efficacy, their activity varies from case to case and from one cycle of therapy to another.

In the treatment of the so-called migrainous variants, there is also indication for histamine desensitization, corticosteroids, and lithium administration. Dimethothiazine is actually preferred for its joint antihistamine and antiserotonin action, and seems to be active in the prophylaxis of classic migraine.

In the above-mentioned migrainous variants (i.e., syndromes bearing possible relationship with both cluster and migraine), in classic and common migraine, and in the so-called mixed headache (headache with vascular and muscle contraction components), a strong pool of pharmacologically active substances can be used: (a) reserpine (which will be more extensively dealt with further on), for its high power in depleting catecholamines; (b) clonidine, a hypotensive agent; (c) dihydroergotamine and methysergide, for their vasoconstrictive action; (d) monoamino oxidase inhibitors (MAO); (e) cyproeptadine and pizotifen, for their joint antihistamine, antiserotonin action; and (f) cinnarizine, a vasoconstriction inhibitor. With regard to the last three compounds, it must be pointed out that every migraine sufferer has a dif-

TABLE 1. *Headache pharmacological therapy: A synoptic attempt*

Tic Douloureux	Cluster Headache	Migrainous Variants	Migraine	Mixed Headaches	Tension Headache	Depression
Carbamazepine anticonvulsant	Histamine desensitization	Dimethothiazine antihistamine + antiserotonin	Reserpine catecholamines depletion		Allylpropylmalonyluria barbiturate	MAO inhibitors
Diphenylhydantoin anticonvulsant	Corticosteroids anti-inflammatory		Clonidine hypotensive		Benzodiazepine tranquilizer	
	Lithium electrical conductivity in CNS		Dihydroergotamine vasoconstrictor		Tryptophan 5-HT precursor	
			Methysergide vasoconstrictor		Amitriptyline antidepressant	
			MAO inhibitors		Imipramine antidepressant	
			Cyproeptadine			
			Pizotifen antihistamine + antiserotonin			
			Cinnarizine vasoconstriction inhibitors			
			Propanolol			
			Pindolol β-adrenergic blockers			
			Nonsteroids anti-inflammatory			
			Aspirin			
			Sulfinpyrazone			
			Dipyrimodale platelet antagonists			

ferent response to each of them. As for the quite recent employment of propanolol and pindolol, they are now widely used beta-adrenergic blockers.

In this powerful pool of substances, antiphlogistic, nonsteroidal agents, such as indomethacin and ketophenylbutazone, must be included. After the individuation of leukotrienes, the antimigraine action of these remedies might be explained. Platelet antagonists, such as aspirin, sulphinpyrazone, and dipyrimodale, should also be noted for their antiaggregating power.

At present, the pathogenetic, platelet hyperaggregating stage of migraine is still much debated and discussed, but no agreement on this point has been reached yet. In this connection, an investigation carried out by our research group and based on the use of the Breddin test (i.e., *in vitro* spontaneous aggregation) on migraine patients, ranging in age from 14 to 52 years and in number proportional to the incidence of migraine in both sexes, tends to confirm the platelet hyperaggregation in migraine. However, the statistical significance (sign test) is on the border line.

In mixed headache and muscle contraction headache, allylpropylmalonylurea, a barbiturate, benzodiazepine, a tranquilizer, and tryptophane, a 5-HT precursor, seem to be the medications of choice.

Amitriptyline and imipramine are largely used, both in tension headache and headache associated with depression, for their antidepressant action. In the latter form, MAO inhibitors find a clear indication.

All these compounds, with the exception of histamine, reserpine, and clonidine, are usually administered at the current dosage.

In this wide range of drugs, a considerable amount of empiricism has to be taken into account because compounds endowed with such different pharmacological activities often prove to be effective in the same headache form. This phenomenon might be explained by the drugs' different mechanisms of action on the various links of the pathogenetic chain of these headaches.

Other antimigraine remedies worthy of mention include (a) lisuride, widely used for its dopaminergic and antiserotonin action; (b) methergoline, a valuable therapeutic agent in migraine associated with high prolactin plasma levels; and (c) sulpiride, used in mixed headache. Reserpine and beta-blockers need to be dealt with more extensively, particularly the former because of its proved efficacy through the years (about 20 in my personal experience with this drug) with the "desperately ill" migraine patient.

Reserpine

The most interesting aspect of reserpine is its profound effect on monoamine storage and metabolism. The first evidence for this is its mechanism of action, causing the release of serotonin from its storage sites in the brain, gastrointestinal tract, and blood platelets. Catecholamines, norepinephrine, and dopamine are also released from their storage sites, centrally and peripherally, by the same alkaloid. In addition, reserpine inhibits the monoamine uptake process in various tissues. A very lipid-soluble compound, reserpine readily crosses the blood-brain barrier and is rapidly metabolized in the body. Because of these good pharmacological presuppositions, it was studied in migraine prophylaxis.

It was first necessary to standardize the cycles of prophylaxis and therapy, lasting about 6 weeks, at pre-fixed, carefully tested small doses, injected intravenously on alternate days, in order to prevent migraine attacks prior to provoking undesirable side effects (e.g., psycho-nervous depression, gastric disturbance) and to enable a statistical evaluation of the results. A comparison of data was then made between the pretherapeutic and posttherapeutic conditions. In cases where the therapeutic cycle had to be repeated more than once in the course of some years, the data of the most effective cycle were evaluated.

Positive, highly significant results were obtained with the above-mentioned regimen. No side effects were observed in the large population investigated.

A double-blind clinical trial was carried out in 1975. The practical difficulty in using placebo on outpatients who had to come to the hospital at least 20 times had obviously reduced the number of controls. Thus only 18 migraine sufferers were included in this study. Reserpine and placebo results were evaluated by means of the McNemar test. Positive, highly significant data were obtained.

It was therefore decided to adopt these therapeutic, standardized cycles of reserpine in the treatment of 37 cases of cluster headache. Reserpine alone was administered to one group of 25 patients. Desensitization with histamine was used on a second group of 18 patients. With a third group of 7 patients, both cycles were adopted at different times.

Supposing that in the "cluster period" untreated patients keep stationary, a nonparametric test (tc) inside treatment, was used in order to evaluate the reported effects by means of marks (from 0 to 3) equivalent to the entity of the effect. The therapeutic activity by means of histamine was also highly significant. The average intensity of effects in the group treated with histamine was lower than in the group treated with reserpine.

In the comparison of activities between the two treatments, the difference of behavior between the two groups was highly significant in favor of reserpine.

Beta-Blockers

With regard to drugs commonly known as beta-blockers, this term refers to agents that selectively antagonize catecholamine effects on specific receptors at the postsynaptic membrane level, called "beta-adrenolytic." Their use in migraine therapy seems to have started when a group of coronary patients with migraine headaches reported improvement in both syndromes after administration of beta-blockers alone.

The pharmacological presupposition of beta-blockers is mainly based on their power to inhibit the extracranial vasodilatation peculiar to the algic phase of migraine.

In recent literature, updated to 1979, the majority of authors [Appenzeller (1) and Diamond and Dalessio (3) among them] approved the use of propanolol for migraine prophylaxis. They report excellent responses in at least one-third of the patients investigated. Lesser or dubious responses in general are reported by others. A minority report patients having as many, or even more, attacks under propanolol administration.

Recent data, collected at the Turin Center for an investigation on propanolol and pindolol activity, seem to be positive. However, there is evidence of a discrepancy between one migraine subject's response to this treatment and another's. It still remains to be explained why the therapeutic results are either excellent or null.

Nadolol, a new beta-blocking agent, has also been recently proposed for the prophylactic treatment of migraine.

COMMENTS

In conclusion, when dealing with the pharmacological therapy of headache, one should always bear in mind that, before adopting any kind of acute or chronic treatment, all possible contraindications and side effects must be considered. In many instances, the individual sensitivity of each patient to anticonvulsant drugs may generate leukopenia and agranulocytosis.

Contraindications might be generally outlined as follows: (a) common antimigraine drugs in glaucoma and ocular hypertonia; (b) phenothiazine in renal disease; (c) reserpine and histamine in gastric ulcer; (d) tranquilizers in latent depression forms; (e) beta-blockers in asthma and abnormal atrioventricular conduction; and (f) lithium, when a lack of responsibility on the patient's part in undergoing periodic controls of blood levels, has been ascertained.

BIOFEEDBACK THERAPY

The necessity of avoiding with the utmost care the side effects caused by long-term medical treatment has induced researchers at the Turin Center to study the therapeutic possibilities and the variety of applications of biofeedback for the cure of headache.

It is well known that biofeedback consists of a technique that allows one to identify and correct peculiar behavior, involuntary muscular movements, and undesirable responses to situational or external stimuli.

For some years, biofeedback was first employed by headache researchers in an attempt to alleviate problems and to relieve the pain of migraine headache patients. Later on, these researchers decided to adopt it mainly in mixed headache and in muscle contraction headache. In a preliminary assessment of the patient, the contraction of the head, neck, shoulder, and upper back muscles is registered by means of electromyography and then a direct relationship between extracranial blood flow and hand temperature is sought and evaluated in vascular headache patients.

In an investigation conducted in 1980 and based on $1\frac{1}{2}$ years' retrospective follow-up, a group of 72 patients examined at the center were treated with EMG biofeedback sessions. These headache sufferers of both sexes ranged in age from 10 to 60 years, were randomly selected, and did not undergo any other kind of therapy. In migraine headache sufferers, autogenic training obtained 77% improvement; this lasted in 86% of the women and in 100% of the men at follow-up. In mixed headache sufferers, autogenic training was successful in 70% of cases; this lasted longer in women than in men (80 and 62%, respectively). In the tension headache group, a long-lasting improvement of 75% in adult men was reduced to 50% in adult women; total relief was achieved in children. In all three groups, the improvement lasted at least until the follow-up visit.

With regard to the parameters for headache severity and frequency, it can be said that, in migraine and mixed headache, a remarkable reduction in pain frequency was obtained in comparison with the reduction in pain severity. Both parameters appeared reduced in tension headache cases.

The therapeutic efficacy of the combined EMG and thermal biofeedback treatment was evaluated in a group of 72 patients, including tension headache sufferers. Only 50% of these patients, treated with both procedures, reported improvement. On a careful check of the results of this investigation, and on the basis of previous accurate diagnosis, the number of improved patients was higher in the tension vascular headache group.

Even though our data are only preliminary, indication for a combined treatment of headache by EMG and thermal biofeedback seems to be confirmed.

Additional research is needed to evaluate the validity of EMG data because EMG therapeutic measures are often affected by many methodological variables, including type of electrodes used, site of application, subject's resistance, differential pain thresholds, and other causal inferences. Sometimes even the interpretation of the results is difficult because not all of the variables are reported in the literature. Furthermore, improved methodology and research design are required to clarify and ascertain relationships and inferences.

At this point, children seem to be the most benefited by the use of biofeedback training, as demonstrated by the total relief obtained in their population. This goal, achieved without the aid of pharmacological treatment, encourages the application of this procedure in children and additional research in view of its improvement.

SURGICAL THERAPY

The surgical attempts to treat migraine headache can substantially lead to two directions: (a) the pathogenetic mechanism at its origin, or at least the nearest possible to its origin, or (b) interrupt the pathways of vascular pain.

These attempts are less important than medical strategies and consist of the following operations: removal of both chains of the cervical sympathetic nerves and ganglions; lower cervical and first thoracic ganglionectomy; perivascular sympathectomy at carotid bifurcation level; resection of the trigeminal nerve; subtotal rhizotomy of the ophthalmic fiber; infiltration of the gasserian ganglion; resection of supraorbital, supratrochlear, occipital, posteroauricular, and greater occipital nerves; intervention on paranasal area cavities; binding of the middle-meningeal artery; and cryotherapy of neural ganglions or of one or more external carotid artery branches. (Most of these destructive procedures rarely produce long-term relief and should *not* be considered.)

CONCLUSION

An extremely large number of valuable therapeutic measures and procedures are at the physician's disposal for the treatment of headache patients. However, it is necessary to insist on a severe control of data. First, we need statistical criteria suitable for the right evaluation of the headache improvement because idiopathic headaches have a peculiar, recurring behavior, sometimes with long-lasting, spontaneous, pain-free periods. Second, we need long follow-up studies because, in some pain-affected subjects, a placebo effect might also be exercised by some therapeutic agents, as well as occurring with the use of placebo.

REFERENCES

1. Appenzeller, O. (Ed.) (1976): *Pathogenesis and Treatment of Headache.* Spectrum Publications, New York.
2. Barolin, G. S. (Ed.) (1969): *Migräne.* Facultas Verlag, Wien.
3. Diamond, S., and Dalessio, D. J. (Eds.) (1978): *The Practicing Physician's Approach to Headache.* Williams & Wilkins, Baltimore.
4. Heyck, H. (Ed.) (1981): *Headache and Facial Pain.* George Thieme Verlag, Stuttgart-New York.
5. Lance, J. W. (Ed.) (1969): *The Mechanism and Management of Headache.* Butterworths, London.
6. Nattero, G. (1972): Le cefalee a grappolo (e/o varianti emicraniche). In: *Cefalee ed Algie Cranio-Facciali di Interesse Otorinolaringoiatrico,* edited by E. De Amicis, pp. 56–77. Pacini Mariotti, Pisa.
7. Nattero, G. (1972): La sindrome emicranica. In: *Cefalee ed Algie Cranio-Facciali di Interesse Otorinolaringoiatrico,* edited by E. De Amicis, pp. 79–128. Pacini Mariotti, Pisa.

8. Nattero, G. (1972): Tension headache. In: *Cefalee ed Algie Cranio-Facciali di Interesse Otorinolaringoiatrico*, edited by E. De Amicis, pp. 130–136. Pacini Mariotti, Pisa.
9. Nattero, G. (1975): Le cefalee. In: *Patologia Medica*, edited by G. Lenti, pp. 1993–2009. Minerva Medica, Torino.
10. Sicuteri, F. (1973): Clinica e terapia delle cefalee essenziali. In: *La Medicina d'Oggi*, edited by A. Beretta Anguissola. Biomedical Press, Torino.
11. Vinken, P. J., and Bruyn, G. W. (Eds.) (1968): *Handbook of Clinical Neurology: Headaches and Cranial Neuralgias*. North-Holland Publishing Company, Amsterdam.
12. Wolff, H. G. (Ed.) (1963): *Headache and Other Head Pain*. Oxford University Press, New York.

Advances in Pain Research and Therapy, Vol. 7,
edited by C. Benedetti et al.
Raven Press, New York © 1984.

Neuralgia: Mechanisms and Therapeutic Prospects

Ulf Lindblom

Department of Neurology, Karolinska Hospital, S-104 01 Stockholm, Sweden

Neuralgia is usually the product of several cooperative peripheral and central mechanisms, whose relative importance varies from case to case. Analysis of the sensory abnormalities that often accompany neuralgia may help to understand the neural dysfunction behind neuralgic pain and may indicate peripheral or central factors that could be the target of treatment. Sensory testing before and after treatment can elucidate the link between allodynia, hyperalgesia, and spontaneous pain. We have observed a differential effect of afferent stimulation on tactile and thermal allodynia. Such effects might be related to the type of therapeutic stimulation, a hypothesis that will be tested by comparing the results of selective stimulation of large and small afferent fibers.

During recent years, there has been a bias toward electrical stimulation and acupuncture, both in research and in clinical application. It seems worthwhile to reanimate less spectacular forms of afferent stimulation, such as vibration and heat, and appraise their therapeutic effects and if they can contribute to our understanding of the mechanisms of neuralgia. A restrictive attitude toward neurolysis and other destructive procedures should be maintained. Medical treatment for neuralgia is hampered by the lack of analgesics, with a specific effect on the processes of nociception and pathologic pain mechanisms.

DEFINITIONS AND DIAGNOSIS

Neuralgia may be defined as "pain in the distribution of a peripheral nerve, often accompanied by signs of nerve dysfunction." The pain may be aching, burning, or lancinating, with superimposed attacks of more severe pain like stabs or lightning. Not infrequently there are paresthesiae, thermal, pins and needles, tingling, and so on, indicating abnormal impulse activity in various types of afferent fibers (34). The paresthesiae may follow the distribution of the affected nerve more precisely than the pain, which may radiate outside its territory. The pain also may be referred to structures or regions not innervated by a particular nerve. Causalgia is a special type of neuralgia following acute traumatic nerve injury, where the pain should include a burning character (*causalgia* = burning pain). Some authors claim that relief by sympathetic block is so typical that it should be a prerequisite for the diagnosis of causalgia (3). The pain in radiculopathy, and in some polyneuropathies (44), is of the same character as in neuralgia.

The most common sign of nerve dysfunction is sensibility abnormalities (21,25). If the affected nerve is mixed, there also may be muscle weakness and atrophy. The signs of nerve dysfunction usually can be taken as evidence of a lesion in the peripheral nerve. Occasionally, the function of the nerve improves when the pain is temporarily or permanently relieved, which indicates that the dysfunction also may be due to a central blocking effect of the pain.

Neuralgia often is associated with signs of increased sympathetic outflow to the affected region. This is generally assumed to constitute one link of a vicious circle with pain and hyperalgesia and may lead to the condition of reflex dystrophy. It is less often pointed out that the change in sympathetic tone may be in the opposite direction, resulting in a warm, dry, and perhaps reddened skin.

Signs of nerve lesion are not a prerequisite for the diagnosis of neuralgia. For instance, in tic douloureux, no sensory disturbance can be demonstrated even with the most refined methods of sensory testing available (25). Whatever the causes are for the pain and trigger mechanism in this condition, they do not affect the normal conductivity and sensory function of the nerve. The only reported exception is a slightly longer latency of the cortical evoked potential in some cases (40). In other neuralgias, disordered sensibility is typical and valuable for the diagnosis because it usually indicates the presence of a nerve lesion as a basis for pain. Examples of such neuralgias are the common herpes zoster neuralgia, meralgia paresthetica, inguinalis neuralgia, saphenous neuralgia, neuralgia in the median, ulnar and sciatic nerves, and some cases of postoperative neuralgia.

There are also less common or well-known conditions with neuralgia, due to entrapment of, for example, the suprascapular nerve, nervus cutaneous antebrachii, ramus cutaneous dorsalis, nervus abdomini superficialis, and nervus tibialis. Even when the cutaneous distribution of the nerve is circumscribed, a close examination may reveal hyperpathia. It is reasonable to assume that nerves innervating deep somatic or visceral structures may cause neuralgia, in analogy with that of cutaneous nerves. But the generally diffuse distribution of deep pain and the virtually complete lack of methods to test the functions of the corresponding nerves leave us with diagnostic uncertainty. In some instances of supposed autonomous nerve neuralgia, associated effector or reflex phenomena may be helpful, such as heart irregularities or cough in glossopharyngeal and vagal neuralgia.

MECHANISMS

General

In research about the mechanisms of neuralgia, experimental pain models in humans or animals are a very important tool. With due ethical consideration, they deserve a wider use and may be further improved. There is a certain limitation in that it has been, and probably always will be, difficult to design a model that imitates or explains all features of a particular clinical pain syndrome (e.g., tic douloureux or causalgia). This emphasizes the importance of using the actual patient as much as possible. Parallel analyses on both patients and experimental models may be the most rewarding approach.

Our knowledge of neuralgia mechanisms primarily is based on comparisons of clinical features with neurophysiologic data from normal animals, or animals in which lesions have been induced to imitiate clinical pain syndromes. Support for a particular hypothesis about the mechanisms sometimes is obtained by the results of pharmacologic tests or therapeutic procedures in patients. All this evidence is more or less indirect, and most probably will remain so because of the restricted possibilities of direct studies of neural mechanisms in patients, and because of the general difficulty in demonstrating the physical basis of sensations. This particularly pertains to central pain mechanisms, where our knowledge today is much less precise than that of peripheral mechanisms, and where we become more speculative the higher up in the nervous system we get.

Ectopic Impulses

Ectopic impulse generators in afferent nociceptive fibers most probably are a significant source of neuralgic pain after peripheral nerve lesions. It appears that seemingly all continuity lesions lead to the formation of neuromas and nerve sprouts (52), which display abnormal excitability and discharge afferent impulses in pain fibers spontaneously, at least for a period of time. Percutaneous microneurography in diseased nerves of awake humans offers the possibility of direct evidence of this mechanism by means of a recent technical innovation with the method (49). There is very convincing experimental evidence for the peripheral basis of radicular pain in the form of ectopic impulses originating in sensitized dorsal root fibers and ganglion cells (15).

Ephaptic Transmission

Ephaptic excitation of pain fibers as a source of clinical pain has been reinforced by recent experiments on neuromas (39) and nerve roots with dysmyelination (38). Ephaptic transmission from tactile or thermal afferent fibers to nociceptive afferents at the site of the lesion also would explain the common finding in neuralgia patients that nonnoxious stimulation of the painful skin area produces pain.

Neural Nociceptors

A special peripheral pain mechanism that might be involved in neuralgia, but which is seldom discussed, would be pain from intraneural nociceptors (45) (M. von During, *personal communication*). Such pain would have the same dull, aching character as deep pain, and might even be referred. Apart from the morphologic demonstration of free nerve endings in peripheral nerves, this mechanism is purely speculative, but the presence of a dull aching pain in some types of nerve lesion, such as neuralgic amyotrophy (6), and the relation between pain and rate of degeneration in some neuropathies (8) are suggestive.

Central Mechanisms

The central consequences of deafferentation and their possible role for neuralgia, as well as for phantom pain and pain after lesions in the central nervous system, have been investigated experimentally during recent years and were reviewed at the Third World Congress on Pain in 1981. It seems safe to assume that denervation hypersensitivity and central hyperexcitability following deafferentation are crucial factors for development of anesthesia dolorosa and similar clinical pain states. The demonstration of interneuronal hyperexcitability, and that it may spread to successively higher levels (29), is an important illustration to the old hypothesis of secondary, central, self-sustaining "pain foci," which is prompted by so many clinical observations. The central effects of deafferentation might be contributory in many cases of neuralgia, but it should be kept in mind that deafferentation per se is not pain-producing, as demonstrated by the vast number of neurologic conditions with deafferentation that are totally painless.

The importance of central mechanisms, even when the primary lesion is in the peripheral nerve, has been emphasized repeatedly in the literature, for example, by Livingston (26), but experimental data that directly support a specific mechanism are lacking. It is generally assumed that disinhibition of nociceptive relays may be one factor, and more complex disturbances have been suggested and given special attributes, such as "pattern generating mechanism" (31). In the clinic, certain features are suggestive of peripheral mechanisms, such as strictly localized pain and hyperalgesia. Other phenomena, such as abnormal aftersensation, may be explained either by peripheral or central afterdischarges (4), whereas symptoms like radiation of pain outside the territory of the affected nerve, widespread hyperesthesia, and recurrence of pain after neurotomy are indicative of central mechanisms. For the clinician, who has to select the most adequate treatment, it should be of great importance to know the relevance of peripheral and central mechanisms in the particular case. Any piece of evidence or new test that would distinguish various mechanisms would be helpful. Diagnostic nerve blocks have not turned out to have the wanted predictive value for the outcome of peripheral neurolysis.

Constitutional Factors

An individual's constitutional disposition may be one important factor for the occurrence of neuralgia. This is suggested by the well-known circumstance that only a fraction of patients with seemingly identical nerve lesions develop chronic pain. A similar, perhaps corresponding, phenomenon appears in experiments with animal "pain" models. Behavioral signs of sensory disturbances appear only in some animals in a uniformly treated group, and the signs may vary in intensity from one animal to another (53). Quite recently, a genetic disposition for pain-prone behavior in rats has been demonstrated (7).

Some features of neuralgia are difficult to understand without assuming that humoral factors are involved. For example, the several hours' long pain relief that is sometimes produced by a few minutes of afferent stimulation or a transitory nerve block is difficult to explain solely in electrophysiologic terms.

DIAGNOSTIC PROCEDURES

Sensibility Tests

It seems possible to get some evidence of the location of the pain-producing dysfunction by relatively simple measurements. As part of the hyperpathic syndrome, nonnoxious stimulation of the aching region may produce pain (allodynia) (17), and noxious stimuli may produce stronger pain than normal (hyperalgesia). These painful responses appear to be more or less intimately linked to the spontaneous pain in neuralgia. They occur together, and effective treatments usually relieve both hyperpathia and spontaneous pain (23,27). It was thought, therefore, that the neural dysfunction that produces spontaneous pain might be elucidated by a close study of the hyperpathic disturbance by means of quantitative sensory tests. These should at least help to describe and define the sensory abnormalities and some of the pain features. This chapter will describe some of the results obtained at the Sensibility Laboratory at Karolinska Hospital in Stockholm, where two major lines of analysis are currently performed. One line is to apply well-defined stimuli to the painful skin area and record the abnormal sensations carefully. Both noxious and nonnoxious stimuli are used, either mechanical (tactile and pinch) or thermal (22). The stimuli are largely modality-specific and can be graded in intensity. They consist either of pulses or of continuous stimulation at a preset and variable rate of change. The pulsed stimuli enable measurement of the latencies of the subjective responses and of evoked potentials. The second line of analysis is to undertake therapeutic manipulations and compare the effect on the spontaneous pain with the effect on the sensory dysfunction. The therapeutic procedures may consist of conditioning afferent stimulation, pharmacological tests, or nerve blocks.

Reaction Times

The reaction times to the painful responses evoked by stimulation of hyperpathic skin in neuralgia patients were different for tactile, cold, and warm stimuli (11). The logical interpretation of this result seems to be that the peripheral pathway of the pain-producing impulses is the regular modality-specific afferents, and that transformation to pain occurs centrally. The results thus indicate that the hyperalgesia, and perhaps the spontaneous pain, is more dependent on central mechanisms than was expected, since peripheral mechanisms are naturally first thought of in patients with peripheral lesions. If this is so, it is less astonishing that measures directed toward peripheral mechanisms may fail, and that the pain may recur after neurolysis and perhaps even become worse because of the ensuing deafferentation.

Conditioning Stimulation

The effect of dorsal column stimulation (DCS) will be used to illustrate sensibility measurements with therapeutic manipulations (23,24). In a case of ulnar nerve neuralgia, there were both tactile and thermal allodynia, as well as spontaneous pain, when the patient was unstimulated. After 20 min of DCS at 60 Hz, which totally blocked the spontaneous pain, the tactile allodynia was replaced by tactile hypoesthesia, but the thermal allodynia persisted. Thus there were residual signs of dysfunction of the sensory modality whose afferent fiber system was not directly stimulated by the DCS. It may be speculated that conditioning stimulation with heat could have the reverse effect.

The pulsed stimuli can also be used to analyze such temporal abnormalities as pathologic summation and adaptation. In neuralgias with hyperpathia, a painful reaction usually recurs on repeated stimulation, even at short intervals. Aftersensations may summate and build up a stronger and more long-lasting pain than that produced by a single stimulus. In contrast to tic douloureux, the evoked pain in peripheral neuralgias is not followed by a clear-cut refractory period. On the other hand, it may be possible to avoid the painful reaction by manipulation with the pulse parameters. Thus gradual increase in pulse strength, or duration, starting from a value that is subliminal for pain, may proceed painlessly up to, and above, stimulus levels that earlier were intolerably painful. The painful response can habituate. Furthermore, a painful response to moderately cold pulses may be eliminated after a series of warm pulses. Thus the pain mechanism can be conditioned by selected types of afferent stimulation, which may vary from patient to patient. Abnormal summation and adaptation phenomena occur in parallel, as revealed by stimuli that are either supra- or subliminal, respectively, for painful responses. Some of these conditioning effects might be involved in conventional therapies like transcutaneous nerve stimulation (TNS) and acupuncture, and it may be worthwhile to explore them further.

TREATMENT

Nerve Blocks

Besides afferent stimulation, somatic or sympathetic nerve blocks with local anesthetics are the first choice treatment of neuralgia. The mechanism of action for the pain relief after a single block, or a series of blocks, when the relief outlasts the local anesthetic effect, will probably remain unrevealed for quite a time. It might be less mysterious if one thinks in terms of neurochemical and humoral effects instead of mere blocking of afferent nerve impulses. Is it possible that substances are released locally by the injections which, via the axoplasmic flow, influence the central nervous system and alter its excitability? This would explain the positive result of blocks distal to the lesion (18,28).

The trauma of surgical or chemical neurolysis might operate through the same hypothetical mechanism for some period of time. It is noteworthy also that neurotomy distal to the lesion may be effective (33,46). The old hypothesis that the nerve block, such as an efferent sympathetic block in causalgia, interrupts a vicious circle is still the subject of experimentation to obtain direct positive evidence. A sympathetic block may be effective even when signs of increased sympathetic tone are absent and when the afferent nerve has been divided. Therefore a retrograde effect seems more plausible (41).

Afferent Stimulation

Much interest has been devoted to acupuncture and TNS during the last decade (1), and some operative mechanisms and indications for clinical use, and in patients with neuralgia, have been established (32). The success rate of TNS in neuralgia is reported to be as high as 30 to 60%. Other forms of afferent stimulation, or "counterirritation," have been investigated sporad-

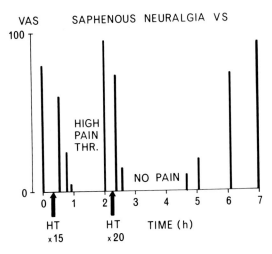

FIG. 1. Pain relief in neuralgia patient following two series of rapid heat applications (HT 15 and 20 times, respectively) in pain area. Note poststimulatory reduction of pain; longer pain-free period after the second, stronger, heat application; and successive recurrence of pain thereafter. VAS = visual analog scale.

ically. Vibration, which is a very efficient way of activating the large afferent fibers, has been shown to increase the threshold for induced pain (14,37,51), and there are some positive reports on the relief of clinical pain (13,35,36,50). Two of these reports include patients with neuralgia (13,36).

In a recent study, ice massage was found to be as effective as TNS in chronic low back pain (30). Heat, which predominantly stimulates unmyelinated fibers, also may have a pain-relieving effect similar to that of TNS (Fig. 1). Controlled heat pulses up to the heat pain tolerance level (45°–55°C) were applied to the pain area of a patient with saphenous neuralgia, using the Marstock stimulator (12). A series of 15 pulses at a rate of 5/min were followed by an hour-long reduction of the spontaneous pain, as rated by visual analog scale. After another series of 20 heat pulses, there was a poststimulatory decline of the spontaneous pain and a totally pain-free period of 2 hr. The threshold of allodynia was markedly increased when the pain was relieved.

A similar effect of heat or other forms of counterirritation, including vibration and electrical stimulation, already was demonstrated by Gammon and Starr in 1941 (13). They pointed out that intermittent stimulation was most effective. It is conceivable that various forms of afferent stimulation, besides TNS and acupuncture, deserve a further systematic analysis and a wider application in neuralgia.

It should be pointed out that afferent stimulation sometimes may worsen the neuralgia, which is not well reported in the literature. In 3 of 11 cases, TNS increased the pain (25). In tic douloureux, TNS or vibration is not adequate because this type of stimulation triggers the attacks (19).

The possibility to manipulate the spontaneous pain and hyperalgesia with afferent stimulation of the pain area emphasizes the potential therapeutic value of preserving the afferent neural channel and that one should be restrictive with neurolytic agents, neurotomy, and rhizotomy. This standpoint is underscored by the relatively high rate of relapses, sometimes severe (anesthesia dolorosa), after such procedures.

Medication

Although nonsteroid anti-inflammatory (aspirin-like) analgesics are widely used in conditions with neuralgia, they are relatively ineffective. This is not surprising since they primarily exert their action peripherally by interfering with the chemical process of nociception and not with pain mechanisms in the nervous system itself. It is noteworthy that none of the anti-inflammatory analgesics were developed and tested for specific antinociceptive effects. Some of them may have a central analgesic effect as well, which has not been explored until lately (5,9). Another point of action for these drugs within the nervous system would be at intraneural nociceptors, which were mentioned above as a possible source of clinical pain in nerve lesions.

The narcotics are virtually the only analgesics whose mode of action on central processes of nociception has been explored. Their well-known suppressive effect on nociceptive-driven interneurons and excitatory effect on endogenous inhibition at nociceptive relays strongly suggest that narcotics would effectively relieve not only acute nociceptive pain but also neuralgia. It is then remarkable how ineffective they are in the latter condition, as well as in other types of neurologic pain. One explanation may be that the action on the central nervous system is complex (54), as is indicated, for example, by the disappearance of the morphine suppression of nociceptive interneurons when the preparation is shifted from spinal to decerebrate (20). Another explanation may be that we are dealing with pathologic pain mechanisms in neuralgia, which are not tested in our experimental models of nociceptive transmission.

The prospect of demonstrating nociception-specific transmitters opens the possibility of developing transmitter blockers for pain relief. There is certainly a need for new analgesics with a different pharmacologic profile than that of, for example, the aspirin-like drugs and a more specific antinociceptive and analgesic activity. This is needed for several conditions with recurrent or lingering pain. Zomepirac is a new, nonaddicting compound that may be a specific analgesic (55), but its efficacy in neuralgia has not yet been appraised. There is still only one example of a specific pharmacologic action in a neuralgic condition, which is becoming classic: anticonvulsants in idiopathic trigeminal neuralgia. Carbamazepine is the most used drug, and the possibility of monitoring the plasma levels of the compound and its metabolites offers a further improvement of this therapy (43,47,48).

Quite recently, glycerin injection into the trigeminal cistern in nonneurolytic doses has been introduced by Hakansson (16) as a new, effective, and apparently specific local treatment. This can be recommended before destructive lesions or surgical procedures are undertaken. Occasionally, paroxysmal pains and neuralgias other than tic douloureux may respond to anticonvulsants (10,42). Generally, however, they are useless in neuralgia secondary to trigeminal or peripheral nerve lesions or herpes zoster infection. This circumstance illustrates that neuralgic pains may be produced by different mechanisms.

It is not within the scope of this chapter to describe medication with psychotropic drugs, or psychologic or surgical methods, which are also very important for the treatment of neuralgia. Generally, I confess the conviction shared by many colleagues that the multidisciplinary approach as originally advocated by Bonica (2) is the optimal way of meeting the very diversified needs of patients with neuralgia, as well as with other types of lingering pain. It is hoped that therapists who monomanically claim that one kind of treatment cures various pains and patients represent a vanishing corps.

REFERENCES

1. Andersson, S. A. (1979): Pain control by sensory stimulation. In: *Advances in Pain Research and Therapy, Vol. 3*, edited by J. J. Bonica, J. C. Liebeskind, and D. C. Albe-Fessard, pp. 569–585. Raven Press, New York.
2. Bonica, J. J. (1974): Organization and function of a pain clinic. In: *Advances in Neurology, Vol. 4*, edited by J. J. Bonica, pp. 433–443. Raven Press, New York.
3. Bonica, J. J. (1979): Causalgia and other reflex sympathetic dystrophies. In: *Advances in Pain Research and Therapy, Vol. 3*, edited by J. J. Bonica, J. C. Liebeskind, and D. C. Albe-Fessard, pp. 141–166. Raven Press, New York.
4. Calvin, W. H. (1979): Some design features of axons and how neuralgias may defeat them. In: *Advances in Pain Research and Therapy, Vol. 3*, edited by J. J. Bonica, J. C. Liebeskind, and D. C. Albe-Fessard, pp. 297–309. Raven Press, New York.
5. Chen, A. C. N., and Chapman, C. R. (1980): Aspirin analgesia evaluated by event-related potentials in man: Possible central action in brain. *Exp. Brain Res.*, 39:359–364.
6. Devathasan, G., and Tong, H. I. (1980): Neuralgic amyotrophy: Criteria for diagnosis and a clinical with electromyography study. *Aust. N.Z. J. Med.*, 10:188–191.
7. Devor, M., and Govrin-Lippmann, R. (1981): Constitutional differences in susceptibility to peripheral nerve pathophysiology and pain. *Pain* (Suppl. 1):91.
8. Dyck, P. J., Lambert, E. H., and O'Brien, P. C. (1976): Pain in peripheral neuropathy related to rate and kind of fiber degeneration. *Neurology*, 26:466–471.
9. Ferreira, S. H., Lorenzetti, B. B., and Correa, F. M. A. (1978): Central and peripheral antialgesic action of aspirin-like drugs. *Eur. J. Pharmacol.*, 53:39–48.
10. Fields, H. L., and Raskin, N. H. (1976): Anticonvulsants and pain. In: *Clinical Neuropharmacology*, edited by H. L. Klawans, pp. 173–184. Raven Press, New York.
11. Fruhstorfer, H., and Lindblom, U. (1984): Sensibility abnormalities in neuralgic patients studied by thermal and tactile pulse stimulation. In: *Somatosensory Mechanisms*, edited by C. V. Euler, O. Franzén, U. Lindblom, and D. Ottoson. Macmillan, London.
12. Fruhstorfer, H., Lindblom, U., and Schmidt, W. G. (1976): Method for quantitative estimation of thermal thresholds in patients. *J. Neurol. Neurosurg. Psychiatry*, 39:1071–1075.
13. Gammon, G. D., and Starr, I. (1941): Studies on the relief of pain by counterirritation. *J. Clin. Invest.*, 20:13–20.
14. Grabois, M., Sharkey, P. S., Lauber, A., and Dimitrijevic, M. R. (1977): Suppressive effects of vibration and electrical stimuli on experimentally induced pain. *Arch. Phys. Med. Rehabil.*, 58:542–543.
15. Howe, J. F., Loeser, J. D., and Calvin, W. H. (1977): Mechanosensitivity of dorsal root ganglia and chronically injured axons: A physiological basis for the radicular pain of nerve root compression. *Pain*, 3:25–41.
16. Håkansson, S. (1981): Trigeminal neuralgia treated by the injection of glycerol into the trigeminal cistern. *Neurosurgery*, 9:638–646.

17. IASP Subcommittee on Taxonomy (1979): Pain terms: A list with definitions and notes on usage. *Pain*, 6:249–252.
18. Kibler, R. F., and Nathan, P. W. (1960): Relief of pain and paraesthesiae by nerve block distal to a lesion. *J. Neurol. Neurosurg. Psychiatry*, 23:91–98.
19. Kugelberg, E., and Lindblom, U. (1959): The mechanism of the pain in trigeminal neuralgia. *J. Neurol. Neurosurg. Psychiatry*, 22:36–43.
20. Le Bars, D., Menetrey, D., and Besson, J. M. (1976): Effects of morphine upon the lamina V type cells activities in the dorsal horn of the decerebrate cat. *Brain Res.*, 113:293–310.
21. Lindblom, U. (1979): Sensory abnormalities in neuralgia. In: *Advances in Pain Research and Therapy, Vol. 3*, edited by J. J. Bonica, J. C. Liebeskind, and D. C. Albe-Fessard, pp. 111–120. Raven Press, New York.
22. Lindblom, U. (1981): Quantitative testing of sensibility including pain. In: *Neurology, Vol. 1: Clinical Neurophysiology*, edited by E. Ståhlberg and R. Young. Butterworth International Medical Reviews, London.
23. Lindblom, U., and Meyerson, B. A. (1975): Influence on touch, vibration and cutaneous pain of dorsal column stimulation in man. *Pain*, 1:257–270.
24. Lindblom, U., and Meyerson, B. A. (1976): Mechanoreceptive and nociceptive thresholds during dorsal column stimulation in man. In: *Advances in Pain Research and Therapy, Vol. 1*, edited by J. J. Bonica and D. Albe-Fessard, pp. 469–474. Raven Press, New York.
25. Lindblom, U., and Verrillo, R. T. (1979): Sensory functions in chronic neuralgia. *J. Neurol. Neurosurg. Psychiatry*, 42:422–435.
26. Livingston, W. K. (1943): *Pain Mechanisms*. Macmillan, New York.
27. Loh, L., and Nathan, P. W. (1978): Painful peripheral states and sympathetic blocks. *J. Neurol. Neurosurg. Psychiatry*, 41:664–671.
28. Loh, L., Nathan, P. W., and Schott, G. D. (1981): Pain due to lesions of central nervous system removed by sympathetic block. *Br. Med. J.*, 282:1–9.
29. Lombard, M. C., Nashold, Jr., B. S., and Pelissier, T. (1979): Thalamic recordings in rats with hyperalgesia. In: *Advances in Pain Research and Therapy, Vol. 3*, edited by J. J. Bonica, J. C. Liebeskind, and D. C. Albe-Fessard, pp. 767–772. Raven Press, New York.
30. Melzack, R., Jeans, M. E., Stratford, J. G., and Monks, R. C. (1980): Ice massage and transcutaneous electrical stimulation: Comparison of treatment for low-back pain. *Pain*, 9:209–217.
31. Melzack, R., and Loeser, J. D. (1978): Phantom body pain in paraplegics: Evidence for a central "pattern generating mechanism" for pain. *Pain*, 4:195–210.
32. Meyerson, B. A. (1983): Electrostimulation procedures. Their effects, presumed rationale, and mechanisms. In: *Advances in Pain Research and Therapy, Vol. 5*, edited by J. J. Bonica, U. Lindblom, and A. Iggo, pp. 495–534. Raven Press, New York.
33. Mitchell, S. W. (1872): *Injuries of Nerves and Their Consequences*. J. B. Lippincott Co., Philadelphia.
34. Ochoa, J. L., and Torebjörk, H. E. (1980): Paraesthesiae from ectopic impulse generation in human sensory nerves. *Brain*, 103:835–853.
35. Ottoson, D., Ekblom, A., and Hansson, P. (1981): Vibratory stimulation for the relief of pain of dental origin. *Pain*, 10:37–45.
36. Ottoson, D., Lundeberg, T., Håkansson, S., and Meyerson, B. (1981): Control of intractable chronic orofacial pain by vibratory stimulation. *Pain* (Suppl. 1):182.
37. Pertovaara, A. (1979): Modification of human pain threshold by specific tactile receptors. *Acta Physiol. Scand.*, 107:339–341.
38. Rasminsky, M. (1978): Ectopic generation of impulses and crosstalk in spinal nerve roots of "dystrophic" mice. *Ann. Neurol.*, 3:351–357.
39. Seltzer, Z., and Devor, M. (1979): Ephaptic transmission in chronically damaged peripheral nerves. *Neurology*, 29:1061–1064.
40. Stöhr, M., Petruch, F., and Scheglmann, K. (1981): Somatosensory evoked potentials following trigeminal nerve stimulation in trigeminal neuralgia. *Ann. Neurol.*, 9:63–66.
41. Sunderland, S. (1976): Pain mechanisms in causalgia. *J. Neurol. Neurosurg. Psychiatry*, 39:471–480.
42. Swerdlow, M. (1980): The treatment of "shooting" pain. *Postgrad. Med. J.*, 57:16–18.
43. Taylor, J. C., Brauer, S., and Espir, M. L. E. (1981): Long-term treatment of trigeminal neuralgia with carbamazepine. *Postgrad. Med. J.*, 57:16–18.
44. Thomas, P. K. (1979): Painful neuropathies. In: *Advances in Pain Research and Therapy, Vol. 3*, edited by J. J. Bonica, J. C. Liebeskind, and D. C. Albe-Fessard, pp. 103–111. Raven Press, New York.

45. Thomas, P. K., and Olsson, Y. (1975): Microscopic anatomy and function of the connective tissue components of peripheral nerve. In: *Peripheral Neuropathy*, edited by P. J. Dyck, P. K. Thomas, and E. H. Lambert, pp. 168–189. Saunders, Philadelphia.
46. Tinel, J. (1918): Causalgie du nerf median par blessure a la partie moyenne du bras; insuffisance de la sympathectomie periartérielle; guerison par la section du nerf au poignet. *Rev. Neurol. (Paris)*, 25:79–82.
47. Tomson, T., and Ekbom, K. (1981): Trigeminal neuralgia: Time course of pain in relation to carbamazepine dosing. *Cephalalgia*, 1:91–97.
48. Tomson, T., Tybring, G., Bertilsson, L., Ekbom, K., and Rane, A. (1980): Carbamazepine therapy in trigeminal neuralgia. Clinical effects in relation to plasma concentration. *Arch. Neurol.*, 37:699–703.
49. Torebjörk, H. E., and Ochoa, J. L. (1981): Intraneural microstimulation. A new method in sensory research. *Pain* (Suppl. 1):42.
50. Trontelj, J. V., Dimitrijevic, M. R., Galloway, B. L., Faganel, J., and Gregoric, M. (1975): Effects of vibration on pain in spinal cord injury patients. Abstract, First World Congress on Pain, Florence, Italy, Sept. 6.
51. Wall, P. D., and Cronly-Dillon, J. R. (1960): Pain, itch, and vibration. *Arch. Neurol.*, 2:365–375.
52. Wall, P. D., and Devor, M. (1978): Physiology of sensation after peripheral nerve injury, regeneration, and neuroma formation. In: *Physiology and Pathobiology of Axons*, edited by S. G. Waxman, pp. 377–388. Raven Press, New York.
53. Wiesenfeld, Z., and Lindblom, U. (1980): Behavioral and electrophysiological effects of various types of peripheral nerve lesions in the rat: A comparison of possible models for chronic pain. *Pain*, 8:285–298.
54. Yaksh, T. L. (1979): Central nervous system sites mediating opiate analgesia. In: *Advances in Pain Research and Therapy, Vol. 3*, edited by J. J. Bonica, J. C. Liebeskind, and D. C. Albe-Fessard, pp. 411–426. Raven Press, New York.
55. Yezierski, R. P., Wilcox, T. K., and Willis, W. D. (1981): The effect of zomepirac sodium on primate spinothalamic tract cells. *Pain* (Suppl. 1):247.

Advances in Pain Research
and Therapy, Vol. 7,
edited by C. Benedetti et al.
Raven Press, New York © 1984.

Recent Advances in Treatment of Trigeminal Neuralgia

Carlo Alberto Pagni

*2nd Chair of Neurosurgery and Aldo Pasetti, Center for Pain Research and
Therapy, University of Turin, 10126 Turin, Italy*

Many treatments for trigeminal neuralgia have been proposed: drug therapy with diphenilhydantoine (2) or carbamazepine (46); block or cutting of trigeminal branches (49); injection of alcohol (5), phenol (22), saline (39), or boiling water (18) into the gasserian ganglion and trigeminal nerve root; mechanical damage to the ganglion and root (23,40); decompression of the root by opening the dural sheets (44); partial or total retrogasserian rhizotomy by subtemporal extradural (7) or transdural (50) route; partial or total juxtapontine rhizotomy by posterior fossa approach (6); selective juxtapontine rhizotomy by transtentorial or posterior fossa route (19,36); and bulbar trigeminal tractotomy (41), among others. Each procedure has advantages and disadvantages, but the continuous effort to find a new and better method of treatment reflects the fact that pathophysiology of trigeminal neuralgia is far from clear and indicates that no method is fully satisfactory.

This chapter reports some current ideas on pathophysiology and treatment of tic douloureux based both on literature and personal experience. My experience stems from two sources: (a) study of 140 cases submitted before 1969 to Frazier's operation by the staff of the Neurosurgical Clinic of the University of Italy, Milan, of which I was a member and (b) study of a personal series of 85 cases treated with various methods and followed between 1970 and 1981 (Table 1; Fig. 1).

VASCULAR DECOMPRESSION OF THE TRIGEMINAL NERVE: JANNETTA'S OPERATION

On the basis of careful observation of the trigeminal root at the pons during posterior fossa approach, Dandy (6) suggested compression or distortion of the root could be the cause of tic douloureux; in some cases a small tumor encroached on the root, and its ablation eliminated the bouts of pain. Moreover, he observed that in almost every additional case of tic douloureux, a large arterial branch (superior cerebellar artery) lay on or under the root that was compressed and distorted. However, he cut the rootlets and did

TABLE 1. *Data on 85 patients with trigeminal neuralgia*

Sex
  Male 31; Female 54
Sides Involved
  Right 48; Left 35; Bilateral 2
Division Involved
  First 6; Second 28; Third 24; First + Second 9; Second + Third 16; All three
  branches 2
Associated Diseases
  Multiple sclerosis 1; Facial spasm 1; Glossopharyngeal neuralgia 1; Familial cases 2
Previous Treatments by Other Physicians

Acupuncture	3	Avulsion of peripheral branches	16
Sympathetic block	1	Cryosurgery of gasserian ganglion	1
Gasserian ganglion block with local anesthetic (LA)	2	Electrocoagulation of gasserian ganglion	1
LA block of peripheral branches	22	Posterior rhizotomy	8
Alcohol block of gasserian ganglion	8	Other	1

  Total: 63 procedures on 47 patients

Patients Not Subjected to Previous Surgery:	38

Treatments Applied by Author on 85 Patients

1. Medical pharmacologic therapy		11
2. Surgical therapy including nerve blocks		75
Surgery on peripheral branches	3	
Gasserian ganglion block with phenol	11	
Gasserian ganglion block with glycerol	1	
Percutaneous electric coagulation of gasserian ganglion and root	23	
Frazier's retrogasserian rhizotomy	7	
Juxtapontine rhizotomy via transtentorial route Total 7; sparing of intermediate fibers 5	12	
Juxtapontine rhizotomy via Dandy's posterior approach	17	
Jannetta's decompressive procedure	1	

not try simply to separate the root from the vessel distorting it. Others (10,36) made similar observations. Another cause of distortion of the root could be, according to Gardner et al. (11), the angulation of the trigeminal root over the petrous ridge, which on the basis of radiographic study in most of the cases seems to be higher on the side of the neuralgia.

Dandy's hypothesis was completely forgotten until recently when Beaver (1) and Kerr (24) demonstrated in tic douloureux changes of the posterior root consisting of disorganization, abnormal proliferation, degeneration, and loss of myelin sheets; eccentricity, hypertrophy, and tortuosity of axons; and modification of Nissl's substance of the gasserian ganglion cells. These observations renewed interest in Dandy's hypothesis.

Gardner (8,9) suggested that the cause of trigeminal neuralgia is in the nerve root. The continued gentle pressure exerted by small tumors, vascular loops, or the apex of the petrous bone causes deterioration of the nerve sheaths so that an artificial synapse develops in the root. Pain paroxysms result from the transaxonal excitation of pain fibers by impulses traveling

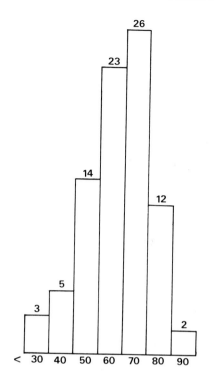

FIG. 1. Age distribution in 85 cases of trigeminal neuralgia.

in the nearby fibers. Afferent impulses resulting from a tactile stimulus activate the trigeminal sensory nucleus and from there pass to a parasympathetic nucleus, which in turn discharges a barrage of impulses to the periphery. As this efferent barrage passes the point of the root where the artificial synapse developed, it excites the naked pain fibers, giving rise to paroxysms of pain. This hypothesis was accepted by many authors who believe the minor damage inflicted to the root during Taarnhoj's procedure is effective in abolishing pain paroxysms in that it disrupts at least temporarily the artificial synapse.

In 1978 (35), I suggested a different pathophysiologic mechanism. The reported changes of the posterior root fibers alter more or less the input to the trigeminal nucleus or to a part of it, but usually do not cause objective sensory loss to crude sensory tests. More accurate techniques reveal a reduced number of pain and touch points or higher threshold of excitation in the painful area (29). Sometimes there is sensory loss even to crude clinical tests (9,45). The consequence of this is a minor deafferentation syndrome. In the cat, discrete partial deafferentation gives rise to localized hyperactivity with burst discharges or a repetitive firing pattern of single cells in the corresponding part of the trigeminal nucleus (3). Light tactile stimulation of nearby nondenervated areas gives rise to prolonged afterdischarges of the totally or partially denervated central neuronal pool (3). Loeser et al. (30)

recorded spontaneous discharges in deafferented neuronal pools of the dorsal horn, which is the homologue of the trigeminal nucleus caudalis in humans (16). My hypothesis is that damage to the posterior root gives rise to partial deafferentation of the trigeminal nucleus. Neuronal hyperactivity ensues, but it is subliminal. Pain attack develops only if paroxysmal afterdischarge is driven by peripheral subliminal or liminal tactile barrage.

The pathophysiologic mechanism of pain paroxysms is identical to that of the seizure in Amantea's reflex epilepsy. The cortical epileptic focus is subliminal and turns to a seizure discharge with clinical signs only when driven by peripheral sensory afferent stimuli (33). If that hypothesis is correct, it could explain all the clinical features of tic douloureux. One feature is its peripheral origin. In addition, like epilepsy, it is an unstable syndrome; its attacks occur at random. Bouts of pain usually are provoked by nonpainful stimuli to discrete trigger zones, by face movements, or by other mild stimuli. Spontaneous attacks probably are triggered by afferents not consciously perceived. There is a refractory period after each paroxysm found in epileptic seizures (27,33). Anticonvulsant drugs stop the bouts of pain (2,25,46). My colleagues and I demonstrated in 1961 that mephnesin blocks driving of interictal epileptic discharges into seizure activity both in human and experimental reflex epilepsy (for a review, see 31). Denervation of the trigger zone and painful facial area prevents afferent impulses from reaching the hyperactive trigeminal neurons in the descending nucleus, thus stopping pain paroxysms. Increasing frequency of pain paroxysms in nontreated patients probably is caused by the progressive increase of deafferentation due to persistence of pressure on the posterior root. After partial section of the posterior root, pain attacks may recur in other divisions; that may be because the process of deafferentation spreads, involving adjacent parts of the nucleus. Finally, definitive abolition of pain attacks follows total juxtapontine root section; it prevents any precipitating afferent impulses from reaching the trigeminal nucleus (36).

Observation of the root near the pons with the operating microscope convinced Jannetta (20,21) that, in every case, a neurovascular contact causes the pain. In about 85% of the cases, the superior cerebellar artery or one of its branches encroaches on the anterosuperior aspect of the root, compressing the second- and third-division sensory rootlets. Less often, the anterior inferior cerebellar artery pushes from below, forward, and upward, on the first-division rootlets (12); a vein courses alongside the nerve (21); a dense arachnoidal annulus constricts the root (36); or an aneurysm or small tumor distorts the root (9,21). Hardy and Rhoton (14) observed a high incidence of neurovascular contacts in patients who did not suffer from trigeminal neuralgia and believe neurovascular contacts observed at operation are merely coincidental.

However, Jannetta (21) was able to achieve total relief from pain in 93% of 411 cases by repositioning the artery away from the nerve, retaining it in its new position by means of a small piece of plastic sponge inserted between the nerve and artery, avoiding section of the root with the attendant sensory loss and possible dysnesthesia and sequelae. The follow-up period in Jannetta's series is now longer than 10 years.

The mechanism by which decompression works, according to Jannetta, is far from clear. If the nerve is not traumatized during the dissection, paroxysmal pain disappears, progressively fading away in the days or weeks that follow the operation. In my opinion, this is the proof that the disappearance of pain is due to the restoration of the normal afferent barrage on the partially deafferented trigeminal nucleus, with disruption of the pathologic hyperactivity.

THERMOCOAGULATION OF GASSERIAN GANGLION AND ROOTLETS

Electrocoagulation Technique

Electrocoagulation of the gasserian ganglion and rootlets was introduced by Kirschner in 1936 (26). It is based on the well-known principle that denervation of the trigger zone or of the area to which pain paroxysms are referred blocks pain attacks. The coagulation was performed with the aid of a stereotactic frame, using a percutaneous technique of inserting an electrocoagulating apparatus generally used for surgery under general anesthesia or anesthetic block of the ganglion. With this technique an "uncontrolled" destruction of the ganglion was achieved, with the obvious risk of destruction of undesired parts of the ganglion and denervation of undesired parts of the face (17,38).

The introduction of neuroleptoanalgesia allowed the performance of electrocoagulation in the semi-awake patient. It was possible to change the position of the needle to destroy the appropriate trigeminal division(s) and to control the resultant sensory defects (37,38). The use of short and low-intensity coagulations avoided the risks of large destructions of the ganglion with the related complications (facial and corneal anesthesia, keratitis, anesthesia dolorosa) (48). In that way, it was possible to perform a nearly "controlled" partial electrocoagulation of the ganglion.

The method was used in very large case series in the German-speaking countries for over 35 years. In skilled hands, it was a safe technique, with the mortality reduced to practically zero; keratitis occurred in about 1.3 to 5% of the cases, painful anesthesia in only 1.5% of the cases, and paresthesia in no more than 10% of the patients. The recurrence rate ranged from 13 to 80% in series with more than 30 years of follow-up (17,32,38); because it was feasible to repeat the procedure, however, about 95% of the patients were relieved without major complications (32,38). Despite these impressive results, this technique was not used widely outside of Germany.

Differential Controlled Thermocoagulation

An improvement of the technique was introduced by White and Sweet (49). They used an electrical generator of a precisely controlled heat source with special probes bearing small thermistors that measured the heat generated. The stimulation of the ganglion and root in the conscious patient allows the control of the exact positioning of the probe in the part of the trigeminal to be destroyed. A radiofrequency current is transmitted from the probe to the surrounding tissues where progressive increase of the temperature is generated. The procedure is based on the assumption that less myelinated fibers for pain (A-delta and C) are more vulnerable to heat than the heavily myelinated A-beta touch fibers. The hypothesis has been confirmed by experimental studies (4,28). Thus the procedure allows a differential destruction of pain fibers (43), and for that it is called *differential controlled thermocoagulation.*

The goals of the procedure are: (a) to denervate only the trigeminal branch(es), including the "trigger zone" or the branch(es) to which paroxysmal pain is referred; (b) to destroy only the thinly myelinated or unmyelinated nociceptive fibers, sparing the thickly myelinated touch fibers; and (c) to decrease the undesired intratrigeminal morbidity (i.e., excessive or inappropriate denervation of branches not involved in pain, thus avoiding anesthesia dolorosa, undesired corneal anesthesia, and keratitis). Technical details to avoid undesired side effects are discussed elsewhere (42,43).

Results seem to be excellent. All those who have used this technique have reported that the procedure works in nearly every patient. Because it may be repeated a few days later if the desired result is not achieved, or as soon as there is recurrence of pain, it is possible to produce short-term pain relief in nearly 100% of the patients. Complications of the procedure are minimal and practically limited to the trigeminal nerve. There is no operative mortality; oculomotor deficit with diplopia was observed in less than 2% of the cases and always was transient. Hearing loss, facial nerve palsy, hemiplegia, and aphasia were not reported. Herpes simplex was observed in about 3 to 15% of the cases. Transient dysphagia and aseptic meningeal reaction, always transient, were observed in a few isolated cases. Sweet (42) reported a late temporal abscess.

Trigeminal morbidity that may develop includes undesired sensory loss outside the involved division in about one-third of the patients. Unintended corneal anesthesia and keratitis was observed in about 1.5 to 5% of the patients, in some cases even if there was preservation of some corneal touch perception; in no case was there loss of sight owing to keratitis. The most consistent side effect was some disagreeable sensation on the face due to sensory loss—crawling, itching, burning, little electric shock-like cramps, stinging, and so on. However, painful anesthesia was reported in less than 2% of the cases. In the series of 484 cases reported by Sweet (42), only six patients (1.2%) experienced painful anesthesia. Only sporadic cases were reported in other series. Masticatory paralysis or weakness occurred in about 20% of the patients. This usually was partial and recovery was gradual or prompt and did not cause significant disability.

As far as long-term results are concerned, there are now large series with follow-ups of more than 10 years. The recurrence rates are as high as following subtemporal retrogasserian rhizotomy and range from 5.8 to 36%. However, because the procedure can be repeated on recurrence of pain in the coagulated branch or the development of pain in other branches, the final success rate reaches 95 to 99% (37,38,42,47). There is usually a direct relation between the persistence of sensory deficit and pain relief. Recurrence is easier if the sensory deficit disappears and sensation of the face recovers.

Currently, controlled percutaneous trigeminal thermorhizotomy seems to be the best and the most widely used method of treating patients with trigeminal neuralgia. It is much preferred to all other methods for the following reasons. Most patients affected by trigeminal neuralgia are elderly. Operative risk is minimal with the percutaneous procedure and mortality rate is zero even though a brief anesthesia is required; therefore, it can be performed regardless of the patient's age. Production of analgesia of the trigger zone and/or of the involved division(s) relieves virtually every patient. Hospitalization is very short, lasting no more than 2 to 3 days; patients can return to active life a few days later. The rate of recurrence is about the same as observed after partial posterior rhizotomy both by subtemporal route (Frazier's operation) or posterior fossa approach (Dandy's operation), or after Sioqvist's operation, but it is lower than following alcoholic nerve block or decompression-compression procedures (for reviews, see 49). Only two procedures seem to have lower rates of recurrence: juxtapontine rhizotomy, total or with preservation of the intermediate fibers (36), and Jannetta's vascular decompression (21). Both, however, entail a certain operative risk (mortality 0.5 to 2%). Moreover, total juxtapontine rhizotomy affords the risk of occurrence of painful anesthesia (34). The procedure may be repeated if pain recurs at long term, with a global success rate of about 95% so that only a few cases are to be submitted to other procedures (37,42,47). Distressing dysesthesia or painful anesthesia, which make the procedure a failure, are experienced by less than 1 to 2% of the patients, a much lower rate than following posterior rhizotomies of alcoholic block (for review, see 34). Only compression-decompression operations give a lower rate of painful anesthesia (for reviews, see 49), whereas Jannetta's operation never provokes it (21). The incidence of keratitis is reduced to about a quarter of that observed with surgical rhizotomies or alcoholic blocks. Finally, extratrigeminal complications that occur after other procedures occur only rarely and usually are transient.

NEW TRENDS

Two new techniques of treating trigeminal neuralgia that seem to produce peristent pain relief without operative risks or undesired side effects have been reported. These will be described briefly.

Bone-Wax Injection

Gleadhill (11) reported he was able to secure complete and permanent relief in 196 of 203 patients by injecting into Meckel's cavity a small mixture of bone-wax, phenol, and myodil. The needle point was placed into the cavity using Hartel's technique (15). Relief was gained in 163 patients by one injection; in 30 after a second injection; and in 3 after a third injection. There were no complications; sensation in the face was normal and the corneal reflex never was affected. The patients were discharged 3 to 4 hr after the procedure. The patients who were not helped subsequently were submitted to alcohol injection or trigeminal rhizotomy. Gleadhill believes that the bone-wax exerts a light pressure on the ganglion and root (blocking the artificial synapse?) and thus produces pain relief. Gleadhill has not published his results elsewhere, but he confirmed the results in a letter 3 years after he made the initial report.

Intracisternal Glycerol Injection

Another method was reported by Hakanson (13). In the course of developing a stereotactic technique for gamma irradiation of the trigeminal ganglion and root, he unexpectedly observed that the intracisternal injection of pure sterile glycerol rendered the patient completely free from the paroxysmal pain without producing any significant sensory loss. He then used the technique in 75 consecutive patients, including 3 of multiple sclerosis; 47 of the patients (63%) had had one or more prior surgical procedures, except neurectomy.

Technique

The patient is positioned in a rotating chair. Under local anesthesia, a thin, disposable lumbar puncture needle is introduced into the trigeminal cistern via the foramen ovale by Hartel's technique. Trigeminal cisternography with metrizamide is performed to ensure the intracisternal position of the needle. This is a necessary guide to the intracisternal injection of glycerol. If trigeminal cisternography fails, the method cannot be used; in fact, cerebrospinal fluid (CSF) could escape the needle even if it reaches the subarachnoid subtemporal space.

After the correct positioning of the needle tip has been verified, the metrizamide is evacuated and the patient is placed in a recumbent position for about 5 min. Then the patient is placed again in the sitting position and pure sterile glycerol in a total volume of 0.2 to 0.4 ml is injected slowly. After injection, the patient's head is kept in a ventrally flexed position for about 1 hr to prevent too rapid escape of the glycerol from the cistern. Glycerol is hyperbaric in front of the CSF so that it remains in the interolateral part of the cistern, which contains the rootlets.

Results

Results of the procedure seem to be excellent (13). After the first injection, 74 of 75 patients became completely pain-free. In the only patient who was unrelieved, a second injection was also unsuccessful. Seventy-three patients were followed up from 2 months to 4 years; 13 had a recurrence; only 4 of them required a second injection, which made them pain-free. Of the patients treated, 64 (86%) derived complete relief, 60 after one injection and 4 after two injections. In 9 patients the pain recurred but it was controlled with low doses of carbamazepine. In 3 patients who had continuous aching pain associated with the typical paroxysms, only the latter type of pain was abolished by the treatment.

In the experience of Hakanson (13), the method is not influenced by previous surgical procedures, such as peripheral-branches alcohol injection, injection of alcohol and phenol in the trigeminal cistern, or bulbar tractotomy. It is not indicated in patients previously submitted to operation on the ganglion or posterior root, such as Taarnhoj's operation or subtemporal rhizotomy, because these cause damage to the trigeminal cistern and thus it is unable to contain the glycerol.

The procedure did not produce any objective sensory loss at crude clinical examination, but about 60% of the patients who had glycerol injection as the first procedure reported a slight numbness on the face that usually faded away in a few weeks. None complained of disagreeable dysesthesia or painful anesthesia. Corneal sensation was preserved in all the cases, although a few had slight impairment of the corneal reflex. No patient developed keratitis. In about 50% of the patients, herpes appeared on the lips. There were no signs of injury to other cranial nerves or masticatory weakness. Thus this technique seems, to date, the best ever proposed; it is highly effective without producing serious complications, damage to the ganglion and root, or trigeminal or extratrigeminal morbidity.

Mechanism

The mechanism by which glycerol abolishes paroxysmal pain is not known. On the basis of some experimental data, Hakanson (13) suggests that glycerol is not a "neurolytic" agent that produces a prolonged nerve block, but may have a delayed effect on the excitatory fiber activity as a result of interference with the resynthesis of proteins, especially in previously demyelinated axons. That could explain why some patients have increase of paroxysms of pain for a few days immediately after treatment. The glycerol thus could reduce activity of a certain number of fibers, and that could be sufficient to reduce the afferent input that usually triggers paroxysms of pain. Another possibility is that the glycerol acts particularly on the denuded axons of the artificial synapse, abolishing the basic mechanism that triggers pain paroxysms (13).

I have used Hakanson's method in a unique case of tic douloureux with total relief at 2-months follow-up. I injected glycerol with phenol 3% in cases of continuous facial pain of unknown origin; there was no sensory facial loss, but pain was unrelieved.

CONCLUSIONS

During the last 10 years, a new era has opened up for treatment of drug-resistant tic douloureux. If the methods of Gleadhill (11) and Hakanson (13) prove effective in other hands, they should be the methods attempted first in every patient. If these methods fail, then percutaneous thermorhizotomy (49), which is nearly devoid of major complications but which still gives a rather high rate of recurrence, should be the method of second choice.

Other operations should be used only if a repeated trial with thermorhizotomy is unsuccessful. In that case, I believe a posterior fossa approach according to Dandy, with the operative microscope, is mandatory. It will be possible to ascertain if there is any compressive lesion (i.e., a small tumor that had escaped neuroradiologic investigations) or any arterial or venous loop distorting the trigeminal root. Eventually the lesion should be removed or an arterial decompression using Jannetta's technique should be performed. If no lesions or arterial compressing loops are found, total trigeminal rhizotomy sparing the motor root should be performed.

ACKNOWLEDGMENT

This paper was supported in part by grant CT790188304 of the National Research Council, Rome, Italy.

REFERENCES

1. Beaver, D. L. (1967): Electron microscopy of the Gasserian ganglion in trigeminal neuralgia. J. Neurosurg., 26:138–150.
2. Bergouignan, M. (1942): Cures heureuses de neuralgies faciales essentielles par le diphenylydantoinate de soude. Rev. Laryngol. Otol. Rhinol. (Bord.), 63:34–41.

3. Black, R. (1970): Trigeminal pain. In: *Pain and Suffering*, edited by B. L. Crue, pp. 119–137. Charles C Thomas, Springfield, Ill.
4. Broggi, G., and Siegfried, J. (1977): The effect of graded thermocoagulation on trigeminal evoked potentials in the cat. *Acta Neuroch. (Wien)*, (Suppl. 24):175–178.
5. Ciocatto, E. (1970): The management of trigeminal neuralgia. In: *Progress in Anesthesiology: The Proceedings of the 4th World Congress of Anaesthesiologists*, edited by T. B. Boulton, R. Bryce-Smith, and M. K. Sykes, pp. 274–275. Excerpta Medica Foundation, Amsterdam.
6. Dandy, W. E. (1934): Concerning the cause of trigeminal neuralgia. *Am. J. Surg.*, 24:447–455.
7. Frazier, C. H. (1925): Subtotal resection of sensory root for relief of major trigeminal neuralgia. *Arch Neurol. Psychiatry*, 13:378–384.
8. Gardner, W. J. (1962): Concerning the mechanism of trigeminal neuralgia and hemifacial spasm. *J. Neurosurg.*, 19:947–958.
9. Gardner, W. J. (1970): Trigeminal neuralgia. In: *Trigeminal Neuralgia: Pathogenesis and Pathophysiology*, edited by R. Hassler and A. E. Walker, pp. 153–174. George Thieme Publishers, Stuttgart.
10. Gardner, W. J., Todd, E. M., and Pinto, J. P. (1956): Roentgenographic findings in trigeminal neuralgia. *Am. J. Roentgenol.*, 76:346–350.
11. Gleadhill, C. A. (1975): Paroxysmal trigeminal neuralgia treated by injection not producing sensory loss: Results of 200 cases. In: *Abstracts of First World Congress on Pain, Florence, Italy, September 5–8, 1975*, p. 92.
12. Haines, S. J., Martinez, A. J., and Jannetta, P. J. (1979): Arterial cross compression of the trigeminal nerve at the pons in trigeminal neuralgia. Case report with autopsy findings. *J. Neurosurg.*, 50:257–259.
13. Hakanson, S. (1981): Trigeminal neuralgia treated by injection of glycerol into the trigeminal cistern. *Neurosurgery*, 9:638–646.
14. Hardy, D. G., and Rhoton, A. L., Jr. (1978): Microsurgical relationships of the superior cerebellar artery and the trigeminal nerve. *J. Neurosurg.*, 49:668–687.
15. Hartel, F. (1914): DieBehandlung der Trigeminusneuralgie mit intrakraniellen Alkoholein-spritzungen. *Deutsch. Z. Chir.*, 126:429–552.
16. Hasser, R. (1970): Dichotomy of facial pain conduction in the diencephalon. In: *Trigeminal Neuralgia: Pathogenesis and Pathophysiology*, edited by R. Hassler and A. E. Walker, pp. 123–138. George Thieme Publishers, Stuttgart.
17. Hubner, B. (1975): Remarks on the techniques of electrocoagulation of the Gasserian ganglion for trigeminal neuralgia. Experience with more than 900 operations performed in over 600 patients from 1952 to 1974. In: *Advances in Neurosurgery, Vol. 3, Brain Hypoxia, Pain*, edited by H. Penzholz, M. Brock, J. Hamer, M. Klinger, and O. Spoerri, pp. 314–315. Springer Verlag, Berlin.
18. Jaeger, R. (1959): The results of injecting hot water into the Gasserian ganglion for the relief of tic douloureux. *J. Neurosurg.*, 16:656–663.
19. Jannetta, P. J. (1967): Arterial compression of the trigeminal nerve in patients with trigeminal neuralgia. *J. Neurosurg.*, 26:159–162.
20. Jannetta, P. J. (1976): Microsurgical approach to the trigeminal nerve for tic douloureux. In: *Progress in Neurological Surgery*, edited by H. Krayenbuhl, P. E. Maspes, and W. H. Sweet, pp. 180–200. Karger, Basel.
21. Jannetta, P. J. (1981): Vascular decompression in trigeminal neuralgia. In: *The Cranial Nerves*, edited by M. Samii, and P. J. Jannetta, pp. 331–340. Springer Verlag, Berlin.
22. Jefferson, A. (1963): Trigeminal root and ganglion injections using phenol in glycerine for the relief of trigeminal neuralgia. *J. Neurol. Neurosurg. Psychiatry*, 26:345–352.
23. Jelasic, F. (1959): Uber die Behandlung der Trigeminusneuralgie mittels mechanischer Kompression des Ganglion gasseri durch das Foramen ovale. *Acta Neurochir. (Wien)*, 7:440–445.
24. Kerr, F. W. L. (1967): Evidence for a peripheal etiology of trigeminal neuralgia. *J. Neurosurg.*, 26:168–174.
25. King, R. B. (1958): The medical control of tic douloureux. Preliminary report on the effect of mephenesin on facial pain. *J. Neurosurg.*, 15:290–298.
26. Kirschner, M. (1942): Die Behandlung des Trigeminusneuralgia (nach Erfahrungen an 1113 Kranken). *Munch. Med. Wschr.*, 89:235–239;263–269.
27. Kugelberg, E., and Lindbom, U. (1959): Studies on the mechanism of pain in trigeminal neuralgia. In: *Pain and Itch Nervous Mechanisms*, edited by Ciba Foundation, Study Group 1, pp. 98–107. Churchill Ltd., London.

28. Letcher, F. S., and Goldning, S. (1968): The effect of radiofrequency current and heat on peripheral nerve action potential in the cat. *J. Neurosurg.*, 29:42–47.
29. Lewy, F. H., and Grant, F. C. (1938): Physiopathologic and pathoanatomic aspects of major trigeminal neuralgia. *Arch. Neurol. Psychiatry*, 40:1126–1134.
30. Loeser, J. D., Ward, A. A., and White, L. E. (1968): Chronic deafferentation of human spinal cord neurons. *J. Neurosurg.*, 29:48–50.
31. Maspes, P. E., Infuso, L., Migliore, A., Marossero, F., and Pagni, C. A. (1961): Emploi de la myanesine associee au metrazol comme methode d'activation en electroencephalographie. *Epilepsia*, 2:318–335.
32. Menzel, J. Piotrowski, W., and Penzholz, H. (1975): Long-term results of Gasserian ganglion electrocoagulation. *J. Neurosurg.*, 42:140–143.
33. Moruzzi, G. (1950): *L'epilepsie Experimentale*. Hermann et Cie, Paris.
34. Pagni, C. A. (1977): Central pain and painful anesthesia. In: *Pain: Its Neurosurgical Management. Part II: Central Procedures*, edited by H. Krayenbuhl, P. E. Maspeas, and W. H. Sweet, pp. 132–257. Karger, Basel.
35. Pagni, C. A. (1978): *Lezioni di neurochirurgia*. Ed. Cortina, Torino.
36. Pagni, C. A., and Maspes, P. E. (1975): Microneurosurgical treatment of trigeminal neuralgia by selective juxtapontine rhizotomy of the portio major sparing the intermediate fibers. In: *Advances in Pain Research and Therapy, Vol. 1*, edited by J. J. Bonica and D. Albe-Fessard, pp. 301–313. Raven Press, New York.
37. Schürmann, K., Butz, M., and Brock, M. (1972): Temporal retrogasserian resection of trigeminal root versus controlled elective percutaneous electrocoagulation of the ganglion of Gasser in the treatment of trigeminal neuralgia. Report on a series of 531 cases. *Acta Neurochir. (Wien)*, 26:33–53.
38. Schürmann, E., and Schürmann, K. (1975): Controlled and partial percutaneous electrocoagulation of the Gasserian ganglion in facial pain. In: *Advances in Neurosurgery, Vol. 3, Brain Hypoxia, Pain*, edited by H. Penzholz, M. Brock, J. Hamer, M. Klinger, and O. Spoerri, pp. 301–313. Springer-Verlag, Berlin.
39. Schwartz, H. G. (1955): Gasserian gangliolysis for trigeminal neuralgia. *South. Med. J.*, 48:189–192.
40. Shelden, C. H. (1966): Deploarization in the treatment of trigeminal neuralgia. Evaluation of compression and electrical methods, clinical concept of neurophysiological mechanisms. In: *Pain: Henry Ford Hospital International Symposium*, edited by R. S. Knighton and P. R. Dunke, pp. 373–386. Little, Brown and Co., Boston, Mass.
41. Sioquist, O. (1938): Studies on pain conduction in the trigeminal nerve. A contribution to the surgical treatment of facial pain. *Acta Psychiatr. Kbh. (Scand)*, (Suppl. 17):139.
42. Sweet, W. H. (1975): Percutaneous differential thermal trigeminal rhizotomy for management of facial pain. In: *Advances in Neurosurgery, Vol. 3, Brian Hypoxia, Pain*, edited by H. Penzholz, M. Brock, J. Hamer, M. Klinger, and O. Spoerri, pp. 274–286. Springer Verlag, Berlin.
43. Sweet, W. H., and Wepsic, J. G. (1974): Controlled thermocoagulation of trigeminal ganglion and root for differential destruction of pain fibers. Part 1: Trigeminal neuralgia. *J. Neurosurg.*, 39:143–156.
44. Taarhos, P. (1952): Decompression of the trigeminal root and the posterior part of the ganglion as a treatment in trigeminal neuralgia. Preliminary communication. *J. Neurosurg.*, 9:288–290.
45. Taarnhoj, P. (1956): Trigeminal neuralgia and decompression of the trigeminal root. *Surg. Clin. North Am.*, 36:1145–1157.
46. Taylor, J. C. (1966): Tegretol in the treatment of trigeminal neuralgia. *J. Neurol. Neurosurg. Psychiatry*, 29:478–479.
47. Tew, J. J. (1976): Percutaneous rhizotomy in the treatment of intractable facial pain (trigeminal, glossopharyngeal, and vagal neves). In: *Current Techniques in Operative Neurosurgery*, edited by H. H. Schmedek and W. H. Sweet, pp. 409–426. Grune & Stratton, New York.
48. Thiry, M. S. (1962): Experience personelle basee sur 225 cas de neuralgie essentielle du trigemineau traites par electrocoagulation stereotaxique du ganglion de Gasser entre 1950 et 1960. *Neurochirugla (Stuttg.)*, 8:86–92.
49. White, J. C., and Sweet, W. H. (1969): *Pain and the Neurosurgeon: A Forty-Years' Experience*. Charles C Thomas, Springfield, Ill.
50. Wilkins, H. (1966): The treatment of trigeminal neuralgia by section of the posterior sensory fibers using the transdural temporal approach. *J. Neurosurg.*, 25:370–373.

Advances in Pain Research
and Therapy, Vol. 7,
edited by C. Benedetti et al.
Raven Press, New York © 1984.

Reflex Sympathetic Dystrophy

*R. Rizzi, *M. Visentin, and **G. Mazzetti

*Department of Anesthesiology, Intensive Care, and Pain Relief and
**Department of Orthopedics, Regional Hospital, I-36100 Vicenza, Italy

There is evidence the burning pain and associated symptomatology following peripheral nerve injuries had been encountered and noted by Paré in the sixteenth century (4,32) and by others subsequently, but it was not until the American Civil War that an accurate description of causalgia as a clinical syndrome was given. In 1864, Mitchell et al. (29) described a number of cases of soldiers who sustained peripheral nerve injuries and who subsequently developed severe burning pain and other symptoms. Eight years later, Mitchell used the term *causalgia* for the burning pain (28). Although he did not use the term to designate a definite clinical syndrome but merely to denote the symptom of burning pain, his description of many cases manifesting this and other associated phenomena served the same purpose and his coinage achieved universal acceptance. A year later, Letievant of France, in an extraordinary monograph, discussed causalgia and related painful disorders with rare insight (21).

Following an indistinct description of the condition by several clinicians in the latter part of the nineteenth century (cf. ref. 4 for review), in 1900 Sudeck (39) published his classic description of the clinical features and radiographic characteristics of posttraumatic bone atrophy in the limb. During World War I, European surgeons reported a number of patients with causalgia following injury to a major nerve. The French surgeon Leriche (18) called attention to the role of the sympathetic system in the genesis of certain painful syndromes following war wounds. In 1915, he performed the first periarterial sympathectomy; soon after, he blocked the appropriate sympathetic chain with procaine to relieve the symptoms. Except for a few scattered reports, causalgia was forgotten until World War II when a large number of reports were published (for reviews, see refs. 4,5).

During the first five decades of this century, there were many reports of patients with symptoms similar to causalgia, but of a lesser degree and caused by factors other than major nerve injury. The following terms were used for these conditions (4,5,8,10,17,22,39):

1. Sympathalgia, algodystrophy, thermalgia, acute peripheral trophoneurosis, reflex nervous dystrophy

2. Neurovascular reflex dystrophy, neurovascular reflex sympathetic dystrophy, neurovascular posttraumatic painful syndrome

3. Posttraumatic sympathetic dystrophy, peripheral neuropathy, ascending neuritis, spreading neuralgia

4. Traumatic angiospasm, traumatic vasospasm, posttraumatic chronic edema

5. Sudeck atrophy or osteodystrophy, posttraumatic painful osteoporosis, posttraumatic painful arthritis or arthrosis, posttraumatic painful syndrome

6. Crush lesion, frostbite, shoulder-hand syndrome (following myocardial infarction and other diseases).

The precipitating factor may have been accidental or surgical trauma or one of a variety of disease states (4,5,9,10,13,14,18,21,38–40,44), but all were characterized by a varying degree of burning, aching pain, vasomotor and other autonomic disturbances, delayed recovery of function, and trophic changes. It was reported that if applied early, sympathetic interruption produced pain relief and disappearance of the pathophysiology. Because of these similarities, Bonica (4) suggested they all be considered under the generic term *reflex sympathetic dystrophy* (RSD). Earlier, Livingstone (22) noted a similarity between minor causalgia and posttraumatic pain syndrome and concluded they presented lesser degrees of the same pathophysiologic process as causalgia. Later Evans (10) used the term *reflex sympathetic dystrophy* for some but not all of the conditions included by Bonica.

Despite widespread and persistent acceptance of this classification, there still has been some confusion because a few researchers included cases not characteristic of RSD. Being from different disciplines, they viewed the symptomatology from their own particular perspectives. For example, Goldberg and Kennedy (12) reported cases of gynecologic cancer patients manifesting causalgia, and they used the terms *causalgia* and *RSD* interchangeably. Based on the response to chemical therapy, it is obvious that some did not fulfill the criteria for RSD. Moreover, some reports of RSD (or causalgia) have shown that ill-defined clinical entities were produced by various etiologies and that these conditions improved after therapies were initiated with totally different mechanisms of action than those of sympathetic interruption. This has led to a lack of homogeneity in the grouping of these conditions. It is noteworthy to mention that Bonica's book (4), in addition to being the most comprehensive volume on the management of pain published at the time, contains as one of its many assets, a systematic classification of pain syndromes. Three decades later, Bonica's classification is being used as the framework for development of a taxonomy by the International Association for the Study of Pain (IASP) (27). [The authors approve the decision of IASP to appoint a subcommittee on taxonomy to prepare definitions and classifications with the aim of avoiding misunderstandings (6,34).]

The purpose of this chapter is to further analyze the classification and compare the pathogenic and clinical pictures of causalgia and RSD, bearing in mind the statement supported by Bonica (4,5) and by Doupe et al. (8) that a positive response to sympathetic blockage is an essential criterion for including any condition in the RSD group.

DEFINITION

According to the IASP definition, causalgia is described as "a syndrome of sustained burning pain after traumatic nerve lesion combined with vasomotor and sudomotor dysfunction and later trophic changes." Causalgia was first used to describe symptoms of burning pain and vasomotor and sudomotor disturbances following injury to nerves by high-velocity missiles, but a large number of cases were described with symptoms similar to causalgia but without peripheral nerve injury, that occurred during peacetime, under the aforementioned various terms. Bonica has insisted (4,5) that due to its historical importance, and because it has such clear-cut and distinctive features, "causalgia" deserves exclusive use of this term, and the rest of the conditions should be considered under the term *reflex sympathetic dystrophy*. On the other hand, he has repeatedly pointed out that the basic mechanisms, pathophysiology, and symptomatology of RSD are similar to those of causalgia and require the same form of therapy to warrant including all of them under the generic term *reflex sympathetic dystrophy*.

Recently Tahmoush (41) used the McGill Pain Questionnaire to test homogeneity in a group of patients with symptoms suggestive of causalgia. All patients presented with continuous burning pain distal to the site of injury, hyperalgesia and allodynia (pain caused by nonnoxious stimuli) in the painful area, and a traumatic event occurring proximal to the painful area within weeks prior to the onset of the pain. Four patients had penetrating missile injuries and evidence of nerve damage; 4 had the onset of burning pain following surgery or trauma; and 3 had no clinical evidence of nerve damage. Tahmoush compared the scores from the McGill Pain Questionnaire for these 8 patients with published values for seven other conditions and found the pain descriptions chosen by patients with burning pain and nerve injury similar to those of patients without nerve injury; also, both of these differed from the reported meaning of the seven other painful conditions. Tahmoush concluded that the population of patients with burning pain, hyperalgesia, and allodynia was homogeneous whether or not a nerve lesion was present and that the underlying basic mechanism, pathophysiology, and diagnosis of both causalgia and the various RSD are the same (41).

Nathan (30) has had extensive experience with this problem and recently discussed the response to sympathetic blockade suggesting the neuropathophysiologic basis of the condition. He pointed out that the syndrome should be called reflex sympathetic dystrophy:

> *dystrophy*, because all of the tissues of the region including muscles and bones eventually waste, and there are abnormal growth features such as ridging of

TABLE 1. *Characteristics of causalgia and other reflex sympathetic dystrophies*

Characteristics	Causalgia	Reflex sympathetic dystrophy
Etiology		
Type	Partial major nerve injury	Accidental trauma: sprain, fracture, dislocation
Mechanisms	High velocity missile or violent injury	Surgical trauma: casts, amputation, chemical irritants
Site	Brachial plexus, median nerve, sciatic nerve	Peripherally in the limbs
Pain		
Latency	Immediate or after several days/weeks	Several days/months delay
Character	Burning, lancinating, spontaneous, continuous; without dermatomeric distribution, aggravated by tactile and emotional stimuli	Burning
Site	Distal	Distal
Sensory disturbances	Hyperpathia, allodynia	Hyperpathia, allodynia
Other symptoms	Alterations: vasomotor, neurovegetative, trophic, psychological	Alterations: vasomotor, neurovegetative, trophic, psychological
Therapy	Sympathetic blockade or surgical sympathectomy	Sympathetic blockade or surgical sympathectomy

the nails or hyperkeratosis of the skin; *sympathetic*, because there are features indicating abnormal sympathetic control such as inappropriate sweating, vasodilation or constriction, because the condition responds to sympathetic blocks, and because it is thought the condition spreads within the sympathetic system distribution; *reflex*, because the condition appears to spread from the lesion into the spinal cord and out via the sympathetic nerves.

Table 1 compares the characteristics of causalgia and reflex sympathetic dystrophy suggested by Bonica (4,5), Nathan (30), the IASP Subcommittee on Taxonomy (34), and Sunderland (40).

MECHANISM AND PATHOGENESIS

Bonica (4,5) reviewed the mechanisms of these conditions that have been proposed since the time of Mitchell. In 1872, Mitchell (28) proposed that "the irritation of a nerve at the point of the wound might give rise to changes in the circulation and nutrition of parts in its distribution, and these alterations might be themselves of a pain-producing nature." Moreover, he believed "nerve injuries may also cause pain which owing to inexplicable reflex transfers in the (spinal cord) centers may be felt in remote tissues outside the region which is contributory to the wounded nerve." A somewhat similar, though more sophisticated, hypothesis was proposed a year later by

Letievant (21) who stated there were three anatomic sites fundamental to the mechanisms: (a) the peripheral nerve and its point of irritation; (b) the spinal centers; and (c) the sensorium. He believed local irritation from an injury produced impulses that were transmitted to the spinal centers where abnormal neural activity developed and spread to adjacent centers if the impulses were strong and sustained. Consequently, in addition to those from the periphery, impulses from the spinal cord adjacent to the disturbed area also ascended to the sensorium and produced abnormal pain. Together, the peripheral and spinal impulses caused the peripheral phenomena associated with the pain.

In the ensuing seven decades, little attempt was made to further elucidate mechanisms of causalgia until 1943 when Livingston published his classic work on pain mechanisms (22). Others had published hypotheses and conceptual formulations on the basic pathophysiology of causalgia and other reflex sympathetic dystrophy. Some suggested, and indeed insisted, the primary site for pain mechanisms was in peripheral tissues (18,19); others believed it was in the peripheral nervous system (8); some suggested involvement of both the peripheral and central nervous system (5,22,30,32,45); others insisted the critical dysfunction was primarily or wholly in the spinal cord (40); and still others invoked higher structures in the neuraxis (26).

Peripheral Hypotheses

These emphasize the following phenomena:

1. Vasomotor balance in the affected area is altered by sympathetic hyperactivity (18,19) with subsequent liberation of algesic substances, thus producing hyperalgesia (14) and establishing and sustaining a vicious circle.

2. At the level of the lesion, electrical synapses (ephapses) are formed between efferent sympathetic and afferent pain fibers, and thus short-circuiting impulses (8). (This does not explain the efficacy of sympathetic block performed distal to the point of lesion, such as regional intravenous blockade with guanethidine.)

3. Noordenbos (32) suggested that high-velocity missiles selectively damaged large myelinated fibers causing loss of their inhibitory effects, thus facilitating the passage of an abnormal pattern of slowly conducted impulses, creating abnormal activity in the neuraxis.

4. Regenerating afferent fibers are stimulated by norepinephrine, touch, and blood flow (42).

Central Hypotheses

Several central hypotheses have been based on a number of considerations. The early observers of causalgia noted that pain and dystrophy spread along the affected limb and beyond it, eventually involving a body-quarter. The proponents of these hypotheses postulate that the nerve lesion creates abnormal activity in the dorsal horn of the spinal cord and/or higher up in the neuraxis. This abnormal activity could spread from the segment of entrance of the damaged fibers to neighboring segments and out along afferent nerves that end in the adjacent posterior segments of the dorsal horn (30). Further evidence of an abnormal state within the central nervous system (CNS) is also suggested by the phenomenon of allodynia. It has been suggested that mechanoreceptors and nociceptors converge on wide-dynamic-range dorsal horn cells in laminae IV to VI to produce an abnormal activity (30).

Sunderland (40) believes causalgia is a functional expression of the intensity of the retrograde neuronal reaction in which pools of dorsal horn neurons convert into foci of abnormal activity. To support this speculation, which he called the turbulence hypothesis, he marshalled well-established neuropathophysiologic evidence. Melzack (26) believes causalgia results from loss of normal sensory input from peripheral tissue to the brainstem reticular formation, which usually exerts a tonic inhibitory influence and which he calls the central biasing mechanism.

Carron (7) believes that to understand the pathophysiology of RSD, it is useful to try correlating the symptomatology with denervation hyperesthesia found in some humans following surgical interruption of the sympathetic chain supplying the extremities (20). In RSD, one can distinguish 3 stages: the "denervation phase" with increased blood flow; the "hypersensitivity phase" with increased sympathetic activity because of a hypersensitivity to circulating catecholamines; and the "reinnervation phase" when sympathetic reinnervation takes place (usually within 18 months) in all but 3 to 5% of the patients.

An unanswered question is why a causalgic syndrome more often develops after a partial rather than a complete nerve injury. A second question is why is there a low percentage of partial nerve lesions followed by this syndrome. Another issue is the role played by the individual's psychologic state at the time of the injury (40,44). Wirth and Rutherford (44) frequently found an altered emotional state; Owens (35) noted that 70% of patients had sympathetic hyperactivity before the injury. We agree with Bonica (5) who, in discussing the two conditions separately, considers the mechanisms and causes of causalgia and RSD to be similar and to involve abnormal activity in various parts of the peripheral and central nervous system.

THERAPY

Most writers have emphasized that the primary therapy is interruption of the sympathetic activity to the affected limb. For many years local anesthetic block of the sympathetic chain supplying sympathetic nerves to the upper or lower limb, if carried out early, proved an effective diagnostic and therapeutic procedure (4,5). Indeed, many writers believe if the condition is promptly diagnosed, treatment with a sympathetic block will prevent progression of the condition to the late phases characterized by trophic changes. In this regard, White and Sweet (43) suggest that in order to rule out emotional factors as being a prominent etiologic role, a placebo block with saline should be done before injecting local anesthetic. If a local anesthetic block of the paravertebral sympathetic chain supplying nerves to the region was effective but gave only transient relief, a sympathectomy should be done.

In 1974, Hannington-Kiff (15) introduced local block of sympathetic nerve endings in the limb with guanethidine administered intravenously using a tourniquet or blood pressure cuff to confine the drug to the affected limb. This technique was first suggested for patients who had previously submitted to sympathectomy in whom a ganglion block with local anesthetic was not considered possible, but, later, Hannington-Kiff (16) used it routinely. Giles (11) reported this technique was helpful in the diagnosis and treatment of reflex sympathetic dystrophy and vascular disease. Later, with the same objective in mind, Benzon et al. (2) injected reserpine and suggested regional intravenous block as an alternative to paravertebral block with local anesthetics. According to Loh and Nathan (23), the results are the same with either procedure.

A number of other therapeutic procedures have been suggested. Transcutaneous electrical stimulation has been reported effective in treating this condition by Richlin et al. (37), but others have noted application of transcutaneous nerve stimulation (TNS) results in increased sympathetic activity (1). Further studies are needed to clarify the role of TNS in treating RSD. Martelete (24) has reported that long-term results of acupuncture are similar to those of sympathetic block. The use of aprotinin is suggested by Noledy (31) in Sudeck's atrophy. Others have suggested beta blockers, corticosteroids, and biofeedback with discrepant results (3,25). Surgical posterior rhizotomy for this syndrome is not a good treatment because, in our experience, it aggravates pain and other symptomatology. Our results obtained with different therapeutic modalities further emphasized how far we are from an exact knowledge of the mechanism of this syndrome.

Personal Cases

During the period from March, 1963 to February, 1983, there have been 2,559 patients referred to our Pain Relief Unit. Of these, only 37 (1.5%) were diagnosed as having reflex sympathetic dystrophy. Of this group, only 16 fulfill the aforementioned criteria of burning pain, hyperesthesia, and allodynia; the rest were classified as "atypical cases." The latter group was further subdivided according to etiopathogenesis as (a) postsurgical; (b) postischemic of the central nervous system; and (c) neuropathies of various

TABLE 2. *Typical reflex sympathetic dystrophy*

Patients' initials	Sex	Age	Lesion	Symptoms	Time of onset after injury[a]		Type of blockade	No. of blocks	Results	
					Pain	Therapy			Immediate	Long-term
MP	M	48	Forearm fracture	Burning pain, atrophy, osteoporosis	2 mo	4 mo	CTSB	7	Very good	
DB	M	34	Brachial plexus avulsion	Burning pain, paresthesia, atrophy, vasospasm	6 mo	5 yr	CTSB	5	Very good	Poor (13 yr)
GE	M	38	Ankle sprain	Burning pain, atrophy, osteoporosis	1 mo	4 mo	LSB	20	Good	
CE	F	67	Shoulder bruise	Shoulder and upper limb burning pain	5 day	24 day	CTSB	18	Good	Good (5 yr)
ZN	F	30	Leg crush	Burning pain, paresthesia, hyperesthesia, allodynia	1 mo	4 mo	Sciatic block	15	Good	Poor (3 yr)
LV	M	32	Exposed fracture	Burning pain, paresthesia, vasomotor disturbance	2 mo	3 mo	LSB	15	Good	
SM	F	58	Advanced cervical arthrosis (operated on foramina enlargement)	Burning painful paresthesia, allodynia	2 mo	18 mo	CTSB	48	Good	Good (11 mo)

ZG	M	70	Metacarpal fracture	Burning pain, paresthesia, atrophy, osteoporosis	1 mo	40 day	CTSB	17	Very good	Very good (7 mo)
CL	M	23	Tibial fracture	Burning pain, edema, atrophy, osteoporosis	2 mo	3 mo	LSB	30	Very good	Fair (5 mo)
BR	M	21	Femoral nerve tear	Burning pain, paresthesia, atrophy, autonomic disturbance	1 yr	2 yr	LSB	20	Good	Fair (9 mo)
VG	M	40	Heel fracture	Burning pain, edema, osteoporosis	1 mo	2 mo	LSB + trigger points	10 8	Poor Good	Fair (2 mo)
PA	F	58	Femoral fracture	Burning pain, hyperalgesia, allodynia	1 mo	3 mo	LSB	10	Good	Poor (2 mo)
GA	M	65	Upper limb crush	Burning pain, atrophy, autonomic disturbance	3 mo	36 yr	CTSB	16	Good	Good (16 mo)
MF	M	60	Forearm tear	Lancinating pain, hypoesthesia, allodynia	10 day	3 yr	CTSB Guanethidine	12 3	Poor Fair	Poor (11 mo)
RM	F	41	Radial fracture	Lancinating pain, allodynia, edema, autonomic disturbance	20 day	7 day	Guanethidine	2	Good	Very good (6 mo)
DR	M	46	Wrist fracture	Burning pain, paresthesia, allodynia	1 mo	6 mo	CTSB	8	Good	Good

CTSB, cervicothoracic stellate block; LSB, lumbar sympathetic block.

TABLE 3. *Reflex sympathetic dystrophy (atypical cases)*

Patients' initials	Sex	Age	Symptoms	Time of onset after injury		Type of blockade	No. of blocks	Results	
				Pain	Therapy			Immediate	Long-term
After Surgical Trauma									
Radical mastectomy									
ZR	F	52	Pain, edema, motor impairment				5	Fair	
TT	F	69	Pain, edema, motor impairment				6	Very good	
GR	F	60	Pain, edema, vasomotor disturbances	3 mo	2 yr	CTSB	13	Good	Poor (18 mo)
MI	F	74	Pain, edema, skin atrophy	20 day	4 yr	CTSB	20	Good	Poor (14 mo)
CL	F	43	Pain, atrophy	10 day	1 mo	CTSB	10	Good	Poor (14 mo)
ME	F	60	Pain, edema, motor impairment	3 yr	7 mo	CTSB	5	Fair	Poor (3 mo)
TR	F	58	Burning pain, paresthesia, hyperesthesia, motor impairment	2 yr	1 mo	CTSB	13	Good	Fair (3 mo)
Surgical ant. and post rhizotomy									
PB	F	62	Pain, edema, atrophy, motor paralysis	10 day	4 mo	CTSB	10	Good	Poor (9 mo)
Hysterectomy									
AR	F	66	Pain, edema, dystrophy, motor impairment	5 day	3 yr	LSB	16	Very good	Good (2 yr)
Lumbar sympathectomy									
LI	F	74	Lancinating pain, allodynia	7 day	3 mo	LSB	12	Very good	Very (4 mo) good

After CNS ischemia

Shoulder-hand syndrome following hemiplegia

RG	M	66	Paresthesia, edema, vasomotor disturbance, osteoporosis	1 mo	6 mo	Suprascapular nerve block	8	Poor	Poor (13 mo)
MF	M	58	Pain, edema, vasomotor disturbance, osteoporosis	15 day	2 mo	CTSB	8	Good	Fair (8 mo)
SI	F	80	Pain, paresthesia, atrophy, osteoporosis	10 day	40 day	CTSB	8	Good	Good (2 mo)
MA	M	41	Pain, edema, vasomotor disturbance, osteoporosis	15 day	2 mo	CTSB	15	Good	Good (2 mo)
RA	F	50	Pain, paresthesia, edema, atrophy	15 day	3 mo	CTSB	10	Good	Good (1 mo)
BG	M	68	Pain, hypoesthesia, atrophy	1 mo	7 mo	CTSB	22	Good	Good (1 yr)
SM	F	67	Pain, paresthesia, vasomotor disturbance	20 day	4 mo	CTSB	16	Good	Poor (3 mo)

Neuropathies of different origin

Unknown

ZR	F	57	Pain and paresthesias		10 mo	Sciatic	16	Good	Poor (9 yr)

Perivenous pentothal injection

CG	F	61	Burning pain, paresthesia	immediate	1 mo	CTSB	1	Worsening of pain	

Diabetic

MR	F	62	Burning pain, paresthesia, edema		1 mo	LSB	10	Poor	Poor (3 mo)

After brachial plexus anesthetic block (axillary)

BG	M	74	Pain and paresthesia along ulnar nerve	7 day	5 mo	Guanethidine	4	Good	Poor (1 mo)

CTSB, cervicothoracic stellate block; LSB, lumbar sympathetic blocks.

origins. Although these subgroups were not considered typical RSD, they were included to ascertain the results of sympathetic block.

Material

All patients were treated with a series of sympathetic blocks using 10 to 15 ml of 0.5% bupivacaine injected by a technique proven to achieve interruption of all the sympathetic fibers to the upper or lower limb. For the upper limb, we used the classic anterior paratracheal technique to block the sympathetic chain from the middle cervical ganglion to the second thoracic ganglion, which although misnamed stellate block is really a cervicothoracic sympathetic block (CTSB) (4). For the lower limb, we used the paravertebral approach to produce blockade of the lumbar sympathetic chain (LSB).

The blocks were repeated every 24 hr until the pain and vasomotor disturbances disappeared, or until a significant number of blocks failed to produce the desired results. Hannington-Kiff (15,16) has cautioned against producing adhesions or scarring in the region of the sympathetic chain consequent to repeated injections. We have not encountered this problem even after a large number of procedures. In 2 patients we performed a sciatic nerve block, but we now consider this approach incorrect because, although the block does interrupt all the sympathetic fibers to the leg and foot, the procedure produces transient anesthesia and motor blockade. In 3 patients we produced intravenous regional sympathetic block with guanethidine. In one case the patient failed to respond to 12 CTSB, and guanethidine produced fair results. One patient who failed to improve with LSB obtained good results with local anesthetic injection of trigger points. We did not consider doing chemical or surgical sympathectomy because these cause prolonged side effects, such as Horner's syndrome after CTSB and lumbar neuralgia after LSB.

Results

The results were classified as follows: (a) poor, no change in symptomatology; (b) fair, some symptoms improved, but the overall results were less than satisfactory; (c) good, overall improvement of the syndrome associated with sporadic pain; and (d) very good, disappearance of all symptoms. The results were evaluated after a series of blocks and followed for varying periods of time.

The results are listed in Tables 2 and 3. In patients with positive results, pain relief was the first to disappear and, soon thereafter, vasomotor disturbances improved. In patients with atrophy of the skin and bones, regression of these pathologic changes required a longer period of time.

Discussion

Our results confirmed those reported by Bonica (4,5), Loh and Nathan (23,30), and others (7–10,18,22,33,35,36,38). When RSD is treated early, sympathetic blocks are effective in relieving the burning pain and other symptoms. The response duration varies from a few hours to several days. In a small number of patients treated with sympathetic block promptly after the onset of the disorder, the pain is permanently relieved with 2 or 3 blocks. In others, a larger series of blocks is necessary. Usually with each subsequent injection, the relief of pain, hyperpathia, and other symptoms become progressively longer. Eventually the patient is permanently cured, thus avoiding the necessity of chemical or surgical sympathectomy. Unfortunately, in many patients, a correct diagnosis is not made by the general practitioner or orthopedic surgeon, and sympathetic block therapy is delayed for months or years. In such cases, the results are less satisfactory, especially regarding improvement of trophic changes. In chronic advanced cases of RSD, sympathetic interruption should be supplemented with an aggressive program of physical therapy, exercise, and, in some instances, psychotherapy. Our results indicate this sympathetic blockade is more effective in "typical" than in "atypical" cases of the syndrome.

Although some patients with causalgia and other RSD may recover spontaneously, most will have a progression of the symptoms and develop trophic changes that eventually become irreversible. For this reason, we agree with Bonica (5) that all patients should be treated early with sympathetic blockade using either local anesthetic or guanethidine as both a therapeutic and prophylactic measure. We therefore also agree with all researchers who favor an immediate and complete intervention with sympathetic blockade associated with proper physiotherapy and psychotherapy.

SUMMARY

In the past, many pain syndromes with the same symptoms as causalgia but less severe and without major peripheral nerve injury have been included under the heading *reflex sympathetic dystrophy*. Although a number of other therapeutic procedures seem to provide some improvement of the symptoms, sympathetic blockade, if applied early, produces complete relief of the burning pain and other symptoms. We therefore share Bonica's opinion that a positive response to sympathetic interruption is a cardinal feature of causalgia and other reflex sympathetic dystrophy, and conditions that do not respond to this therapy should not be included in this syndrome.

REFERENCES

1. Abrams, S. E. (1976): Increased sympathetic tone associated with transcutaneous nerve stimulation. *Anesthesiology*, 45:575–577.

2. Benzon, H. T., Chomka, C. M., and Brunner, E. A. (1980): Treatment of reflex sympathetic dystrophy with regional intravenous reserpine. *Curr. Res. Anesth. Analg*, 59:500–502.

3. Blanchard, E. B. (1979): The use of temperature biofeedback in the treatment of chronic pain due to causalgia. *Biofeedback Self Regul.*, 4:183–188.

4. Bonica, J. J. (1953): *The Management of Pain*. Lea & Febiger, Philadelphia.

5. Bonica, J. J. (1979): Causalgia and other reflex sympathetic dystrophies. In: *Advances in Pain Research and Therapy*, Vol. 3, edited by J. J. Bonica, J. C. Liebeskind, and D. Albe-Fessard, pp. 141–166. Raven Press, New York.

6. Bonica, J. J. (1979): The need of a taxonomy. *Pain*, 6:247–248.

7. Carron, H. (1983): Discussion on sympathetic block in pain syndromes. In: *Pain Therapy*, edited by R. Rizzi and M. Visentin, Elsevier/North Holland, Amsterdam.

8. Doupe, J., Cullen, C. H., and Change, C. G. (1944): Post-traumatic pain and the causalgia syndrome. *J. Neurol. Neurosurg. Psychiatry*, 7:33–48.

9. Drucker, W. R., Hubay, C. A., Holden, W. D., and Bukovnic, J. A. (1959): Pathogenesis of post-traumatic sympathetic dystrophy. *Ann. J. Surg.*, 94:454–465.

10. Evans, J. A. (1947): Reflex sympathetic dystrophy: report on 57 cases. *Ann. Intern. Med.*, 26:417–426.

11. Giles, K. E. (1978): Intravenous guanethidine in the diagnosis and treatment of reflex sympathetic dystrophies and vascular disease: A clinical and laboratory study using radioactive xenon blood flow measurements and thermography. Abstract from the Second World Congress on Pain, 29.

12. Goldberg, M. I., and Kennedy, S. F. (1979): Reflex sympathetic dystrophy. Recognition and management in gynecologic oncology. *Gynecol. Oncol.*, 8:288–295.

13. Goldner, J. L. (1980): Causes and prevention of reflex sympathetic dystrophy. *J. Hand Surg.*, 5:295–296.

14. Hallin, R. G., and Torebjork, H. E. (1978): Observation of hyperalgesia in the causalgia syndrome. *Abstract from the Second World Congress on Pain*, 48.

15. Hannington-Kiff, J. G. (1974): Intravenous regional sympathetic block with guanethidine. *Lancet*, 2:1019–1020.

16. Hannington-Kiff, J. G. (1979): Relief of causalgia in limbs by regional intravenous guanethidine. *Br. Med. J.*, 2:367–368.

17. Homans, J. (1940): Minor causalgia: A hyperesthetic neurovascular syndrome. *N. Engl. J. Med.*, 222:870–874.

18. Leriche, R. (1916): De la causalgie envisagee comme une nevrite du sympathique et son traitement par la denudation et l'escision des plexus nerveux periarteriees. *Presse Med.*, 24:178–180.

19. Lewis, T. (1942): *Pain*. Macmillan, New York.

20. Litwin, M. S. (1962): Post-sympathectomy neuralgia. *Arch. Surg.*, 84:591–595.

21. Letievant, E. (1873): *Traite de Sections Nerveuses*. J. B. Bailliere et fils, Paris.

22. Livingston, W. K. (1943): *Pain Mechanism: A Physiological Interpretation of Causalgia and its Related States*, pp. 83–113. Macmillan, New York.

23. Loh, L., and Nathan, W. (1978): Painful peripheral states and sympathetic blocks. *J. Neurol. Neurosurg. Psychiatry*, 41:664–671.

24. Martelete, M. (1983): Therapy of causalgia and reflex sympathetic dystrophy. In: *Pain Therapy*, edited by R. Rizzi and M. Visentin, Elsevier Biomedical Press, Elsevier/North Holland, Amsterdam.

25. May, V., and Glowinski, J. (1979): Algoneurodystrophie, Traitement par les betabloquants. *Nouv. Presse Med.*, 8:1095.

26. Melzack, R. (1971): Phantom limb pain: implications for treatment of pathologic pain. *Anesthesiology*, 35:409–419.

27. Merskey, H. (1983): Development of a universal language of pain syndromes. In: *Advances in Pain Research and Therapy*, Vol. 5, edited by J. J. Bonica, U. Lindblom, and A. Iggo, pp. 37–52. Raven Press, New York.

28. Mitchell, S. W. (1872): *Injuries of Nerves and Their Consequences*. Smith Elder, London.

29. Mitchell, S. W., Morehouse, G. R., and Keen, W. W. (1864): *Gunshot Wounds and Other Injuries of Nerves*. J. B. Lippincott, Philadelphia.

30. Nathan, P. W. (1980): Involvement of the sympathetic nervous system in pain. In: *Pain and Society*, edited by H. W. Kosterlitz and L. Y. Terenius, pp. 311–324. Verlag Chemie, Deerfield Beach, Fla.

31. Noledy, L. (1978): Considerazioni sull'uso dell'aprotinina nel trattamento del morbo di SUDECK post-traumatico. *Chir. Organi. Mov.* 64:353–357.
32. Noordenbos, W. (1959): *Pain*. Elsevier/North Holland, Amsterdam.
33. Omer, G., and Thomas, S. (1971): Treatment of causalgia: review of cases at Brook General Hospital. *Tex. Med.*, 67:93–96.
34. Pain terms: A list of definitions and notes on usage (1979). *Pain*, 6:249–252.
35. Owens, J. C. (1957): Causalgia. *Ann. Surg.*, 23:636–643.
36. Procacci, P., Francini, F., Zoppi, M. and Maresca, M. (1975): Cutaneous pain threshold changes after sympathetic blocks in reflex dystrophies. *Pain*, 1:167–175.
37. Richlin, D. M., Carron, H., and Rowlingson, J. C. (1978): Reflex sympathetic dystrophy: Successful treatment with TEN. *J. Pediatr.*, 93:84–86.
38. Sternschein, M. J., Myers, S. J., Frewin, D. B., and Downey, J. A. (1975): Causalgia. *Arch Phys. Med. Rehabil.*, 56:58–63.
39. Sudeck, P. (1900): Uber die akute entzundlike knockenatrophie. *Arch. Klin. Chir.*, 62:147–156.
40. Sunderland, S. (1976): Pain mechanism in causalgia. *J. Neurol. Neurosurg. Psychiatry*, 39:471–480.
41. Tahmoush, A. J. (1981): Causalgia: Redefinition as a clinical pain syndrome. *Pain*, 10:187–197.
42. Wall, P. D., and Gutnick, M. (1974): Ongoing activity in peripheral nerves: The physiology and pharmacology of impulses originating from a neuroma. *Exp. Neurol.*, 43:580–593.
43. White, J. C., and Sweet, W. H. (1969): *Pain and the Neurosurgeon: A Forty-Year Experience*, pp. 87–109. Charles C. Thomas, Springfield, Ill.
44. Wirth, F. P., and Rutherford, R. B. (1970): A civilian experience with causalgia. *Arch. Surg*, 100:633–638.
45. Zimmermann, M. (1979): Peripheral and central nervous mechanisms of nociception, pain, and pain therapy: Facts and hypotheses. In: *Advances in Pain Research and Therapy*, Vol. 3, edited by J. J. Bonica, J. C. Liebeskind, and D. Albe-Fessard, pp. 3–32. Raven Press, New York.

*Advances in Pain Research
and Therapy, Vol. 7,*
edited by C. Benedetti et al.
Raven Press, New York © 1984.

Treatment of Myofascial Pain Syndromes

Anders E. Sola

*Department of Anesthesiology and Pain Service, University of Washington
Medical School. Seattle, Washington 98195*

Throughout medical history there have been references to numerous painful entities such as fibrositis, myalgia, myositis, and psychogenic rheumatism (3,13,14,20,21,26,29). The International Association for the Study of Pain prefers the term *myofascial pain syndromes* to describe these entities.

The most prominent complaint of myofascial syndromes is pain. This may be associated with fatigue, stiffness, limited range of motion, increased sensitivity to cold or chilling, and increased emotional response such as irritability and depression. Disturbed, non-rapid eye movement (nonREM) sleep patterns are common (19). Prolonged feelings of helplessness and despair are not uncommon, and myofascial pain is often associated with a premature sense of aging.

Myofascial syndromes occur with many other conditions and can intensify any pain phenomenon. They are also physical disturbances that can be treated in their own right and are characterized by the presence of highly localized, exquisitely sensitive, tender areas that can be identified by palpation. These are the trigger points. They usually are located within or near the pain reference pattern but may also be outside of it. In many patients, trigger point therapy is the key to control or reduce pain (2,22,27).

PHYSIOLOGY OF TRIGGER POINT PHENOMENON

The exact physiology of the trigger point phenomenon has not been identified; however, we know pain sensations are initiated or reinforced at these points, and treatment can disrupt the continuous cyclic pattern that produces and exacerbates pain. Research data suggest that trigger points are associated with a lowering of the pain threshold, are often associated with previous injury or overuse of muscle, and are particularly vulnerable to stressful stimuli (1,5,8,17). In addition, the presence of trigger points is influenced by genetics, personality, and physiologic status of the individual (Fig. 1).

Although trigger points can be observed clinically, the histologic evidence to substantiate their importance and mechanisms of influence is scant. Phys-

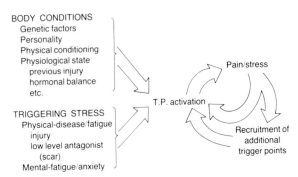

FIG. 1. Stress and body conditions. A variety of stress-inducing stimuli may be implicated in the onset of myofascial pain. The power of these stimuli to induce pain is moderated by the genetics, personality, conditioning, and physiologic state of a particular individual. Once established, however, a painful event may sustain itself despite control or elimination of the initiating stimuli.

iologic dysfunctions attributed to trigger point disturbances have been reported by Edagawa and Friedmann (7). More recent studies (13) show that muscle tissue taken from areas of tenderness in patients with primary fibromyalgia had a "moth-eaten" appearance. Adenosine triphosphate and phosphocreatine were much reduced in the patients with fibromyalgia; lactate values were normal, but glycogen concentrations were below normal, leading investigators to conclude that this may represent either a primary metabolic disturbance or overload secondary to muscle tension.

The mechanism can be described as follows. When a trigger point "fires" in response to a stimulus, impulses sent to the central nervous system result in physiologic changes such as muscle tension and vasoconstriction (Fig. 2). The local ischemia or increased vascular permeability that follow bring about changes in the extracellular environment near the trigger point, release of algesic agents, and osmotic and pH changes, all of which increase the sensitivity or activity of nociceptors in the area. This further increases sympathetic activity, and a cycle is established, producing continuous pain (Fig. 3).

As the patient becomes fatigued, additional trigger points flare up—first in the immediate area and then in areas more remote from the original point. Both the duration and spread of myofascial pain can be explained by cycles of responses, including well-defined pathways such as motor reflexes and less well-known autonomic feedback cycles and changes in the microenvironment of tissue (32). Autonomic concomitants often seen in association with trigger points include decreased electrical skin resistance, pilomotor reaction in the reference area, and vasodilation with dermatographia and skin temperature changes. I have also noted hypoesthesia in the involved extremities, local and general fatigue, fine tremor, muscle shortness, and weakness (24).

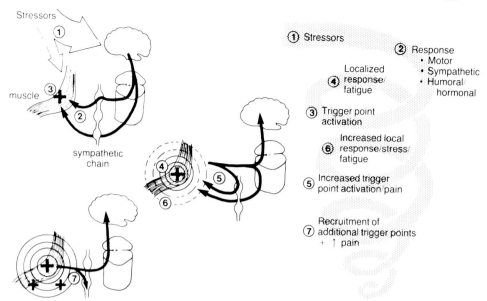

FIG. 2. The primary role. The individual, subjected to the physical and emotional stresses of daily living (*1*), responds with defense mechanisms that include various physiologic changes, such as splinting and bracing of muscles, vasomotor changes, increased sympathetic discharge, and hormonal and other humoral changes in the plasma and extracellular fluids (*2*). A particular point in a braced, stressed muscle or fascia that is more sensitive than the surrounding tissue—perhaps due to previous injury or genetic mandate—fatigues and begins to signal its distress to the central nervous system (*3*). A number of responses may result. The most readily understood involves the motor reflexes. Various muscles associated with the trigger point become more tense and begin to fatigue. Sympathetic responses lead to vasomotor changes within and around the trigger point. Local ischemia after vasoconstriction or increased vascular permeability after vasodilation may lead to changes in the extracellular environment of the affected cells, release of algesic agents (bradykinins, prostaglandins), osmotic changes, and pH changes, all of which may increase the sensitivity or activity of nociceptors in the area. Sympathetic activity may cause smooth muscle contraction in the vicinity of nociceptors, increasing their activity (*4*), which contributes to the cycle by increasing motor and sympathetic activity. This in turn leads to increased pain (*5*). The pain is shadowed by growing fatigue, adding an overall mood of distress to the patient's situation and feeds back to the cycle (*6*). As tense muscles in the affected area begin to fatigue in an environment of sympathetic stimulation and local biochemical change, latent trigger points within these muscles may also begin to fire, adding to the positive feedback cycle and spreading the pain to these adjacent muscle groups. The stress of pain and fatigue, coupled with both increased muscle tension and sympathetic tone throughout the body (conceivably with ipsilateral emphasis through the sympathetic chain), may lead to flare-ups or trigger points in other muscles remote from the initial area of pain (*7*).

NATURE OF COMPLAINT

As trigger point therapy is a relatively recent therapeutic modality, most of the patients who now are seen for treatment have a history of persistent pain or pain that has defied diagnosis. The initial complaint may be headache, neck pain, joint pains, backache, or sciatica-like pain in the buttocks and

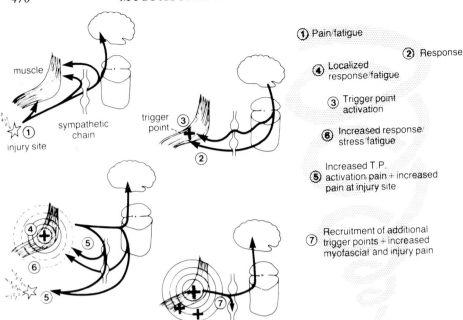

FIG. 3. The secondary role. Myofascial pain generated secondary to painful stimuli such as trauma, ligamental injury, facet lesions, or nerve root lesions follows the same course as myofascial pain due to nonpainful stress stimulators. In this situation, fatigue, muscle tension, and, perhaps, splinting, sympathetic activation, and extracellular fluid change in response to the painful stimulus lead to the initial myofascial pain. Subsequent events duplicate the primary course. In addition, the cyclic responses accompanying trigger point involvement may feed back on the initial pain stimulus. Conditions such as phantom pain, painful scars, or trauma to peripheral tissues often may stimulate trigger points in the segment and subsequently be affected. Thus conditions such as increased stimulation and increased levels of algesic agents in the blood may act with the increased emotional stress to the individual to prolong and intensify the pain and dysfunction at the site of injury.

lower extremities. Pain initiated or intensified by hyperactivity of trigger points can affect any part of the musculoskeletal structure.

In many cases, the patient has recently had a thorough medical evaluation that disclosed no positive findings to explain the pain. In other cases, the pain has been explained as a concomitant of a known condition or by association with a broad diagnostic category such as bursitis and sciatica. For some patients the pain experience is so nonspecific or so widely manifested that its etiology has been dismissed by more traditional clinicians as being psychosomatic in origin or having a strong psychosomatic component. Since living with pain has an effect on personality, it is difficult before treatment to determine if the pain is causing the personality disturbances or if psychologic needs are initiating or increasing pain.

One particular description of myofascial pain is extremely common when the pain experience is of long duration. The patient will suggest that one entire side of the body seems to be involved. He or she may be extremely aware of headache, neck, or shoulder pain, but also will remark on diffuse pain in the arm and some discomfort in the lumbar area, hip, and leg on the involved side. Some patients are more aware of the lower trunk or leg pain but will report gradiations of discomfort from mild to intense in the upper areas on the same side of the body.

Examination will confirm slight to moderate hemihypoesthesia, with all trigger points hyperactive compared to those in the contralateral muscles. Apparently what begins as a localized hyperactivity has the potential for generalizing to other segmental points and intensifying to severe sympathetic disturbance of one entire side of the body.

INJURY POOL CONCEPT

When a patient experiences pain of longer duration or higher intensity than that commonly associated with current medical concepts, the clinician should be alerted to possible activation of an "injury pool." This consists of prior injuries that may have been managed appropriately but resulted in localized abnormal metabolism, degenerative changes, or both. It also may include surgeries and injuries that were subclinical or asymptomatic.

In a thought-provoking paper, Gunn (11) suggests that peripheral pain disturbances often have their origin with a preexisting radiculopathy arising in sympathetic nerve fibers in the spinal root within the spinal canal and at the intervertebral foramina, resulting in a denervation supersensitivity with secondary myofascial disturbances and clinically observable trophic changes. However, sympathetic disturbances also remain after injuries not involving compromised nerves at the foramina. Wall and Devor (31) "investigated the dorsal root ganglion as a source of ectopic afferent impulses and the possibility that its discharge is exaggerated in the aftermath of a peripheral nerve lesion." This work concludes,

> It is generally presumed that afferent signals received by the spinal cord in normal animals arise exclusively in sensory nerve endings. The results described here show that . . . the dorsal root ganglion constitutes a second source of afferent impulses. . . . We have now shown that nerve injury also induces dorsal root ganglion cells to increase their tendency to discharge and bombard the spinal cord with ectopic sensory signals. Furthermore, individual axons may contain two loci of generation of afferent impulses, one in the periphery (sensory endings or neuroma) and the other in the dorsal root ganglion.

The dorsal root ganglia are described as contributing to a low level, spontaneous background discharge that is increased by slight mechanical pressure on the ganglion, as well as by nerve injury.

These findings are consistent with our clinical observations that the body seems to have a physiologic memory that recalls previous sympathetic disturbances, particularly in the same spinal nerve segments or in ipsilateral muscles. This is seen more clearly in young individuals who are likely to incur musculoskeletal injuries without involving the vertebral column.

Indications for Trigger Point Therapy

The main indication for trigger point therapy is pain that may range from a slight nagging pain to a sharp burning pain aggravated by movement. The pain may be intense and continuous or it may disappear at night. Morning stiffness is quite commonly associated with myofascial pain syndromes. Trigger point treatment is also useful to reduce pain associated with trauma because it speeds recovery and return to normal activity. It is sometimes useful to inject tight, shortened skeletal muscles without evidence of trigger points, as their condition suggests segmental reflex disturbance.

For some patients, treatment can reduce the pain to a level where a primary disease entity can be unmasked. A trial period of trigger point therapy may be indicated when a diagnosis is uncertain. When myofascial pain is secondary to a condition such as degenerative vertebral disease, nerve root lesions, or nerve compression, the patient usually will not respond to injection treatment, although at times some amelioration of pain occurs. Patients with hip and low back pain associated with late pregnancy are commonly relieved with this treatment, as are some patients diagnosed as having bursitis and sciatica; these terms are used broadly and may include many patients who actually have myofascial disturbance.

Contraindications for Trigger Point Therapy

Trigger point therapy is contraindicated for patients with systemic illness, particularly fever. It is not advisable to treat patients who have missed a meal, who show signs of alcohol intake, or who state that they do not feel well enough. The patient should be alert at the time of treatment because cooperation is essential. Treatment is also contraindicated for any patient with a high anxiety or emotional stress level in whom treatment might precipitate an emotional crisis.

The medical history should screen for patients who report hypersensitivity, syncopal reactions to injections, or possible allergic reactions to drugs of the caine family. Patients with fair skin, light or red hair, and blue eyes seem to have a greater tendency toward these reactions and may experience more intense flare-ups and pain after treatment. As a precaution, these patients should be treated in a recumbent position and should not receive injections at more than a few trigger points at the first visit. Administration of 50 to 75 mg of pentobarbital intravenously 5 min before local injections is sufficient to avoid psychogenic reactions that might otherwise limit the number of trigger points that can be treated at one session.

Examination Procedure

When dealing with patients in pain, the experienced practitioner will add significant information to the formal history-taking and examination through observation. The physician should observe the way the patient approaches the examining table, ease of movement while assuming the requested position, and efforts to limit movement or favor any part of the body.

In taking the history, the quality of the patient's voice may be more significant than the words in determining the amount and duration of pain. The voice gives clues to the amount of energy or fatigue, frustration, anxiety, or depression. Strident, impatient, and whining tones are also measures of the psychologic temperature of the patient. How much is said, or left unsaid, is as important as the appropriateness of the responses. Facial expression, on the other hand, often masks one's true feelings.

One of the best ways to measure the pain level throughout the entire treatment schedule is to monitor the voice. Pain impairs function and is intimately related to stress. It is also clear that the endorphins and enkephalins released as responses to stress have functions other than those suggested by their opiate-like activities. There is strong speculation that they play some role in the function of the brain related to mood, emotion, and behavior (10). This type of continued observation and intense listening is a very difficult, tiring chore for the busy physician, but in view of its diagnostic and therapeutic importance, it is worth the effort.

Many patients will be able to describe precisely where pain is experienced and the events associated with its onset. In myofascial pain, the symptoms are more commonly experienced in muscles innervated by the anterior division of the spinal cord segment, and the patient may be unaware of involvement of the posterior division pathways. A good clinical approach is always to examine all muscles associated with both the anterior and posterior divisions of the nerves that supply the affected muscle(s).

Muscles are examined in both relaxed and stretched positions, and any suspicious areas are compared with the contralateral muscle group. The examiner should not discontinue the search when the first trigger point is identified, but should continue in a systematic way to note all involved areas.

Skin texture, color, and temperature also provide evidence of myofascial disturbance. Often the patient describes a dry, itchy sensation that may be accompanied in chronic cases by an "orange peel" appearance when the skin is gently squeezed. This is associated with subcutaneous edema (12). The condition may be ipsilateral or segmental involving both sides. Minimal to moderate swelling of the extremities may be present in conjunction with these findings.

Examination of Head, Neck, Upper Limbs, and Upper Torso

Examination of the head, neck, upper torso, or upper extremities usually is done with the patient seated on the examining table. Beginning with the painful areas identified by the patient, the clinician proceeds to use fingertip palpation along the entire length of the involved muscles. Pressure on a trigger point usually will elicit a distinct pain reaction from the patient.

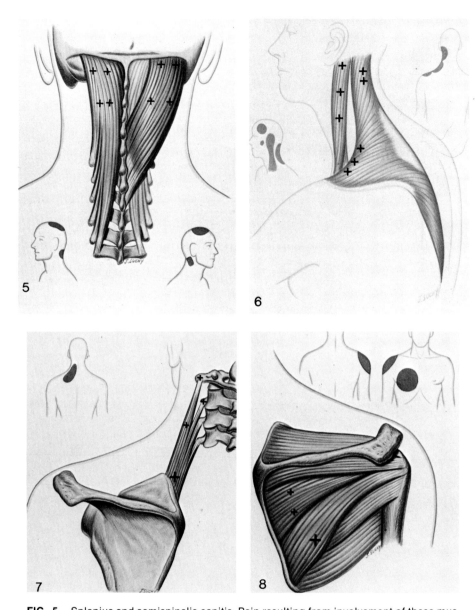

FIG. 5. Splenius and semispinalis capitis. Pain resulting from involvement of these muscles may be located over the muscles themselves. However, both the splenius and semispinalis can mediate pain to the head and face, and are commonly involved in headache. Occasionally, dizziness will accompany involvement of these muscles. Because trigger points are difficult to pinpoint in these muscles, patient cooperation in pointing out positions of maximum tenderness is extremely helpful.

FIG. 6. Trapezius and sternocleidomastoid. The trapezius is a frequent source of muscle pain and headache, especially at the angle of the neck or the muscle's occipital insertions where trigger points are most commonly located. When injecting trigger points at the angle of the neck, care must be taken to avoid the apical pleura. The sternocleidomastoid muscle is often a source of neck pain and headache. Also, dizziness and ipsilateral ptosis, lacrimation, and reddening of the conjunctiva have been reported in

Patients complaining of pain in the temporomandibular joint (TMJ) area, but with no clinical evidence of organic disease or structural abnormalities, are often classed as having psychosomatic complaints. However, TMJ pain, jaw pain, facial pain, unilateral tinnitus, pain deep in the ear, and trismus can all be caused by active trigger points. When clinically significant pain of this type is caused by skeletal muscle, it is almost always referred some distance from the source (6). Domnitz et al. (6) reporting on four cases referred to a department of oral surgery, successfully identified and treated trigger points in the sternocleidomastoid, digastric muscle, buccinator muscle, temporalis, and masseter regions, as well as in the TMJ area. Location of the trigger points and needling reproduced the pain experienced in various facial areas. In all cases, reported injection of anesthetic (0.5 to 1% lidocaine) eliminated the hypersensitive trigger point, alleviating pain of months-to-years duration. The procedure for examination and treatment has been developed and described in detail elsewhere (22,30).

A typical examination for the complaint of shoulder pain would include the following steps. After examination and range of motion have ruled out cervical lesions, the arthritides, shoulder tendonitis, and capsulitis, the patient is examined for myofascial trigger points. The patient should be positioned in such a way that the muscles can be examined in both a relaxed and stretched condition. Any suspicious areas are compared with the contralateral muscle group (Figs. 5–8).

The entire surface of the posterior scapula, scapula, and periscapular muscles is palpated for masses, tightness, or ropiness, paying particular attention to teres minor and major on the lateral border of the scapula, the supraspinatus and infraspinatus on the posterior aspect of the scapula, the rhomboid major and minor on the medial aspect of the scapula, and trapezius and levator scapulae muscles, which are invariably involved. Occasionally the serratus anterior and the subscapularis muscles have sensitive trigger points. One should not forget the erector spinae muscles. Postcervical and upper thoracic spinal muscles are examined to the midthoracic region. The

---

association with this muscle's involvement. Trigger points are most commonly located at occiput insertion in the upper two-thirds of the muscle, and often on its sternal and clavicular origins. The pain pattern may involve the muscle or refer to the ear region, the face, and the frontal area.

FIG. 7. Levator scapulae. Painful sensitive foci may occur at the origin on the superior medial aspect of scapula, along the entire flat muscle belly, or on the insertions on the transverse processes of the first four cervical vertebrae. Invariably, it is involved in chronic cervical conditions, as well as in torticollis. The pain usually is referred to the posterior cervical region, the posterior scalp, and the area around the ear. The levator scapulae muscles are supplied by the posterior division of the nerve.

FIG. 8. Infraspinatus. This muscle, a prominent member of the rotator cuff, is involved in many types of shoulder lesions. Careful palpation is necessary to locate trigger areas. It is useful to search the entire muscle along the length of the muscle bundles as well as across the "grain." Related pain is usually located on the posterior and lateral aspect of the shoulder and, occasionally, may return to the anterior chest. All of the scapular muscles are frequently involved, either singly or in concert with each other.

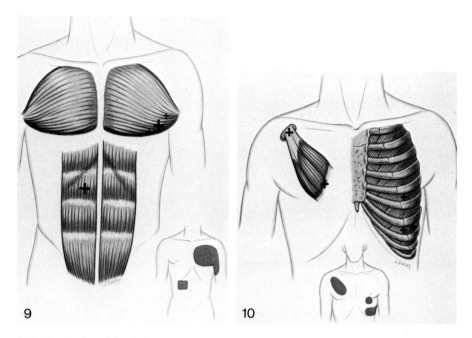

FIG. 9. Rectus abdominis and pectoralis major. The rectus abdominis muscles are common sites of anterior abdominal pain. The trigger points are best located with the patient supine with head and neck flexed so the abdominal rectus muscles are under tension. These trigger points often flare-up after abdominal surgery and can be one of the chief constituents of postoperative pain. They commonly are found in all segments of the abdominal rectus muscle and the pain usually is localized over the involved site of the muscle. The pectoralis major muscles are a frequent site of myofascial pain in the area of the muscle insertion on the anterior medial shoulder. The inferior belly of the muscle is a common area of trigger points; however, the entire muscle must be searched diligently. The clavicular part of this muscle usually refers pain to the uppermost part of the muscle. On occasion, there is some referral into the arm.

FIG. 10. Pectoralis minor and intercostal muscles. In the pectoralis minor, pain is deep and sharply circumscribed over the outline of the muscle when involved. Trigger points are most common near the origin and insertion of the muscle. The intercostals should be examined for chest pain routinely by palpating the intercostal spaces with the fingers because they often are involved after chest surgery or trauma. In treating chest pain, when intercostal blocks are not successful, care must be taken on injection to avoid entry into the pleural space. Pain from the exterior intercostal muscle usually is localized near the site of the trigger point and emphasized during inspiration.

longissimus, splenius, and semispinalis muscles extend from the C2 to the T6 level. Trigger points in these muscles not only cause neck pain but can influence shoulder pain. If a decisive trigger point is not located, the search is continued along the deltoid, triceps, and particularly the pectoral muscle groups (Figs. 9 and 10).

Whether or not upper torso examination reveals presence of clinical trigger points, the patient should be asked about pain in the lower back, hip, and lower extremities, especially on the ipsilateral side. Much therapeutic time can be wasted if this is not done because trigger points in these areas could affect treatment of head and neck and the upper trunk and extremities.

Lower Torso Examination

Examination of the lower torso usually is accomplished with the patient lying prone. Again, muscles are examined in both a relaxed and stretched condition. Trigger points in the gluteus medius may be the most important in the lower extremity because they can cause widespread lower back discomfort. It is uncommon for a patient to have pain in the gluteal area without also having sensitive trigger points elsewhere. A common interaction between the gluteal area and the cervical area may be expressed as headache or cervical pain. Trigger points in the erector spinae and gluteal area also can cause pain in the lower extremities.

The trigger points most commonly are located along the iliac shelf, and the entire shelf should be examined along the ridge under the anterior superior spine, and 1 to 2 inches below the iliac crest. When trigger points are found along the iliac crest, the tensor fascia lata, gluteal muscles, erector spinae, and quadratus lumborum all may be involved at the same time (Fig. 11).

The quadratus lumborum is also implicated in many painful conditions. J. Travell (*personal communication*) referred to this muscle as the "joker" because it is one of the most common causes of undiagnosed low back pain because it is covered by the erector spinae, it is difficult to palpate, and not much has been written about its role. Hyperactive trigger points in the quadratus lumborum can cause pain on deep inspiration (12th rib pain), can accentuate pain associated with abdominal surgery and scar tissue, and can contribute to pain referred as far as the head and neck area. Trigger points are most commonly located on the 12th rib, at the iliac crest, and along the lateral border of the entire muscle.

Examination of Lower Extremities

After examination of the upper and lower trunk, a systematic survey of the large groups of the thigh and the flexors and dorsiflexors of the ankle should be completed, covering the anterior and posterior divisions of spinal nerve segments. The same applies to upper extremities, with particular emphasis on flexors and extensors of the wrist and elbow and the supinator and pronator muscles, all of which are capable of causing pain (Figs. 12–14).

INJECTION THERAPY TECHNIQUES

Before treatment, an equipment tray is prepared containing a small (5-ml) syringe, a 26 ga. needle, alcohol for preparation of the injection site, and the solution of choice for local injection. I have obtained good results using normal physiologic saline for both moderate and severe pain (22–26). How-

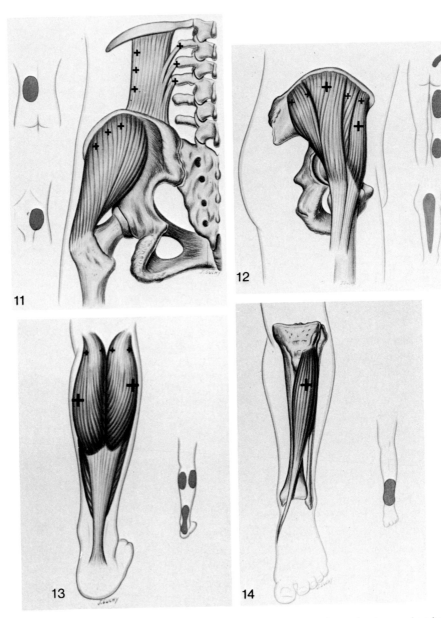

FIG. 11. Quadratus lumborum and gluteus medius. The quadratus lumborum has been referred to as the "joker" in the lower back syndrome and deserves this title. It is a hip hiker and lateral flexor of the spine. In addition, it assists respiratory function by anchoring the 12th rib for the pull of the diaphragm and often signals its distress on deep inspiration with pain of the 12th rib. Pain can be local or referred to the anterior abdominal wall and may accentuate postoperative pain or painful abdominal scars over the lower quadrant. Trigger points occur on the 12th rib, the iliac crest, and along the lateral border of the entire muscle. The trigger points in the gluteus medius may well be

ever, when a patient has a low pain threshold or is in severe pain, the use of 0.5% lidocaine or 1% procaine is advised unless contraindicated by known sensitivity.

It is preferable to have the patient lie on a table, even for head, neck, and upper torso injections, to prevent syncopal reactions. Gorrell (9) states that "location is not a contraindication to injection . . . if the underlying anatomic structure is understood. A sharp slender needle may be introduced into myofascial tissues without harm and without regard to the depth of injection in muscle provided sterile technic is followed."

The hypersensitive point is located and the area prepared for injection. The syringe is filled and 0.5 to 2.0 ml of solution is injected using a "fanning" technique with the needle repeatedly withdrawn part way and redirected. This assures maximum coverage of the trigger point area. If too much fluid is injected, the patient may feel achiness the next day. Immediately after injections, a moist hot pack is applied to the area temporarily to relieve local discomfort.

Few complications are associated with injections; however, it is appropriate to watch for signs of fainting. One monitoring technique is to touch the patient's skin with the back of your hand to detect excessive sweating. When local anesthetics are used in the injection rather than normal saline, the risk increases slightly; however, it is minimal if patients have been screened for allergies and excessive drug quantities and if intravenous injections are avoided. If the patient becomes faint or if there is any sign of complications, the injection should be stopped immediately. A few people have a hyperreaction to the injection several hours after treatment, usually during the night. Mild analgesics are provided or recommended to be used as necessary.

---

the most critical in the lower extremity. Activity of these trigger points often involves those in the quadratus lumborum, the tensor fasciae latae, and other gluteal muscles, thus inducing widespread lower back discomfort. There is also interaction between the trigger points of the gluteus and those in the cervical area, sometimes involving this remote muscle in cervical pain and headache. Although this muscle seldom causes pain without involving other muscles, the pattern most often attributed to the gluteus medius is along the iliac crest and into the posterior thigh and calf and is a common cause of hip pain in the later stages of pregnancy and simulates sciatica. The trigger points most commonly are found along the iliac shelf. With extensive involvement, the entire gluteal ridge, including the gluteal minimus and maximus muscles from the sacroiliac joint to the anterior superior spine, may contain painful trigger points.

FIG. 12. Tensor fasciae latae. This muscle is easy to examine, and it is easy to locate the common trigger points that are present in the muscle belly. Pain is usually referred to the lateral aspect of the thigh as far as the knee.

FIG. 13. Gastrocnemius/soleus. Myofascial pain related to this muscle is felt behind the knee, over the muscle bellies, and along the achilles tendon near the heel. Trigger points usually are found on the medial and lateral margins of the muscle group and along the midline of the group. These trigger points often flare-up when a patient is experiencing vascular problems of the lower extremities.

FIG. 14. Anterior tibialis. Pain in the anterior ankle usually is experienced when the trigger points of this muscle flare-up, although in severe cases the entire muscle may be painful. Trigger points are found most commonly in the upper one-third of the muscle, and pain is referred to the anterior part of the leg and into the dorsal part of the ankle.

Treatment of Trigger Points in Upper Torso

Myofascial pain is commonly associated with a number of muscles in the scapular area: the rhomboids, serratus anterior, subscapularis muscles, infraspinatus, and, at the superior edge, the levator scapular muscle. When injecting these scapular and periscapular muscles, extreme care should be taken to stabilize the scapula because the pleura is close to the injection site.

The patient should lie prone on a table with arms along the sides and a pillow under the chest to round the shoulders, facilitating injection. A small pillow may be used to rest the forehead. Landmarks should be carefully noted, and the patient should be warned not to move the shoulders. The rhomboids, serratus anterior, teres major-minor, and latissimus dorsi are easily treated.

The levator is best injected at an oblique angle to the muscle because patients often flinch during injection and deep injection could puncture the pleura. If painful areas exist on the lower medial border, placing the patient's hand behind his or her back will cause a "winging" of the scapula, allowing easier and safer injection with a laterally directed needle. Even the under-surface of the scapula can be reached in this way.

When injecting the infraspinatus, it must be remembered that the inferior apex of the scapula moves easily, and this could allow the injection to miss the inferior aspect totally and puncture the pleura. The patient must be warned not to move the shoulder or arm. I identify the superior and medial borders as landmarks and often hook a thumb on the medial border to stabilize it. Care must also be taken when treating the trapezius, as the apical pleura is higher than expected in some individuals.

The lateral and anterior intercostals are treated more easily by having the patient's arm positioned over the head. Localized muscle spasms may be very small, $\frac{1}{4}$ inch or less in width, and can be located by combing the ribs with the fingertips. A smaller needle, 27 gauge or less, is used, and is carefully inserted at an angle. The patient is less likely to tense up and change position if he or she has closed eyes and is not trying to watch the treatment procedure.

Treatment of Trigger Points in Lower Torso

Treatment of trigger points in the lower torso is generally uncomplicated because of the greater muscle bulk. The quadratus lumborum deserves special care because of the underlying kidneys and is best approached with the patient lying on his or her side on the plinth. The lateral margins of the muscle mass can then be identified.

Treatment of Extremities

The main concern of treatment to the extremities is to localize the trigger point. When it has been identified, injection is generally safe and easy. Bleeding into tissues may occur after injection, particularly in tight compartments of the forearm. If this should occur, treatment is followed with application of cold packs and compression rather than the warm packs normally recommended.

ADJUNCTIVE THERAPY

Follow-up treatment for patients with myofascial pain may include one or more of the following: repeated injection therapy, adjunct physical therapy, and special techniques such as intermittent cervical or lumbar traction, manipulation, relaxation techniques, ultrasound, periosteal stimulation (16), electrical stimulation, massage (especially deep friction), and coolant sprays using Travell's and Simons' techniques or ice packs (30). Cases involving minimal nerve damage may require 2 to 3 months of treatment with traction. The use of home traction units is not recommended for a medically or emotionally compromised individual unless supervised. Therapeutic exercises are prescribed routinely. I have found hyperextension exercises particularly useful for low back pain in addition to the routine flexion exercises (18).

SUMMARY

Myofascial pain is not a life-threatening entity, and the physiologic and historical findings to substantiate a patient's pain complaints are often meager. Approaches based on clinical observations are viewed with some apprehension by persons trained in scientific disciplines. For these reasons, many physicians are uncomfortable with treating myofascial pain. It is a neglected and ignored area. Yet the clinical evidence shows that persons can be relieved of debilitating and disabling pain through treatment approaches that have not been well studied. To deny their effectiveness because of a lack of understanding of why and how they work is to withhold potential relief through a therapeutic measure that is both medically safe and cost-effective.

Trigger point therapy is not a cure-all. However, when used in a comprehensive program of diagnosis, treatment, and management, it can provide dramatic pain relief for patients in whom hyperactive points in myofascia are a primary factor perpetuating pain. It can reduce pain when a myofascial pain cycle has been established secondary to other painful stimuli.

ACKNOWLEDGMENT

The author acknowledges the assistance of L. Dahm of the Educational Resources Center of the University of Washington in development and preparation of the manuscript, and Jim Suchy for the illustrations.

REFERENCES

1. Axelsson, J., and Thesleff, S. (1959): A study of supersensitivity in denervated mammalian skeletal muscle. *J. Physiol. (Lond.)*, 147:178.
2. Bonica, J. J. (1954): *Management of Pain*. Lea & Febiger, Philadelphia.
3. Bonica, J. J. (1957): Management of myofascial pain syndrome in general practice. *JAMA*, 164:732–738.
4. Bray, E. A., and Sigmund, H. (1941): The local and regional injection treatment of low back pain and sciatica. *Ann. Intern. Med.*, 15:840–852.
5. Cannon, W. B., and Rosenblueth, A. (1949): *The Supersensitivity of Denervated Structures*, Macmillan, New York.
6. Domnitz, J. M., Swintak, E. F., Schriver, W. R., and Shereff, R. H. (1977): Myofascial pain syndrome masquerading as temporomandibular joint pain. *Oral Surg.*, 43:11–17.
7. Edagawa, N., and Friedmann, L. W. (1981): *The Treatment of Disordered Function*. Exposition Press, Smithtown, N.Y.
8. Fink, B. R., and Cairns, A. M. (1982): A bioenergetic basis for peripheral nerve fiber dissociation. *Pain*, 12:307–317.
9. Gorrell, R. L. (1950): Musculofascial pain. *JAMA*, 142:557–600.
10. Guillemin, R. (1980): Beta lipoprotein and endorphins. In: *Implications of Current Knowledge, Neuroendocrinology*, edited by B. T. Kriege and J. C. Hughes, pp. 67–74. Sinauer Associates, Inc., Sunderland, Mass.
11. Gunn, C. C. (1980): Prespondylosis and some pain syndromes following denervation supersensitivity. *Spine*, 5:185–192.
12. Gunn, C. C., and Milbrandt, W. E. (1978): Early and subtle signs in low-back sprain. *Spine*, 3:267–281.
13. Henriksson, K. D., Bengtsson, A., Larsson, J., Lindstrom, F., and Thornell, L. E. (1982): Muscle biopsy findings of possible diagnostic importance in primary fibromyalgia (fibrositis, myofascial syndrome). *Lancet*, 2:1395.
14. Kraft, G. H., Johnson, E. W., and Laban, M. W. (1961): The fibrositis syndrome. *Arch. Phys. Med.*, 43:704–709.
15. Kraus, H. (1970): *Clinical Treatment of Back and Pain*. McGraw-Hill, New York.
16. Lawrence, R. M. (1978): New approach to the treatment of chronic pain: Combination therapy. *Am. J. Acupuncture*, 6:59–62.
17. Lomo, T. (1976): The role of activity in the control of membrane and contractile properties of skeletal muscle. In: *Motor Innervation of Muscle, Chapter 10*, edited by S. Thesleff. London Academic Press, New York.
18. McKenzie, R. (1980): *Treat Your Own Back*. Spinal Publications, New Zealand.
19. Moldofsky, H., and Scarisbrick, P. (1976): Induction of neurasthenic musculoskeletal pain syndrome by selective sleep stage deprivation. *Psychosom. Med.*, 38:35–44.
20. Simons, D. G. (1975): Muscle pain syndromes: Part I. *Am. J. Phys. Med.*, 54:289–311.
21. Simons, D. G. (1976): Muscle pain syndromes: Part II. *Am. J. Phys. Med.*, 55:15–42.
22. Sola, A. E. (1981): Myofascial trigger point therapy. *Resident Staff Phys.*, 27:38–46.
23. Sola, A. E. (1984): Trigger point therapy. In: *Clinical Procedures in Emergency Medicine*, edited by J. R. Roberts and J. R. Hedges. Saunders, Philadelphia (*in press*).
24. Sola, A. E. (1984): Upper extremity pain. In: *Textbook of Pain*, edited by R. Melzack and P. D. Wall, Churchill-Livingstone, Edinburgh (*in press*).
25. Sola, A. E., and Kuitert, J. H. (1955): Myofascial trigger point in the neck and shoulder girdle. *Northwest Med.*, 54:980–984.
26. Sola, A. E., and Williams, R. L. (1956): Myofascial pain syndromes. *Neurology*, 6:91–95.
27. Travell, J. (1960): Temporomandibular joint dysfunction. *J. Prosthet. Dent.*, 10:745–763.

28. Travell, J. (1976): Myofascial trigger points. In: *Advances in Pain Research and Therapy, Vol. 1*, edited by J. J. Bonica and D. Albe-Fessard, pp. 919–926. Raven Press, New York.
29. Travell, J., and Rinzler, S. H. (1952): The myofascial genesis of pain. *Postgrad. Med.,* 11:425–434.
30. Travell, J., and Simons, D. G. (1983): *Myofascial Pain and Dysfunction: The Trigger Point Manual*. Williams & Wilkins, Baltimore.
31. Wall, P. D., and Devor, J. (1983): Sensory afferent impulses originate from dorsal root ganglia as well as from the periphery in normal and nerve injured rats. *Pain*, 17:321–339.
32. Zimmermann, M. (1979): Physiological mechanisms in chronic pain. In: *Pain and Society*, pp. 283–298. (Report of Dahlem Workshop, Berlin, November 21–30, 1979) Verlag, Chemie Weinheim and Deerfield Beach, Florida, Basle, 1980.

*Advances in Pain Research
and Therapy, Vol. 7,*
edited by C. Benedetti et al.
Raven Press, New York © 1984.

Management of Low Back Pain

Harold Carron

*Department of Anesthesiology, University of Virginia Medical Center,
Charlottesville, Virginia 22908*

Each year millions of people experience acute or chronic low back pain, consuming a disproportionate part of health care resources throughout the civilized world. In many instances of acute pain and in most of those with recurrent or chronic low back pain, treatment may not be effective and the result may be a progressive physiologic and psychologic deterioration. Added to the pain are those additional stresses relating to work, social, and economic factors that tend to enhance the disability and impair the quality of life. While accurate statistics on the incidence of back pain are difficult to assess, in the United States alone it is estimated that one in 8 to 10 people will suffer from acute back disorders annually, 10% of these will require medical attention, and about 200,000 surgical explorations of the back will be performed for the relief of pain and disability.

The causes of low back pain are many and relate to infectious, degenerative, and malignant disease. Of greatest importance to society, however, are those low back disorders of musculoskeletal origin in patients in whom continued physical exertion during employment causes aggravation of the pain and increasing disability.

Published studies would suggest that most of the western cultures suffer a high incidence of back pain. A Swedish study by Hult (9) found that 60% of a sample of men ranging in age from 25 to 65 had suffered at least one episode of low back pain. Of this study population, 16% had been incapacitated for periods ranging from 6 weeks to 6 months, and 79% had had one or more bouts of low back pain. English studies would indicate that back pain is a significant social problem responsible for a high incidence of physician contact and increasing evidence of disability.

In the United States, in 1977–1978, there were about 15 million workers who suffered from major and minor injuries to the lower back. It has been estimated by Bonica (1) that, in 1980 alone, acute and chronic disorders of the back resulted in 165 million days of work lost due to low back pain. Low back pain is among the most common causes of disability in persons 18 years of age or older. It is estimated that among this group over 10 million have mild to moderate functional limitation. Three million have severe functional limitation. Over four million are not able to work at all; the rest have severe limitation in their capacity for productive activity. Estimated costs of health care for low back pain in the United States in 1980, according to Bonica (1), approached 25 billion dollars annually.

With these data in mind, and with the realization that with an increasing aging population the incidence of degenerative changes producing low back disability will consistently increase, it is essential that long-range plans be made for prevention of low back disability as well as improvement of function of those suffering from the physical, social, and emotional deterioration incident on chronic low back pain.

Among the most pressing social problems is the impact of low back pain on industrial productivity and the costs of industrial injury. Several characteristics of patients sustaining industrial low back injuries would tend to bear out the assumption that, in many instances, low back disability serves as a means of avoidance of unpleasant working conditions, job dissatisfaction, boredom of repetitive work manipulations, and continued heavy labor with advancing age. It has been shown that the closer the compensation payments for disability approximate the original income, the more protracted the disability. It also has been demonstrated that the period of disability shortens when the expected duration of compensation is limited as opposed to being open-ended.

In one group of patients reported by Johnson (10) from Washington state, almost 80% of patients sustaining low back injuries had complaints unsupported by physical findings, 60% were on dependency-inducing drugs, and 50% had sustained previous back injury. Of this group, there were a significantly large number who were overweight, had incomes less than the average wage, and were in nonsupervisory jobs. In this particular study, 16% of low back injuries were responsible for work time loss of 181 days or more, representing 84.6% of all time loss compensation.

EVALUATION

History

A careful and detailed history is essential for the differential diagnosis of low back disorders and for the identification of the psychosocial and economic factors influencing the attendant disability. The multiplicity of examinations to which the low back pain patient is subjected often leads to learned behavior of physician-expected responses. It is, therefore, essential that the examining physician not be confused by such learned behavior in determining the degree of physiologic derangement.

Information as to the onset of pain may help differentiate among systemic, traumatic, or degenerative processes (14). Long-standing chronic, low back discomfort without radicular signs is suggestive of either developmental abnormality or a degenerative process. The acute onset of low back pain secondary to excessive lifting, straining, or direct trauma followed shortly by the development of radicular pain in the lower extremity suggests lumbar disc extrusion. The spontaneous onset of pain without trauma in the middle-age to elderly patient may be a manifestation of a metastatic process to the lumbar spine.

The patient also should be questioned as to factors that influence the pain. Nerve root entrapment is characterized by dermatomal pain produced by coughing, sneezing, or straining at stool, or by prolonged sitting or standing. Most degenerative processes will produce pain on any activity, but the patient will be comfortable in the sitting or recumbent position. Most musculoskeletal pain is relieved by rest, but lumbar pain due to metastatic disease is unchanged with position or activity. Arthritic pain is worse on arising in the morning and improved with activity. All patients who have undergone laminectomy or fusion will, on occasion, undergo mechanical stresses that may cause low back pain and/or radiculopathy.

Complaints of dysesthesia, anesthesia, or motor weakness should be elucidated to determine whether they are global or dermatomal in nature. Low back pain associated with dysesthesias and pain in the lower extremities below the knee suggest either alcoholic or diabetic neuropathy. In these conditions, pain is usually bilateral.

With nerve root irritation, the initial complaint is usually a pain in the "hip" area that progresses distally, whereas sensory defects primarily are appreciated distally (6). Hip pain should be differentiated from low back pain by its aggravation through step climbing or internal or external rotation of the leg and by the absence of increased pain with impulse maneuvers.

An occupational history will reveal factors that aggravate the low back pain as well as delineate work satisfactions and work requirements that may be hazardous, overly difficult, and nonrewarding.

Physical Examination

The physical examination should consist of systemic, functional, and neurologic evaluations. Low back pain can result from aortic aneurysm with occlusion of the lumbar vessels or peripheral vascular disease producing low back pain through impairment of gait. Pelvic and rectal examination may reveal an oncologic basis for the low back pain.

For a complete musculoskeletal examination, the patient must be inspected unclothed in the standing position to determine the presence of scoliosis, lordosis, leg-length inequalities, and other postural deformities that may result in undue stress at the sites of nerve root emergence from the lumbar spine (13). The back should be inspected for muscle tenderness and spasm and the extremities for tenderness as well. Sagging of the inferior fold of the buttock occurs with S1 root lesions. With flexion of the trunk, nerve root irritation will produce deviation to the affected side. Degeneration changes with posterior joint lesions may be detected as the patient resumes the normal erect posture. At that time, the patient may tuck the pelvis under the spine, while flexing the knees and hips. Lateral movements are essentially unaffected by most lesions causing low back pain.

Spinal stenosis produces a constellation of clinical findings that are fairly characteristic of that condition. Uphill walking is easier than downhill. Sitting relieves pain. Bicycling is not impaired. There is increased pain on arising in the morning. A neurogenic intermittent claudication is often present. There are multiple radicular and bilateral findings on electromyography, with frequent involvement of higher radicular elements.

Heel walking toward and toe walking away from the examiner will reveal lesions of the L5 and S1 dermatomes, respectively. Squatting and resuming the erect position will elicit hip or knee pain if pathology in those areas is present. The patient should be requested to perform reverse straight leg raising in the erect position, since L3–L4 nerve root compression will provoke L4 dermatomal distribution pain.

With the patient supine on the examining table, the abdomen should be checked for masses or abnormal pulsations and the peripheral vessels for competence. The legs should be measured from the anterosuperior iliac spine to the superior border of the medial malleolus. Differences in leg lengths in excess of 2 cm may be sufficient to impair gait and produce postural back strain. Thigh and calf measurements should be at 15 cm cephalad from the lower border of the patella and 10 cm below the inferior border, respectively. At this point of the examination, all of the joints of the lower extremity should be manipulated to determine limitation of motion or duplication of pain complaints. A Patrick test should be performed, placing the heel of one foot on the patella of the opposite leg and then depressing the knee. Hip pathology as a basis for low back pain will be reproduced by this maneuver, as will internal and external rotation of the flexed knee at the hip joint.

Straight leg raising and the Lasègue maneuver should be performed. At the point at which the patient complains of radicular pain, foot flex or head lift should be performed. Both of these maneuvers produce increased stretch on the sciatic nerve and nerve root entrapment will increase, rather than decrease, the pain. Therefore, these movements should be performed with negative questioning (e.g., "Does this relieve the pain?"). With the Lasègue maneuver, the thigh is flexed to 90 degrees at the trunk with the knee bent. In a patient with nerve root entrapment, this should not produce discomfort. With extension of the knee, however, radicular pain will be elicited if there is nerve root entrapment. Straight leg raising also should be checked with the patient sitting. With the examiner seated in front of the patient, the patient is requested to extend the legs and flex the feet so that the soles of the feet can be examined for corns, calluses, or other abnormalities that might produce altered weight bearing. In the patient without nerve root entrapment, there will be no pain with this particular maneuver; in the patient with nerve root entrapment, the patient will lean back and away from the affected side on extension of the knees.

Neurologic examination should include the cranial nerves and sensory-motor examination of the upper extremity to rule out central neurologic disease or cervical spondylosis as a basis for the patient's pain. Sensory examinations should be performed with both light touch and pin prick; motor function should be assessed for all lumbar and first sacral dermatomes; and attempts should be made to relate dermatomal complaints to sensory changes in the extremity. Patellar reflexes should be elicited while the patient is sitting, ankle reflexes with the patient prone with knees flexed, and the tensor fascia femoris reflex with the Babinski maneuver. With an S1 lesion, this latter reflex will be absent.

The patient should be observed unobtrusively while undressing and dressing, since unobserved function may be different from that elicited during physical examination. Learned behavior that the patient associates with the particular disability results from repetitive examinations, and it may be necessary to observe the patient's gait as he or she leaves the facility to assist in determination of limitation of function.

Psychologic Evaluation

The psychosocial and economic aspects of low back pain are often of greater magnitude than the physical aspects in producing the degree of disability observed. Social factors involved are work dissatisfactions, as previously discussed, physical requirements of the patient's occupation, and lack of work opportunities. Secondary gain and familial interactions to the patient's pain all influence the degree to which the patient's physical impairment is related to total disability. It may be necessary to perform psychologic testing on pain patients, particularly after several months of chronic pain. These patients tend to fall within the same grouping of psychologic responses on tests such as the Symptom Check List-90 and the Minnesota Multiphasic Personality Inventory, with elevations in the scales of somatization, depression, and hysteria. Of these, somatization and depression are the most commonly found disorders. Depression may be perpetuated and aggravated by the use of depressant, narcotic, and muscle relaxant medications. It is imperative that all of these nonphysical factors be investigated in depth, particularly in those patients in whom the physical findings are inconsistent with the patient's complaints.

Special Studies

Special studies should be performed as required in the patient with low back pain. Although radiography will show the presence of degenerative changes and neoplastic involvement of the skeleton, radiographic findings cannot always be correlated with physical complaints or findings. Radiography is probably indicated for (a) severe back pain following significant trauma, (b) patients over age 50 with a history of pain without trauma, (c) obvious spinal deformity, (d) suspicion of ankylosing spondylitis, or (e) persistence of pain after treatment (14).

Of great diagnostic value and minimally invasive (in suspected nerve compression by disc, fracture, or osteoarthritis) is electromyography (EMG), preferably performed on the paravertebral muscles in the nonoperated back or on the peripheral musculature of the patient who has previously undergone laminectomy. Characteristically, nerve root lesions produce denervation changes in the muscles supplied by a single nerve root (11). With most root compression, not all of the supplied muscles will show denervation. As a peripheral nerve exits an intervertebral foramen, it divides into anterior and posterior primary divisions. The anterior division innervates the limb and the anterior and lateral trunk. The posterior division innervates the paraspinal muscles and the back. The segmental pattern of innervation is best defined in the deep paraspinal muscles, with the root level corresponding with the vertebral body adjacent to the muscle tested. After laminectomy, however, denervation of the paravertebral muscles occurs and EMG studies must be performed on peripheral musculature. Characteristic denervation changes are positive waves, reinnervation potentials polyphasic in character, and fibrillation potentials on needle insertion. Denervation changes rarely are seen less than 3 weeks after injury and reinnervation changes occur only after several months. Denervation and reinnervation changes in the muscles may persist even though there is no evidence for continuing injury. This diagnostic technique is accurate in about 85% of patients with back pain and/or radicular symptoms, and generally will assist in delineating the level of involvement (15). Myelography should only be done where surgical intervention is being contemplated for disk rupture or nerve root compression and should never be used as a routine diagnostic procedure. Its purpose is to rule out a neurogenic cause for the clinical picture and to localize the level of nerve root compression. Abnormal findings in disk herniation and rupture include deformity of the nerve roots, root sheaths, and of the neural sac.

Myelography is more specific than EMG in outlining the level and extent of nerve root entrapment, but may be less diagnostic in demonstrating hypertrophic osteophytic impingement on nerve roots.

Additional studies that may be of value are epidural venography and computed tomography scans. Epidural venography is particularly useful in the nonoperated back in detecting disk herniation at the L5–S1 level, where the dural sac is narrow and the epidural space is large. Venography will demonstrate a more lateral herniation where the nerve roots are no longer invested by arachnoid. Venography demonstrates the spinal epidural venous plexus where disk herniation produces deformity or nonfilling of the internal or intervertebral veins.

Computed axial tomography is most useful in the diagnosis of suspected spinal stenosis, intraabdominal tumors as a cause of back pain, or in the diagnosis of the extent, rather than the level, of disk herniation. The high resolution scanner can determine the presence of compression in the lateral recesses of the vertebral bodies. Radionuclide bone scan will detect neoplastic or inflammatory disease before radiographic changes can be observed.

Thermography has come into vogue as a diagnostic tool in evaluating pain, but current methods of interpretation are not yet statistically accurate and thermography does not replace other methods of evaluation (12). Thermography, a method of measuring heat or infrared radiation, reflects the cutaneous blood flow only and is not an accurate representation of the flow through underlying tissues. Generally, it represents the degree of cutaneous vasoconstriction or vasodilation, which, in turn, is a reflection of sympathetic activity.

In acute vascular trauma, temporary paralysis of sympathetic fibers may result in increase in cutaneous blood flow. This may be mimicked by any inflammatory process, the use of vasodilator drugs, heat, rebound from cold, or vascular (tourniquet) occlusion.

At a later stage of sympathetic denervation, the sympathetic receptors become hypersensitive to circulating catecholamines. Therefore, decrease in cutaneous blood flow may be seen as a "cold" area on thermography and can occur as a response to injury, cold, emotional upsets, vasoconstrictor drugs, tension, and exercise. After surgery on the nerve roots, it is possible for the thermogram to show "hot" or "cold" areas, depending on the extent to which sympathetic fibers are damaged during nerve root exploration.

It is not possible thermographically to date an injury with a high degree of accuracy because sympathetic stimulation or denervation responses vary with the type and extent of the injury. Thermographic changes also can reflect changes in sympathetic tone that result from spontaneously occurring medical disorders, such as osteoarthritis and other degenerative changes that cause impingement on nerve roots. Diabetes mellitus also may produce abnormalities unrelated to trauma.

Thermography is not necessarily diagnostic of trauma but may assist in the evaluation of chronic pain disorders by identifying sympathetic activity as a concomitant to other physical findings. To use thermography as the sole determinant of chronic pain due to trauma is to approach the problem in a simplistic manner.

Assumptions based on thermography are fraught with the hazard that self-induced trauma cannot be differentiated from trauma in the immediate or remote past.

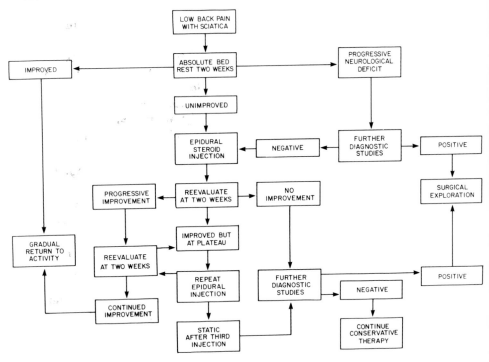

FIG. 1. Sequential therapy for low back pain and sciatica. Conservative treatment. (From Carron, ref. 3, with permission.)

TREATMENT MODALITIES

Conservative Management of Acute Low Back Pain

The first treatment for acute low back pain should be conservative, with a minimum 2- to 3-week period of absolute bed rest on a hard mattress. Pelvic traction during this period is of little value other than to maintain the patient in bed because distraction of the lumbar spine by acceptable weights is not possible. For acute muscle spasm accompanying acute back pain, ice massage is far more effective than heat, and analgesics should be administered on a schedule rather than on a demand basis. Gentle manipulation of flexion, extension, and rotation of the trunk, as well as stretching, may be useful in relieving muscle spasm. As improvement occurs, the patient should be instructed in modified Williams exercises. Return to full activity should be gradual (Fig. 1).

If "hard signs" of nerve root compression are present, such as radicular distribution of pain, impulse discomfort, positive EMG or myelographic findings, sensory deficits consistent with pain complaints, motor weakness, and depressed or absent reflexes, the patient can be treated with epidural steroid blocks (8). The use of epidural steroids is based on decreasing the edema and inflammation of a nerve root compressed by a herniated disk. The epidural steroid (50 mg of triamcinolone diacetate or 80 mg of methylprednisolone) combined with 3 to 5 ml of 1% lidocaine should be injected epidurally at the site of nerve root entrapment. The local anesthetic is used as a "marker" to indicate that the epidural space has been entered. The patient is then instructed to perform straight leg raising. Improvement of pain indicates an effective block and the patient is instructed in knee-to-chest flexion exercises to be performed on a regular basis.

The patient should be seen again in 2 weeks. At that time, if improvement has been noted and is continuing, no further injection is done, but the patient is followed at another 2-week interval. If, during the previous 2 weeks, the patient has improved but has reached a plateau in pain relief, the steroid injection is repeated. If, however, no sustained improvement is noted at the 2-week interval, no further injections are done and further investigative procedures (e.g., EMG, myelogram, venogram) are performed. After one or two blocks in the patient with acute herniated disks, significant changes will be noted in the level and duration of pain, sensory and motor deficits will decrease, and reflex changes will be reversed. If, however, the patient sustains immediate improvement of pain after block and remains comfortable for 4 to 5 days but then returns to previous symptomatology, or if he or she demonstrates "breakthrough" of the pain on straight leg raising beyond 90 degrees immediately after block, the possibility of central extrusion of an intervertebral disk should be entertained; myelography is indicated.

The safety of the procedure is attested to by the relative dearth of complications and the large series of reported successes. Animal studies by Delaney et al. (4) have shown that at least a single injection of tramcinolone has no neurolytic effect on the meninges, spinal cord, or nerve root sleeves.

Another conservative measure consists of facet block for those patients with limitation of function and muscle spasm in the back without radicular symptoms. Edgar (5) studied the nerve supply of the facet joints and found that the medial branch of the posterior ramus of the spinal nerve gave off small filaments to the facet joints. He stimulated the lumbar facet joints with hypertonic saline and was able to reproduce radicular pain. He then injected a series of patients with local anesthetic alone or with a depot steroid and reported 66% improved at 48 hr, with about 50% improvement at 1-year follow-up. The technique may be useful in relieving the spasm and rapidly improving function. The procedure is performed under biplaner fluoroscopy.

The procedure is performed by inserting a fine needle into both the superior and inferior facets at the level of suspected irritation as well as one level above and below. Local anesthetic in small volumes is injected at each facet, and relief is prompt. Exercise programs should be instituted immediately after the block in order to maintain mobility and prevent recurrence of muscle spasm. More permanent destruction of the filaments can be obtained through the use of phenol blocks, radiofrequency rhizolysis (16), or by cryotherapy (2).

TABLE 1. *Protocol for conservative
treatment of chronic back pain*

Somatic pain modulation
  Epidural or facet blocks
  Transcutaneous electrical stimulation
  Trigger point injections
Pharmacological
  Nonsteroid, nonnarcotic analgesics
  Tricyclic antidepressants
  Phenothiazines
Physical reconditioning
  Exercise program
  Graded activity schedule
  Vocational retraining
Psychological
  Relaxation training
  Biofeedback
  Counseling

The unoperated chronic back pain patient with radiculopathy and attendant chronic pain should be treated with pain modulation through epidural blocks, facet block, or transcutaneous electrical stimulation (Table 1). Investigations by Shealy et al. (17) on electrical stimulation for relief of pain led to the use of the dorsal column stimulator for pain relief. In developing screening techniques to identify suitable patients, they found that noninvasive transcutaneous stimulation was effective in 80% of pain patients. More recent studies would indicate somewhere between 30 and 60% improvement, particularly in patients with denervation dysesthesias or degenerative disk disease. The electrodes may be applied paravertebrally or along the course of the sciatic nerve. A progressive exercise program should be instituted, providing first stretching and then muscle strengthening.

Pharmacologic Management

Antidepressants, scheduled nonsteroidal anti-inflammatory drugs, and antianxiety drugs should be added to the regimen. The anxiety associated with acute back pain often leads to depression when the pain becomes chronic. Depression is manifested by disturbance of the circadian rhythm, alterations in life-style, loss of interest in social and sexual activities, and drug abuse. Perhaps the most useful pharmacologic agents in the management of chronic back pain and depression are the tricyclic antidepressants. The depressed patient with high residual anxiety state and sleep disturbances will respond best to the serotonin reuptake inhibitors (doxepin, amitriptyline, nortriptyline), whereas the patient with low psychomotor activity responds better to the norepinephrine reuptake inhibitors (imipramine, amoxapine). These drugs have the additional advantage of producing analgesia through descending modulating systems.

Nonsteroidal anti-inflammatory analgesics should be prescribed on a scheduled basis to prevent, rather than treat, pain. Their anti-inflammatory action is useful in decreasing nerve root edema and inflammation by prostaglandin synthesis inhibition.

When considerable anxiety persists, the use of the phenothiazines should be considered. Because of the possibility of development of tardive dyskinesia with this group of drugs, pulsed therapy with 2 to 3 weeks' withdrawal every 3 months is recommended.

Psychologic Therapy

Psychologic intervention in the treatment of low back pain should be directed at teaching the patient to accept limitations imposed by the pain and coping mechanisms to learn to function despite it. The patient must learn to control the pain rather than vice versa.

Relaxation training, autosuggestion, and biofeedback are all useful techniques in decreasing the awareness and responses to pain. This training by mental health professionals provides the time and opportunity for other psychotherapeutic measures.

Patients with chronic low back pain without "hard signs," including those who are suffering from the residuals of low back and leg discomfort after laminectomy, also should be treated conservatively, but nerve blocks are not indicated. Trigger point injections, however, may be helpful, as might transsacral nerve blocks for pain limited to the lumbosacral area or upper sacrum.

Of importance in the rehabilitation of the chronic back pain patient is the physician's involvement in the patient's socioeconomic problems to help solve compensation, social security disability, and other litigation issues. The physician should be honest in the evaluation of the patient's potential for either return to work or permanent disability. It may be necessary to contact employers recommending changes in employment or limitation of physical activities.

Neurosurgery

There is little place today for neurosurgery in the treatment of either acute or chronic back pain except in the patient with disk extrusion into the central canal or progressive neurologic deficit including bladder and bowel dysfunction. Under these conditions, laminectomy should be prompt after appropriate diagnostic procedures.

Most authors report good results of 30 to 85% after lumbar disk surgery via laminectomy. In 1978, Williams (18) developed a technique of microlumbar diskectomy in which he performed the procedure through a 2.5-cm incision, avoided laminectomy and facet trauma, used no electrocautery in the epidural space, approached the disk through blunt penetration of the annulus instead of by scalpel incision, and did not curette the disk space. Goald (7) subsequently reported on 803 patients with previously unoperated backs in whom he performed microlumbar diskectomy for disk herniation. He reported good results, defined as ability to work without narcotic drugs, in 90.7% of patients after the initial operation. An additional 7.3% achieved a good result from reoperation. Long-term follow-up was not reported, however.

SUMMARY

Conservative therapy is the keynote in the management of low back pain and sciatica. Duration of pain and disability may be decreased markedly by early intervention with multimodal therapy. Invasive surgical procedures should be reserved for those patients with disks extruded into the spinal canal or any instance of progressive neurologic deficit despite adequate therapy.

REFERENCES

1. Bonica, J. J. (1982): The nature of the problem. In: *Management of Low Back Pain*, edited by H. Carron and R. McLaughlin, pp. 1–16. John Wright-PSG, Inc., Littleton, Mass.
2. Brechner, T. (1981): Percutaneous cryogenic neurolysis of the articular nerve of Luschka. *Regional Anesth.*, 6:18–22.
3. Carron, H. (1982): Epidural steroid therapy for low back pain. In: *Chronic Low Back Pain*, edited by M. Stanton-Hicks and R. Boas. Raven Press, New York.
4. Delaney, T. J., Carron, H., Rowlingson, J. C., Butler, A., and Jane, J. J. (1980): Effect of epidural steroids on nerve roots and meninges. *Anesth. Analg.*, 59:610–614.
5. Edgar, M. S. (1973): The applied anatomy of lumbar facet innervation. Orthopedic Conference, Rancho Los Amigos Hospital. Presented September 8, 1973.
6. Finnesa, B. E. (1980): *Low Back Pain*. Lippincott, Philadelphia.
7. Goald, H. J. (1982): Microlumbar discectomy. *Resident and Staff Physician*, 28:60–64.
8. Goebert, H. W., Jullo, S. J., Gardner, W. J., and Wasmuth, C. E. (1960): Sciatics: Treatment with epidural injections of procaine and hydrocortisone. *Cleve. Clin. Q.*, 27:191–197.
9. Hult, L. (1954): Cervical, dorsal, and lumbar spinal syndromes: A field investigation of a nonselected material of 1200 workers in different occupations with special reference to disc degeneration and so-called muscular rheumatism. *Acta. Orthop. Scand.*, (Suppl.):17.
10. Johnson, D. (1982): Unpublished data, 1978 in Carron, H.: Compensation aspects of low back claims. In: *Management of Low Back Pain*, edited by H. Carron and R. McLaughlin. John Wright-PSG, Inc., Littleton, Mass.
11. Johnson, E. W., and Melvin, J. L. (1971): Value of electromyography in lumbar radiculopathy. *Arch. Phys. Med. Rehabil.*, 52:238–243.
12. Karpman, H. L., Knebel, A., Semel, C. J., and Cooper, J. (1970): Clinical studies in thermography. II. Application of thermography in evaluating musculoligamentous injuries of the spine–a preliminary report. *Arch. Environ. Health*, 20:412–417.
13. Keim, H. A. (1973): Low back pain. In: *Clin. Symp.* 25(3).
14. Macnab, I. (1978): *Backache*. Williams & Wilkins, Baltimore.
15. Shea, P. A., Woods, W. W., and Werden, D. H. (1950): Electromyography in diagnosis of nerve root compression syndrome. *Arch. Neurol. Psychiatry*, 64:93–104.
16. Shealy, C. N. (1975): Percutaneous radiofrequency denervation of spinal facets. Treatment for chronic back pain and sciatica. *J. Neurosurg.*, 43:448–451.

17. Shealy, C. N., Mortimer, J. T., and Roswick, J. B. (1967): Electrical inhibition of pain by stimulation of the dorsal columns: preliminary clinical report. *Anesth. Analg.*, 46:489–491.
18. Williams, R. W. (1978): Microlumbar discectomy: A conservative surgical approach to the virgin herniated lumbar disc. *Spine*, 3:175–182.
19. Wood, P. H. N. (1976): Epidemiology of back pain. In: *The Lumbar Spine and Back Pain*, edited by M. Jayson. Grune & Stratton, New York.

*Advances in Pain Research
and Therapy, Vol. 7,*
edited by C. Benedetti et al.
Raven Press, New York © 1984.

Advances in the Management of Cardiac Pain

Vittorio Pasqualucci

*Second Department of Anesthesiology and Pain Therapy, Ospedale Policlinico,
06100 Perugia, Italy*

Effective relief of severe or very severe pain associated with acute myocardial infarction remains an important and pressing task for physicians (4–6). This importance stems from the following considerations. Myocardial infarction is one of the most frequent causes of severe or very severe acute pain. Although most physicians usually treat the pain effectively, in all too many instances it is not completely relieved. This is due to improper administration of systemic (narcotic) analgesics—the most frequently used therapy—and/or the ineffectiveness of these drugs in relieving the pain completely. Equally important, systemic analgesics do not beneficially affect the associated pathophysiology and produce well-known, adverse side effects. Therefore it is desirable to complement or substitute narcotics with other therapeutic modalities that, though usually available, are not well known and/or not considered by general physicians and cardiologists. These include inhalation analgesia; various techniques of regional analgesia that specifically and completely interrupt nociceptive pathways from, and sympathetic pathways to, the heart; and intraspinal narcotics.

To underscore the importance of promptly relieving the pain and fully appreciate the value of alternative therapy, it is desirable to first describe the pathophysiology of nociception and acute pain in general and those of pain of myocardial infarction in particular. This is followed by a summary of the advantages, disadvantages, and side effects of (a) narcotics administered systemically via intravenous or intramuscular route, (b) inhalation analgesics, (c) cervicothoracic sympathetic block with local anesthetics, (d) segmental epidural block, and (e) intraspinal narcotics. Finally a summary of results obtained in a controlled clinical study of the effects of intraspinal narcotics on respiration is presented to provide evidence that this method does not produce respiratory depression, provided excessive doses of narcotics are avoided.

BIOLOGY AND PATHOPHYSIOLOGY OF MYOCARDIAL INFARCTION PAIN

It has long been widely appreciated that pain of acute injury or disease, such as myocardial infarction, has the important biologic function of signaling to the patient that something is wrong and of prompting the patient to limit activity and to seek medical counsel. Pain is also used by physicians as a diagnostic aid. Moreover, the tissue damage initiates local biochemical changes and segmental and suprasegmental reflex responses that are intended to help the organism maintain homeostasis during the initial phase of the disease. Bonica (4–7) has repeatedly emphasized that what has not been recognized or fully appreciated is that once the pain and associated responses have served their biologic function, they must be promptly terminated because persistent reflex responses often become abnormal and aggravate the pathophysiology.

In the chapter on postoperative pain (*this volume*), Benedetti and Bonica describe, in some detail, the local biochemical changes and reflex responses that are likely to occur in the postoperative period following injury to viscera and somatic tissue inherent in intraabdominal operations. There is impressive evidence that a variety of tissue injuries, including myocardial infarction, produce a similar set of physiologic and pathophysiologic responses with only minor variations (49). The following is a brief overview of the pathophysiology of acute myocardial infarction previously described by Bonica (5–7), and is intended to provide the background for evaluation of various modalities.

Tissue damage from myocardial ischemia and mechanical changes of the ventricles consequent to an acute infarct produce local biochemical changes and stimulate vagal and sympathetic afferents to produce pain and reflex responses. Local biochemical changes consequent to cellular damage include liberation of intracellular algogenic ("pain-producing") substances, such as potassium ions (K^+), lactic acid, serotonin, histamine, and bradykinin, which directly excite C nociceptive afferents and, possibly, the prostaglandins that sensitize these fibers (51,52,65). There is also evidence that cardiac A-delta nociceptive afferents are stimulated directly by unphysiologic motion of the ischemic myocardium and are probably sensitized by the algogenic substances, becoming mechanosensitive (64,65). Cardiac vagal afferents are mechanoreceptors that may also become sensitized consequent to myocardial infarction and provoke abnormal reflexes.

The reflexes elicited by acute myocardial infarction involve afferents and efferents of both cardiac vagi and cardiac sympathetic nerves that produce symptomatology characteristic of vagovagal reflexes and sympatho-sympathetic reflexes (4,64). Under normal conditions these two extrinsic neurogenic controls of cardiac function have reciprocal neural organization so that stimulation of sympathetic afferents not only elicits increased action of sympathetic efferents but also simultaneously reduces the discharge of vagal efferents, and vice versa. However, under pathophysiologic conditions, this typical response is disturbed. Consequently, in most patients with acute myocardial infarction there is overactivity of both systems. The one that will predominate is determined by many interrelated factors including the presence and intensity of pain and the size and location of the infarct: sympathetic overactivity predominates in cases of anterior infarction; parasympathetic overactivity predominates in patients with diaphragmatic lesions (58,64).

The potential danger of abnormal vagovagal reflexes is the Bezold–Jarisch effects of severe bradycardia, atrioventricular block, peripheral vasodilation, and consequent severe hypotension that may progress to cardiogenic shock. The concurrent sympathetic hyperactivity increases myocardiac contractility and may be considered an important mechanism to oppose ventricular dilatation and cardiogenic shock. On the other hand, these potentially protective sympathetic reflexes may prove detrimental by imposing increased oxygen consumption to the myocardium (64). Moreover, there is animal experimental evidence that the α-adrenergic portion of the sympathetic nervous system can exert a vasoconstrictor effect on the coronary vessels with consequent decrease in both coronary blood flow and myocardial oxygen supply (2,16,17). Although evidence in humans is limited, it has been shown that in patients with coronary artery disease, the vasoconstrictor tone may be augmented to the point of angina (33). Clinical evidence also has demonstrated the important role that sympathetic hyperactivity may play in the pathophysiology of myocardial infarction (23,34) and fatal cardiac arrhythmia (28,42). Finally, in addition to the sympathosympathetic reflexes, stimulation of sympathetic afferents by mediating nociceptive (pain) impulses can elicit widespread cardiac, vascular, and hormonal changes.

Nociceptive impulses generated by tissue injury of myocardial infarction are transmitted to the spinal cord dorsal horn via sympathetic afferents and not via the vagi nerves. On reaching the dorsal horn, nociceptive impulses are subjected to modulating influences coming from the periphery, from local interneurons, and from supraspinal descending control systems, which together with other factors determine their further transmission. Some of the nociceptive impulses pass to the anterior and anterolateral horn cells and thus initiate segmental (spinal) reflex responses. Other nociceptive impulses are transmitted to neurons, the axons of which pass predominantly to the opposite anterolateral quadrant and ascent cephalad, thus conveying these impulses to the brainstem to provoke suprasegmental reflex responses and to the brain to produce cortical responses.

Segmental (Spinal) Reflexes

Segmental (spinal) reflexes may, and often do, enhance nociception and produce alteration of ventilation, circulation, and gastrointestinal and urinary function. Thus stimulation of somatomotor cells results in increased skeletal muscle tension, which decreases chest wall compliance and initiates positive feedback loops that generate nociceptive impulses from the muscle (65). Stimulation of sympathetic preganglionic neurons in the anterolateral horn of the spinal cord causes an increase in heart rate, stroke volume, and consequently, cardiac work and myocardial oxygen consumption; as previously mentioned, this may increase the risk of serious cardiac arrhythmia. Moreover, if coronary vasoconstriction develops and occurs in vessels, perfusing myocardial tissue adjacent to the infarcted muscle, it may make previously healthy myocardial tissue ischemic and previously ischemic tissue necrotic. Since these cardiac effects occur in animals who have had vagotomy and C1 spinal section, they are produced by truly segmental spinal reflexes (30,64). In addition, sympathetic hyperactivity causes decreasing gastrointestinal tone that may progress to ileus and a decrease in urinary function that reduces urinary output.

Suprasegmental Reflex Responses

Suprasegmental reflex responses result from nociceptive-induced stimulation of medullary centers of ventilation and circulation, of hypothalamic (predominantly sympathetic) centers and neuroendocrine function, and some limbic structures. These responses consist of hyperventilation, increased neural sympathetic tone, and increased secretion of catecholamines and other endocrines (12,49,53,54,59). The increased neural sympathetic tone and catecholamine secretion add to the effects of spinal reflexes and further increase cardiac output, peripheral resistance, blood pressure, cardiac workload, and myocardial oxygen consumption. In addition to catecholamine release there is an increased secretion of cortisol, ACTH, glucagon, and other catabolically-acting hormones with a concomitant decrease in the anabolically-acting hormones insulin and testosterone. This type of endocrine secretion, characteristic of the stress response, produces widespread metabolic effects, including increased blood glucose, plasma cyclic AMP, free fatty acids, blood lactates, and ketones, as well as generalized increased metabolism and oxygen consumption. The endocrine and metabolic changes result in substrate utilization from storage to central organs and injured tissue and lead to a catabolic state with a negative nitrogen balance. The degree and duration of these endocrine and metabolic changes are related to degree and duration of tissue damage, and many of these biochemical changes last for days (3).

Cortical Responses

Cortical responses include not only the perception of pain as an unpleasant sensation and a negative emotion but also initiation of psychodynamic mechanisms of anxiety, apprehension, and fear. The intense anxiety and fear that invariably develops in patients with acute myocardial infarction through cortical stimulation greatly enhances the hypothalamic responses characteristic of stress. Indeed, cortisol and catecholamine responses to anxiety may exceed the hypothalamic responses provoked directly by nociceptive impulses (19). Moreover, anxiety may cause cortically mediated increased blood viscosity (44), clotting time (15), fibrinolysis (35), and platelet aggregation (10,63).

Thus it is obvious that segmental and suprasegmental reflexes, anxiety, and psychologic stress greatly increase the workload of the heart and its oxygen consumption. Moreover increased blood clotting and the possible coronary vasoconstriction may further decrease the already compromised arteriosclerotic coronary circulation and markedly increase the discrepancy between oxygen supply and oxygen demand, possibly extending the infarction. One or more of these responses may be a critical factor in the cause of the death of the patient. It is, therefore, essential to promptly and effectively relieve the pain, anxiety, and mental stress, and decrease the aforementioned reflex responses.

There is ample laboratory and clinical evidence for the beneficial effect of interrupting afferent and efferent sympathetic pathways in patients with acute myocardial infarction. Nearly half a century ago, three groups of investigators demonstrated that sympathetic denervation of the heart significantly reduced the size of experimentally induced myocardial infarction, and the mortality of animals in the study group compared to a control group (13,32,43). More recent laboratory studies have confirmed the earlier results. In animal studies, Schwartz and Stone (45) showed that surgical sympathectomy increased the endocardial/epicardial blood flow ratio, thus improving the perfusion to the myocardium and endocardium. Even more impressive beneficial effects were noted in dogs by Klassen et al. (26) in which acute myocardial infarction was induced experimentally, and subsequent sympathetic denervation was achieved with epidural blockade. Other animal studies have shown that sympathetic denervation has a protective effect against cardiac arrhythmias of myocardial infarction (42,55). On the clinical side, the protective role of the beta-blocking drugs toward arrhythmias in the early stage of acute myocardial infarction, is well established (21,34).

THERAPY OF ACUTE MYOCARDIAL INFARCTION PAIN

Since the medical therapy of acute myocardial infarction is well known by cardiologists and general physicians, discussion in this section will be limited to the effective and sustained relief of pain, and possibly interruption of abnormal reflex mechanisms. For the latter objective, it is essential to consider the predominant reflex response.

Systemic Analgesics and Related Drugs

Acute severe pain of myocardial infarction is most frequently managed with morphine or other potent narcotic analgesics administered intravenously, intramuscularly, or a combination of the two methods. In addition, anxiolytic agents and sedatives are used for patients with severe anxiety and apprehension. The predominance of this form of therapy was impressively demonstrated by an extensive international survey that revealed this method was used by 86% of clinicians (9). These drugs are widely used for acute pain because they are readily available, relatively easy to administer, and inexpensive, and when properly administered, they provide good (but not always complete) pain relief. Although most experienced cardiologists use these drugs properly, many house officers and other physicians do not (6,11,31). A survey of 130 house officers in two hospitals in New York City revealed these physicians overrated the potency and duration of narcotics and had an exaggerated fear of addiction (31). Often the error is in administering insufficient amounts of the selected drug by the wrong route.

Patients with severe or very severe pain should be given narcotics intravenously in increments of small to moderate doses (e.g., 3–5 mg morphine or equivalent dose of other narcotics, diluted in 5 ml of saline) given slowly and repeated at 15- to 20-min intervals until the patient experiences good pain relief. This method may be combined with continuous infusion technique of administering narcotics. Since infusion of therapeutic doses may require from 3 to 4 hr to reach the minimum analgesic concentration, it should be started at the same time as the intravenous incremental technique; after 3 or 4 hr, this method is terminated. Of course, the intravenous route requires more time and effort on the part of the nursing and medical staff and, consequently, the intramuscular route is used more frequently.

It deserves emphasis, however, that recent studies of the pharmacokinetics and analgesic efficacy of narcotics showed clearly that the minimal analgesic concentration of narcotics is not achieved until the second or third injection of the usual therapeutic dose (1). Moreoover, this method produces peaks and valleys in the blood concentration of the analgesics and does not provide sustained analgesia. Another option is to use a system that permits "on demand" analgesia, known as PACAT (patient-controlled analgesic therapy). (For a lucid discussion of these various methods, see C. Benedetti et al., *this volume.*)

The disadvantage of systemic narcotic analgesics is that even when properly administered, they often do not produce complete relief of severe or very severe pain and do not eliminate abnormal reflex responses. Moreover, they are associated with such well-known adverse side effects as nausea, vomiting, and circulatory depression reflected by a decrease in heart rate and peripheral resistance (41). Ample analgesic doses (10 mg) of morphine, given intravenously to patients with acute myocardial infarction, caused arterial hypotension, an increased dead space, and an increase in alveolar arterial oxygen tension difference.

These circulatory alterations are especially detrimental to patients with acute myocardial infarction who already have bradycardia, arterial hypotension, and cardiac dilatation. Intravenous morphine given to patients with acute myocardial infarction complicated by left ventricular failure caused a significant reduction in heart rate, blood pressure, and cardiac index (29,41,50). In such patients it is essential to exercise extreme caution: the use of small intravenous doses given at more frequent intervals, the concomitant use of atropine to offset bradycardia, and the monitoring of circulatory function frequently or continuously in patients in the intensive care unit. In patients manifesting excessive sympathetic activity, narcotics should be complemented with thorazine for its sedative and hypotensive effect. If cardiac arrhythmia is present, beta-blocking agents should be used. Hydroxozine may also be considered as an adjunct to narcotics because of its strong anxiolytic and antiemetic effect and because it potentiates the analgesic action of narcotics (20).

Inhalation Analgesia

The use of nitrous oxide and oxygen to treat acute pain was first described by Klikovich over a century ago (27). In 1881 he reported the use of a mixture of 80% N_2O and 20% O_2 on several patients with acute myocardial pain with a good outcome. These results were overlooked for over 70 years, and this method was not given clinical trial in patients with myocardial infarction until 15 years ago. Parbrook (36) in a review paper on the therapeutic use of nitrous oxide in oxygen analgesia summarized the good results obtained by different authors in treating patients with myocardial infarction. More recently, Kerr et al. (25) reported on a double-blind trial of patient-controlled nitrous oxide/oxygen analgesia in myocardial infarction with an Entonox Demand Apparatus which delivers a mixture of 50% N_2O and 50% O_2. They found that severe myocardial pain is effectively relieved by this method, at least for a short period of time.

Advantages

The advantages of inhalation analgesia include rapid action (analgesia and often amnesia is obtained within 5–7 min); absence of the deleterious hemodynamic, respiratory, renal, and hepatic effects; mild anticoagulant action; and the patient can self-administer the agent. Lack of hemodynamic effects makes this method especially useful in patients with severe arterial hypotension. The method is complemented with atropine if bradycardia is present, and/or beta blockers if arrhythmia occurs. Because of rapid analgesia, this method can be used in conjunction with intramuscular narcotics to provide relief during the initial period until the narcotic reaches an effective analgesic plasma concentration. It may also be used subsequently to potentiate the analgesic action of the narcotic. To obtain optimal results the patient must be instructed on how to use the equipment and monitored for a period of time both to assure effective administration and to evaluate the analgesic efficacy.

Disadvantages

The disadvantages of inhalation analgesia are that time is required to observe the patient until effective pain relief is achieved and sustained; nitrous oxide in a concentration of 50 to 60% does not provide complete relief of severe or very severe pain in all patients; it cannot be continuously administered for over 24 to 48 hr due to its leukopenic effect; and, importantly, this method does not decrease the abnormal segmental and suprasegmental neuroendocrine responses. Furthermore, N_2O should be given with caution in patients with abdominal distension since it may aggravate the symptoms due to its diffusion effect; in patients with nausea, it may increase the symptoms.

Cervicothoracic Sympathetic Block

In patients with severe or very severe excruciating pain that does not respond to narcotics, cervicothoracic sympathetic block should be considered, provided a person capable of executing it carefully and promptly is readily available (4,7). Indeed, under such circumstances, this procedure may be used initially in patients with very severe pain. In contrast to narcotics, the regional analgesic block produces complete pain relief, and since it prevents the nociceptive impulses from reaching the neuraxis, it eliminates the segmental, suprasegmental, and cortical responses to noxious stimulation and the aforementioned consequent deleterious effects. Moreover, it interrupts the efferent sympathetic pathways to the heart. These effects are especially important in patients with myocardial infarction who manifest excessive sympathetic activity. The beneficial effects of sympathetic denervation of the heart in significantly reducing the size of experimentally induced myocardial infarction mortality of animals have already been cited.

Physicians skilled in this technique can carry it out in less than 5 min and by using thin needles, it is virtually painless. Injection of 12 to 15 ml of a local anesthetic via the anterior paratracheal technique using a 25-gauge or 22-gauge 5-cm needle and advancing the needle until its bevel is in the proper fascial plane (just anterior to the fascia of the precolli muscles) results in diffusion of the solution from the fourth or fifth cervical to the fourth or fifth thoracic vertebral level. Figure 1 shows the pattern of diffusion of the local anesthetic demonstrating that it will block the paravertebral sympathetic

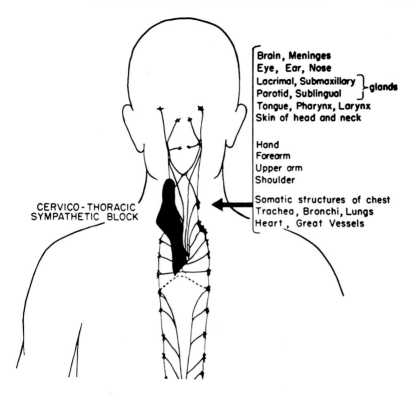

Fig. 1. Diffusion of local anesthetics injected in the vicinity of the stellate ganglion. Note that the drug diffuses from the middle cervical to the fifth thoracic sympathetic ganglia and thus blocks all afferents from, and sympathetic pathways to, the heart (as well as all sympathetic fibers to the head, neck, upper extremity, chest, and its other viscera). (From J. J. Bonica, ref. 7a, with permission.)

chain (and any anomalous sympathetic fibers) from the middle cervical ganglion to the fifth thoracic ganglion, which contain all of the sympathetic afferents from, and sympathetic efferents to, the heart. Patients who are very nervous and anxious should be given a small dose (50–75 mg) of thiopental 45 sec prior to puncturing the skin. This interval permits this drug to have the maximum effect on the brain and is sufficient to produce amnesia and sedation for the 3 to 4 min required to complete the procedure.

In patients with severe pain predominant on one side (most often the left), a unilateral block usually suffices. If the pain is bilateral, it is best to block the side with the most severe pain first; after an interval of 20 to 30 min, the procedure can be carried out on the other side. Allowing this interval of time will minimize the impact on the heart of complete sympathetic denervation. Moreover, this, together with the use of a dilute solution of local anesthetics, will virtually eliminate the risk of systemic toxicity provided the drug is not accidentally injected intravenously. Using 0.25% bupivacaine (Marcaine) as the anesthetic solution produces analgesia and sympathetic interruption within 5 to 10 min lasting from 6 to 8 hr, and 0.75% lidocaine (Xylocaine®) will produce a block within 4 to 6 min lasting from 3 to 4 hr.

This procedure is most useful in patients manifesting sympathetic over-activity. In addition to interruption of efferent sympathetic fibers, the local anesthetic has an antiarrhythmic effect that is especially useful in patients with severe pain and cardiac arrhythmia. On the other hand, in patients manifesting predominantly parasympathetic hyperactivity of bradycardia and arterial hypotension, it should be used with great care and administered only after the heart rate has been restored to near normal with atropine and after the blood pressure has been restored with appropriate therapy. In such cases, cervicothoracic sympathetic block is still useful to produce complete pain relief and to counteract any concurrent sympathetic stimulation of the heart.

The advantages of cervicothoracic sympathetic blocks have already been alluded to. Although no studies have been done on patients with myocardial infarctions, numerous other studies (see refs. 7, 24, for review) have im-pressively demonstrated the efficacy of regional analgesia in minimizing or completely eliminating the segmental and suprasegmental neuroendocrine responses provoked by surgical or accidental trauma, or injury associated with visceral disease. The disadvantages of this method are that it can be used only if an anesthesiologist or a physician skilled and experienced in the technique is available and can only be used in a hospital, preferably in the coronary intensive care unit.

Segmental Epidural Block

Epidural block limited to the upper five thoracic segments and the last cervical segment produces complete denervation of not only the cardiac sympathetic afferents and efferents but also the somatic sensory fibers and, if high concentrations are used, the somatic motor fibers. To achieve an-algesia and sympathetic blockade limited to these segments without con-current motor block, 4 to 6 ml of 0.25% bupivacaine or 1% lidocaine is injected in the epidural space at the T2-3 intervertebral level (4,8). Although this can be achieved with a single dose injected through a needle, it is best to introduce a plastic catheter into the epidural space because this permits repeated injection and thus provides sensory and sympathetic blockade for several days or even longer (4,8).

The advantage of this procedure over cervicothoracic sympathetic block is that it interrupts nociceptive impulses from the chest wall, which may occur in patients with acute myocardial infarction. Bromage (8), an out-standing authority on epidural block, has demonstrated that this procedure obviates or minimizes decreased chest wall compliance that may be pro-voked by segmental somatomotor hyperactivity. In collaboration with Klas-sen et al. (26), Bromage studied the effects of segmental epidural block in three groups of dogs; in one group, myocardial infarction was induced. In that group they observed a significant decrease in left atrial pressure and a decrease in heart rate after epidural block. This led them to believe that these hemodynamic changes would act to decrease myocardial oxygen consumption. Very importantly, the acute sympathectomy redistributed coronary blood flow to the endocardium, with an improvement in the endocardial/epicardial ratio, in dogs with both infarcted and uninfarcted hearts. The improvement in distribution to the endocardium was particularly striking at low flow rates after acute infarction. They concluded that sympathetic blockade achieved with epidural analgesia might be a useful adjunct in the treatment of acute myocardial infarction through improved endocardial blood flow and a decrease in the determinants of myocardial oxygen consumption. Bromage (8) also emphasized the value of epidural block in eliminating the severe pain of myocardial infarction.

The theoretical adverse effects of complete sympathetic denervation of the heart and consequent loss of inotropism and chronotropism are apparently not clinically significant. Although this may be true in patients with acute myocardial infarction manifesting abnormal sympathetic response, the complete denervation in patients with severe bradycardia and hypotension may prove deleterious unless prophylactic measures are used. A disadvantage of this procedure for routine use is similar to that of cervicothoracic block, i.e., the need to have a person with extensive experience and skill to administer the procedure and the need to closely monitor the patient's circulation. Moreover, extreme caution must be carried out to obviate such complications as systemic toxic reactions and extensive subarachnoid block consequent to penetration by the catheter of the dura arachnoid, which occasionally occur even after the first, second, or third injection produces epidural block.

Intrathecal Morphine

Intrathecal morphine was proposed and clinically applied by Wang (56,57) in 1977 based on the experimental work by Yaksh and Rudy (62). Subsequently this (subarachnoid) technique and, later, epidural injection of narcotics were given extensive clinical trials for the relief of acute postoperative and posttraumatic pain, cancer pain, and various other types of acute and chronic pain syndromes. Since L. Jacobson (*this volume*) and Yaksh (61) have reviewed the extensive literature, it will not be repeated here. Suffice it to state that it is generally agreed this method has the following advantages:

1. It provides rapid, intense, and prolonged analgesia.
2. The dose used for subarachnoid injection is much smaller (about one-tenth or less) than that used for intramuscular injection.
3. Most importantly, it is not associated with any adverse side effects on circulation, function of the autonomic nervous system, or skeletal muscle

tone, and, with rare exceptions, has no depressant effects on respiration [see L. Jacobson, *this volume*, and Yaksh (61) for detailed discussion].

In 1977, these considerations prompted my colleagues and me to begin applying this method to relieve pain in patients with acute myocardial infarction. Initially we carried out a controlled clinical trial on 19 patients admitted to the cardiology service of our hospital with the clinical diagnosis of acute myocardial infarction. These patients were randomly assigned to two groups: group A consisted of 10 patients and group B consisted of 9 patients. Patients in group A received a single dose of 0.5 mg morphine diluted in 1 ml normal saline injected, with slight barbotage, in the lumbar subarachnoid space. (Lumbar puncture was performed at L4–3 or at L3–2 level.) The patients in group B received the standard analgesic treatment by our cardiologists consisting of repeated injections of morphine or pentazocine, mostly intramuscularly and occasionally (approximately 30% of the time) intravenously. The average dose of narcotic given during the first 24 hr after admission to the hospital was 23 ± 3 mg for morphine and 64 ± 6 mg for pentazocine. We evaluated the pain relief induced by the two methods using the visual analogue scale of Scott–Huskisson.

The patients in group A who received subarachnoid morphine had statistically significantly less pain than the patients of group B, especially 12 hr after administration of the drug. Figure 2 depicts curves of pain scores in the two groups of patients. Since these data were collected and subsequently reported (39), we have treated an additional 98 patients with severe pain of acute myocardial infarction with intrathecal morphine with similar beneficial effects (37,38,40). Similar results were also published by others (46). These results prompted the following conclusions:

1. A single dose of 0.5 mg morphine injected into the subarachnoid space produced effective relief of pain of acute myocardial infarction that was more rapid in onset, more intense, and of longer duration during the first 24 hr than that obtained with total doses of morphine 40 times larger administered intramuscularly or intravenously.

2. The differences in pain scores were statistically significant.

3. For patients with acute myocardial infarction pain, the subarachnoid route is preferred to the epidural route because it is simpler and more rapid to execute, and one administration is usually sufficient.

4. No depression of respiration or circulation occurred in patients receiving intrathecal morphine.

5. The only adverse side effects noted were a tendency toward urinary retention in some patients.

6. Like other laboratory and clinical reports, our data demonstrate that morphine has no adverse effects on the spinal cord or cerebrospinal fluid.

7. The procedure is not painful and does not add to the patient's psychologic stress, provided it is carried out by a skilled and experienced phy-

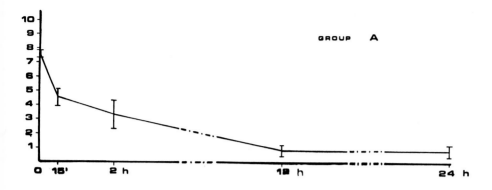

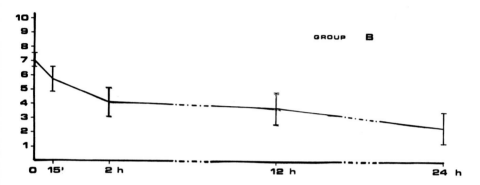

Fig. 2. Analgesic effect: Pain scores (represented on vertical axis with 0 for no pain and 10 the most excruciating pain) of patients treated with intrathecal morphine (group A) and those treated with parenteral morphine (group B). Mean scores ± SE for 2 or more doses administered are shown. The differences at 15 min are highly significant ($p < 0.025$) and at 12 hr are highly significant ($p < 0.005$).

sician who effectively prepares the patient psychologically and, if necessary, with sedatives.

Some of these points regarding circulation and respiration deserve amplification.

Effects on Circulation and Respiration

It deserved reemphasis that our data confirmed those of others regarding an absence of depression of circulatory function following subarachnoid or epidural administration of morphine and, indeed, following the use of numerous other narcotics. The absence of circulatory depression is due to the lack of impairment of sympathetic and parasympathetic nervous system function. This is in contrast to epidural subarachnoid injection of local anesthetics that produce sympathetic block and, if sufficiently extensive, cause arterial hypotension. Moreover, the lack of circulatory depression consequent to intrathecal morphine also is an advantage over intramuscular or intravenous administration of morphine, or other narcotics, which as previously mentioned, may decrease heart rate, cardiac index, and arterial pressure.

The lack of respiratory depression consequent to subarachnoid morphine noted in our patients has been reported by Yaksh (61) and confirmed by many clinical reports (see L. Jacobson, *this volume*). Analysis of such parameters as tidal volume, minute volume, and maximum expiratory flow demonstrated the lack of depression. Indeed, some researchers (22) reported improvement of these parameters in patients with multiple fractured ribs and postoperative pain, as one may expect as a result of the pain-relieving action of the procedure. To further study the effects of morphine and respiration, we conducted a clinical experiment aimed at the evaluation of the effects of spinal morphine and compared these with the effects of an equal dose of drugs injected intravenously (40).

Methods and Results

We studied 10 subjects who gave informed consent, all suffering from pain caused by cancer of the lung and, therefore, not in the best ventilatory condition. The methodology used precluded the application of the various tests to patients with myocardial infarction (47,48). Moreover, because we wished to continue the use of intraspinal narcotics in managing such patients for a prolonged period of time, we selected the continuous epidural route rather than giving repeated subarachnoid injections.

Two milligrams of preservative-free morphine chlorate diluted in 10 ml of normal saline was injected in 5 patients through an epidural catheter inserted in the upper thoracic or lower cervical levels. The other 5 patients received the same dose of morphine intravenously. The two groups of patients were homogeneous with regard to age and respiratory functions (Table 1). The following parameters were evaluated:

1. Minute ventilation (V_e) and correlated indices; tidal volume (V_t) and average respiratory rate (RR).
2. $P_{0.1}$ occlusion pressure measured at the mouth during the first 100 msec of inspiration against closed airway. This measures the output of the respiratory centers which is projected on the entire inspiratory musculature and is not influenced by alterations in the mechanics of respiration (60).
3. V_t/T_i ratio between tidal volume and inspiratory time (mean inspiratory flow rate). These parameters measure the *drive* of the respiratory center that is the constant increase of the inspiratory activities associated with the stimulation of the alpha motoneurons. These parameters are influenced by alteration of the respiratory mechanics.
4. T_i/T_{tot} ratio between inspiratory time and total time. It is an index of the mechanism of temporal regulations of respiration.

TABLE 1. *Comparison of two patient groups given morphine via different routes*

Group given morphine epidurally				Group given morphine intravenously			
No. Patient	Age	Pa_{O_2}	Pa_{CO_2}	No. Patient	Age	Pa_{O_2}	Pa_{CO_2}
1 P.G.	61	82	36	1 R.G.	73	73	35
2 B.G.	71	71	40	2 R.E.[a]	51	70	34
3 A.D.[a]	50	72	44	3 M.A.[a]	61	73	41
4 B.B.[a]	47	68	39	4 S.R.	62	102	38
5 C.G.[a]	65	63	44	5 V.O.[a]	52	75	33
Mean	59	71	41	Mean	60	79	36
SE	4.5	3.1	1.2	SE	4.0	5.9	1.4

[a] Hypoxemic conditions.

Measurements of these parameters were obtained before and 5,15,30,45, and 60 min after morphine administration. Arterial blood gasses were obtained at 30 and 60 min after morphine administration. The results of this study are summarized in Figs. 3 and 4.

It should be noted that although epidural morphine caused no statistically significant reduction in any of the parameters studied, intravenous morphine caused a statistically significant reduction of $P_{0.1}$, V_t/T_i, and V_e 5 min after

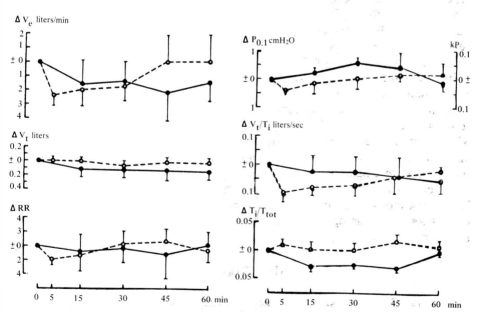

Fig. 3. Changes in minute ventilation (V_e), tidal volume (V_t), respiratory rate (RR), occlusion pressure ($P_{0.1}$), mean inspiratory flow (V_t/T_1), and the inspiratory to total time ratio (T_i/T_{tot}) in 5 patients after 2 mg of epidural morphine (*solid circles*) and in 5 patients after 2 mg of intravenous morphine (*open circles*). Mean values ± SE are shown; $p < 0.05$ (see text).

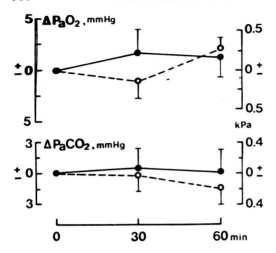

Fig. 4. Changes in Pa_{O_2} and Pa_{CO_2} after 2 mg of epidural morphine (*solid circles*) and intravenous morphine (*open circles*). Mean values ± SE are shown; $N = 5$.

injection and of V_t/T_i 15 min after administration. The statistically insignificant reduction of V_e noted after epidural morphine follows the slight reduction of T_i/T_{tot}. Since there is neither a reduction in the $P_{0.1}$, which instead seems to increase, nor in the average inspiratory flow (V_t/T_i), decrease of V_e in this group of patients is not associated with a depressive action on the respiratory center but instead must be associated with pain reduction.

From the results of the study, we conclude that 2 mg of epidural morphine produces effective analgesia without significantly depressing the respiratory center. The early significant respiratory depression that occurred with the same dose of drug injected intravenously, without obtaining a measurable degree of analgesia, suggests the advantage of the epidural route over a systemic administration of the drug.

Our clinical results and the results of the study, as well as the reports of many others (see L. Jacobson, *this volume*), make it difficult to explain the cases of marked respiratory depression that progress to apnea, in some instances, after injection of intraspinal morphine (14,18). Careful examination of these reports leads us to conclude that, in all cases, the amount of morphine given was definitely excessive and/or was administered in conjunction with one or more agents—other opiates, pancuronium bromide, and/or local anesthetics—injected in the subarachnoid space to potentiate the effects of intrathecal morphine. The same comments apply to reports of respiratory depression following epidural morphine or intrathecal/epidural injection of other opiates.

SUMMARY

Effective therapy of severe or very severe pain and the associated pathophysiologic reflex responses consequent to acute myocardial infarction remain a challenge for cardiologists and general physicians alike. Although the classic therapy of systemic (narcotic) analgesics remains the most frequently employed method of therapy, because narcotics are easy and simple to administer and usually effective, alternate methods should be considered in patients who do not respond to these drugs. These include inhalation analgesia, block of the cervicothoracic sympathetic chain, segmental epidural analgesia, and, most importantly, intrathecal injection of morphine in small doses. These represent important alternative methods that may be used as a complement or as a substitute for narcotics.

On the basis of the results obtained from a controlled clinical trial, and subsequent extensive use in patients with acute myocardial infarction, the present author considers intrathecal morphine a highly effective and refined method of therapy, not only because it produces prompt, intense, and sustained analgesia but also because it is not associated with adverse effects on circulation and respiration. These results confirm those of other authors who have used intrathecal and/or epidural narcotics as an effective form of therapy of acute and chronic pain.

REFERENCES

1. Austin, K. L., Stapleton, J. V., and Mather, L. E. (1980): Multiple intramuscular injections: A major source of variability in analgesic response to meperidine. *Pain*, 8:47–62.
2. Berne, R. M., DeGeestand, H., and Levy, M. N. (1965): Influence of the cardiac nerves on coronary resistance. *Am. J. Physiol.*, 208:763–769.
3. Bessman, F. P., and Renner, V. J. (1982): The biphasic hormonal nature of stress. In: *Pathophysiology of Shock, Anoxia and Ischemia*, edited by R. A. Cowley, and B. F. Trump, pp. 60–65. Williams & Wilkins, Baltimore.
4. Bonica, J. J. (1953): *The Management of Pain*, pp. 1310–1340. Lea and Febiger, Philadelphia.
5. Bonica, J. J. (1979): Important clinical aspects of acute and chronic pain. In: *Mechanisms of Pain and Analgesic Compounds*, edited by R. F. Beers and E. G. Bassett, see also his discussion, pp. 97–105, pp. 13–31. Raven Press, New York.
6. Bonica, J. J. (1980): Pain research and therapy: Past and current status and future needs. In *Pain and Discomfort*, edited by J. J. Bonica and L. Ng, pp. 1–16. Elsevier/North Holland, Amsterdam.
7. Bonica, J. J. (1980): *Sympathetic Nerve Blocks for Pain Diagnosis and Therapy*, Vol. 1, pp. 46–50. Breon Laboratories.
8. Bromage, P. R. (1978): *Epidural Analgesia*, pp. 643–647. W. B. Saunders, Philadelphia.
9. Brusa, R. (1962): *L'infarto miocardico: incheista internazionale*, Vol. II. Minerva Medica Ed., Torino.
10. Cash, J. D., and Allan, A. G. E. (1967): The effect of mental stress on the fibrinolytic reactivity. *Br. Med. J.*, 2:545–548.
11. Chapman, C. R., and Bonica, J. J. (1983): *Current Concepts of Acute Pain*, pp. 1–44. Upjohn Co.
12. Christensen, N. J., and Videbaek, J. (1974): Plasma catecholamines and carbohydrate metabolism in patients with acute myocardial infarction. *J. Clin. Invest.*, 54:278–283.
13. Cox, W. V., and Robertson, H. F. (1936): The effect of stellate ganglionectomy on the cardiac function of intact dogs and its effect on the extent of myocardial infarction and on cardiac function following coronary artery occlusion. *Am. Heart J.*, 12:285–300.
14. Davies, G. K., Tolhurst-Cleaver, C. L., and James, T. L. (1980): Respiratory depression after intrathecal narcotics. *Anaesthesia*, 35:1080–1083.
15. Dreyfuss, F. (1956): Coagulation time of the blood, level of blood eusinophyles and thrombocytes under emotional stress. *J. Psychosom. Res.*, 1:252–257.
16. Feigl, E. O. (1967): Sympathetic control of the coronary circulation. *Circ. Res.*, 20:262–271.

17. Feigl, E. O. (1975): Control of myocardial oxygen tension by sympathetic coronary vasoconstriction in the dog. *Circ. Res.*, 37:88–95.
18. Glynn, C. J., Mather, L. E., Cousins, M. J., Wilson, P. R., and Graham, J. R. (1979): Spinal narcotics and respiratory depression. *Lancet*, 2:356–357.
19. Hume, D. M. (1969): The endocrine and metabolic response to injury. In: *Principles of Surgery*, edited by S. E. Schwartz, pp. 3–42. McGraw-Hill, New York.
20. Hupert, C. (1978): Treatment of postoperative pain—Analgesic potentiation. *Hosp. Pract.* (Special Report), 13:27–31.
21. Jewitt, D. E., Mercer, C. J., and Shillingford, J. P. (1969): Practolol in the treatment of cardiac arrhythmias due to acute myocardial infarction. *Lancet*, 2:227–230.
22. Johnston, J. R., and McCaughey, W. (1980): Epidural morphine. A method of management of multiple fractured ribs. *Anaesthesia*, 35:155–157.
23. Khan, M. I., Hamilton, J. T., and Manning, G. W. (1973): Early arrhythmias following experimental coronary occlusion in conscious dogs and their modification by beta-adrenoceptor blocking drugs. *Am. Heart J.*, 86:347–358.
24. Kehlet, H. (1982): Modifying effect of general and regional anesthesia on the endocrine metabolic response to surgery. *Reg. Anaesth.* 7(4s):38–48.
25. Kerr, F., Hoskins, M. R., Brown, M. G., Ewing, D. J., Irving, G. B., and Kirby, B. J. (1975): A double-blind trial of patient-controlled nitrous oxide/oxygen analgesia in myocardial infarction. *Lancet*, 1:1397–1400.
26. Klassen, G. A., Bramwell, R. S., Bromage, P. R., and Zborowska-Sluis, D. T. (1980): Effect of acute sympathectomy by epidural anesthesia on the canine coronary circulation. *Anesthesiology*, 52:8–15.
27. Klikovich, S.: Cited in Parbrook (36).
28. Kliks, B. R., Burgess, M. J., and Abildskov, J. A. (1975): Influence of sympathetic tone on ventricular fibrillation threshold during experimental coronary occlusion. *Am. J. Cardiol.*, 36:45–49.
29. Lal, S., Savidge, R. S., and Chabra, G. P. (1969): Cardiovascular and respiratory effects of morphine and pentazocine in patients with myocardial infarction. *Lancet*, 1:379–381.
30. Malliani, A., Schwartz, P. J., and Zanchetti, A. (1969): A sympathetic reflex elicited by experimental occlusion. *Am. J. Physiol.*, 217:703–709.
31. Marks, R. M., and Sachar, E. J. (1973): Undertreatment of medical inpatients with narcotic analgesics. *Ann. Intern. Med.*, 78:173–181.
32. McEachern, C. G., Manning, G. W., and Hall, G. E. (1940): Sudden occlusion of coronary arteries following removal of cardiosensory pathways. *Arch. Intern. Med.*, 65:661.
33. Mudge, G. H., Grossman, W., Mills, R. M., Jr., et al. (1976): Reflex increase in coronary vascular resistance in patients with ischemic heart disease. *N. Engl. J. Med.*, 295:1333–1337.
34. Mueller, H. S., Ayers, S., Religa, A., et. al. (1974): Propranolol in the treatment of acute myocardial infarction. *Circulation*, 49:1078–1087.
35. Ogston, D., McDonald, G. A., and Fullerton, H. W. (1962): The influence of anxiety in tests of blood coagular ability and fibrinolytic activity. *Lancet*, 2:521–523.
36. Parbrook, G. D. (1968): Therapeutic use of nitrous oxide. *Br. J. Anaesth.*, 40:365–372.
37. Pasqualucci, V. (1980): Il dolore cardiaco. *Farmaci*, 4:725–737.
38. Pasqualucci, V., Moricca, G., and Solinas, P. (1979): The antalgic treatment in acute coronary thrombosis: A new method (abstract). *International Symposium on Pain*, Sorrento, June 11–15.
39. Pasqualucci, V., Moricca, G., and Solinas, P. (1981): Intrathecal morphine for the control of the pain of myocardial infarction. *Anaesthesia*, 36:68–69.
40. Pasqualucci, V., Sorbino, C. A., Grassi, V., Paoletti, F., Tantucci, C., and Bifarini, G. (1981): Influenza della morfina per via peridurale alta sull'attivita del centro respiratorio: comportamento della pressione di occlusione e del pattern del respiro (abstract). *5th Congresso Naz. A.I.S.D.*, Perugia, 7–9 May.
41. Samuel, I. O., Dundee, J. W. (1975): Circulatory effects of morphine. *Br. J. Anaesth.*, 47:1025–1026.
42. Schaal, S. F., Wallace, A. G., and Sealy, W. C. (1969): Protective effect of cardiac denervation against arrhythmias of myocardial infarction. *Cardiovasc. Res.*, 3:241–244.
43. Schauer, G., Gross, L., and Blum, L. (1937): Hemodynamic studies in experimental coronary occlusion. IV. Stellate ganglionectomy experiments. *Am. Heart J.*, 14:669–676.

44. Schneider, R. A. (1950): The relation of stress to clotting time, relative viscosity and certain biophysical alterations of the blood in normal tensive and hypertensive subjects. In: *Life Stresses and Bodily Disease*, edited by H. G. Wolff, S. G. Wolf, and C. C. Hare, pp. 818–831. Williams & Wilkens, Baltimore.
45. Schwartz, P. J., and Stone, H. L. (1977): Tonic influence of the sympathetic nervous system on myocardial reactive hyperemia and on coronary blood flow distribution in dogs. *Circ. Res.*, 41:51–58.
46. Sciandra, G., and Piazza, A. (1981): La morfina per via intratecale e peridurale. *2nd Corso Superiore di Aggiornamento in Terapia Antalgica*, Asolo, 24–26 June.
47. Sorbini, C. A., Grassi, V., Boschetti, E., Dottorino, M., and Muiesan, G. (1976): Occlusion pressure ($P_{0.1}$). Variability in normal subjects during rebreathing-induced hypercapnia. *Bull. Eur. Physiopathol. Respir.*, 12:237–241.
48. Sorbini, C. A., Grassi, V., Montanari, G., Corbucci, G. G., and Tantucci, C. (1981): Breathing pattern during exercise in runners. *Pharmacol. Res. Commun.*, 13:287–299.
49. Strange, R. C., Vetter, N., Rowe, M. J., and Oliver, M. F. (1975): Plasma cyclic AMP and total catecholamines during acute myocardial infarction in man. *Eur. J. Clin. Invest.*, 4:115–120.
50. Timmis, A. D., Rothman, M. T., Henderson, M. A., Geal, P. W., and Chamberlain, D. A. (1980): Haemodynamic effects of intravenous morphine in patients with acute myocardial infarction complicated by severe left ventricular failure. *Br. Med. J.*, 281:980–982.
51. Uchida, Y., and Murao, S. (1974): Potassium-induced excitation of afferent cardiac sympathetic nerve fibers. *Am. J. Physiol.*, 226:603–609.
52. Uchida, Y., and Murao, S. (1974): Excitation of afferent cardiac sympathetic nerve fibers during coronary occlusion. *Am. J. Physiol.*, 226:1094–1098.
53. Valori, C., Thomas, M., and Shillingford, J. P. (1967): Free noradrenalin and adrenalin excretion in relation to clinical syndromes following myocardial infarction. *Am. J. Cardiol.*, 20:605–617.
54. Vetter, N. J., Strange, R. C., Adams, W., and Oliver, M. F. (1974): Initial metabolic and hormonal responses to acute myocardial infarction. *Lancet*, 1:284–289.
55. Vik-mo, H., Ottesen, S., and Renck, H. (1978): Cardiac effects of thoracic epidural analgesia before and during acute coronary artery occlusion in open chest dogs. *Scand. J.Clin. Lab. Invest.*, 38:737–746.
56. Wang, J. K. (1977): Analgesic effect of intrathecally administered morphine. *Reg. Anaesth.*, 2:3–8.
57. Wang, J. K. (1979): Pain relief by intrathecally applied morphine in man. *Anesthesiology*, 50:210–214.
58. Webb, S. W., Adgey, A. A. J., and Pantridge, J. F. (1972): Autonomic disturbance at onset on acute myocardial infarction. *Br. Med. J.*, 3:89–92.
59. Wilmore, D. W., Long, J. M., Mason, A. D., and Pruitt, B. A., Jr. (1976): Stress in surgical patients as a neurophysiologic reflex response. *Surg. Gynecol. Obstet.*, 142:257–269.
60. Withelaw, W. A., Derenne, J.Ph., and Milic-Emili, J. (1975): Occlusion pressure as a measure of respiratory center output in conscious man. *Respir. Physiol.*, 23:181–199.
61. Yaksh, T. L. (1981): Spinal opiate analgesia: characteristics and principles of action. *Pain*, 1:293–346.
62. Yaksh, T. L., and Rudy, T. A. (1977): Studies on the direct spinal action of narcotics in the production of analgesia in the rat. *J. Pharmacol. Exp. Ther.*, 202:411–428.
63. Zahavi, J., and Dreyfuss, F. (1971): Adenosine diphosphate-induced platelet aggregation in myocardial infarction and ischemic heart disease. *Second Congress of the Society of Thrombosis and Hemostasis*, Oslo, July 13, 1971.
64. Zanchetti, A., and Malliani, A. (1974): Neural and psychological factors in coronary disease. *Acta Cardiol. [Suppl.] (Brux)*, 20:69–93.
65. Zimmermann, M. (1979): Peripheral and central nervous mechanisms of nociception, pain, and pain therapy: Facts and hypotheses. In: *Advances in Pain Research and Therapy, Vol. 3*, edited by J. J. Bonica, J. C. Liebeskind, and D. G. Albe-Fessard, pp. 3–32. Raven Press, New York.

Advances in Pain Research
and Therapy, Vol. 7,
edited by C. Benedetti et al.
Raven Press, New York © 1984.

Muscular Pain in Chronic Occlusive Arterial Diseases of the Limbs

*Marco Maresca, **Giuseppe Nuzzaci, and †Massimo Zoppi

*Department of Medical Therapy, **Department of Cardiovascular Diseases, and
†Department of Rheumatology, Institute of Clinical Medicine, University of
Florence, I-50134 Florence, Italy

According to a well-known and classic concept derived from Lewis et al. (8), intermittent claudication is due to an inadequate supply of arterial blood to contracting muscles and thus results in the rapid accumulation of algogenic substances. When this inadequate supply becomes absolute, rest pain arises. Other factors for rest pain may be the development of inflammation and necrosis. This concept was partly revised in recent years. In this chapter, we discuss some diagnostic criteria and some therapeutic measures to be used.

DIAGNOSTIC CRITERIA

It is generally accepted that the arterial pressure ratio of the ankle to the arm (ankle-to-arm pressure index) and the absolute value of the ankle arterial pressure are more useful in assessing the degree of lower limb ischemia than blood flow measurements. Within certain limits, during rest, the flow in normal subjects and in subjects with arterial occlusion is the same for the development of collateral pathways. The resistance offered by the collateral vessels is considerable and, consequently, there is a pressure drop across these vessels. A normal rate of flow often is maintained, however, because of a compensatory decrease in the resistance of the vascular beds in muscles and skin.

Another useful test is based on measurements of the calf blood flow during reactive hyperemia. If the arterial inflow to a muscle of a normal limb is suddenly occluded so that blood flow ceases, the release of the occlusion is associated with a marked and rapid increase in flow that is considerably above the resting control value (reactive hyperemia). This increased flow rate returns quickly to the control levels. In a limb with occlusive arterial disease, the peak hyperemic response to a period of occlusion is delayed in onset and reduced in magnitude, and the duration of the hyperemia is prolonged. These abnormalities result from the increased resistance to flow offered by the pathologically narrowed arteries and the collateral circulation (10).

An ankle-to-arm pressure index of 0.5 at rest and 0.15 after exercise indicates severe ischemia (6). It has been ascertained that a critical value of the arterial pressure is 50–60 mm Hg (80 mm Hg in diabetics). Subjects with rest pain show an arterial pressure below that value. It is important to note that, if this is true, the inverse is not true; that is, not all the subjects with reduced pressure values have pain. In subjects who die from different causes, it is not uncommon to observe severe stenosis or complete occlusions of the main arteries of the lower limbs without a history of pain. In a subject with a complete occlusion of the popliteal artery, who during life did not suffer from calf pain, we observed a greatly enlarged and hyperplastic (superior) artery of the knee that probably was sufficient to cover all the circulatory needs of the limb. Above the mentioned critical values, there is no correlation between pressure and maximal walking distance (MWD) before the onset of pain. For instance, it is possible to observe subjects with an MWD of 600 to 700 m with an arterial pressure near the critical values, and subjects with an MWD of 50 to 100 m with an arterial pressure of only slightly below normal.

To understand these apparently contradictory observations, we have to consider individual differences, i.e., the degree of denervation, the presence of myalgic spots, the activation of reflex arcs, and the training to walk.

The Degree of Denervation

Large myelinated fibers are damaged more readily by ischemia than are small unmyelinated C fibers. This selective destruction of large fibers is responsible for an unbalanced input, with predominance of discharge from the small fibers that conduct pain sensation. Other factors that may contribute to this partial denervation include the concomitant presence (a) of metabolic disturbances that can damage the peripheral nerves, such as diabetes or chronic alcoholism, or (b) of lesions of the sciatic nerve and its roots caused by pressure from a protruded intervertebral disk. At the extreme limits we may observe claudication without overt signs of arterial occlusion. This pseudo-claudication syndrome, which was described in cases of compression of the cauda equina by hypertrophic ridging or a herniated lumbar disk (14), was observed by us in three subjects without afferent occlusive arterial diseases; two were diabetics and the other had no afferent disease.

The Presence of Myalgic Spots

A typical myalgic spot is found in all patients with claudication pain. These myalgic spots are located in the calf at the junction between the soleus muscle and the Achilles tendon. These myalgic spots act as trigger points that evoke pain radiating on the posterior surface of the leg. Individual differences not due to the degree of the occlusion are responsible for the development and importance of these trigger points. These include: (a) inherited factors such as the "fibrositic diathesis" that is characterized by a facility to develop myofascial pain; (b) exposure to cold; and (c) other physical agents such as trauma and infectious foci.

The Activation of Reflex Mechanisms

An important mechanism for pain and dystrophy that occur in these patients is the activation of abnormal somatosympathetic reflexes. This mechanism is similar to the "vicious circle" mechanism described for reflex sympathetic dystrophy (2,9,11). The onset of a vicious circle of impulses from the periphery to the central nervous system and back to the periphery, which plays a very important role in posttraumatic arteriopathies, is facilitated by, for example, trauma, painful scars, and concomitant phlebitis. The abnormal efferent sympathetic activity may contribute to the pain and dystrophies through different mechanisms: vasomotor changes, fast and slow changes in permeability of microvessels and in tissues inhibition, release of active substances, direct control of some enzymatic reactions, or direct modulation of sensory receptors (12).

Walking Exercise

Training in walking exercise acts per se to determine the capacity for walking (7,13). To explain this concept, which also has important consequences for therapy, we mention our unpublished investigation on 8 men ranging in age from 45 to 72 (mean, 57 years) who suffered from femoropopliteal or femoral occlusive arterial diseases. None of the subjects had cardiac or pulmonary disorders. The subjects walked up on a treadmill with a 1 in 12 gradient at a velocity of 3 km/hr every day for 12 days. The MWD before the onset of the inhibiting pain was recorded. Before the training period and at the 6th and 12th days of training, we measured in the painful limb: (a) the ankle-to-arm pressure index, using an ultrasound transducer based on the Doppler effect; and (b) the total arterial flow of the calf by means of strain-gauge plethysmography during reactive hyperemia after a complete occlusion of the blood inflow to the limb for 5 min, obtained with a pneumatic cuff put around the thigh. We recorded the flow value obtained 10 sec after the interruption of the ischemia.

Figure 1 shows in a simplified manner the changes of the MWD during the 12 days of training. It is interesting to note that, at the beginning of the training, the MWD was about the same in all the subjects (about 250 m) but increased about 500% in 4 subjects defined "good walkers," that is, subjects

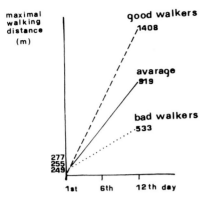

FIG. 1. Maximal walking distance of good and bad walkers during 12 days of physical training.

who (for work or as hobby) had the habit to walk. The increase was smaller but still significant (about 150%) in 4 subjects who led a sedentary life and who were defined "bad walkers." The reactive hyperemia at the end of the training showed a significant increase ($p < 0.0025$) in comparison with the starting value in the group of good walkers. In the group of bad walkers, the changes were not significant (Fig. 2). The ankle-to-arm pressure index did not change in either group during the training.

The increase of the MWD at the end of the training is not due to an increase of the perfusion pressure because the ankle-to-arm pressure index did not change. The increase of the MWD after the training may be partly due to an improvement of the local circulation in the good walkers, as indicated by the increase of the reactive hyperemia, which is a very reliable index of the circulatory response of tissues to ischemia. In the group of bad walkers, the increase of the MWD probably is due exclusively to a better adaptation of the tissues to ischemic work without significant changes of the reactive hyperemia.

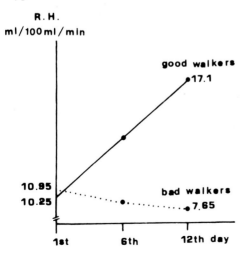

FIG. 2. Reactive hyperemia (R.H.) of good and bad walkers during 12 days of physical training.

COMMENTS ON THERAPY

These observations suggest criticism of many clinical studies that tend to demonstrate a positive effect of vasodilating drugs on the MWD. There are theoretical and practical reasons against the use of vasodilating drugs in the occlusive arterial diseases. Muscular flow largely is regulated by local metabolites that induce a maximal vasodilation during ischemia. Cutaneous flow, instead, is regulated mainly through the activity of the efferent sympathetic nerves, so the vasodilation induced by drugs almost exclusively is exerted on cutaneous vessels that are constricted on the ischemic limb. This pharmacologic activity of vasodilating drugs may divert flow from the ischemic muscle to skin or from the ischemic bed to a normal one (e.g., to the opposite leg), worsening the ischemic condition of the affected muscle (4).

In our opinion, vasodilators are indicated only in some patients with rest pain. Rest pain is not due to the same mechanisms as claudication pain. Claudication pain is mainly muscular and is felt in different areas of the lower limbs, but mainly in the calf. Rest pain is felt mainly during the night because of the physiologic decrease of the arterial pressure and probably because of the reduced inhibitory influence of the central nervous system. It often is accompanied by ulcers and gangrene. This frequently excruciating pain is mainly of cutaneous and also of tendinous and bony origin. In these cases, vasodilator drugs may exert a beneficial effect by relieving rest pain. Other reasons for the improvement sometimes exerted by vasodilators are: (a) their α-adrenergic blocking activity, which interrupts a vicious circle of impulses, which is often an important cofactor, especially in subjects with a low MWD and a perfusion pressure that is only slightly reduced; and (b) their placebo effect; the induced cutaneous flush often is seen as beneficial by the subjects.

The improvement obtained with the classic therapy of intraarterial infusion of acetylcholine is not due to the vasodilation because acetylcholine is inactivated rapidly by cholinesterase. It is probably due to the fibrinolytic activity, which reduces recent thrombi.

Similar considerations may be given to block of the sympathetic activity achieved temporarily with a local anesthetic (reversible block) or for prolonged periods with chemical or surgical sympathectomy (nonreversible block). Some authors insist that surgical sympathectomy must be avoided in intermittent claudication because it does not improve the muscular blood flow; the increase of flow is exerted mostly on the skin (5). We believe it is necessary to differentiate reversible and nonreversible blocks. After nonreversible blocks, an increased sensitivity to circulating amines may develop within a few days. This denervation hypersensitivity may induce a worsening of dystrophy with a reduction of the MWD and eventually the appearance of ulcers in the extremity.[1] Reversible blocks, instead, may induce a reset of an unbalanced system toward a more physiologic steady state. The relief of pain and improvement in the dystrophic changes may last for a long period.

We have observed good results with a series of 10 to 20 reversible blocks of the lumbar sympathetic chain in many subjects with slightly reduced arterial pressure of the ankle and an MWD of 50 to 100 meters, and in subjects with very active myalgic spots. The block is indicated also in patients with rest pain, without skin lesions, or with very small periungual ulcers.

SUMMARY

From the aforementioned comments and concepts, it is easy to understand that, in many cases, pain in occlusive arterial diseases is a symptom that must be treated with local blocks of trigger points, anti-inflammatory agents such as aspirin-like drugs, or, in severe rest pain, narcotics. In many patients, walking exercise is enough per se to improve the walking capacity of the patients. These simple therapies often are enough to reduce or to relieve pain for many years, and consequently they must be considered the first therapeutic approach in atherosclerotic occlusive arterial disease.

REFERENCES

1. Boas, R. A., Hatangdi, V. S., and Richards, E. G. (1976): Lumbar sympathectomy: A percutaneous chemical technique. In: *Advances in Pain Research and Therapy, Vol. 1,* edited by J. J. Bonica and D. G. Albe-Fessard. Raven Press, New York.
2. Bonica, J. J. (1953): *The Management of Pain.* Lea & Febiger, Philadelphia.
3. Cousins, M. J., Reeve, T. S., Glynn, C. J., Walsh, J. A., and Cherry, D. A. (1979): Neurolytic lumbar sympathetic blockade: duration of denervation and relief of rest pain. *Anaesth. Intensive Care,* 7:2,121–135.
4. Gillespie, J. A. (1959): The case against vasodilator drugs in occlusive vascular disease of the legs. *Lancet,* 2:995–997.
5. Gillespie, J. A. (1960): Late effects of lumbar sympathectomy on blood-flow in the foot in obliterative vascular disease. *Lancet,* 1:891–894.
6. Juergens, J. L., and Bernats, P. E. (1980): Atherosclerosis of the extremities. In: *Peripheral Vascular Diseases,* edited by J. L. Juergens, J. A. Spittel Jr., and J. F. Fairbairn 2nd, pp. 253–293. Saunders, Philadelphia.
7. Larsen, O. A., and Lassen, N. A. (1966): Effect of daily muscular exercise in patients with intermittent claudication. *Lancet,* 2:1093–1096.
8. Lewis, T., Pickering, G. W., and Rothschild, P. (1931): Observations upon muscular pain in intermittent claudication. *Heart,* 15:359–383.
9. Livingston, W. K. (1943): *Pain Mechanisms. A Physiologic Interpretation of Causalgia and its Related States.* Macmillan, New York.
10. McGrath, M. A., Verhaeghe, R. H., and Shepherd, J. T. (1980): The physiology of limb blood flow. In: *Peripheral Vascular Diseases,* edited by J. L. Juergens, J. A. Spittel Jr. and J. F. Fairbairn 2nd, pp. 83–105. Saunders, Philadelphia.
11. Nathan, P. W. (1980): Involvement of the sympathetic nervous system in pain. In: *Pain*

---

[1] Boas et al. (1) and Cousins et al. (3) have reported excellent results with chemical sympathectomy achieved with 7 to 10% phenol in Conray 60 in providing prolonged relief of rest pain and improvement of skin ulcers in patients with arteriosclerosis obliterans (*Editors*).

and Society, edited by H. W. Kosterlitz and L. Y. Terenius, pp. 311–324. Verlag Chemie, Weinheim.

12. Procacci, P., Francini, F., Zoppi, M., and Maresca M. (1975): Cutaneous pain threshold changes after sympathetic block in reflex dystrophies *Pain*, 1:167–175.

13. Skinner, J. S., and Strandness, D. E. Jr. (1967): Exercise and intermittent claudication. II. Effect of physical training. *Circulation*, 36:23–29.

14. Snider, E. N. Jr., Mulfinger, G. L., and Lambert, R. W. (1975): Claudication caused by compression of the cauda equina. *Am. J. Surg.*, 130:172–175.

*Advances in Pain Research
and Therapy, Vol. 7,*
edited by C. Benedetti et al.
Raven Press, New York © 1984.

Cancer Pain: Basic Considerations

Costantino Benedetti and John J. Bonica

*Department of Anesthesiology, University of Washington, Seattle, Washington
98195*

For over three decades, Bonica and his colleagues (7–14) have repeatedly emphasized that proper control of cancer pain has long been and continues to be one of the most important and pressing issues of modern society in general and in the field of oncology and the health care systems of many countries in particular. This importance stems from the following considerations. Annually, cancer pain afflicts nearly 800,000 Americans and some 18 million patients worldwide. Although the drugs and other therapeutic modalities currently available are effective in relieving the pain of most cancer patients when properly used, they are often inadequately applied. Consequently, many patients spend their last weeks and months of life in great discomfort, suffering, and disability that preclude a quality of life vital to them.

The objective of this chapter is to present an overview of: (a) the magnitude of the problem, including its importance, incidence, and prevalence; and the physiologic and psychologic effects of cancer pain; (b) the current status of its therapy and the reasons for existing deficiencies; (c) the most important cancer pain syndromes and the possible mechanisms; and (d) the basic principles in managing patients with cancer-related pain. This chapter is an update of previous reports (8,9) including chapters in books edited by Bonica (11) and by Moossa (13).

MAGNITUDE OF THE PROBLEM

Importance

Pain is the most dreaded complication of cancer among the millions of persons who develop cancer worldwide. Once the patient accepts and somewhat adjusts to the shocking news of the presence of cancer, one of the greatest problems is the fear of excruciating pain and suffering the patient believes will inevitably ensue. A survey carried out by Aitken-Swan (1) in Britain revealed that pain ranked next to incurability among the factors people feared about cancer. Epidemiologic studies carried out by Daut and Cleeland (18) at the University of Wisconsin and by Greenwald et al. (26)

at the University of Washington, sponsored by the National Cancer Institute of the United States, revealed the general public believes cancer to be much more painful than it actually is. This has been generated in part by the fact that a significant percentage of patients with advanced cancer do develop moderate to severe pain and, in many patients, the pain has been and continues to be inadequately managed. In recent years these facts have come to the attention of the general public and this, in turn, has generated fear and apprehension about cancer pain and the inability of many health professionals to relieve it effectively.

Incidence and Prevalence

The incidence and prevalence of pain associated with cancer throughout the world cannot be defined with accuracy simply because no national or international epidemiologic studies have been carried out. However, one can gain some insight by extrapolating data derived from local studies on the incidence and prevalence of cancer pain to the data on the incidence and prevalence of cancer and cancer deaths published by the American Cancer Society and the World Health Organization (WHO). On the basis of 1979 cancer statistics cited by Stjernward (47), chief of the cancer unit of WHO, it is estimated that worldwide the incidence (new cases) of cancer is 16 million, the prevalence (new and old cases) is 37.1 million, and there are 6.9 million deaths from cancer, representing 10% of all deaths throughout the world. Moreover, in developed countries in Europe and North America and in parts of the world where major infectious diseases and nutritional problems are no longer leading causes of death, cancer is responsible for 20% of the total deaths. A study of data published by WHO and the American Cancer Society (2) reveals that age-adjusted death rates per 100,000 population for selected cancer sites were similar in some 50 countries, including all the Western European countries, Canada, and many Central and South American countries, Australia, New Zealand, Japan, and Singapore. Using these data, and data derived from a number of surveys carried out in specific hospitals in the United Kingdom, the United States, Canada, Italy, Israel, Brazil, and a few other countries, it is possible to compute an estimation, albeit a crude one, of the prevalence of cancer-related pain.

United Kingdom

Surveys carried out in the United Kingdom include one by Wilkes (56), who in 1974 reported that of nearly 300 patients in an English provincial city who were admitted to a 25-bed unit used for the care of dying cancer patients, pain was the major symptom in 58%. It occurred in 82% of patients with cervical cancer, in 75% of patients with gastric cancer, and in 45 to 60% of patients with cancer of the lungs, rectum, and breast. Twycross (50) reviewed the records of the patients admitted each year and found that over 84% required diamorphine (heroin) for severe pain during their hospital stay. In still another British survey of 276 cancer patients who received terminal care, Parkes (40) found that, among those given care in hospitals, 38% had moderate pain and 22% had severe or very severe pain; among patients managed in the home, the figures were 21 and 48%, respectively. Still other British reports include those of Aitkin-Swan (1), who found an incidence of approximately 50%; of Hinton (28), who reported pain to have been experienced by 67% of 82 patients with terminal cancer; and of Cartwright et al. (15), who reported that 87% of patients who died from cancer had pain before death.

United States

Surveys done in the United States include those carried out by Foley et al. (22) at the Memorial Sloan-Kettering Cancer Institute. In a survey of 540 patients, pain was experienced by: 85% of patients with primary bone tumors; 80% with cancer of the oral cavity; 75% of men and 70% of women with cancer of the genitourinary system; 52% of patients with breast cancer; 45% of patients with cancer of the lung; 20% of patients with lymphoma; and 5% of patients with leukemia. In a subsequent survey of 397 patients, about 38% had pain related to cancer, but this rose to 60% among the terminally ill patients in the hospital. Norton and Lack (36), associated with two American hospices, reported pain was a significant symptom in 75% of 100 cancer patients managed in their homes. Kornell (34), a member of our cancer pain study group, noted that 86% of patients with advanced cancer reported pain and these patients ranked pain as the most distressing symptom they experienced. Oster et al. (37) reported that 72% of the patients with terminal cancer experienced pain.

Epidemiologic studies carried out by Daut and Cleeland (18) and Greenwald et al. (26,27) provide an even more comprehensive overview of the prevalence of pain and its impact on the patient. Daut and Cleeland (18) studied 667 patients, including 289 with cancer of the breast, 48 with cancer of the prostate, 127 with cancer of the colon-rectum, 91 with cancer of the cervix, 27 with cancer of the corpus uteri, and 85 with cancer of the ovary. Each group was also subdivided into those that had no metastases (nm) and those in whom metastases were present (mp). The incidence of pain in the nm and mp groups respectively was as follows: breast 40 and 64%; prostate 30 and 75%; colon-rectum 40 and 47%; cervix 35 and 0%; uterine corpus 14 and 40%; ovary 39 and 49%. An important finding of this survey was that a significant percentage of patients reported a surprisingly high frequency of pain as a symptom when the cancer was first diagnosed. The percentages were as follows: breast 39%; prostate 45%; colon-rectum 42%; cervix 18%; ovarian 49%; and uterine corpus 22%. These investigators also noted that cancer patients with moderate to severe pain (visual analog scale rating of 5 or more on a 0–10 scale) reported significant interference with their activity and enjoyment of life. Moreover, among terminal patients who had severe pain, 70% reported that the pain disrupted their sleep.

Greenwald and associates (26,27) at the University of Washington studied 390 cancer patients including 179 with cancer of the lung, 15 with cancer of the pancreas, 157 with cancer of the prostate, and 39 with cancer of the cervix. Each of the four groups was subdivided into three subgroups depending on the stage of malignancy: group 1 with local lesion only; group 2 with regional spread; and group 3 with distant spread. The percentage of patients who reported any pain with each of these three stages was as follows: lung 80/70/68%; pancreas 100/90/100%; prostate 65/62/66%; uterine cervix 65/40/100%. Among these groups, continuous pain during the preceding week was experienced by a third of the patients with cancers of the lung, prostate, and cervix, and by 100% of the patients with cancer of the pancreas. The percentage of patients who reported severe pain the week preceding the interview was as follows: lung 55%; pancreas 85%; prostate 35%; and cervix 33%. The percentage of lung and prostate cancer patients reporting continuing pain increased steadily from stage 1 through 3 but those with the other two cancers did not evidence a steady increase in pain by stage. The overall incidence of pain among the entire group with various stages of disease was a mean of 63%.

Canada

Turnbull (49) studied the prevalence and characteristics of pain in 280 patients with recurrent cancer of the lung referred to the British Columbia (Canada) Cancer Control (Institute) Agency for Palliative Therapy. At the time that the patients were first seen at the Institute and a diagnosis of an incurable lesion had been made, 71% had pain that had the characteristics of five pain syndromes. At the end of palliative therapy pain was still present in 45%, and during the last two months of life 65% of the patients had significant pain.

Italy

In Italy there have been four published reports of surveys on the incidence and prevalence of cancer pain. Pannuti and associates (38) of the Division of Oncology, Malpighi Hospital, Bologna, Italy, reported that in one series of 291 patients with advanced solid tumors, moderate to severe pain was experienced by nearly 64% of the patients. The incidence of moderate to severe pain with specific lesions was as follows: 68% with breast cancer; 67% with stomach cancer; 60% with prostatic cancer; 58% with intestinal and with lung cancer; 55% of patients with kidney tumors; and by nearly half of those who had head and neck cancer. In another study of 324 patients with advanced cancer managed in their service in a 3 ½ year period, Pannuti et al. (39) noted that 88% had moderate to severe pain for more than 15 days at some stage of the disease. The incidence of pain in patients with specific tumors was a follows: 100% with cancer of the ovary and with cancer of the cervix; 95% with cancer of the rectum and with cancer of the breast; 85% with cancer of the lung and with cancer of the colon; and 75% with stomach cancer. Moreover, 15 days before death, pain was present in patients with bone metastases in 80% of patients with primary lung tumors, in 77% of patients with breast cancer and 67% with other tumors. Similar figures for soft tissue metastases were 67, 73, and 50% respectively; with visceral metastases, they were 50, 59, and 56%. They reported that these patients averaged 3 months of survival time with pain, that with commonly used antiplastic chemotherapy, pain relief occurred in only 23% of patients whereas with high doses of medroxyprogesterone acetate (MAP) pain relief occurred in 68% of the patients. Apart from patients with ovarian cancer, there was a consistent tendency for the incidence of pain to decrease from the first admission to 15 days before death, presumably due to anticancer therapy.

In another study in Italy, Ventafridda and Gallucci (*personal communication*) reported that in patients with cancer of the lung, the incidence of pain was 91% in patients under 54 years, 86% in patients 55 to 64 years, and 65% in patients 65 years or older. A retrospective study performed at the Department of Pediatric Hematology and Oncology of the Gaslini Children's Hospital in Genoa by Cornaglia and Massimo in collaboration with Benedetti and Bonica (17) revealed that pain was experienced by over 50% of children with neoplasms. Of 910 charts reviewed, 814 had complete data that allowed evaluation regarding the presence or absence of pain in these patients: 54.6% suffered moderate to severe pain requiring narcotic medication sometime during the course of the disease. We found however, a wide spread of the incidence of pain depending on the type of neoplasm: Ewing's sarcoma caused pain the highest number of patients (89%), and bone tumors caused pain in 67 to 75% of the patients, while retinoblastoma pain was present in only 20% of the children. This study also shows that pain was present in 46.6% of children when the neoplasm was first diagnosed (see Table 1).

Israel

In a survey of cancer patients carried out in Brazil, M. Martelete (1982, *personal communication*) found that 80 to 90% of patients with advanced cancer had moderate to severe pain. Birkhahn (3) conducted a survey of the general cancer population in Israel and found that about 40% of patients with various stages of the disease experienced moderate to severe pain. Front and associates (23) of the Rambam Medical Center, Haifa, did a pro-

TABLE 1. *Incidence of pain in children with neoplastic diseases*

Type of neoplasia	No. of charts with data on pain	No. of patients with pain (%)	No. of patients with pain at diagnosis of neoplasia (%)
Ewing's sarcoma	18	16 (88.9)	16 (88.9)
Astrocytoma	6	5 (83.3)	5 (83.3)
Soft tissue neoplasia	17	14 (82.4)	13 (76.5)
Medulloblastoma	15	12 (80.0)	11 (73.3)
Ovarian neoplasia	9	7 (77.8)	7 (77.8)
Other brain neoplasia	16	12 (75.0)	11 (68.7)
Osteosarcoma	4	3 (75.0)	3 (75.0)
Histiocytosis X	32	22 (68.8)	18 (56.2)
Non-Hodgkin's lymphoma	60	35 (68.6)	27 (45.0)
Acute nonlymph. leukemia	53	36 (67.9)	26 (49.0)
Bone neoplasia	3	2 (66.6)	2 (66.6)
Rhabdomyosarcoma	35	22 (62.9)	19 (54.3)
Miscellaneous	53	31 (58.5)	25 (47.2)
Acute lymphatic leukemia	278	160 (57.6)	128 (46.0)
Neuroblastoma	93	51 (54.8)	42 (45.2)
Wilms' tumor	53	20 (37.7)	14 (26.4)
Testicular neoplasia	4	1 (25.0)	1 (25.0)
Endocrine neoplasia	4	1 (25.0)	1 (25.0)
Hodgkin's lymphoma	51	12 (23.5)	9 (17.6)
Retinoblastoma	10	2 (20.0)	1 (10.0)
Totals (averages)	814	464 (57.0)	379 (46.6)

spective study of 190 patients with cancer and found that of 66 patients with bone metastasis, 68% had pain. Although there were 155 sites of skeletal metastasis, pain was associated with only 50 sites.

The data summarized in Tables 2 and 3 indicate that varying degrees of pain is experienced by about 20 to 50% of patients when the lesion is diagnosed, by 30 to 40% of patients with intermediate stages of the disease, and by 55 to 90% of patients with advanced or terminal cancer, depending on the specific types of neoplasm. Careful study of the published reports also suggests that: (a) of cancer patients with pain, in 60 to 80% it is moderate to severe; (b) the pain generally is severe or very severe in an overall average of 60 to 65% of patients with advanced cancer and higher in the terminal phases of the disease; and (c) in most cancer patients, the pain is of two or more types and/or etiologies (7,12,18,52).

Bonica and his colleagues (9–11,14) have used these data and data published by the American Cancer Society and WHO to estimate the prevalence of moderate to severe pain among the cancer population in the United States and worldwide. To estimate the number of American patients with advanced cancer with moderate to severe pain, they have used the middle of the range

TABLE 2. *Prevalence of cancer-related pain: Average data[a]*

Country	Author (ref.)	No. of patients	Stage of disease	Percent with pain
Canada	Turnbull (49)	280	Advanced	71
Israel	Birkham (3)	168	All stages	39
	Font et al. (23)	66	Advanced	70
Italy	Pannuti et al. (38)	291	Advanced	64
	Pannuti et al. (39)	324	Advanced	88
	Ventafridda (*personal communication*)	145	Terminal	73
United Kingdom	Aiken-Swan (1)	200	Terminal	52
	Cartwright et al. (15)	215	Final year	87
	Hinton (28)	82	Terminal	67
	Parkes (40)			
	Hospital care	100	Terminal	60
	Home care	65	Terminal	70
	Twycross (52,54)	500	Terminal	80
	Wilkes (56)	300	Terminal	71
United States	Daut and Cleeland (18)	286	Nonmetastatic	36
		381	Metastatic	60
	Foley (19)	540	All stages	29
	Foley (19,21)			
	All stages	397	All stages	38
	Terminal	39	Terminal	60
	Greenwald et al. (26)	390	All stages	63
	Norton and Lack (36)	100	Advanced	75
	Kornell (34)	39	Advanced	86
	Oster et al. (37)	43	Terminal	72
	Pollen and Schmidt (41)	42	Advanced	55

[a] Includes pain produced by direct tumor involvement, by cancer therapy, or by the debilitating effects of the disease.

TABLE 3. *Prevalence of cancer-related pain: Percent of specific lesions[a]*

Lesions	Percent	Lesions	Percent
Bone	70–85	Small intestine	60–70
Ovary/cervix	70–100	Prostate	70–75
Colon/rectum	50–95	Lung	60–85
Stomach	70–75	Oral cavity	70–80
Breast	52–95	Urinary organs	60–75
Pancreas	70–100	Larynx	55–70
Uterus	40–70	Lymphoma	20
Biliary	65–80	Leukemia	5

[a] Includes pain produced by direct tumor involvement, by cancer therapy, or by the debilitating effects of the disease. Data on lymphoma and leukemia from Foley (19,21). Other data from Daut and Cleeland (18), Foley (19,21), Greenwald et al. (27), Pannuti et al. (38,39), Pollen and Schmidt (41), Turnbull (49), Ventafridda (*personal communication*), and Wilkes (56).

TABLE 4. *Prevalence of cancer pain in USA (1981 estimates)[a]*

Stage/type of cancer	No. of patients (1,000s)	Prevalence of pain (% of patients)	Patients with pain (1,000s)
Advanced			
Lung	105	73	77
Colon/rectum	56	73	41
Breast	37	75	27
Stomach	22	73	16
Pancreas	22	85	19
Prostate	22	73	16
Lymphomas	22	20	4
Ovary/cervix/corp.	22	75	17
Urinary organs	17	68	12
CNS	10	70	7
Oral/pharynx	9	75	7
Liver/biliary	9	73	7
Larynx	4	62	2
Bone	2	80	2
All other	61	20	12
Subtotal	420	63	266
Intermediate-Therapy/			
other	1,500(?)	35	525
Total	1,920	41	791

[a] Rounded to nearest unit.

for each specific lesion (e.g., 73% for cancer of the lung, 75% for cancer of the colon/rectum and breast, 73% for prostate cancer) and multiplied this figure by the number of deaths due to each cancer type estimated for 1981 (2). They also used 35% for the presence of moderate to severe pain in the prevalence group. These computations shown in Table 4 suggested that, of the 420,000 Americans estimated to have died from cancer in 1981, 266,000 (63%) had moderate to severe pain; of the remaining 1.5 million patients in the prevalence group, 515,000 had moderate to severe pain. This gives an overall average of about 780,000 Americans who experienced moderate to severe pain due to cancer or cancer therapy that year. Using the same type of computation, they estimated that annually moderate to severe pain is experienced by 4 million patients who die from cancer worldwide and 14 million patients in the prevalence group, for a total of 18 million patients.

Effects of Cancer Pain

Persistent cancer pain and suffering, like nonmalignant chronic pain, has serious physiologic and psychologic impact on the patient and the family. The physical deterioration of cancer patients is even more severe than in the case of nonmalignant chronic pain because they have greater problems with sleep disturbance and with lack of appetite, nausea, and vomiting (7,9,10,14,19,26). Daut and Cleeland (18) found that cancer patients with moderate to severe pain (visual analog scale rating of 5 or more on a 0 to 10 scale) reported significant interference with their activity and enjoyment of life. Moreover, 60 to 65% of patients with advanced cancer pain reported that pain disrupted their sleep. Similar effects were experienced by the cancer patients studied by the University of Washington group (26).

Cancer patients also develop greater emotional reactions to pain consisting of anxiety, depression, hypochondriasis, somatic focusing, and neuroticism than patients with nonmalignant chronic pain (4–6,16,57). Woodforde and Fielding (57) examined cancer patients with and without pain using the Cornell Medical Index and found patients with pain were significantly more emotionally disturbed than those without pain, responded less well to cancer treatment, and died sooner. The causes of emotional morbidity were depression, hypochondriasis, and psychosomatic symptoms. These, together with intractable pain, represent symptomatology indicative of a state of helplessness or inability to cope with disease, damage to the body, and the threat to life—responses to having a progressive and potentially fatal illness. Bond (5) found that cancer patients with pain had elevated levels of hypochondriasis and neuroticism, whereas pain-free cancer patients had low levels. He further noted that the scores of patients with high levels of emotionality fell after the pain was relieved by percutaneous cordotomy. This led Bond to conclude that personality factors are distorted by severe pain and that its relief results in restoration toward normality.

Many patients with cancer pain, knowing the causative factors are unremovable, cannot give meaningful purpose to the pain and develop feelings of hopelessness and despair. These feelings, like the sleeplessness, spiral to greater proportions as the patient is subjected to surgical operations, chemotherapy, radiation therapy, and/or other anticancer treatment. Each time the patient experiences hope; if the therapy fails, disappointment and gradually increasing bitterness, anger, and resentment follow. Some patients with advanced cancer develop intense fear of abandonment to a condition of unrelieved suffering.

The social effects of uncontrolled cancer pain are equally devastating. In many patients pain becomes the central focus of their lives and the lives of their families. The fact that most patients with advanced cancer must stop working causes not only economic but also emotional stress and a feeling of dependency and uselessness. The physical appearance and behavior produced by the patient's pain and suffering stresses the family emotionally; this in turn is perceived by the patient and consequently aggravates the pain and suffering. Some patients with severe intractable pain become so discouraged and desperate as to contemplate suicide.

PAST AND CURRENT STATUS OF CANCER PAIN CONTROL

Various sources of information suggest that, like chronic pain in general, cancer pain all too frequently has been and continues to be improperly managed. A study by Marks and Sachar (35) of Montefiore Hospital in New York revealed that physicians prescribed amounts of narcotic analgesic for patients with moderate to severe pain due to cancer (and other medical disorders) that were about 50 to 65% of the doses established as effective and nurses administered as little as 20 to 30% of the (inadequate) amount prescribed. For example, for patients with severe pain due to abdominal cancer, cancer of the pancreas, and lymphosarcoma, 50 mg of meperidine every 4 hr was prescribed and yet patients received only 50 to 75 mg of meperidine per day. Consequently, in most patients, moderate to severe pain persisted after the narcotic therapy.

Parkes (40) found that among patients cared for in the hospital who had severe or very severe pain, it remained unrelieved during the terminal stage of the disease. Moreover, of patients managed at home, the incidence of unrelieved severe or very severe pain during the terminal phase increased nearly sixfold over that experienced during the period before the terminal phase of the disease. These figures suggest that pain control was inadequate in the hospital and even worse in the home. Parkes noted that this was in contrast to treatment at St. Christopher's Hospice, where pain control is effectively carried out: the incidence of severe and unrelieved pain was 36% during the preterminal period, but this dropped to 8% during the terminal phase of the disease.

Aitkin-Swan (1) reported that of the 52% of patients with significant pain for a continuous period of time before death, the pain was relieved "to a certain extent" in 18%, whereas the rest had "distressing pain" until death. Hinton (28) reported that in half of the 82 cancer patients with pain, the pain remained unrelieved until death. Other British clinicians reporting unrelieved cancer pain include Cartwright et al. (15) and the problem of unrelieved cancer pain was the subject of an editorial comment by Saunders (45). Turnbull (49) reported that, at the end of palliative therapy, 45% of the patients with lung cancer had pain and two-thirds of the patients died with unrelieved pain. Pannuti et al. (38,39) reported that chemotherapy resulted in remission of pain in only 15% of the patients, and that 2 weeks before death pain was present in 80% of patients with bone metastases, 76% of patients with solid tumors, 67% of patients with soft tissue tumors, and 50% of patients with head and neck cancer. V. Ventafridda and Gallucci (1983, *personal communication*) reported that in 145 patients who died from cancer of the lung, 40% of those treated in the hospital and over half of those treated in the home had unrelieved pain due to insufficient or total lack of narcotic therapy.

At a workshop on cancer pain sponsored by WHO and the Floriani Foundation of Milan, Italy, oncologic authorities from Brazil, India, Israel, Japan, and Sri Lanka reported that of 433 cancer patients treated for pain, 30% had complete or almost complete relief, 40% had only partial relief, and 30% had no relief (46). Greenwald et al. (26) found that during and after cancer therapy, patients continued to have significant pain as follows: pain was present during and after surgical therapy in 85% of the patients with cancer of the lung, in 100% of the patients with cancer of the pancreas, in 57% of the patients with cancer of the prostate, and in 70% of the patients with cancer of the cervix. The statistics for those receiving chemotherapy were 60% with lung cancer and 50% with prostate cancer; after radiation therapy pain was present in 50% with lung cancer, 75% with prostate cancer, and 60% with cervical cancer.

For over three decades Bonica has studied the reasons for inadequate cancer pain control at regular intervals and has repeatedly found these can be arbitrarily listed in two major categories: (a) great voids in the knowledge of the mechanism and pathophysiology of cancer pain, simply because there has been little or no basic research in this field; and (b) improper application of the knowledge and therapeutic modalities that have been available. Since these have been discussed and detailed previously (9–12,14), and since the chapters that follow this consider the proper application of pharmacologic and other therapeutic modalities, no further comments will be made here except to stress one point: We have a variety of drugs and other therapeutic modalities that, if properly applied, provide effective pain relief for most cancer patients. For proper application of these various modalities, it is essential to adhere to certain principles of diagnosis, to identify the cause and mechanism of the pain, and to apply the method or methods more suitable under the circumstances.

BASIC PRINCIPLES OF DIAGNOSIS AND THERAPY OF CANCER PAIN

The objective of a cancer pain control program is to provide the patient with maximum pain relief with a minimum of adverse side effects or aggravation of the existing pathophysiology. Indeed, effective relief of pain should improve the physiologic, psychologic, and emotional state, and thus the quality of life of the patient. Obviously, the primary method of pain relief is to cure the patient by eliminating the tumor with one or more anticancer modalities, but unfortunately we are far from achieving this goal in the majority of patients. This is particularly true in patients with recurrent or metastatic cancer in the advanced or terminal stage of the disease. In such instances, the management of pain revolves around three methods: (a) temporarily decreasing or eliminating the tumor with anticancer therapy; (b) symptomatic relief of the pain without affecting the tumor; or (c) most frequently, a combination of methods. It deserves strong emphasis that while the patient is undergoing therapy intended to cure or diminish the lesion to relieve symptoms, it is essential to use concomitantly various systemic analgesics and adjuvant drugs or other forms of symptomatic therapy to provide respite from the pain during the treatment. The combined use of anticancer therapy and symptomatic pain relief (32,50–52,54) will obviate useless, depressing, and demoralizing pain and suffering the patient and family would otherwise incur while the patient is being subjected to definitive therapy.

Selection of the optimal method of pain relief to be used depends on: (a) an accurate diagnosis of the cancer pain syndrome, i.e., the site, mechanism, intensity, and other characteristics of the pain; (b) the chronology of the oncologic process, including the type of neoplasm, grade of differentiation, site of current or probable future spread or metastasis, and types and responses to previous therapies; (c) the physical and psychologic condition of the patient and his or her decision as to which method is to be used after the advantages, disadvantages, side effects, and complications of each method are discussed with the patient and the family; (d) the drugs, equipment, and other resources available and practical for use; and (e) most importantly, the knowledge and skill of the available personnel to apply each method expertly.

Diagnostic Evaluation

A detailed history of the pain complaint is an essential first step in making a diagnosis. Information should be obtained on the date and characteristics of the pain at the onset, during its course since the condition was diagnosed, and at the time the patient is seen for the pain diagnosis and therapy. It is important to consider the location and distribution of the pain and its possible spread, its quality, its severity, and any time characteristics, i.e., whether it is continuous or recurs periodically for minutes or hours or if it occurs in brief bouts of lancinating pain. To measure the intensity of the pain, one might use the visual analog scale, but for a more comprehensive evaluation of not only intensity but also quality and affective aspects of pain, it may be desirable to use the McGill Pain Questionnaire or a simpler modification of it. It is also important to elicit information about associated symptomatology, including sensory phenomena such as paresthesia, dysesthesia, and numbness, and whether muscle weakness and visceral dysfunction have developed. The patient should be asked to indicate what factors aggravate the pain and what conditions relieve it. What does position, such as lying, standing, or sitting, do to the pain? What are the effects of physical and social activities and how is the pain affected by medication, sleep, and emotional status? Finally, it is important to ascertain the impact of pain on physical activities, sleep, and work.

It is also essential to obtain a general medical and family history. Since most patients with cancer pain present a complex array of physical, psychologic, behavioral, and affective manifestations, a psychosocial and psychologic evaluation is mandatory. The social history should include age, sex, marital status and family, education, religion, medication intake, and cultural and ethnic backgrounds. It is also important to determine the influence of environmental factors on the pain and the impact pain has on patient interactions with spouse, family, and friends and on social activities. The psychologic evaluation should include a psychologic history and determination of the presence and degree of anxiety, depression, hypochondriasis, and neuroticism. This may require the application of various simple psychometric tests such as the Minnesota Multiphasic Personality Inventory, the Beck Depression Inventory, and the Profile of Mood States.

A careful examination of the painful region and general physical, neurologic, and orthopedic examinations are also essential to acquire objective data and substantiate the clinical history. A detailed neurologic examination is particularly useful to differentiate local pain from referred pain, and to differentiate pain due to peripheral-nerve involvement from pain due to plexus or cord involvement. For example, in a patient with low back and radicular symptomatology in L5–S1 distribution, together with an absent ankle jerk, it is likely that nerve roots, rather than the plexus, are involved.

Various diagnostic tools may be essential to determine the mechanisms of pain. Since plain radiographs have limitations, it may be necessary to supplement them with bone scan and tomography. In addition to the usual laboratory examination, special biochemical procedures may be necessary. Cisternal and lumbar myelography and cerebrospinal fluid cytology are sometimes necessary to determine the etiology of the pain. A variety of specific nerve blocks can play an important role in ascertaining the mechanisms and pathways of cancer pain, thus helping to diagnose the cancer pain syndromes.

Evaluation of all therapeutic modalities currently available for the relief of cancer pain is crucial in selecting the most effective therapy. It is essential to know not only the analgesic efficacy and advantages, but also the limitations and disadvantages of each procedure. Only with such knowledge integrated with the information obtained from the history and physical examinations is it possible to determine the best method (or methods) to relieve each patient's pain. It deserves reemphasis that complex cancer pain problems require a multidisciplinary team effort in evaluating the patient and in developing the most appropriate therapeutic strategy.

CANCER PAIN SYNDROMES

The information obtained from the history, physical examination, and laboratory evaluation permits the physician to make a correct diagnosis of the pain syndrome or syndromes involved. This diagnosis is important in deciding the therapeutic modality or modalities to be used because various syndromes respond differently to various therapies (7,11,14,21,26,53). Pain syndromes that develop in cancer patients can be divided into five major groups: (a) those caused by direct tumor involvement; (b) those associated with cancer therapy; (c) those due to the debilitating effects of the disease; (d) those totally unrelated to the cancer; and (e) a combination of two or more of these types.

In one study, Foley (19) found that, among the cancer pain population, pain was due to direct tumor involvement in 78%, to cancer therapy in 19%, and was unrelated to cancer in 3%. In another study involving outpatients, she (20) found the incidence of these three groups to be 62, 29, and 10% respectively, suggesting that in ambulatory patients with treatable cancer, cancer therapy plays a more important role than the cancer itself in producing pain. In a prospective survey of 100 cancer patients admitted to Sir Michael Sobell House in Oxford, Twycross (51) found that 80 of the patients had more than one pain, 34 had four or more sources of pain, and the total number of pains experienced by these 100 patients was 303. Of 91 patients with pain caused by the cancer, 50 had pain caused by other factors, whereas in only 41 was the pain caused by the cancer alone. He noted that, in addition to pain caused by the cancer or cancer therapy, 42 patients also had pain unrelated to the neoplasm, e.g., arthritis, myofascial syndromes, or low back pain. These findings emphasize the importance of making a correct diagnosis of the etiology and possible mechanisms of the pain, and also the fact that the physician must focus attention on the whole patient rather than on the cancer-related problems.

In this chapter only those syndromes due to direct tumor involvement and those produced by or associated with cancer therapy will be considered. The syndromes described in the text and summarized in Table 5 are based on the classification first proposed by Bonica (7,8) three decades ago and a number of syndromes more recently described by Foley (19–22) and by others (24,25,31,33,42,43,48). A few comments on basic mechanisms of pain that may be operative in various types of tumors will preface the discussion of tumor-related and therapy-related pain.

Mechanisms of Cancer Pain

The mechanisms of chronic cancer pain, like those of other types of chronic pain, are unknown. Presumably they involve prolonged dysfunction of the neurologic and/or psychologic substrates of pain. From a therapeutic viewpoint, it is useful to classify these mechanisms arbitrarily into four categories depending on the site and type of their pathology: peripheral, peripheral-central, central, and psychologic (14).

Peripheral mechanisms are operative when the pathophysiology of the tumor causes either persistent noxious stimulation or sensitization or both of the high threshold receptors known as nociceptors that are endings of some A-delta and C fibers involved in transmission of nociceptive (pain) information. With some lesions, stimulation, sensitization, or both involves the axon of these nociceptor-afferent units. Sensitization of the nociceptors of these units results from liberation of certain algesic or pain-producing substances that follows tissue injury or is part of the response to inflammation.

Peripheral-central mechanisms are operative when the tumor or therapy, or both, severely damage or destroy peripheral nerves or nerve roots. This results in loss of normal sensory input, or deafferentation, that in turn produces abnormal firing patterns of neurons in the somatosensory system in the neuraxis (55). Central mechanisms are operative when the tumor or cancer therapy damages the spinal cord and/or brainstem and cause "central" pain.

Psychologic mechanisms are operative when emotional stress or psychopathology is the primary cause of chronic pain. Although anxiety and depression may play an important role in cancer pain, it is unusual for pain to be due primarily to psychologic factors. On the other hand, emotional stress may initiate and sustain psychophysiologic (respondent) mechanisms producing myofascial pain syndromes with trigger areas or cause excessive muscle tension that may be a source of muscle pain. Moreover, in some patients, favorable environmental factors may enhance operant mechanisms and reinforce "pain behavior."

Pain Syndromes Associated with Direct Tumor Involvement

Tumor Invasion of Bone

Bone invasion by either primary or metastatic tumors is the most common cause of pain in patients with cancer (9,10,19,21,24,25,52). Pain may be the presenting complaint as, for example, in patients with multiple myeloma, or it may represent the first sign of metastatic disease, as occurs in patients with carcinoma of the breast or prostate. Pain may be located at the site of the lesion as occurs with rib tumors or may be referred to a distant area of the body such as knee pain associated with metastatic hip disease and sacroiliac pain associated with metastasis at the L1 vertebral body. The pain, usually constant and progressive in severity, is believed to be caused by peripheral mechanisms, especially sensitization of nociceptors by prostaglandins. The most common sites of metastasis are the spine, base of the skull, pelvis, and long bones, although the ribs, shoulder, scapula, and sternum are not infrequently involved.

Tumor Compression or Infiltration of Peripheral Nerves or Plexuses

This is the second most frequent cause of pain in cancer patients (7,11,14,19,21,25). Sudden compression by metastatic fracture of a vertebra or other bone adjacent to nerve roots or nerves is often accompanied by sharp neuralgic pain projected to the distribution of the nerve or nerves involved and is a manifestation of a mechanical radiculopathy or neuropathy. Progressive infiltration, compression, or both of nerve roots, nerve plexuses, or peripheral nerves by enlarging tumor, enlarged lymph nodes, and/or bone

TABLE 5. *Pain syndromes in cancer patients*

Primary etiology	Pathophysiology	Characteristics of pain	Other symptomatology
Pain due to direct tumor involvement *Tumor Invasion of Bone* Vertebral body metastases Subluxation of atlas	Metastasis of odontoid process of axis → fracture of atlas → compression of spinal cord or brainstem	Severe neck pain radiating to back and top of skull, aggravated by flexion and other movements	Progressive sensory, somatomotor, and autonomic dysfunction beginning in upper extremity
C7-T1 metastases	Cancer of breast and lung → hematogenous spread or more frequently tumor originating in brachial plexus or paravertebral space → spread to adjacent vertebra & epidural space	Constant, dull, aching pain in paraspinal area radiating to both shoulders; unilateral radicular pain with radiation to shoulder & medial (ulnar) aspect of limb	Tenderness on percussion of spinous process; paresthesia & numbness in ulnar distribution of limb; progressive weakness of triceps & hand; Horner's syndrome indicating sympathetic involvement
L1 metastases	Frequent site of metastasis from breast, prostate, or other tumors	Dull, aching pain in midback with reference to regions of one or both sacroiliac joints and superior iliac crest; radicular pain with girdle-like distribution anteriorly or to both paraspinal areas in the sacroiliac region	Possible numbness & weakness in the back; pain exacerbated by lying or sitting & relieved by standing
Sacral metastases	Another frequent site of metastasis from breast, prostate, or other tumors	Dull, aching pain in the low back or coccygeal region exacerbated by lying or sitting & relieved by walking	Perianal sensory loss & bowel & bladder dysfunction & impotence
Base of the skull Jugular foramen	Metastasis to jugular foramen with involvement of cranial nerves IX–XII	Occipital pain with reference to the vertex & one or both shoulders & arms, exacerbated by head movement	Tenderness of occipital condyle & often ptosis, hoarseness, dysarthria, dysphagia & neck & shoulder weakness

Clivus syndrome	Metastasis to clivus of sphenoid bone & basilar portion of occipital bone	Progressively severe vertex headache exacerbated by neck flexion	Dysfunction of lower (VII–XII) cranial nerves, which begins unilaterally but extends bilaterally
Sphenoid sinus	Metastasis to the sphenoid sinus on one or both sides	Severe bifrontal headache radiating to both temples with intermittent retro-orbital pain	Nasal stuffiness or sense of fullness in the head associated with diplopia
Other bone involvement			
Pelvis	Metastasis from breast, prostate, or other tumors	Dull, aching pain in sacrum, hips, or pubis	Extension to sacral plexus with consequent motor, sensory, and/or autonomic changes
Long bones	Metastasis from breast, prostate, or other tumors	Dull, aching, severe pain localized to site of tumor that may be referred (e.g., reference to knee from hip metastasis); pathologic fracture produces severe pain on movement	
Tumor Involvement of Nerves, Plexus, or Spinal Cord			
Peripheral, cranial, or spinal neuropathy	Infiltration, compression, or damage to nerve	Dull, aching, burning pain associated with bouts of lancinating pain in distribution of affected nerve or nerves; hyperpathia	Hypesthesia, dysesthesia, motor, and/or autonomic dysfunction & reflex changes
Brachial plexus	Infiltration, compression, or damage of brachial plexus by metastatic tumor of lower cervical & upper thoracic vertebra or Pancoast tumor	Progressively more severe, dull, aching pain which is first located in the shoulder & arm & later extends to medial part of scapula & arm, elbow, forearm, & hand	Paresthesia, dysesthesia, hypesthesia; subjective numbness & progressive muscle weakness in C7, C8, & T1 distribution, often Horner's syndrome & anhidrosis of the ipsilateral face
Lumbosacral plexus	Infiltration, compression, or damage of lumbar & sacral plexus by cancer of the prostate, bladder, uterus, cervix, or colon from extension of tumor into adjacent lymph nodes & bone	Radicular pain either in groin & anterior thigh (L1, 2, & 3 nerve involvement) or down the posterior aspect of leg to the heel (L5, S1, & S2 distribution) or dull, aching midline pain in the perianal area (S2, 3, 4 distribution)	Paresthesia followed by numbness & dysesthesia & progressive motor & sensory loss in the areas supplied by the involved nerves

Continued

TABLE 5. (Continued)

Primary etiology	Pathophysiology	Characteristics of pain	Other symptomatology
Reflex sympathetic dystrophy	Infiltration, compression, or damage of major nerve or plexuses → sprouting/damage to nerve membrane sensitive to norepinephrine/pressure/stress	Severe burning pain not limited to a segmental or peripheral nerve distribution; aggravated by touch & emotional stress	Hyperalgesia, vasomotor, & sudomotor disturbances & other symptomatology of causalgia; complete pain relief with sympathetic block
Leptomeningeal carcinomatosis	Tumor infiltration of the cerebrospinal leptomeninges with or without invasion of the meninges of the brain	Pain in 40% of patients of 2 types: headache, with or without neck stiffness; and pain in the low back & buttock regions	Malignant cells in cerebrospinal fluid, elevated protein, & low glucose
Epidural spinal cord compression	Tumor compression of cervical, thoracic, or lumbosacral parts of spinal cord & involvement of vertebra or roots of spinal nerves	Local dull, aching pain, & tenderness in the region of involved vertebral body or radicular pain which is unilateral with cervical or lumbosacral compression & bilateral with thoracic cord compression	Depend on site of epidural compression, include motor weakness progressing to paraplegia, sensory loss, & loss of bowel & bladder function
Tumor Involvement of Viscera			
Obstruction of hollow viscus or of ductal system of solid viscus	Contraction of smooth muscle under isometric conditions → intense distention of smooth muscles	Diffuse, poorly localized, dull, aching, or colicky pain referred to abdominal wall or chest wall	Dyspnea & cough with thoracic viscera; abdominal distention, nausea, vomiting with abdominal visceral pathology
Rapid tumor growth in solid viscus	Rapid growth of hepatic, splenic, or kidney tumors → rapid distention & stretching of investing fascia → stimulation of mechanical nociceptors	Dull, aching, poorly localized pain referred to midline (liver) or in one side in lower thoracic & upper lumbar segments	Symptomatology of visceral dysfunction
Other Types of Tumor involvement			
Tumor involvement of blood vessels			
Infiltration	Perivascular lymphangitis & vasospasm	Burning pain in the areas supplied by the affected vessels	Signs of vasoconstriction or ischemia

Obstruction of large vein	Venous engorgement → progressive edema → distention of fascial compartments & soft tissue	Severe headache with obstruction of veins to head; pain in limbs with obstruction in axilla or pelvis	Edema & cyanosis of affected part
Obstruction of large artery	Ischemia in tissues with liberation of algesic substances	Progressively severe, burning pain	Paresthesia, pallor of affected part
Necrosis/ulceration of muscus membrane	Necrosis, infection, & inflammation of mucus membrane → algesic substances → lowering of nociceptors' threshold	Excruciating local or referred pain depending on site of lesion	Signs of infection or inflammation
Syndromes associated with cancer therapy *Postsurgical Syndromes* Postthoracotomy, postmastectomy, postradical neck resection	Partial injury or complete severance of nerves during operation → damage to nerve membrane or neuroma formation, which becomes hypersensitive to pressure & norepinephrine → abnormal sensory input to CNS (peripheral-central mechanisms)	Continuous, burning or dull, aching pain with occasional bout of lancinating pains in the areas supplied by affected nerves, aggravated by touch, movement, or emotional stress with catecholamine release	Dysesthesia, hyperesthesia in the scar area with hypesthesia in the surrounding zone
Postamputation pain	Persistent nociception in stump & loss of sensory input to neuraxis → deafferentation (peripheral-central mechanism)	Constant aching or burning pain in stump or in phantom limb or cramping "proprioceptive" pain characterized by abnormal position of missing part of limb, also lancinating pain	Sudomotor & vasomotor changes in stump
Postchemotherapy Pain Peripheral neuropathy	Symmetrical polyneuropathy caused by vinca alkaloids (peripheral mechanism)	Constant burning pain in the hand and/or feet	Dysesthesia & paresthesia
Steroid pseudorheumatism	Diffuse myalgias & arthralgias caused by withdrawal of steroid medication (peripheral mechanism)	Diffuse pain & tenderness in affected muscles & joints	Fatigue & general malaise; these & the pain disappear with reinstitution of steroid medication

Continued

TABLE 5. (Continued)

Primary etiology	Pathophysiology	Characteristics of pain	Other symptomatology
Aseptic necrosis of bone	Aseptic necrosis of humoral head or femoral head as complication of chronic steroid therapy (peripheral mechanism)	Dull, aching pain in the shoulder or knee	Limitation of joint movement with inability to use arm or hip joint → frozen shoulder or impaired hip
Mucositis	Drug produces biochemical changes in mucus membranes & other structures (peripheral mechanisms)	Severe, excruciating pain in mouth, throat, nasal passages, and gastrointestinal tract	Difficulty or inability to eat, drink, or even talk
Postradiation Therapy Pain			
Radiation fibrosis of brachial or lumbosacral plexus	Radiation-induced fibrosis of connective tissue surrounding plexus & consequent injury to nerve structures develops 6 mo to 20 yr following therapy → deafferentation (peripheral-central mechanisms)	Progressively increasing, severe, diffuse, burning pain in a part or the entire limb which occurs after other symptomatology	Numbness, paresthesia, dysesthesia, & motor weakness in distribution of C5 & C6 in the upper limb or in lower limb
Radiation myelopathy	Damage to spinal cord → Brown-Sequard syndrome progresses to complete transverse myelopathy (central pain)	Pain that is localized or referred to peripheral structures	Dysesthesia & other symptomatology of myelopathy
Painful peripheral nerve tumors	Radiation induces nerve sheath tumors 4–20 yrs after therapy	Progressively severe, burning, aching pain in distribution of involved nerves	Progressive neurologic deficit
Postherpetic neuralgia	Induced by radiation or after herpes zoster in the area of tumor pathology	Continuous burning pain associated with intermittent lancinating pain	Dysesthesia, hypesthesia, and hyperaphia
Pain due to cancer-induced debility (constipation, bed sores, gastric distention, rectal or bladder spasm)			
Muscle Spasm or Myofascial Pain Syndromes	Related to specific lesions	Local or referred pain depending on site of pathophysiology	Related to the specific pathophysiology
Pain unrelated to cancer (arthritis, osteoporosis, migraine, etc.)	Pathology of affected parts	Local pain in affected part or referred pain	Related to the specific pathophysiology

metastasis produce neuralgic pain that is often constant and burning in character. It is associated with hyperpathia, hyperesthesia, and dysesthesia in the area of sensory loss and, at times, reflex changes and motor dysfunction.

The pain and symptoms caused by tumor infiltration of the brachial plexus and the lumbar and lumbosacral plexuses are summarized in Table 5. Frequently, superior pulmonary sulcus (Pancoast) tumor extends into the epidural space and produces symptoms of spinal cord compression. Constant, burning pain associated with hyperpathia, hyperesthesia, and dysesthesia is also often associated with intrathoracic or retroperitoneal tumors that compress nerves in the paravertebral area. Metastatic tumors in ribs often involve intercostal nerves, in which case pain is the earliest symptom, followed by progressive sensory loss distal to the site of compression. Initially the pain is due to peripheral mechanisms, but soon the abnormal sensory input produces pathophysiologic changes in the spinal cord, creating a peripheral-central mechanism. This is likely to develop when the tumor severely damages or destroys the nerve, thus producing deafferentation pain. Some patients develop causalgia-like pain and other symptoms of reflex sympathetic dystrophy that can be dramatically relieved with regional sympathetic blockade (7,29).

Tumor Involvement of the Neuraxis

Cerebral metastasis from systemic cancer is a common cause of diffuse headache in cancer patients. The pain is worse in early morning, gradually decreases in intensity by late afternoon, and is often associated with hemiparesis and other central nervous system symptoms. Metastasis to the spinal cord and brainstem may produce "central pain," but more often produces neurologic signs, varying according to the site of the metastasis (24).

Epidural spinal cord compression develops from metastasis of one or more vertebral bodies with consequent encroachment on the spinal cord, or is due to extension of the tumor through the intervertebral foramen into the spinal canal as often occurs with Pancoast tumor. Epidural spinal cord compression is a common cause of local dull aching back pain and tenderness in the region of the affected vertebra often associated with radicular pain and later with neurologic signs (24).

Severe Obstruction of Viscera

Severe obstruction of the stomach, intestine, biliary tract, ureters, uterus, or urinary bladder causes intense contractions of the smooth muscles under isometric conditions (i.e., when the exit of the viscus is obstructed) and produces visceral pain (7,11). The pain is characteristically diffuse and poorly localized and is referred to dermatomes supplied by the same spinal cord segments supplying the affected viscus. A similar mechanism probably operates in oncologic processes that obstruct the outflow of ductal systems of the pancreas, liver, and other solid viscera. In all these conditions, persistent obstruction produces progressively greater contractions and finally intense distention with consequent progressively greater pain. The pain is due solely to peripheral mechanisms created by persistent nociceptor stimulation or sensitization of nociceptors or both.

Infiltration and Occlusion of Blood Vessels

Infiltration of blood vessels by tumor cells resulting in perivascular lymphangitis and vasospasm may produce diffuse burning or aching pain that does not have a peripheral nerve distribution. Partial or complete occlusion of a blood vessel by an adjacent tumor produces venous engorgement, ischemia, or both. Venous engorgement results in edema in all structures supplied by the obstructing vessels. This in turn causes distention of fascial compartments and other pain-sensitive structures, resulting in progressively more severe pain. Examples are the progressively more severe headache consequent to obstruction of the veins draining blood from the head; the pain and edema in an upper limb seen with cancer of the breast that obstructs venous return from the limb; or lower limb pain and edema caused by obstruction of the venous return by tumor and enlarged lymph glands in the pelvis. Ischemia produced by obstruction of a major artery possibly causes cellular breakdown with production of algesic substances that lower the nociceptors' threshold.

Other Etiologies/Mechanisms of Cancer Pain

Rapid distention and stretching of the investing pain-sensitive fascia or periosteum stimulate mechanical nociceptors and produce pain (7). This process is probably responsible for pain associated with growing tumors of liver, spleen, certain types of kidney tumors, or growing tumor of bone. Each of these processes produces distention of the investing pain-sensitive structure, with consequent stimulation of mechanical nociceptors. If the pain-inducing tumor is in a superficial somatic structure, the pain is sharp and relatively well localized; if the tumor is situated in deep somatic structures or viscera, the pain is dull, poorly localized, and usually referred to dermatomes receiving the same nerve supply as the involved structure.

Necrosis, infection, inflammation, and ulceration of mucous membranes caused by cancer (or cancer therapy) produce pain that is frequently excruciating, and is likely to occur with cancer of the lips, mouth, oropharynx, face, and tumors of the gastrointestinal and genitourinary tracts. The inflammatory reaction produces algesic substances that lower the threshold of nociceptors so that innocuous stimuli produce excruciating pain usually localized in the region.

Pain Syndromes Associated with Cancer Therapy

Postsurgical Pain Syndromes

Postthoracotomy pain

A small percentage of patients who undergo thoracotomy for removal of lung cancer or other neoplasms develop pain in the distribution of the intercostal nerves that may be partially injured or completely severed (7,11,14,19,21). The pain usually begins 1 to 2 months after the operation and is characterized by constant pain in the area of sensory loss, with occasional bouts of lancinating "shock-like" pains. Dysesthesia in the scar area with hypesthesia in the surrounding zone are often prominent symptoms. The proximal portion of severed nerves regenerate and produce small neuromata. In partially damaged nerves there is damage to the nerve membrane. The neuroma and damaged membrane are hypersensitive to pressure and norepinephrine (55), and consequently light touch, movement of the part, or emotional stress, which usually increases catecholamines, exacerbates the pain. Moreover, lateral and anterior flexion also exacerbate the pain. As a result, some patients may develop a concomitant frozen shoulder and consequent limitation of motion, disuse atrophy of the arm, and a true reflex sympathetic dystrophy.

Postmastectomy pain

A small but significant number of patients who have undergone radical mastectomy develop pain in the posterior arm, axilla, and anterior chest wall due to damage to the intercostobrachial nerve, the lateral cutaneous branch of T2, and damage to other upper thoracic nerves (7,21). The pain, usually developing 1 to 2 months after the operation, has a tight, constricting, burning character located in the posterior arm and axilla, which radiates across the anterior chest wall and is often associated with hyperesthesia and hyperalgesia, making wearing of a bra or underclothes uncomfortable. The pain is also exacerbated by arm movement; patients often posture the arm in a flexed position close to the chest wall, and consequently incur a high risk of developing a frozen shoulder.

Other postsurgical syndromes

A number of patients who undergo radical neck dissection develop constant burning pain, dysesthesia, and lancinating pain in the region of the neck (7,21). The physiopathologic process is similar to that of other postsurgical neuropathies. Following amputation of a limb, the patient may develop pain in the stump and/or pain in the phantom limb (7). Stump pain is usually constant and burning in character, whereas pain in the phantom limb may be either burning or cramping "proprioceptive" pain such as might be caused by abnormal positioning of the distal part of a limb.

In all these postsurgical pain syndromes, peripheral-central mechanisms are usually operative. Initially, the peripheral nociceptive dysfunction predominates, but eventually the disturbance in the neuraxis plays the most important role.

Postchemotherapy Pain Syndromes

Peripheral neuropathy

Painful dysesthesia following treatment with the vinca alkaloid drugs such as vincristine and vinblastine occurs as part of a symmetrical polyneuropathy that usually develops with the doses of the drug required to achieve an antineoplastic effect (21,43). Dysesthesias are commonly localized to the hands and feet and characterized by burning pain exacerbated by noxious stimuli. Children frequently develop more diffuse generalized myalgia and arthralgia, often beginning with jaw pain and progressing to a symmetrical polyneuropathy that includes cranial nerve dysfunction.

Steroid pseudorheumatism

This condition occurs following withdrawal of steroid medication (44), and is characterized by diffuse pain and tenderness in muscle and joints, fatigue, and malaise, all of which disappear with resumption of steroid medication.

Aseptic necrosis of bone

Necrosis of the head of the femur or the humerus or both with consequent pain in the knee or shoulder joint, respectively, occurs as a complication of chronic steroid therapy in cancer patients (21,30). The pain is deep, dull, aching in character, constant, and often very severe. The pain is often the presenting symptom, followed by radiographic changes several weeks to months after its onset. Patients experience limitation of joint movement and a progressive inability to use the arm. Although it occurs most commonly in patients with Hodgkin's disease, it may also occur in any patient on chronic steroid therapy. A bone scan is the most useful diagnostic procedure and is usually positive before changes in the plain films appear.

Mucositis

Mucositis occurs in the mouth, throat, nasal passages (11) and gastrointestinal tract and results from toxicity of certain chemotherapeutic agents that produce biochemical changes in mucous membranes and other pain-sensitive structures. The consequent excruciating pain is difficult to relieve even with topical anesthetics and may interfere with eating, drinking, and even talking.

Postradiation Therapy Pain

Radiation fibrosis of the brachial and lumbosacral plexus is a cause of progressively severe intractable pain associated with numbness and paresthesia, usually in the C5–C6 distribution on the lower limb, associated with lymphedema in the arm and radiation skin changes. Brachial plexus fibrosis can be differentiated from tumor infiltration or damage of the plexus because the tumor usually involves the lower portion of the plexus and does not present with lymphedema and radiation skin changes (33). Other postradiation complications include myelopathy, pain-peripheral nerve tumors, and postherpetic neuralgia, which may represent a complication of radiation therapy or may occur following herpes zoster that has developed in the area of tumor pathology (21–23).

REFERENCES

1. Aitken-Swan, J. (1959): Nursing the late cancer patient at home. *Practitioner*, 183:64–69.
2. American Cancer Society (1981): *Cancer Facts and Figures*. American Cancer Society, New York.
3. Birkhahn, D. (1982): Data presented at WHO Workshop on Cancer Pain Relief, Pomeiro, Italy, October 14–16.
4. Bond, M. R. (1971): The relation of pain to the Eysenck Personality Inventory, Cornell Medical Index and Whitely Index of Hypochondriasis. *Br. J. Psychiatry*, 119:671–678.
5. Bond, M. R. (1979): Psychologic and emotion aspects of cancer pain. In: *Advances in Pain Research and Therapy, Vol. 2*, edited by J. J. Bonica and V. Ventafridda, pp. 81–88. Raven Press, New York.
6. Bond, M. R., and Pearson, I. B. (1969): Psychologic aspects of pain in women with advanced cancer of the cervix. *J. Psychosom. Res.*, 3:13–19.
7. Bonica, J. J. (1953): *Management of Pain*. Lea & Febiger, Philadelphia.
8. Bonica, J. J. (1954): The management of pain of malignant disease with nerve blocks. *Anesthesiology*, 15(March):134; (May):280–301.
9. Bonica, J. J. (1978): Cancer pain: A major national health problem. *Cancer Nur. J.*, 4:313–316.
10. Bonica, J. J. (1979): Cancer pain: Importance of the problem. In: *Advances in Pain Research and Therapy, Vol. 2*, edited by J. J. Bonica and V. Ventafridda, pp. 1–12. Raven Press, New York.
11. Bonica, J. J. (1980): Cancer pain. In: *Pain*, edited by J. J. Bonica, pp. 335–362. Raven Press, New York.
12. Bonica, J. J. (1980): Pain research and therapy: Past and current status and future needs. In: *Pain, Discomfort and Humanitarian Care*, edited by L. K. Y. Ng and J. J. Bonica, pp. 1–46, Elsevier/North Holland, Amsterdam.
13. Bonica, J. J., and Benedetti, C. (1984): Management of cancer pain. In: *Comprehensive Textbook of Oncology*, edited by A. R. Moossa, M. C. Robson, and S. C. Schimpff. Williams & Wilkins, Baltimore. (*in press*).
14. Bonica, J. J., and Ventafridda, V. (Eds.) (1979): *Advances in Pain Research and Therapy, Vol. 2*. Raven Press, New York.
15. Cartwright, A., Hockey, L., and Anderson, A. B. M. (Eds.) (1973): *Life Before Death*. Routledge & Kegan Paul, London.
16. Chapman, C. R. (1979): Psychologic and behavioral aspects of pain. In: *Advances in Pain Research and Therapy, Vol. 2*, edited by J. J. Bonica and V. Ventafridda, pp. 45–58. Raven Press, New York.
17. Cornaglia, G., Massimo, L., Haupt, R., Melodia, A., Benedetti, C., and Bonica, J. J. (1984): Incidence of pain in children with neoplasms. (*in preparation*).

18. Daut, R. L., and Cleeland, C. S. (1982): The prevalence and severity of pain in cancer. *Cancer*, 50:1913–1918.
19. Foley, K. M. (1979): Pain syndromes in patients with cancer. In: *Advances in Pain Research and Therapy, Vol. 2*, edited by J. J. Bonica and V. Ventafridda, pp. 59–78. Raven Press, New York.
20. Foley, K. M. (1979): The management of pain in malignant origin. In: *Current Neurology, Vol. 2*, edited by H. R. Tyler and D. M. Dawson, pp. 279–302. Houghton Mifflin, Boston.
21. Foley, K. M. (1981): *The Management of Cancer Pain, Vol. 1*. Hoffman-LaRoche, Inc., New Jersey.
22. Foley, K. M., Woodruf, J. M., Ellis, F., and Posner, J. B. (1975): Radiation-induced malignant and atypical schwannomas. *Neurology*, 25:354.
23. Front, F., Schneck, S. O., Frankel, A., and Robinson, E. (1979): Bone metastases and bone pain in breast cancer: Are they closely associated? *JAMA*, 242:1747–1748.
24. Gilbert, P. W., and Krem, T. H. (1978): Epidural spinal cord compression from metastatic tumor: Diagnosis and treatment. *Ann. Neurol.*, 3:40–51.
25. Greenberg, H. S. (1981): Metastases to the base of the skull: Clinical findings in 43 cases. *Neurology*, 31:530–537.
26. Greenwald, H. P., Bonica, J. J., and Chapman, C. R. (1982): Team Management of Pain in Cancer Patients. Proceedings of the XIII International Cancer Congress, Abstract No. 2508, p. 191, Seattle, Washington, September 8–15.
27. Greenwald, H. P., Francis, A., Bergner, M., Perrin, E. B., and Bonica, J. J. (1982): Incidence and natural history of pain in four cancer sites. Proceedings of the XIII International Cancer Congress, Abstract No. 2808, p. 191, Seattle, Washington, September 8–15.
28. Hinton, J. M. (1963): The physical and mental distress of the dying. *Q. J. Med. M. S.*, 32:1–21.
29. Hubert, C. (1978): Recognition and Treatment of Causalgic Pain Occurring in Cancer Patients. *Abstracts of the Second World Congress on Pain, p. 47*. International Association for the Study of Pain, Seattle, Washington.
30. Ihde, D. C., and DeVita, V. T. (1975): Osteonecrosis of the femoral head in patients with lymphoma treated with intermittant combination chemotherapy (including corticosteroids). *Cancer*, 36:1585–1588.
31. Jellinger, K., and Strum, K. W. (1971): Delayed radiation myelopathy in man. *J. Neurol. Sci.*, 14:389–408.
32. Kanner, R. M., and Foley, K. M. (1981): Patterns of narcotic drug use in a cancer pain clinic. *Ann. NY Acad. Sci.*, 362:161–172.
33. Kori, S. H. (1981): Brachial plexus lesions in patients with cancer: 100 cases. *Neurology*, 31:45–50.
34. Kornell, J. A. (1980): *Pain in Advanced Cancer Patients*. Thesis for M.A. of Nursing, School of Nursing, University of Washington, Seattle, Washington.
35. Marks, R. M., and Sachar, E. J. (1973): Undertreatment of medical inpatients with narcotic analgesics. *Ann. Intern. Med.*, 78:173–181.
36. Norton, W. S., and Lack, S. A. (1980): Control of symptoms other than pain. In: *Continuing Care of Terminal Patients: Proceedings of the International Seminar on Continuing Care of Terminal Cancer Patients*, edited by R. G. Twycross and V. Ventafridda, pp. 167–178. Pergamon Press, New York.
37. Oster, M. W., Vizel, M., and Turgeon, M. S. (1978): Pain of terminal cancer patients. *Arch. Intern. Med.*, 138:1801–1802.
38. Pannuti, E., Martoni, A., Rossi, A. P., and Piana, E. (1979): The role of endocrine therapy for relief of pain due to advanced cancer. In: *Advances in Pain Research and Therapy, Vol. 2*, edited by J. J. Bonica and V. Ventafridda, pp. 145–166. Raven Press, New York.
39. Pannuti, E., Rossi, A. P., and Marraro, D. (1980): Natural history of cancer pain. In: *Continuing Care of Terminal Patients: Proceedings of the International Seminar on Continuing Care of Terminal Cancer Patients*, edited by R. G. Twycross and V. Ventafridda, pp. 75–89. Pergamon Press, New York.
40. Parkes, C. M. (1978): Home or hospital? Terminal care as seen by surviving spouse. *J. R. Coll. Gen. Prac.*, 28:19–30.
41. Pollen, J. J., and Schmidt, J. D. (1979): Bone pain in metastic cancer of prostate. *Urology*, 13:129–134.
42. Posner, J. B. (1979): Neurological complications of systemic cancer. *Med. Clin. North Am.*, 63:783–800.

43. Rosenthal, S., and Kaufman, S. (1974): Vincristine neurotoxicity. *Ann. Intern. Med.,* 80:733–738.
44. Rotstein, J., and Good, R. A. (1957): Steroid pseudorheumatism. *Arch. Intern. Med.,* 99:545–555.
45. Saunders, C. M. (1978): Editorial note to relief of pain. In: *The Management of Terminal Disease*, edited by C. M. Saunders, pp. 65–66. Yearbook Publishers, Chicago.
46. Stanley, K. (1982): *Analysis of Cancer Pain*. Questionnaire Data. Presented at WHO Workshop on Cancer Pain Relief, Pomeiro, Italy, October 14–16.
47. Stjernward, J. (1982): Cancer. *World Health*, (September–October) pp. 2–7.
48. Stoll, B. A., and Andrews, J. T. (1966): Radiation-induced peripheral neuropathy. *Br. J. Med.,* 1:834–837.
49. Turnbull, F. (1979): The nature of pain that may accompany cancer of the lung. *Pain,* 7:371–375.
50. Twycross, R. G. (1975): The use of narcotic analgesics in terminal illness. *J. Med. Ethics,* 1:10–17.
51. Twycross, R. G. (1978): Relief of pain. In: *The Management of Terminal Disease*, edited by C. M. Saunders, pp. 65–92. Yearbook Publishers, Chicago.
52. Twycross, R. G. (1982): Controlling pain in cancer patients. *Mod. Med. (Lond.),* 8:2–13.
53. Twycross, R. G., and Ventafridda, V. (1980): *The Continuing Care of Terminal Cancer Patients*. Pergamon Press, New York.
54. Twycross, R. G., and Wald, S. J. (1976): Long-term use of diamorphine in advanced cancer. In: *Advances in Pain Research and Therapy, Vol. 1*, edited by J. J. Bonica and D. C. Albe-Fessard, pp. 653–661. Raven Press, New York.
55. Wall, P. D., and Gutnick, M. (1974): Ongoing activity in peripheral nerves: The physiology and pharmacology of impulses originating from a neuroma. *Exp. Neurol.,* 43:580–593.
56. Wilkes, F. (1974): Some problems in cancer management. *Proc. R. Soc. Med.,* 67:23–27.
57. Woodforde, J. M., and Fielding, J. R. (1975): Pain and cancer. In: *Pain, Clinical and Experimental Perspectives*, edited by M. Weisenberg, pp. 332–336. Mosby, St. Louis.

*Advances in Pain Research
and Therapy, Vol. 7,*
edited by C. Benedetti et al.
Raven Press, New York © 1984.

Use of Systemic Analgesic Drugs in Cancer Pain

V. Ventafridda

Division of Pain Therapy, National Cancer Institute, 20133 Milan, Italy

For optimal results in managing patients with pain of advanced cancer, it is essential that the physician have full knowledge of the three main groups of therapies currently available for this purpose. The first group, specific anticancer treatments, consists of radiation therapy, chemotherapy, hormone therapy, and palliative surgery.

The second group, noninvasive therapies, includes (a) systemic analgesics and related drugs; (b) psychologic techniques such as progressive relaxation, biofeedback, behavior modification, hypnosis, and other cognitive behavioral interventions; (c) neurostimulating techniques; and (d) physical therapy.

The third group, invasive therapies, includes (a) transient regional analgesia achieved by injection of local anesthetics into the subarachnoid or extradural space or near one or more peripheral nerves; (b) regional analgesia achieved by intraspinal injection of narcotics; (c) prolonged regional analgesia achieved by injection of neurolytic agents; and (d) ablative neurosurgical techniques, some that entail open operations to interrupt pain pathways permanently, such as spinal or cranial rhizotomy; spinothalamic, medullary, or mesencephalic tractotomy; control thermocoagulation to produce percutaneous cordotomy or thermorhizotomy; and stereotactic procedures to destroy pain pathways in the midbrain or to place stimulator electrodes deep in the brain to produce brain stimulation analgesia.

In order to decide the technique, method, or combination of methods best for the particular patient, it is necessary for the physician to know the indications, advantages, disadvantages, side effects, complications, and contraindications of each of these various techniques (4,20,21). In regard to anticancer treatment, it is well known that some systemic tumors, lymphomas, and particularly Hodgkin's lymphomas are highly chemosensitive and often undergo complete regression and cure after proper treatment with chemotherapy. Similarly, other tumors with histologically differentiated cells, such as breast cancer in the intermediate stage (T1, M1), respond very positively to new types of combined chemotherapy; many types of bony metastasis respond to radiation therapy (14). Surgery is used to decrease or eliminate the tumor cells either temporarily or permanently or to bypass obstruction of a hollow viscus or large blood vessel. As there is no reason why the patient should continue to suffer from pain while undergoing anticancer therapy, the pain must be managed with systemic analgesics.

In the event anticancer therapy is ineffective or not indicated, the patient's pain must be controlled with one of the other modalities. Before proceeding with antalgic therapy, it is essential for the physician to: (a) carry out an assessment of the quantification of the pain before and after therapy; (b) integrate noninvasive treatment and particularly analgesic drugs with invasive therapies so that they complement one another since no single treatment is ever sufficient for prolonged periods; and (c) recognize that pain is never constant because its location and intensity vary according to the type of nociceptive stimulation produced by a specific neoplastic process.

BASIC CONSIDERATIONS

Evaluation of the Patient and the Pain

No antalgic therapy should be undertaken without a careful evaluation of the patient's physical, psychologic, and emotional status achieved through a detailed history and comprehensive physical and psychosocial assessment (4,21).

A careful history of the pain complaint is an essential first step in determining the most effective therapy. It is important to ascertain the location, distribution, intensity, quality, and time characteristics of the pain (i.e., whether it is continuous or occurs in bouts) and what factors aggravate and relieve it (e.g., effects of coughing, straining, walking, standing, lying down, emotional stress). It is also important to elicit information about associated phenomena including sensory deficits, muscle weakness, and visceral dysfunction, and to obtain a history of the oncologic process to determine the mechanisms and pathophysiology of the pain.

A comprehensive psychologic and social evaluation is essential to develop the most effective therapeutic strategy. This should include a general psychologic and behavioral assessment and the application of appropriate psychometric tests to detect anxiety, depression, mood changes, and other emotional effects of pain accurately. Evaluation of the alteration of personalities should be carried out using such psychometric tests as the Minnesota Multiphasic Personality Inventory and the Hamilton test. Psychosocial evaluation should include determination of cultural background, religious beliefs, interaction with spouse and family unit, social activities, and the impact of these on the pain and vice versa (i.e., impact of the pain on social activities, and interaction with spouse, family, and friends). It is also important to assess the number of hours spent in sleeping, standing, sitting, lying, and the activity of life (5,10).

A careful examination of the painful region and general physical, neurologic, and orthopedic examinations are also essential to acquire objective data and substantiate the clinical history. A detailed neurologic examination is particularly useful in differentiating local pain from referred pain and in differentiating pain due to peripheral nerve involvement from pain due to plexus or cord involvement. The examination should exclude pain due to pathologic fracture, which is best treated with mechanical stabilization, and pain due to some acute cause such as intestinal obstruction. It is also important to determine what specific anticancer therapies have been carried out or are being carried out and their side effects as well as what other antalgic therapy has been used previously and what its effects were.

Various diagnostic tools may be essential to determine the pathophysiology of the pain. As is well known by oncologists, radiographs have limitations in depicting bone metastasis and, therefore, it is usually necessary to supplement them with coned-down views, bone scanning, tomography, and computed tomography scan, in that order. In addition to the usual laboratory examination, special biochemical procedures may be necessary. Cisternal and lumbar myelography and cerebrospinal fluid cytology are sometimes necessary. Diagnostic/prognostic nerve blocks can play a unique role in ascertaining the mechanism and pathways of cancer pain.

The intensity and quality of the pain are assessed by the patient's description in response to the physician's question using Scott and Huskisson's visual analog scale consisting of a bar 10 cm long with 0 being no pain and 10 being the most excruciating intolerable pain (17). In addition, at the National Cancer Institute of Milan, Italy, we use a self-descriptive record in which the patient marks the hours of pain every day, expressed in a scale with five key words that have a certain coefficient. By multiplying the hours by their coefficient and summing up the obtained values, we get a score that is significantly related to the patient's evaluation of pain (22). This evaluation is carried out by specially trained paramedical personnel because the therapist should not take part in the evaluation of the pain to avoid a biased interpretation of the response to therapy. The weekly self-descriptive record and a data record give a concise picture of the physical and behavioral conditions of the patient through numerical data easily computerized (25). This type of evaluation usually takes at least 50 to 60 min.

In the evaluation as well as the management of the patient, relatives are encouraged and, indeed, requested to take active part. Recruitment of relatives to the pain therapy team is one of the first and most important tasks of the pain therapist. Although in most cases at the beginning of treatment patients are able to go to the pain clinic unaccompanied, it is best to have one of the relatives present for the latter to obtain a good insight into the therapy. Later, when the patient is confined to bed at home, the relative's collaboration becomes essential.

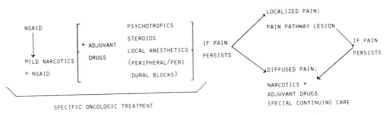

FIG. 1. Therapeutic strategy in advanced cancer pain.

Therapeutic Strategy

Once evaluation of the patient and assessment of the pain are completed, progression of the therapeutic strategy for controlling pain in patients with irreversible cancer should be carried out according to the schema depicted in Fig. 1. During the time the patient is receiving specific anticancer therapy intended to cure the disease or decrease the lesion to provide pain relief, it is essential to use concomitantly various noninvasive antalgic techniques. These include nonsteroidal anti-inflammatory drugs (NSAID), narcotics, psychotropic drugs, steroids, and/or regional analgesia achieved with a local anesthetic or intraspinal narcotics. The combined use of anticancer therapy and symptomatic pain relief will eliminate useless, depressing, and demoralizing pain and suffering the patient and family would otherwise incur while the patient is being subjected to definitive oncologic therapy.

If the pain persists after an adequate trial of oncologic therapy, it must be controlled symptomatically by one or more of the methods mentioned above. If the pain is localized, an ablative neurosurgical procedure such as percutaneous cordotomy or thermorhizotomy should be considered. It is important to appreciate that within 5 to 12 weeks every invasive treatment will require small doses of narcotics. This is due to the recurrence of the pain and/or dysesthetic effects of the neurosurgical operation (21). On the other hand, if the pain is diffuse, ablative neurosurgical techniques are rarely indicated nor should they be considered during the terminal stages of the disease. Under these conditions, the mainstay of therapy is the use of systemic analgesics and related drugs.

Principles of Analgesic Therapy

The administration of systemic analgesics, alone or more frequently in combination with one or more adjuvant drugs, constitutes the most practical and widely used method of relieving cancer pain. These include: (a) nonnarcotic analgesics such as aspirin and other NSAID; (b) narcotic agonists and antagonists; and (c) a heterogeneous group of adjuvant drugs that includes corticosteroids, tricyclic antidepressants, anxiolytic agents, phenothiazines, and other central-acting agents that have some analgesic effects.

Use of these drugs is widespread as they are readily available, inexpensive, simple to administer, and, if properly used, reasonably effective in relieving the pain. Proper use requires thorough knowledge of the pharmacology, including the mechanisms of action, pharmacokinetics, pharmacodynamics, dosage range, optimal route of administration, time of onset and duration of action, side effects, and possible complications and how to prevent these or treat them promptly if they occur. It is especially important to know well the dose of each drug that is less than analgesic, the dose of analgesia, and the dose level at which toxicity develops.

In order to obtain optimal results with this major method of pain control, it is essential to adhere to certain specific rules pertaining to their administration.

1. Select the most effective drug or combination of drugs based on the intensity, quality, and duration of the pain. For mild pain (1 to 3 on the visual analog scale), pain may be managed with aspirin or other NSAID alone or in combination with adjuvant drugs; moderate pain (4 to 6 on the visual analog scale) can usually be managed with NSAID and a weak narcotic such as codeine; severe pain (above 7 on the visual analog scale) is best relieved with a potent narcotic used alone or in combination with NSAID and/or adjuvant drugs.

2. The drugs should be administered by mouth unless this route is contraindicated due to vomiting or other gastrointestinal disorders.

3. Use tablets or preparations that contain a single drug. Avoid tablets containing drug combinations because this precludes individualizing the dose of each ingredient in the tablet.

4. Titrate the correct dose of the drug(s) to the needs of each particular patient.

5. Administer the drug at fixed intervals to prevent recurrence of pain and consequent anxiety and fear.

6. Prevent or treat side effects by employing adjuvant drugs or switch to a less toxic drug of the same class.

7. When the drug is no longer effective, use a more powerful analgesic.

8. In case of persistent severe pain or recurrence of pain, use adjuvant drugs combined with nerve blocks or intraspinal narcotics.

9. As previously mentioned, use analgesics or adjuvant drugs or both during specific oncologic therapy until a maximum analgesic action is produced and as a complement to ablative neurosurgical techniques.

NONNARCOTIC ANALGESICS

Management of mild to moderate pain with aspirin or other nonnarcotic analgesics should be tried before considering the use of narcotics. Moreover, nonnarcotic analgesics are uniquely effective in treating moderate to severe pain due to bone metastases, many of which induce the production of pros-

TABLE 1. *Main nonsteroidal anti-inflammatory drugs*

Type of drug	Daily dosage	Analgesia	Side effects
Acetylsalicylic acid	650 × 5 by mouth	+ +	Gastritis, ipoacusia, ulcers
Lysine acetylsalicylate	1000 × 5 i.v.	+ + +	Gastritis, ipoacusia, ulcers
Indomethacin	50 × 3 by mouth	+ +	Gastritis, disphoria, ulcers
Meglumin indomethacinate	75 × 2 i.m.	+ + +	Gastritis, disphoria, ulcers
Propionic acid derivates (naproxen, ketoprofen, indoprofen)	200 × 5 by mouth	+ +	Gastralgia
Paracetamol	500 × 5 by mouth	+	—

+, minimal; + +, moderate; + + +, strong.

taglandins that cause osteolysis and lower the threshold of nociceptors (3,4,15,26). Since aspirin and NSAID are potent prostaglandin synthetase inhibitors, they produce specific analgesic and anti-inflammatory effects and, in some instances, have antitumor effects in patients with bone metastasis. There is also some evidence that they antagonize or inhibit prostaglandins in the central nervous system and thus increase the analgesic action of narcotic drugs. In high doses they also may produce an antiproliferative action, at least as demonstrated *in vitro* (18). These drugs are also useful in relieving pain caused by: (a) mechanical compression of muscles or tendons (without nerve involvement), as occurs with fibrosarcoma, sarcoma, or swelling of lymph glands; (b) mechanical distention of subcutaneous tissue, as occurs in neoplastic lymphangitis; (c) mechanical distention of the pleura or peritoneum, as occurs in rapidly growing intrathoracic or intraabdominal tumors; and (d) inflammation and stiffness of joints or muscles resulting from anticancer therapy (4).

Table 1 lists the nonnarcotic analgesics in common use and their characteristics. In contrast to narcotics, tolerance and physical dependence do not develop to aspirin and other nonnarcotic analgesics, but these drugs do produce adverse side effects, particularly disturbances of the gastrointestinal tract, hemostasis and coagulation, electrolyte balance, carbohydrate metabolism, protein binding, and clinical manifestation of a hypersensitivity. Of these drugs, aspirin is considered by many oncologic pain specialists to be the drug of choice and acetaminophen (paracetamol) the best alternative to aspirin. The combined use of aspirin with another nonnarcotic analgesic is inadvisable because aspirin lowers the available concentration of the second drug by displacing it from plasma protein.

Acetylsalicylic acid derivatives and other NSAID cause lesions of the gastric mucosa and, because many patients already have inflammation of gastric tissue due to chemotherapy, it is important to use these drugs with caution. The irritating effect on gastric mucosa is particularly strong with aspirin, less with indomethacin and phenylpropionic acid derivatives, and almost nil with drugs such as diflunisal and paracetamol (6).

A retrospective study carried out by the Pain Therapy Division of the National Cancer Institute of Milan on 765 patients treated with different analgesic drugs revealed that NSAID alone can produce good (albeit not complete) pain control in more than 50% of the patients, but that after 5 weeks analgesia persisted in only 25% of the patients (24). Since more than 60% of the patients examined prior to initiating pain therapy revealed that their pain was of high intensity on the visual analog scale, the study impressively demonstrated that the anti-inflammatory drugs can, under certain conditions, control pain of high intensity (24).

If pain persists, the therapist must add a weak narcotic to the nonnarcotic analgesic therapy. Codeine sulphate and dextropropoxyphene are weak narcotics that are effective when combined with NSAID. Codeine sulphate must be administered in dosages of 65 mg combined with 250 mg of aspirin or paracetamol. The typical formula for this combination is 65 mg codeine sulphate, 250 mg acetylsalicylic acid, and 60 mg of caffeine. Dextropropoxyphene should be administered in doses ranging from 50 to 120 mg three times a day combined with 25 to 50 mg of indomethacin or paracetamol.

ADJUVANT DRUGS

Two groups of drugs are adjuvant to the beneficial effects of anti-inflammatory drugs and should be employed in pain therapy. These are psychotropic drugs and steroids.

Psychotropic Drugs

These drugs have an important role in managing cancer pain because of the high percentage of emotional problems present in cancer patients. The main groups of these compounds are the neuroleptics, anxialytics, and antidepressants (Table 2). The antalgic action of this last group, the tricyclic compounds, is very useful at high dosages for pain caused by nervous tissue lesions or by deafferentation (26). The administration of 75 to 100 mg amitriptyline at night combined with the use of 2 to 3 mg of fluphenazine (antianxiety agent) during the day has proven very effective in relieving phantom limb pain, postherpetic neuralgia, and many forms of deafferentation pain. According to some authors, the analgesic action is due to blocking the reuptake of serotonin in the central nervous system and also to blocking synthesis of all prostaglandins (1). In addition to elevating mood and increasing sedation, they assure a good night's sleep. In some patients the atropine-like

TABLE 2. *Main psychotropic drugs*

Group	Drug	Analgesia
Neuroleptics	Chlorpromazine Levopromazine	+ + + (associated with narcotics)
Anxiolytics	Diazepam Lorazepam Fluphenazine	+ (associated with antidepressants)
Antidepressants	Imipramine Amitriptyline	+ + + (in pains due to nervous tissue lesions at high doses) + + (at low doses associated with NSAID or SAID)

effect due to central reduction of the parasympathetic output restricts continuous use of the tricyclic compounds.

Steroids

Corticosteroids enhance or produce analgesia by preventing the release of prostaglandins and commonly stimulate appetite and elevate mood. Although these agents are not as effective as aspirin in relieving bone pain, they seem to be more effective in relieving pain associated with extensive soft tissue infiltration in relatively circumscribed areas, such as head and neck cancer, pelvic malignancies, or massive hepatic metastases. These drugs are also highly effective in relieving pain caused by tumor infiltration of the brachial or lumbosacral plexus or epidural spinal cord compression or severe headache caused by increased intracranial pressure. The study by Gilbert et al. (9) carried out on patients with epidural metastasis established that, with high doses of dexamethasone (96 mg/day in decreasing doses for 15 days), it was possible not only to obtain pain remission but also reduction of the incidence of decompressive laminectomies.

Medroxyprogesterone acetate has a practical application in hormone-dependent tumors such as cancer of the breast, prostate, endometrium, and kidney. This compound administered at very high dosages has an antalgic effect not only because of the steroid activity per se but also due to the chemical hypophyseal block obtained from its administration. In advanced breast cancer with pain that is intractable to specific treatment, the oral administration of 3 g/day for 2 weeks followed by 2 g/day for the following month reduces pain in more than 50% of the cases (7,14). Treatment should be stopped if no results are obtained in the first 2 weeks. Nausea, vomiting, and fluid retention causing hypertension, edema, and cardiac failure are the main side effects. Therefore, this drug is contraindicated in patients with severe cardiac, liver, or kidney disease, as well as those with lung congestion or diabetes.

TABLE 3. *Strong oral narcotic analgesics*

Drug	Typical starting dose (mg)[a]	Potency ratio to oral morphine[b]	Duration of analgesic action (hr)
Morphine	5–10	1	4–5
Methadone	5–10	3–4	6–8
Pethidine	50–100	⅛	2–3
Buprenorphine	0.2	60–80	2–6

[a] These doses are usually adequate but in a small minority a higher dosage may be necessary.
[b] Potency relative to morphine.

Therapy for pain of advanced hormone-dependent cancers should begin with medroxyprogesterone acetate before undertaking any other treatment of pain pathways and before considering hypophysectomy (neuroadenolysis). Localized pain may be relieved by combining this drug therapy with local anesthetic infiltration of the trigger areas or with peripheral blocks, or it may be combined with epidural infusion of local anesthetics and corticosteroids (8).

NARCOTIC ANALGESICS

Morphine and other potent narcotic analgesics are the most frequently used methods for the relief of moderate to severe cancer pain because, as previously mentioned, they are readily available, simple to administer, and effective when properly used (Table 3). Unfortunately, in many instances, patients are given inadequate amounts of narcotics and the pain persists. Several studies have demonstrated that many physicians (including oncologists) and nurses have inadequate knowledge of the pharmacology of narcotics and consequently underestimate the effective dose, overestimate the duration of action, and have serious misconceptions about respiratory depression and addiction. This is further aggravated by the fear of addiction on the part of patients and their relatives and consequently they frequently hesitate to take these drugs or do so infrequently. As will be emphasized below, these are not valid reasons for underdosing patients because, when properly administered, narcotics do not produce clinically significant respiratory depression, and addiction rarely occurs.

Pharmacology

Although all narcotics share the propensity for analgesia, each drug varies in potency, efficacy, and degree and type of adverse side effects. Therefore, to obtain optimal results in cancer patients, it is essential for the physician to know their pharmacology thoroughly, including mechanism of action, pharmacodynamics, dosage range, time of onset and duration of analgesia, side effects, and other characteristics (4). It is now well established that the mechanisms by which these drugs produce analgesia and other effects is by binding to specific opiate receptors in the peripheral and central nervous system of which three specific types are known: (a) mu receptors mediate supraspinal analgesia, euphoria, respiratory depression, and physical dependence; (b) kappa receptors mediate spinal analgesia, miosis, and sedation; and (c) sigma receptors mediate euphoria, hallucination, and respiratory and vasomotor stimulation. The degree of binding to each of these specific receptors is different for each drug and is thus responsible for the variation in potency and in adverse side effects.

Narcotic analgesics also may be classified according to the manner in which they interact with the opiate receptors. Morphine is the prototype of the pure narcotic agonists, which bind and activate the receptors and thus block transmission of nociceptive information, whereas the narcotic antagonists are drugs that block or reverse the effects of morphine and other agonists by more strongly binding to the opiate receptors. Within the latter category are the pure (total) antagonists such as naloxone and a series of antagonists with analgesic action (i.e., partial agonists/antagonists). The latter group affords the advantage of being narcotic analgesics with a lower rate of tolerance development and physical dependence than occurs with the pure agonist, but they also have the disadvantage of producing hallucination and dysphoria in a significant percentage of patients. On the basis of their pharmacologic effects and the characteristics of the abstinence syndrome, two subclasses of partial agonists/antagonists are recognized: (a) the nalorphine-like drugs, which include pentazocine, butorphanol, and nalbuphine, and (b) the morphine-like drugs, partial agonists/antagonists of which buprenorphine is the most promising drug for managing cancer pain patients.

Morphine is the best potent narcotic to treat moderate to severe cancer pain because of its availability and low cost and because, given in optimal doses, it produces effective analgesia for 3 to 5 hr. It has long been considered a standard of reference against which all narcotics are compared. The plasma half-life of morphine is similar to the duration of analgesia. This is in contrast to methadone, which has a longer half-life than the duration of analgesia. Although the parenteral/oral potency ratio is said to be 1:6, some investigators have found that, when the oral form is taken in solution at regular intervals, the ratio can be as low as 1:3. The effective oral dose of morphine varies considerably and ranges from as little as 2.5 mg to more than 200 mg, depending on the age and nutritional state of the patient, the intensity of the pain, and the presence of the disease (Table 4). However, most patients with moderate to severe cancer pain obtain effective analgesia with oral doses ranging from 10 to 30 mg.

Methadone is a synthetic narcotic analgesic that is considered an alternative to morphine in patients who have persistent intolerance to the stan-

TABLE 4. *Initial dosages of morphine by mouth, depending on the previous medication*

Previous medication	Initial dosage of morphine (mg)	Dosage increment (mg)
NSAID	5	2.5
Weak narcotics (pentazocine, codeine, dextropropoxifene)	10	5
Narcotics (3 vials or more per day)	20	10

dard agent. The effects of methadone are similar to those of morphine but it has a higher parenteral/oral potency ratio and a much longer half-life (17 to 24 hr) than morphine and produces analgesia that lasts from 6 to 8 hr. Although the longer half-life and longer duration of action facilitate the achievement of sustained (plateau) analgesia after 4 to 7 days of administering effective doses at fixed intervals, it also tends to accumulate in plasma that accounts for side effects seen with this agent.

Meperidine is a synthetic narcotic analgesic that has a slightly better oral/parenteral potency ratio than morphine but produces analgesia lasting only 2 to 3 hr. It is not as good as morphine in relieving very severe pain. Moreover, it has a relatively high incidence of undesirable central nervous system effects, such as tremor, twitching, agitation, and occasionally convulsions when doses exceed 300 mg every 3 hr. Patients receiving chronic meperidine therapy may develop multifocal myoclonal seizures due to accumulation of its active metabolite normeperidine.

Pentazocine is a widely used antagonist/agonist of the nalorphine type for the relief of moderate cancer pain, but it offers little advantage over other potent narcotics and produces psychomimetic effects in a significant percentage of patients. Nalbuphine and butorphanol offer the advantages of lower incidence of tolerance and physical dependence than the potent agonists, but these advantages are offset by the fact that they are available only for parenteral use. Buprenorphine has a potency ratio to oral morphine of 60:80 and produces analgesia in 2 to 6 hr. Some patients with severe cancer pain are relieved on a 6-hr regimen of sublingually administered buprenorphine.

Side Effects and Complications

Clinical trials have shown that administered in equianalgesic doses to the general population, all potent narcotics produce similar incidences and degrees of side effects. On the other hand, certain patients develop one or more of the adverse effects to greater degrees compared with the general population. In any case, each patient receiving narcotic therapy should be closely monitored for the development of adverse side effects and complications (2,4).

Constipation is the most frequent and uncomfortable side effect of narcotics. Therefore, with the onset of narcotic therapy, measures should be instituted to assure the patient a regular bowel regimen by administering cathartics, stool softeners, and fluids. Untended constipation can lead to frank bowel obstruction.

Nausea and vomiting are other very annoying side effects that can be prevented or effectively treated by giving one of the potent antiemetics such as hydroxyzine, prochlorperazine, or haloperidol. In a vomiting patient, the administration must be done only by the parenteral route and then by the oral route. Peridural or intrathecal infusion by catheter should then be considered. In that case we must remember that the daily dosage should be reduced to about 1/50 of the oral dose (23). Excessive sedation, drowsiness, confusion, and/or dizziness and unsteadiness may develop during the initial few days of proper narcotic therapy but usually clear in 3 to 5 days. Patients in whom persistent sedation and drowsiness occur can be managed with the concomitant use of amphetamines or by reducing the dose and increasing the frequency of the narcotic or both to assure the patient of sustained analgesia.

Provided the doses of potent narcotics are titrated to achieve adequate pain relief, clinically significant respiratory depression does not occur because pain is a powerful respiratory stimulant and thus counteracts the narcotic-induced depression. On the other hand, respiratory depression occurs when the drug is given in excessive doses or when adequate doses are administered too frequently. Severe depression can develop in debilitated patients who are given methadone too frequently with consequent rapid buildup of plasma levels.

Tolerance is a normal pharmacologic response to chronic narcotic therapy, characterized by the development of resistance to the analgesic effects and other actions of the drug. The early sign of tolerance is the patient's complaint that the duration and/or degree of analgesia has decreased. Tolerance is treated by increasing the frequency or dose of the drug or both (20). This means that it is necessary to increase the dosage to obtain the same analgesic effect, as well as the respiratory depression, stipsis, and other toxic phenomena. Keep in mind that the doses required to depress the respiratory centers are much higher than those required to remove pain. The dosage limit of the drug preceding toxicity increases with the dosage needed to obtain an analgesic effect (27). It is important to consider the plasmatic half-life when choosing the opiate because if the half-life has a longer duration than the analgesic effect, the toxic phenomena can be easily pointed out in the chronic administration (11). Although cross-tolerance among narcotics occurs, it is not complete; therefore, switching to an alternative narcotic often results in adequate pain relief.

Physical dependence is the other physiologic response to the pharmacologic effects of chronic narcotic use and is characterized by development of the abstinence syndrome on the abrupt withdrawal of the drug. It can be prevented by slowly tapering the dose of narcotic and can be effectively treated by reinstituting the drug in doses of about 25 to 40% of the previous daily dose. In any case, it is important to emphasize that the problem of physical dependence is not a valid reason for not giving sufficient doses of narcotics to patients with advanced cancer pain.

Addiction is a term used interchangeably with such terms as *drug abuse* or *physical dependence* but should be limited to describing psychologic dependence and must be distinguished from the normal pharmacologic responses of tolerance and physical dependence. Addiction or psychologic dependence is characterized by an abnormal behavior pattern of drug abuse, by craving of a drug for other than pain relief, by becoming overwhelmingly involved in the procurement and use of the drug, and by the tendency to relapse after withdrawal. As previously mentioned, fear of addiction has been the primary factor for underdosing with narcotics in patients with cancer pain and other severe pain. In fact, narcotic addiction occurs rarely or not at all in patients receiving narcotics to relieve acute or chronic pain including cancer pain. Therefore, the fear of addiction should be dispelled among physicians, nurses, and patients and should never be considered as reason for not giving ample doses of narcotics for the therapy of severe cancer pain.

Principles of Narcotic Use

To obtain optimal results with the use of narcotics for the relief of severe cancer pain, it is essential to adhere to certain basic principles. The first is to select the most appropriate drug and determine its optimal dose and route of administration for each patient on the basis of the: (a) intensity and duration of the pain; (b) physical, nutritional, and mental status of the patient; (c) pharmacologic action and side effects of each drug; and (d) optimal route of administration. Whatever the narcotic drug given and the route of administration, a cardinal rule is to give the patient sufficient amounts of narcotics to provide satisfactory and sustained pain relief with minimal side effects. This requires an effective dose of the drug be given at fixed intervals to produce continuous pain relief.

Generally, narcotic analgesics with longer duration of action such as morphine given by mouth are preferable because they produce longer analgesia and therefore require administration at less intervals, obviate needle injections, and facilitate the achievement of sustained analgesia. Most importantly, a degree of self-care and independence is maintained as the patient is not constantly relying on someone else for the next dose. Although the onset of analgesia is slower with oral administration than with parenteral administration, it is of no importance once the patient has achieved sustained analgesia. Extensive clinical trials by Saunders (16) and her staff since 1967, carried out at St. Christopher's Hospice in London, as well as by Twycross

(19,20), Mount (13), and others who have worked in hospices, have clearly demonstrated that oral narcotics are effective in relieving moderate to severe pain in 85 to 90% of patients with advanced cancer. This compared with effective pain relief ranging from 65 to 81% reported by other institutions (12,13,19). The difference is due to the fact that, in St. Christopher's and other hospices, patients are not treated with the usual hospital approach; symptom control and the needs of each particular patient are emphasized. This care is carried out by a highly specialized staff together with the relatives of each patient (16).

To determine the optimal dose and frequency of administration of morphine, it is necessary to titrate the patient's pain with the drug over a period of days and to monitor and evaluate carefully the analgesic action of each dose. Initially, a base-line evaluation is carried out by carefully noting the degree and duration of pain relief following the first two or three doses. If these doses produce inadequate pain relief, subsequent doses are increased in increments of 50% of the initial dose until satisfactory analgesia is achieved. On the other hand, if the initial dose produces adequate analgesia but is associated with respiratory depression, undue sedation, or other adverse side effects, the subsequent doses are decreased.

It deserves reemphasis that one of the most important principles of narcotic therapy for cancer pain should be to administer these drugs at fixed intervals on an around-the-clock basis, including awakening the patient from sleep. This technique provides even, sustained analgesia and thus avoids the peaks-and-valleys effect that causes the patient to have periods of pain, a condition that provokes anxiety and is conducive to the development of "abnormal pain behavior." In addition, giving narcotics at regular intervals to provide sustained analgesia decreases the incidence and magnitude of tolerance to these drugs.

Oral Morphine

The aforementioned experiences in hospices as well as the experience we have had at the National Cancer Institute of Milan suggest that oral morphine is one of the most important recent advances in cancer pain therapy. For optimal results with oral morphine, the following principles must be observed.

Selection of Patients

Patients must be selected according to the following criteria: (a) patients should be those with far advanced neoplastic disease who have severe bilateral or diffuse pain that cannot be managed with other analgesic therapeutic modalities; (b) patients must not have serious central nervous system dysfunction; (c) patients must not have obstruction or dysfunction of the gastrointestinal tract; and (d) patients must be willing and able to cooperate, particularly in regard to self-administering the drugs at the specified intervals.

Choice of Solutions

The choice of the solution to be used will be according to the patient's taste and the quantity needed for effective relief. Usually we prescribe 2 to 5‰ solutions made up either with distilled water or associated with syrup and small doses of alcohol. The volume should not exceed 5 to 15 ml for any single administration. Morphine must be preserved in dark glass bottles away from light and heat to avoid the formation of pseudomorphine.

Control of Adverse Side Effects

As previously mentioned, various side effects should be prevented or promptly treated once they develop. Nausea and vomiting are prevented by the use of potent antiemetics given by mouth or, if this is not possible, intravenously. The antiemetics we use most commonly are metoclopramide given in doses of 2 mg/kg/day intravenously, and also prochlorperazine and haloperidol. Since the addition of phenothiazine to morphine may increase drowsiness as well as analgesia and may cause extrapyramidal signs, care must be exercised in using these drugs. The prevention and treatment of drowsiness and constipation have already been mentioned in the previous section.

Induction of Analgesia

Induction of effective analgesia is perhaps the most difficult phase of managing patients with cancer pain with narcotics. Initiation of the treatment must be preceded by adequately informing the patient and relatives about the plasma half-life and duration of analgesia and emphasizing the importance of taking the drug every 4 hr. This is especially important for patients who are to be managed in the home. For such patients, oral morphine is prescribed in an initial dose of 5 or 10 mg and the patient is instructed to take the drug every 4 hr without fail. The patient should be advised that if after 24 hr of drug intake the degree of analgesia remains inadequate, the dose should be increased by 50% and if the pain is excessive, extra doses are prescribed. The first and last dose of the day are "anchored" to the patient's waking and bedtime. The best times to give additional doses during the day are generally 10:00 a.m., 2:00 p.m., and 6:00 p.m. because at these intervals there is an optimum balance between duration of analgesia efficacy and the incidence and severity of side effects. The prescription of $1\frac{1}{2}$ to 2 times the therapeutic dose at bedtime will obviate a dose in the middle of the night. It is important to emphasize that the dosage of morphine can be increased to 100 mg or more every 4 hr.

In patients who are elderly, very young, in poor nutritional states, or have renal or hepatic dysfunction, small initial dosages should be used. Aging produces changes in the pharmacodynamics of the narcotics and causes an increased response; malnutrition gives rise to change in body composition and function. Since most narcotics and their metabolites are excreted by the kidney, special care should be exercised in prescribing and administering narcotics to patients with liver or renal dysfunction.

Maintenance

Once a degree of effective analgesia has been achieved during the induction phase, maintenance of good pain relief must be assured. Since some patients develop tolerance rather rapidly, the dose should be increased to achieve effective analgesia while keeping adverse side effects at a minimum. According to Twycross (19), the tolerance levels of many patients tend to drop after a few weeks. We, as well as other workers, have found that the majority of patients can experience effective and sustained pain relief with average doses ranging from 25 to 35 mg.

Adjuvant Drugs

As previously mentioned, a number of adjuvant drugs enhance the analgesic action of morphine and other potent narcotics and may decrease the adverse side effects of the opiates. In bone pain, NSAID such as aspirin, or corticosteroids such as prednisolone or medroxyprogesterone, should be combined with the morphine. Tricyclic antidepressant drugs must be used with caution, starting with a low dose, because these compounds may induce sleep or cause confusion when combined with morphine. Tranquilizers such as lorazepam and diazepam are particularly effective in assuring a good night's sleep.

Organization

Perhaps the most important phase of effective therapy of cancer pain with morphine or other opiates is to have a well-organized section of pain therapy composed of medical and paramedical staff who are specially trained in managing these patients. For one thing, it is absolutely essential to monitor the patient every 4 hr systematically and to titrate the dose of morphine or other narcotic according to the needs of the patient. The team should be able to carry out this type of monitoring either in the palliative care unit or at home if there is a clinical care program. Since the administration of morphine represents only one part of the total patient care, it is necessary for the pain team to determine whether other pain therapies such as radiotherapy, physiotherapy, occupational therapy, or block of nociceptive pathways are indicated.

Management of cancer patients' needs in palliative care units of hospitals requires that the usual hospital routines be avoided, particularly those concerning meals, temperature monitoring at fixed hours, and so on. The relatives should be admitted at any time. Once pain control is achieved, the patients may be sent home to the care of their families, but they should be followed by specially trained nurses with coordination by the palliative unit.

ACKNOWLEDGMENT

The author is grateful to the Floriani Foundation for assistance in the preparation of the manuscript.

REFERENCES

1. Akil, H., and Liebeskind, J. C. (1975): Monoaminergic mechanisms of stimulation produced analgesia. *Brain Res.*, 96:279.
2. Baines, M. L. (1978): Control of other symptoms. In: *The Management of Terminal Disease*, edited by C. M. Saunders, pp. 99–118. E. Arnold Publishers, London.
3. Bennett, A., Charlier, E. M., McDonald, A. M., Simson, J. S., Stamford, I. F., and Zebro, T. (1977): Prostaglandins and breast cancer. *Lancet*, 2:624–626.
4. Bonica, J. J., and Benedetti, C. (1984): Management of cancer pain. In: *Textbook of Oncology*, edited by A. R. Moossa, M. C. Robson, and S. C. Schimpff. Williams & Wilkins, Baltimore (*in press*).
5. Calman, K. C. (1978): Physical aspects. In: *The Management of Terminal Disease*, edited by C. M. Saunders, pp. 33–43. E. Arnold Publishers, London.
6. Caruso, I., Fumagalli, M., Montrone, F., Vernazza, M., Bianchi-Porro, G., and Petrillo, M. (1978): Controlled double-blind study comparing acetylsalicylic acid and diflusinal in the treatment of osteoarthritis of the hip and/or the knee: Long term gastroscopic study. In: *Diflunsial in Clinical Practice*, pp. 63–73. Futura Publishing, Mt. Kisco, New York.
7. De Conno, F., and Ventafridda, V. (1984): Trattamento antalgico con il MAP nel carcinoma avanzato della mammella (*in press*).
8. De Conno, F., Sanzerla, E., Fochi, C., Zanini, M., and Ventafridda, V. (1983): Modulazione del dolore lombare nel paziente neoplastico. In: *Il Dolore di Origine Lombare*, pp. 331–337. CIC Gruppo Editoriale Medico, Rome.
9. Gilbert, R. W., Kim, J. H., and Posner, J. B. (1978): Epidural spinal cord compression from metastatic tumor: Diagnosis and treatment. *Ann. Neurol.*, 3:40–51.
10. Karnofsky, D. A., and Burchenal, J. H. (Eds.) (1949): *The Clinical Evaluation of Chemotherapeutic Agents in Cancer*, edited by C. M. McLeod. Columbia University Press, New York.
11. Lewis, B. J. (1979): The use of opiate analgesics in cancer patients. *Cancer Treat. Rep.* 63:341–342.
12. Melzack, R., Ofiesh, J. G., and Mount, B. M. (1978): The Brompton mixture: Effects on pain in cancer patients. In: *Psychosocial Care of the Dying Patient*, edited by C. Garfield, pp. 386–395. McGraw-Hill Book Company, New York.
13. Mount, B. M. (1980): Narcotic analgesics. In: *Continuing Care of Terminal Cancer Patients*, edited by R. G. Twycross and V. Ventafridda, pp. 97–116. Pergamon Press Ltd., Oxford.

14. Pannuti, F., Martoni, A., Rossi, A. P., and Piana, E. (1979): The role of endocrine therapy for relief of pain due to advanced cancer. In: *Advances in Pain Research and Therapy, Vol. 2*, edited by J. J. Bonica and V. Ventafridda, pp. 145–165. Raven Press, New York.
15. Powles, T. J., Alexander, P., and Millar, J. L. (1978): Enhancement of anticancer activity of cytotoxic chemotherapy with protection of normal tissues by inhibition of prostaglandins synthesis. *Biochem. Pharmacol.*, 27:1389–1392.
16. Saunders, C. W. (Ed.) (1978): *The Management of Terminal Disease*. E. Arnold Publishers, London.
17. Scott, J., and Huskisson, E. C. (1976): Graphic representation of pain. *Pain*, 2:175–184.
18. Strausser, H. R., and Humles, J. L. (1975): Prostaglandin synthesis inhibition: Effect on bone change and sarcoma tumor induction in BALB/c mice. *Int. J. Cancer*, 15:724–730.
19. Twycross, R. G. (1977): Choice of strong analgesic in terminal cancer: Diamorphine or morphine? *Pain*, 3:63–104.
20. Twycross, R. G. (1978): Relief of pain. In: *The Management of Terminal Disease*, edited by C. M. Saunders, pp. 65–92. E. Arnold Publishers, London.
21. Ventafridda, V., and De Conno, F. (1983): Multimodal approach in management of cancer pain. In: *Proceedings 13th International Cancer Congress, Part D—Research and Treatment*, pp. 17–25. Alan R. Liss, New York.
22. Ventafridda, V., De Conno, F., Di Trapani, P., Gallico, S., Guarise, G., Rigamonti, G., and Tamburini, M. (1983): A new method of pain quantification based on a weekly self-descriptive record of the intensity and duration of pain. In: *Advances in Pain Research and Therapy, Vol. 5*, edited by J. J. Bonica, U. Lindblom, and A. Iggo, pp. 891–896. Raven Press, New York.
23. Ventafridda, V., Figluizzi, M., Tamburini, M., Gori, E., Parolaro, D., and Sala, M. (1979): Clinical observation on analgesia elicited by intrathecal morphine in cancer patients. In: *Advances in Pain Research and Therapy, Vol. 3*, edited by J. J. Bonica, J. C. Liebeskind, and D. Albe-Fessard, pp. 559–565. Raven Press, New York.
24. Ventafridda, V., Fochi, C., De Conno, F., and Sganzerla, E. (1980): Use of nonsteroidal antiinflammatory drugs in the treatment of pain in cancer. *Br. J. Clin. Pharmacol.*, 10:343–346.
25. Ventafridda, V., Pietrojusti, E., and Rambaldi, S. (1982): The experience of a pain clinic in terminal cancer patients. Proceedings 13th International Cancer Congress, Seattle, Abstract 3329.
26. Ventafridda, V., Sganzerla, E., and Fochi, C. (1979): Considerazioni sull'uso di sostanze psicotrope ad azione antidepressiva in terapia antalgica. *Minerva Med.* 70:667–674.
27. Vere, D. W. (1978): Pharmacology of morphine drugs used in terminal care. In: *Topics in Therapeutics, Vol. 4*, pp. 75–83. Pitman Medical, London.

*Advances in Pain Research
and Therapy, Vol. 7,*
edited by C. Benedetti et al.
Raven Press, New York © 1984.

Treating Cancer Pain as a Disease

Theresa Ferrer-Brechner

*Department of Anesthesiology, Oncology Pain Management, Jonsson
Comprehensive Cancer Center, University of California, Los Angeles,
California 90024*

The general principles involved in the total management of patients with cancer-related pain consist of: (a) the understanding of the pathophysiology involved with each type of pain syndrome; (b) the provision of pain-directed modalities that will provide consistent pain relief commensurate with the patient's life expectancy, with minimal side effects; (c) the expert orchestration of various pain-directed modalities to suit the changing goals of the patient as the disease progresses; and (d) the education of the patient and the patient's family regarding maximum use of resources and decision making for choices of therapy.

Since Bonica has introduced the concept of multidisciplinary approach to the management of chronic pain (6), pain clinics have mushroomed throughout the world; they are most prevalent in the United States. Bonica (7) has repeatedly stated that the multidisciplinary concept should also be applied to cancer pain, yet the emphasis of most of the clinics has been on chronic noncancer pain. Although patients with chronic noncancer pain and those with chronic cancer pain syndromes both suffer from prolonged, intractable pain, and both require a systematic, multidisciplinary approach, distinct differences between the two groups exist and need to be recognized.

Chronic nonmalignant pain syndromes are associated with difficulty in identifying distinct pathophysiologic reasons for pain, whereas pain associated with cancer is usually associated with easy identification of somatic causes. Pain associated with cancer is also characterized by acute exacerbations, according to the progression of the disease. Concomitant symptoms such as nausea and vomiting, constipation, and anorexia need to be dealt with before successful pain relief can be obtained.

In designing programs for the management of cancer-related pain, it is important to deemphasize the use of behavior modification, popular with chronic nonmalignant pain management, and to include adequate use of narcotic and nonnarcotic analgesics, reinforcement of coping with death and dying, and use of various neuroablative procedures. The general principles in designing a program aimed toward the total management of patients with cancer-related pain should include: (a) identification of the cause of pain;

TABLE 1. *UCLA outpatient cancer pain clinic incidence of pain syndromes*

	N	Percent
Direct tumor invasion	74	61.7
Bone metastasis	34	18.3
Neural invasion	19	15.8
Visceral invasion	21	10.0
Therapy-related	37	30.8
Postsurgical	20	16.6
Postchemotherapy	6	5.0
Postherpetic	7	5.8
Postradiation	5	4.2

$N = 120$.

(b) identification of the degree of psychologic distress; and (c) orchestration of pain-relief modalities that can decrease the pain threshold, modulate the pain pathway, or interrupt the pain pathway.

BASIC CONSIDERATIONS

Identifying the Cause of Pain

The pain syndromes associated with cancer have been categorized (6,18), and are summarized by C. Benedetti and J. J. Bonica (*this volume*). Identifying the cause of pain is extremely important in understanding how pain relief can be obtained commensurate to the known characteristics of the primary tumor or its metastatic lesions. In addition, certain analgesics may be efficacious for a specific type of primary or metastatic lesion. An example is the specific use of L-DOPA for estrogen-receptive breast or prostate cancer with bone metastasis (28b).

During 1981–1982, a survey of 120 patients referred to the UCLA Cancer Pain Clinic indicated that pain secondary to tumor invasion occurred in 61.7% of patients. Bone metastasis was the most common (18.3%), followed by neural invasion (15.8%) and visceral invasion (10%) (Table 1).

Almost one-third of the patients had pain secondary to cancer-directed therapy and not due to tumor invasion. Under this category, 16.6% of patients had postsurgical pain, 5.8% due to postherpetic neuralgia, 5% due to chemotherapy, and 4.2% due to radiation injury. Patients with pain secondary to tumor-directed therapy are distinct from patients having pain due to direct tumor extension in that they usually have stable or arrested disease and are expected to have a long life expectancy. Therefore, their treatment consists of a program somewhat similar to a chronic noncancer pain program, except that monitoring for signs of recurrent disease must be ensured by regular visits to the oncologist. Treatment consists of time contingent,

TABLE 2. *UCLA outpatient cancer pain clinic site of primary tumor*

	N	Percent
Breast	26	21.7
Colon	18	15.0
Lung	17	14.2
Cervix and uterus	12	10.0
Urinary system	12	10.0
Lymph and blood	8	6.6
Primary bone	6	5.0
Head and neck	6	5.0
Malignant melanoma	6	5.0
Liver and pancreas	6	5.0
CNS	3	2.5

N = 120.

oral, nonnarcotic, or mild narcotic analgesics and adjuvant drugs; noninvasive somatic therapy; and physical and psychologic rehabilitation.

For patients with pain secondary to direct tumor invasion, disease is usually progressive; cancer-directed therapy has usually been exhausted. The treatment is aimed toward tailoring of narcotic and nonnarcotic analgesics, using invasive somatic therapy such as chemical or neurosurgical ablation, and increasing the patients' and their families' coping skills in dealing with the issue of dying.

The most common sites of primary tumor in the 120 patients studied are listed in Table 2, indicating that breast, colon, and lung cancer were the most common. Since breast cancer is associated with multiple bone metastasis, postmastectomy pain syndrome, and neural compression from lymphatic spread, it is not surprising to find it to be the tumor most commonly associated with the highest incidence of pain.

Understanding the characteristics of the primary tumor is of paramount importance in planning the timing of various pain-relieving modalities. For example, the management of patients with slowly growing tumor such as colon cancer is different from that of rapidly growing tumor such as lung cancer. For slowly growing tumors, the program for pain relief should be designed toward the expectation of long and recurrent exacerbations of pain and behavioral changes that accompany chronic pain. For rapidly growing tumors, the program should be designed toward the expectation of progressively intense pain and behavioral changes characteristic of acute pain.

Identifying Psychologic Distress

Cancer pain management is complicated by the necessity of attending to both physiologic and emotional aspects of patient care. As in chronic, nonmalignant pain, ambiguous physiologic and psychologic characteristics often confront the physician treating cancer pain (3–5,27,35). However, in the case of cancer pain, the life-threatening nature of cancer compounds the psychologic and social stress experienced by patients and family members (1,4,8).

Attention has been focused on an interdisciplinary approach to cancer pain (7,11,26). Careful medical and psychosocial assessment is advocated as an initial step in formulating a comprehensive treatment plan oriented to the individual patient (34). Such an approach is necessary because pain threshold, personality characteristics, and social behavior influence the degree to which patients perceive and process painful impulses and the manner in which each person reacts to pain secondary to malignancy (3,4).

Other researchers in this field have drawn attention to psychosocial dimensions of cancer pain. Psychosomatic disturbance, pain complaint behavior, and acceptance of a sick-role status are important factors contributing to the cancer patient's pain experience (30). Cancer pain cannot be studied adequately without considering the meaning of pain to the associated illness, the setting in which pain occurs, and the response of people to whom requests for care and attention are directed. Woodford and Fielding (43) demonstrated that there was significantly greater personality disturbance in a sample of cancer patients with intractable pain when contrasted to a matched group of cancer patients without pain. Contributing to patients' emotional morbidity were high levels of depression, psychosomatic symptoms, hypochondriasis, and anxiety.

An important factor in cancer pain research is the influence of progression of disease on patients' pain experience and psychosocial functioning. Moderate to severe pain occurs with greatest frequency in patients with metastatic cancer (6,7,37). Unremitting pain interferes with adaptive coping behavior and increases a patient's sense of helplessness and hopelessness in the face of approaching death and separation from family and friends. Current reports in the literature support the notion that an association exists between advancement of cancer, psychosocial disturbance, and heightened subjective experience of pain (3,26).

Several psychologic profile studies performed on our group of cancer patients (21) indicate: (a) heightened experience of pain resulting from progression of the disease associated with increased psychologic distress, as evidenced by abnormally high scores of hysteria, depression, and hypochondriasis scales of the MMPI-168; (b) significant reduction in psychologic distress after treatment in patients successfully treated compared with patients with unsuccessful treatment outcome; (c) significant findings not observed between pretreatment scores of MMPI-168 and Health Locus of Control and treatment outcome, therefore demonstrating the futility of such tests in predicting treatment outcome; and (d) social functioning as measured by the marital adjustment scale not related to treatment outcome. Both successful and nonsuccessful pain treatment outcome groups had equally distressed marital relations.

TABLE 3. *Phases of cancer pain treatment*

Phase I: Elevate pain threshold
  Pharmacologic tailoring
    Nonnarcotic and narcotic analgesics
    Adjuvant drugs: antidepressants, anxiolytic
    Control of side effects
  Nonpharmacologic approach
    Identify degree of coping skills
    Psychologic techniques to increase analgesia: hypnosis, guided imagery
Phase II: Modulate pain pathway
  Central stimulation (periventricular gray)
  Spinal cord stimulation (dorsal column stimulation)
  Peripheral stimulation (transcutaneous electric nerve stimulation, acupuncture)
Phase III: Interruption of pain pathway
  Anesthetic techniques
    Peripheral nerve blocks
    Autonomic blocks
    Spinal and epidural blocks
  Neurosurgical techniques
    Preganglionic rhizotomy
    Myelotomy
    Chordotomy
    Thalamotomy
    Hypophysectomy

In another study, we found that when compared with chronic noncancer pain patients, cancer patients perceived their pain as more unpleasant and had significantly higher scores in the sensation subscale of the McGill Pain Questionnaire. Both groups had similar scores in the affective and evaluative subscales. Cancer patients also had significantly higher expectations for pain relief than did chronic benign pain patients (3).

It is obvious that report of pain perception is highly influenced not only by the sensory experience but also by the patient's psychologic variables such as personality profile, expectation, anxiety, and mood. These factors can influence a cancer patient's attitude toward reporting pain, and therefore must be given serious consideration as an integral part of the total management of the patient with chronic cancer pain.

ORCHESTRATION OF PAIN RELIEF MODALITIES

To orchestrate the appropriate choice and timing of various modalities effectively, one must identify specifically: (a) the cause of the pain complaint; (b) the patient's and family's goals; and (c) the various pain relief modalities available to a specific clinic.

Various modalities can be categorized according to whether they provide pain relief by attacking the pathology directly, by elevating the pain threshold, by modulating the pain pathway, or by interrupting the pain pathway (Table 3). The list of available modalities under each category will vary in each institution but the principle in using one or more of these modalities depends on the rapid or slow progression of the disease, the presence of generalized or localized pain, and the risk-benefit ratio as it applies to the individual patient. One cannot overemphasize the need for individualizing the treatment program and the need for frequent alteration of treatment program to parallel the progression of the disease. Unlike chronic noncancer pain, pain management for cancer patients continues until the patient's demise.

To establish the feasibility of using tumor-directed therapy as a means of providing pain relief, the patient must be evaluated thoroughly by both oncologist and clinical algologist (pain physician). Tumor-directed therapy, such as radiation or chemotherapy, often diminishes pain during the early stages of the disease by diminishing the tumor. However, during the more advanced stages of the disease, further diminution of the tumor is no longer feasible by tumor-directed therapy. At this stage, pain becomes the disease entity in itself and further modalities must be aimed at treating pain as a disease. This transition need not occur before pain management is initiated, as the patient might begin to have intractable pain before exhaustion of tumor-directed therapy. However, the transition from tumor-directed to pain-directed modalities is often difficult for patients and their families to accept. Therefore, to ensure compliance and an intelligent decision-making process, the pain physician must delicately explain this transition to the patient and the patient's family.

Phases of Pain Treatment

To demonstrate the orchestration of various pain modalities available to our cancer pain program, Fig. 1 illustrates the phases of pain management, using analgesic tailoring, peripheral stimulation, and neural interruption. The facility consists of an oncology outpatient clinic located in the UCLA Bowyer Multidisciplinary Cancer Clinic to allow access to both cancer clinic and pain management facilities. The multidisciplinary cancer clinic facility contains well-equipped examining rooms, pharmacy, clinical laboratories, basic radiology, procedure room, and recovery room. In this facility, initial physical and psychologic evaluation, laboratory tests, radiography, neural blocks, and follow-up visits take place. The Pain Management Center, located in another area, provides services for biofeedback, behavior conditioning, and peripheral stimulation-induced analgesia. The Oncology Outpatient Pain Clinic is held 2 days a week, but the team is also available for inpatient consultation. Meeting weekly, the primary team consists of a pain management physician, psychologist, oncologic nurse, analgesic study nurse, pharmacist, public health educator, and volunteers, all primarily interested in the management of cancer-related pain. Proximity to oncologists allows ready access to oncologic consultation.

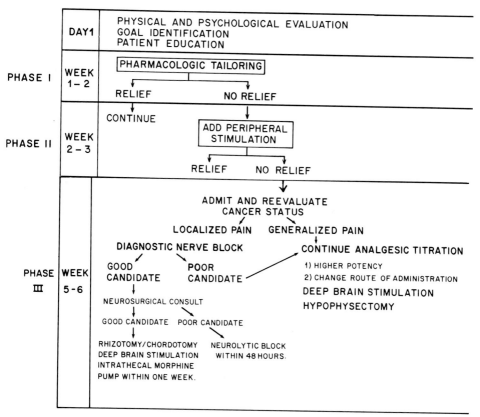

FIG. 1. Management of cancer-related pain. Suggested phases of treatment program utilizing treatment modalities available through the UCLA Cancer Pain Clinic.

The program was established as a satellite of the Pain Management Center, the aim of which was to focus primarily on the management of patients with cancer-related pain. To examine the efficacy of the program, various pain scales, goals for pain relief, and activities were identified on entry to the clinic and weekly for 6 to 8 weeks. Psychologic support was given according to each patient's needs during the entire 6 to 8 weeks. Acceptable pain relief was defined as an analog figure equal to or less than the acceptable pain relief goal and more than 50% reduction of visual analog scales of pain intensity. Acceptable goal was defined as the return to desired goal activities.

Evaluation of the Patient

Before noting the results, it is important to discuss briefly the different phases of treatment, as illustrated in Fig. 1. On entry to the cancer pain center, the first visit is devoted to physical and psychologic evaluation, goal identification, and patient education. To minimize the time spent in the clinic

TABLE 4. *Subjects' profile on analgesic study entry*

Age	31–74 years
Sex	18 males; 12 females
Staging	83% in stage IV
More than 3 sites of metastasis	63%
Past antitumor therapy	86% surgery
	60% chemotherapy
	76% radiation
Current antitumor therapy	33% chemotherapy
	3% radiation
Karnofsky's activity scale	$>74\%$
	$<26\%$

for accomplishing a complete evaluation, a self-history questionnaire and psychologic tests are sent to the patients before the first visit. The questionnaires are designed primarily to gather information useful in planning the treatment program. Data include information on onset of cancer, onset of pain, to what factor does patient attribute the occurrence of pain, previous chemotherapy, surgery, or radiation, sites of metastasis, sites of pain, and review of systems.

Such data are eventually informative in classifying the types of patients being referred to a specific clinic. In reviewing a group of patients who recently completed an analgesic study, we found that 83% of patients referred had stage IV disease, and 60 to 86% had received anticancer therapy, and 63% had more than 3 sites of metastasis (Table 4). This indicates that, in our institution, most patients are referred to the pain center when they are in advanced disease. Therefore, further investigation should include how the patient's pain problem was managed before the time of referral or whether pain problems before referral are significant at all.

Psychologic Evaluation

Part of the evaluation also should include semiquantitative scales that would indicate base-line levels of pain intensity, mood, and psychologic distress. Such tests must be brief enough to allow repeated testing during each patient visit as well as to indicate how the patient is responding to treatment. Tests we use consist of usual analog scales of pain intensity, pain relief, Derogatis Brief Symptom Inventory (12), and the McGill Pain Questionnaire (25). Using such scales also diminishes the time spent during each clinic visit in eliciting meaningful information regarding treatment response.

Neurologic Evaluation

During the first visit, a complete neurologic examination should be done carefully to document existing neural compression. A thorough review of plain radiographs, computed tomography (CT) scans, and tomograms usually reveals the cause of pain. Knowledge of the base-line and periodic neurologic examinations will help alert the pain physician when new or progressive neural compression occurs. A typical example is the occurrence of impending cord compression, characterized initially by escalating pain and later by subtle motor weakness. The pain physician must be alert to the diagnosis of such syndromes, as only prompt treatment with high-dose steroids and radiation therapy could prevent paraplegia or quadriplegia. During the past year, 4 out of 50 patients referred to the cancer pain clinic because of escalating pain were found to have impending cord compression. Thorough neurologic examination during their first visit resulted in prompt referral for appropriate oncologic treatment.

Educational Program

Education of the patient and the family in an organized manner on the function of the cancer pain management clinic is also part of the initial evaluation. In our clinic, we use a slide-tape presentation explaining the role of the cancer pain clinic, the interdisciplinary approach, and appropriate use of analgesics, transcutaneous electric nerve stimulation (TENS), and neural blockage. Such organized patient education can increase the compliance of the patient and the family toward the use of time-contingent analgesic intake, as well as help them in decision making (40).

Goal Identification

Goal identification is an important step in planning the treatment program. Most patients with advanced cancer are unable to identify goals in terms of the pain treatment program. In an attempt to semiquantitate goals, we ask the patients to identify pain relief goals by asking: "If we are able to take away some of your pain, what percentage of pain intensity level (100% being the worst pain you have experienced) would be acceptable to you?" Activities goal is also identified by asking the question: "If we are able to take away your pain significantly, what would you like to be able to do that you can't do now because you have pain?" These goals are recorded on entry to the clinic and reassessed periodically whenever a treatment modality is applied. The overall goal of the pain physician is to provide pain relief by applying modalities with the highest chance of success but with minimal side effects. To achieve this endpoint, we have found that applying a "ladder approach" of treatment modalities provides the optimum method of providing pain relief with minimal side effects.

PAIN TREATMENT MODALITIES

The three phases of treatment consist of: (a) pharmacologic tailoring; (b) peripheral stimulation; and (c) anesthetic neural blockade or neurosurgical intervention. This ladder approach rules out patients who will obtain pain relief with less invasive, lower risk intervention and will identify patients who will need more invasive, higher risk intervention within a reasonable period of time.

Pharmacologic Tailoring

Pharmacologic tailoring involves the effective use of narcotic and non-narcotic analgesic, use of adjuvant drugs to counteract depression and anxiety, and treatment of side effects accompanying any cancer-pain-directed treatment. Although this subject is dealt with elsewhere, reiteration of the principles of pharmacologic tailoring is necessary: (a) individualize the type of drug, dose, frequency, and route of administration; (b) educate the patient and close relatives on the basic pharmacology of the analgesic chosen, since they are the primary monitors of patient response; (c) prescribe medications on a time-contingent, around-the-clock regimen to maintain a continuous and effective serum analgesic level; (d) titrate to an acceptable analgesic level with tolerable side effects; (e) use the oral route as long as possible; and (f) establish a communication line for patients to report efficacy and side effects.

One effective method of increasing the analgesic effect of narcotic analgesic without increasing CNS side effects is by combining a peripherally acting nonnarcotic analgesic. In a recent study of patients with chronic cancer pain we have demonstrated in a double-blind, complete crossover study that the addition of ibuprofen (Motrin) to methadone (Dolophine) resulted in a statistically significant difference in pain intensity and pain relief that persisted through the entire 4 hr of study (Fig. 2). The analgesic effect was more profound in patients with bone pain than in patients with visceral or tissue involvement (Fig. 3), probably because of the antiprostaglandin effect of nonsteroidal anti-inflammatory drugs when combined with narcotic analgesics. Care must be taken that studies be carried out in cancer patients with chronic pain and not acute pain because the analgesics are primarily used for the management of chronic pain.

Medications to decrease anxiety and depression are necessary adjuvants in the management of cancer pain (38). As mentioned earlier, the highest score on the MMPI-168 applied to the cancer patients with pain referred to our clinic is depression (20). In contrast to psychiatric patients, the dose of antidepressents used for cancer patients is 15 to 20% of the usual dose. Antianxiety agents given for prolonged periods of time can aggravate reactive depression. If a prolonged use of anxiolytic agents is necessary, an

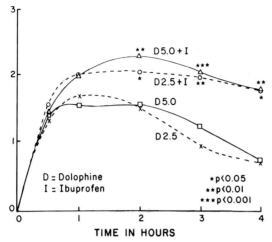

FIG. 2. Results of double-blind complete crossover study in chronic cancer pain patients showing statistically significant pain relief with dolophine alone versus addition of ibuprofen 600 mg to dolophine.

antianxiety drug with some antidepressant effect such as alprazolam (Xanax) may be more appropriate (10).

Central and Peripheral Stimulation

Although peripheral and central stimulation is used widely for the alleviation of chronic noncancer pain, its use for chronic cancer pain is limited.

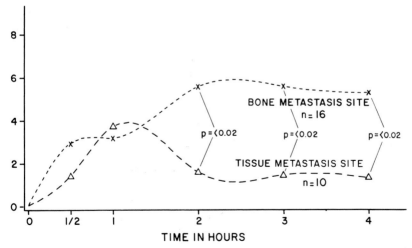

FIG. 3. Mean pain intensity differences by metastasis site. Results of double-blind complete crossover study showing efficacy of dolophine 5.0 plus ibuprofen in patients with bone metastasis.

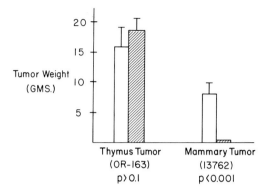

FIG. 4. Tumor weight differential between PAG-stimulated (*open bars*) and nonPAG-stimulated (*striped bars*) groups at sacrifice. Prolactin sensitive tumor growth in rats receiving PAG stimulation is statistically larger than control. There was no difference in the groups with prolactin insensitive tumor. PAG = Periqueductal gray. (From Ferrer-Brechner et al., ref. 16, with permission.)

Release of endogenous opiates by periventricular gray (PVG) stimulation has been effective in midline and bilateral cancer-related pain (28). Recent studies, however, question the opioid mechanism of PVG stimulation since no difference was found between sham and real stimulation in patients with chronic noncancer pain, even when a presurgical i.v. morphine test indicated naloxone reversal of morphine analgesia (41). In our experience, cancer patients referred to the clinic are already on medium- to high-potency narcotic, thus invalidating the use of i.v. morphine test as a predictor of a successful outcome with deep brain stimulation (DBS). Since most patients have advanced disease on referral to the pain center, one has to consider the risk-benefit ratio of surgery and anesthesia in patients with advanced disease.

Deep brain stimulation is also associated with increased hormone serum release. Growth hormone and prolactin increase after DBS (19). Such hormonal changes may have an effect on the growth of tumors sensitive to the released hormones. In a recent animal study (Fig. 4), we have shown that DBS in the rat is associated with a statistically significant increased weight of prolactin-sensitive mammary tumor but not that of prolactin-insensitive thymus tumor (16). We also found that stimulation, and not the mere placement of electrodes, is necessary for enhanced mammary tumor growth (15). Exogenous opiate administration does not seem to have this effect and there was no difference in tumor size when opiate or prolactin blockage was attempted (15). These studies may indicate caution on the use of DBS in patients with prolactin-sensitive tumors until further studies clarify the presence or absence of any adverse effects of DBS on tumor growth.

Peripheral stimulation has a limited use in the cancer patient. Since most patients referred for pain management are already taking narcotic analgesic, release of beta-endorphins with low-frequency, peripheral stimulation loses effect when applied to chronic cancer pain patients. Transcutaneous electric nerve stimulation was found to be maximally effective during the first 10 days, decreasing to 11% after 1 month (39). Our experience is similar in that few of our patients obtain pain relief with TENS alone and that pain relief is limited in duration. High-frequency TENS stimulation seems to be more effective for patients taking narcotic analgesic, although well-controlled studies on the effect of peripheral stimulation are lacking in this particular group of patients.

Neural Blockade

Interruption of a nociceptive pathway, considered the "panacea" for permanent pain relief in cancer patients, is probably the most popular form of treatment in these patients. Neural interruption, achieved by chemical neurolysis or surgery, dates back to 1900 (6). Various neurolytic substances have been injected in an attempt to block accessible plexuses and nerves "permanently." Before chemical neurolysis is attempted in the patient with cancer-related pain, it is important to consider various physiologic factors inherent in the cancer patient. These factors may influence the decision to attempt neurolysis: inadequate platelet count, decreased circulating volume, compromised pulmonary function from localized or metastatic lung disease, and tumor encasement of nerves or plexuses. These factors can all influence the risks and result of the intended neural blockade. Before any intrathecal or epidural block, a myelogram with or without CT scans is almost imperative for ruling out any epidural or intradural tumor encroachment that may influence the outcome of the neurolytic block, especially if the solution is deposited in the intrathecal or epidural space.

Before an intrathecal neurolysis, at least two diagnostic blocks with a local anesthetic must be done to predict the result of chemical neurolysis and the possible side effects, including unpleasant sensation, loss of bowel and bladder function, and profound motor loss. Of 33 cancer patients in our center who received diagnostic nerve blocks before intended neurolysis, 3 patients experienced unacceptable side effects and 2 patients did not obtain acceptable pain relief because of neural encasement by tumor. Only when 75% pain relief occurs with diagnostic block do we proceed with chemical neurolysis. Any unavoidable side effect must be one that could be handled by both patient and family. For example, any motor loss must be avoided in patients whose motor function is necessary to continue functioning in a capacity that is extremely important to the individual patient. Loss of bladder and bowel function may further devastate the dignity of some patients, and therefore its possibility must always be explained before the performance of a neurolytic block involving the sacral roots. The results and side effects of phenol injection have been reviewed (6,42).

Various agents applied for neural blockade include local anesthetics, hypertonic saline, opiates, phenol, alcohol, and ammonium sulfate. The choice is governed by the duration of block discomfort on injection and the purpose of the block. For diagnostic blocks, we prefer to use lidocaine or bupivacaine in concentrations necessary for sensory block. For neurolysis, phenol is preferred because in our experience there is less pain on injection compared with alcohol or ammonium sulfate. For intrathecal injection, 4% phenol in absolute glycerol is used, whereas for epidural injection, 10% phenol in 10% glycerol is preferred because of ease of injection through the epidural catheter (13). Only for neurolytic celiac plexus block do we use 50% alcohol because volumes up to 50 ml are necessary to achieve a successful block (36). Such large volumes of phenol can result in renal damage.

Ablative Neurosurgical Procedures

We found that the most rational use for diagnostic neural blockade is to outline the dermatomal distribution of localized pain and to predict the usefulness of neurosurgical procedures as outlined in the previous flow chart. However, meticulous attention to detail and accuracy of needle placement is of paramount importance (14). If a patient is a good candidate for neural interruption, neurosurgery consultation must be sought immediately to determine the feasibility of using procedures such as chordotomy (33), rhizotomy (2), DBS (28), or implantation of intrathecal or epidural morphine pump (31).

For intractable generalized pain, use of more potent narcotics given intramuscularly or intravenously, hypophysectomy, originated by Moricca (see Chapter by G. Gianasi, *this volume*) for generalized bone pain (17,22–24), and DBS (32) may all be considered. The important principle is the persistent search for a pain-relieving modality with the lowest risk-benefit ratio.

RESULTS OF THE PROGRAM

Using the described program, the results from the first 120 patients indicate that acceptable pain relief goal was achieved in 75.3% during the 6-week program. However, only 50% of the patients with acceptable pain relief were able to perform their goal activities (Fig. 5). Most of these patients who achieved their goal activities belong to the group with stable and not progressive disease. Pharmacologic tailoring for 2 weeks was successful in achieving acceptable pain relief in 20% of patients. However, when either peripheral-stimulation-produced analgesia, neural block, or higher-dose narcotics were added, acceptable pain relief increased to a total of 75.3% by the end of the program (Fig. 6).

In analyzing the number of patients receiving neural interruption, 38% underwent diagnostic nerve blocks; of this group, 85% were candidates for neural ablation. Of this group, 3 eventually proceeded to have chordotomy and 2 had DBS. Of the rest, 40 received neurolytic block with either phenol or alcohol. It is important that the choices of therapy be presented to the patient and solution sought within a week of the diagnostic nerve block.

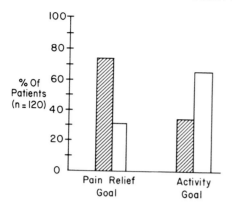

FIG. 5. Successful treatment outcome in patients with cancer pain, comparing pain relief and achievement of activities. *Open bars* indicate failure; *striped bars* indicate success.

In categorizing the results as influenced by the type of pain syndrome, we found that our program is successful with most pain syndromes but was least successful in the management of radiation-induced pain syndromes. Successful pain relief was achieved in 81.8% of patients with bone metastasis and only 40% in patients with postradiation pain.

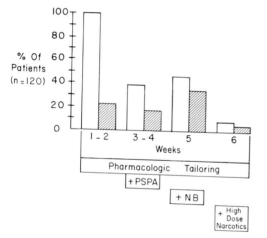

FIG. 6. Acceptable pain relief in patients with cancer pain during various phases of treatment over a period of 6 weeks. *Open bars* indicate percentage of patients receiving treatment; *striped bars* indicate percentage with acceptable pain relief. PSPA = Peripheral-stimulation-produced analgesia; NB = neural block.

CONCLUSION

This initial study indicates that the total management of chronic intractable cancer pain requires a persistent orchestration of various treatment modalities in a pain clinic setting distinct from that used for the chronic noncancer-type pain. Various phases of treatment include the adequate and tailored use of narcotic and nonnarcotic analgesics, neural stimulation, or neural ablation. These phases of treatment must be pursued until acceptable pain relief is obtained with the lowest risk involved.

REFERENCES

1. Bahnson, C. B. (1975): Psychologic and emotional issues in cancer: The psychotherapeutic care of the cancer patient. *Semin. Oncol.*, 2:293–310.
2. Barrash, J. M., and Leavens, M. E. (1973): Dorsal rhizotomy for the relief of intractable pain of malignant tumor origin. *J. Neurol.*, 38:755–757.
3. Bond, M. R. (1976): Pain and personality in cancer patients. In: *Advances in Pain Research and Therapy, Vol. 1*, edited by J. J. Bonica and D. Albe-Fessard, pp. 311–316. Raven Press, New York.
4. Bond, M. R. (1979): Psychologic and emotional aspects of cancer pain. In: *Advances in Pain Research and Therapy, Vol. 2*, edited by J. J. Bonica and V. Ventafridda, pp. 81–88. Raven Press, New York.
5. Bond, M. R., and Pearson, I. B. (1969): Psychological aspects of pain in women with advanced carcinoma of the cervix. *J. Psychosom. Res.*, 13:13–19.
6. Bonica, J. J. (1953): *Management of Pain*. Lea & Febiger, Philadelphia.
7. Bonica, J. J. (1982): The management of cancer pain. *Acta Anesthesiol. Scand. [Suppl.]*, 74:75–82.
8. Chapman, C. R. (1979): Psychologic and behavioral aspects of cancer pain. In: *Advances in Pain Research and Therapy*, edited by J. J. Bonica and V. Ventafridda, pp. 45–56. Raven Press, New York.
9. Cohen, R. S., Brechner, T., and Reading, A. E. (1982): A survey of the subjective parameters of pain in cancer patients. *Am. Pain Soc. Abstr.*, 18.
10. Cohn, J. P. (1981): Multicenter double-blind efficacy and safety study comparing alprazolam, diazepam and placebo in clinically anxious patients. *J. Clin. Psychiatry*, 42:347–351.
11. Cole, R. (1975): The problem of pain in persistent cancer. *Med. J. Aust.*, 1:682–687.
12. Derogatis, L. R. (1978): *Brief Symptom Index*. Johns Hopkins University, Baltimore.
13. Ferrer-Brechner, T. (1981): Epidural and intrathecal phenol neurolysis for cancer pain: Review of rationale and techniques. *Anesth. Rev.*, 8:14–20.
14. Ferrer-Brechner, T., and Brechner, V. (1976): Accuracy of needle placement during diagnostic and therapeutic nerve block. In: *Advances in Pain Research and Therapy, Vol. 1*, edited by J. J. Bonica and D. Albe-Fessard, pp. 679–683. Raven Press, New York.
15. Ferrer-Brechner, T., Joo, S., and Motyka, D. (1982): Is growth of prolactin-sensitive tumor after morphine administration influenced by prolactin and opiate antagonists? Abstr American Pain Society Third General Meeting, Miami Beach, Florida, October 29–31.
16. Ferrer-Brechner, T., Motyka, D. and Sherman, J. (1983): Growth enhancement of prolactin-sensitive mammary tumor by periaquaductal grey stimulation. *Life Sci.*, 32:525–530.
17. Fitzpatrick, J. M., Gardiner, R. A., and Williams, J. P. (1981): Pituitary ablation in the relief of prostatic carcinoma. *Br. Med. J.* 284:75–76.
18. Foley, K. M. (1979): Pain syndromes in patients with cancer. In: *Advances in Pain Research and Therapy, Vol. 2*, edited by J. J. Bonica and V. Ventafridda. Raven Press, New York.
19. Foley, K. M., Kaiko, R. F., Inturrisi, C. D., Posner, O. P., Li, C. H., and Houde, R. W. (1978): *Pain Abs.*, 1:17.
20. Gitelson, J., Brechner, T., and McCreary, C. (1981): Psychological predictors of response to treatment for cancer pain. Abstr. Third World Cong on Pain Internat. Assoc. for the Study of Pain, Edinburgh.
21. Gitelson, J. S., Brechner, T. F., McCreary, C., and Dong, T. (1980): Psychological aspects of cancer pain: Correlation with response to standard medical treatment for relief of pain. *Am. Pain Soc. Abstr.*, 25.
22. Katz, J., and Levin, A. B. (1977): Treatment of diffuse metastatic cancer pain by instillation of alcohol into the sella turcica. *Anesthesiology*, 46:115–121.
23. Lipton, S., Miles, J., and Williams, N. (1978): Pituitary injection of alcohol for widespread cancer pain. *Pain*, 5:73–82.
24. Lloyd, J. W., Rawlinson, M. A., and Evans, P. J. (1961): Selective hypophysectomy for metastatic pain. A review of ethyl alcohol ablation of the anterior pituitary in a regional pain relief unit. *Br. J. Anaesth.*, 53:1129–1133.
25. Melzack, R. (1975): The McGill Pain Questionnaire: Major properties and scoring methods. *Pain*, 1:277–299.

26. Melzack, R., Ofiesh, J. G., and Mount, B. M. (1976): The Brompton mixture: Effects on pain in cancer patients. *Can. Med. Assoc. J.*, 115:125–129.
27. Merskey, H., and Boyd, D. (1978): Emotional adjustment and chronic pain. *Pain*, 5:173–178.
28. Meyerson, B. A., Boethius, J., and Carlsson, A. M. (1978): Percutaneous central grey stimulation for cancer pain. *Appl. Neurophysiol.*, 41:57–65.
28b. Minton, J. P. (1974): The reponse of breast cancer to L-Dopa. *Cancer*, 33:358–363.
29. Moricca, G. (1974): Chemical hypophysectomy for cancer pain. In: *Advances in Neurology, Vol. 4*. edited by J. J. Bonica. Raven Press, New York.
30. Pilowsky, I., and Bond, M. R. (1969): Pain and its management in malignant disease: Elucidation of staff-patient transactions. *Psychosom. Med.*, 31:400–404.
31. Poletti, C. E., Cohen, A. M., and Todd, D. P. (1981): Cancer pain relieved by long-term epidural morphine with permanent indwelling system for self-administration. *J. Neurosurg.*, 55:581–584.
32. Richardson, E. C., and Skil, H. (1977): Pain reduction by electrical brain stimulation in man. *J. Neurosurg.*, 47:178–183.
33. Rosomoff, H. F., Carral, F., and Brown, J. (1965): Percutaneous radiofrequency cervical cordotomy technique. *J. Neurosurg.*, 23:639.
34. Shimm, D. S., Logue, G. L., Maltbie, A. A., and Dugan, S. (1979): Medical management of chronic cancer pain. *JAMA*, 241:2408–2412.
35. Sternbach, R. A. (1974): *Pain Patients: Traits and Treatment*. Academic Press, New York.
36. Thompson, G. E., Moore, D. C., and Bridenbaugh, L. D. (1977): Abdominal pain and alcohol celiac plexus nerve block. *Anesth. Analg. (Cleve.)*, 56:1–5.
37. Turnbull, F. (1971): Pain and suffering in cancer. *Can. Nurse*, 67:28–30.
38. Ventafridda, V., Sganzeria, E. P., and Fochi, C. (1979): Use of psychotropic substances with antidepression action in pain control. *Minerva Med.*, 70:667–674.
39. Ventafridda, V., Sganzeria, E. P., and Fochi, C. (1979): Transcutaneous stimulation in cancer pain. In: *Advances in Pain Research and Therapy, Vol. 2*, edited by J. J. Bonica and V. Ventafridda. Raven Press, New York.
40. Weinstock, E. (1983): Value of patient education in an outpatient cancer pain clinic. *Am. Pain Soc. Abstr.*, Chicago, November 11–13.
41. Wolskie, P. J., Gracely, R. H., and Greenberg, R. P. (1982): Comparison of effects of morphine and deep brain stimulation on chronic pain. *Am. Pain Soc. Abstr.*, p. 36.
42. Wood, K. (1978): The use of phenol as a neurolytic agent. A review. *Pain*, 5:205.
43. Woodford, J. M., and Fielding, J. R. (1970): Pain and cancer. *J. Psychosom. Res.*, 14:365–370.

Advances in Pain Research
and Therapy, Vol. 7,
edited by C. Benedetti et al.
Raven Press, New York © 1984.

Hormones and Pain: Clinical Management of Pain in Disorders of the Breast

N. Deshpande

*Imperial Cancer Research Fund, Lincoln's Inn Fields,
London WC2A 3PX, England*

Although almost all women suffer from some form of breast discomfort and pain during their reproductive life, the problem is not given any serious attention until the diagnosis of carcinoma in the breast is made or until they start suffering from intractable pain due to cancer metastases. In this chapter, I would like to try to redress this imbalance and review the literature on the treatment of pain in both noncancer and cancer patients. Until recently, breast pain in a noncancerous patient was usually thought to be psychosomatic in origin; therefore investigations into the causes of such complaints were related mainly to studying the psychologic makeup of the patient. It is true that, in a minor proportion of cases, the main cause of the phantom pain is the fear of breast cancer, and these patients are merely seeking reassurance. However, in most cases, breast pain can be attributed to well-defined physiopathologic causes; these patients need and deserve proper diagnosis and treatment.

CAUSES OF PAIN IN DISORDERS OF THE BREAST AND DIAGNOSIS

If one excludes cases in whom the pain is of psychosomatic origin, breast pain is generally divided into six categories: (a) cyclical pronounced mastalgia, usually defined as premenstrual breast pain associated with breast nodularity; (b) ductectasia or periductal mastitis; (c) Tietze syndrome, in which pain is associated with a tender and enlarged costochondral junction; (d) trauma; (e) sclerosing adenosis; and (f) cancer (14). It is worth considering each of these conditions in some detail before going on to treatments available for them.

In any breast clinic, most patients who complain of breast pain suffer from the syndrome of pronounced cyclic mastalgia. Breast pain either is felt or is exacerbated during the premenstrual period and is easily distinguished from the minor discomfort experienced by many women during this period by both its intensity and persistence. In most cases, patients are unable to pinpoint the site of pain, but a few indicate it is in the upper and outer quadrant of the breast. In about half the cases, pain is felt bilaterally. Mammograms of the breast usually reveal fibroadenosis either with or without cysts, and this seems to be the main cause of the complaint.

About 20 to 30% of patients suffer from ductectasia/periductal mastitis. In this condition there is no clear discernible pattern. The pain appears randomly and, in some cases, the intensity increases during the premenstrual period. The site(s) of pain is more localized in that patients are able to pinpoint it consistently in the subareolar, nipple, or inner quadrant area of the breast. In most cases, coarse calcification or flame-shaped shadows are seen on mammograms at or near the site of pain, and these features are accompanied by dilated ducts elsewhere in the breast or in the contralateral gland.

Up to 10% of patients suffer from Tietze syndrome, in which pain is associated with a tender and enlarged costochondral junction. The pain is chronic without any clear pattern. Many patients feel that the pain is in the chest wall rather than in the breast. Radiologic examination of the breast shows no abnormalities, and this in itself is helpful in the diagnosis of the syndrome. Trauma or sclerosing adenosis is observed as a cause of pain in a tiny minority of patients.

In patients with trauma, pain is localized at the site of the surgical scar or previous injury and in some cases at the site of incision for breast drainage. In patients undergoing breast biopsy, pain usually is observed if there is evidence of hematoma. Sclerosing adenosis is observed as the cause of pain in a few cases. This is easily diagnosed because patients observe pain over a period of several years. Pain due to carcinoma of the breast will be discussed in a separate section.

NONHORMONAL TREATMENTS FOR BREAST PAIN IN NONCANCEROUS PATIENTS

Patients suffering from some of the above complaints have been treated by breast surgery with variable success. For example, in sclerosing adenosis, the results of excision are unpredictable in that pain relief is observed in some, but not all, patients. In failed cases, many surgeons prefer to perform a subsequent mastectomy. Excision of the subareolar duct system and wedge in patients suffering from periductal mastitis have proved beneficial in terms of pain relief in most cases. Similarly, excision of the painful scar relieves pain in patients suffering from trauma. Patients suffering from pain due to Tietze syndrome have not been treated successfully by surgery, and some clinicians are referring these patients for long-acting intercostal nerve block. Cyclical pronounced mastalgia can be treated successfully by nonsurgical treatments.

HORMONAL TREATMENTS IN THE RELIEF OF BREAST PAIN

From puberty onward, various functions of the human breast are controlled by a variety of hormones. For example, during each menstrual cycle, under the influence of pituitary and ovarian hormones, breast size increases due to development of stromal tissue and an extensive ductal system. Similarly, after parturition, lactation is strictly under the influence of pituitary lactogenic hormones. As a result of this, any abnormal functioning of the breast is immediately attributed to pathophysiologic changes in the endocrine environment and is investigated in terms of alterations in plasma concentrations of various hormones. Such studies have revealed that, in patients with benign diseases of the breast, plasma concentrations of progesterone in the luteal phase of the menstrual cycle were significantly lower than those found in normal women of comparable age (16), indicating that the development of benign breast lesions in these patients might be attributed to an inadequate luteal phase of the menstrual cycle.

In another study, Cole et al. (4) observed that patients with benign breast tumors had higher plasma titers of prolactin than age-matched controls. A logical extension of such findings is to treat patients with drugs that will correct the hormonal imbalance in the hope that this will alleviate the condition. Such hypotheses suffer from certain drawbacks. First, the plasma concentrations of a hormone vary manyfold in a large sample of the general population so that disease/nondisease comparisons depend on the sample size and process of selection of patients for inclusion in the study. Second, it is quite possible under certain circumstances that the abnormalities observed in plasma hormone concentrations might be the result rather than the cause of the disease, and therefore correcting the imbalance might not be the right approach in these cases. Finally, even if a treatment relieves breast abnormalities by correcting the hormonal imbalance, it may affect other functions of these hormones to such an extent that it would be unethical to treat patients with such drugs. Because of these and other considerations, there are very few successful treatments based on hormonal or antihormonal drugs. In the following section, I will present some recent data on two such treatments.

BROMOCRIPTINE IN THE MANAGEMENT OF NONCANCEROUS DISORDERS OF THE BREAST

Whether prolactin plays any major role in the induction and/or maintenance of breast lesions remains unclear. However, there are many publications in which its involvement in disorders of the human breast has been postulated (for references, see 12). Therefore it is argued that treatments based on the drugs that either inhibit the release of the hormone from the pituitary, or block its action(s) at the target site(s) might be useful in at least some of these disorders. Bromocriptine (2Br-alpha-ergocryptine) (CB-154) is a long-acting dopaminergic drug that suppresses prolactin secretion from the pituitary. It has been used in the treatment of breast disorders. Schulz et al. (15) treated 15 patients suffering from mastodynia with a 5 mg/day dose of bromocriptine and observed a complete response in 10 and a partial response in 3 patients. A similar response rate to bromocriptine treatment in 7 patients with fibrocystic disease has been reported by Martin-Comin et al. (9). A slightly different dosage was administered to 23 patients with fibroadenosis or fibrocystic disease by Mussa and Dogliotti (12). They treated these patients with 2.5 mg of the drug every 8 hr and observed that 21 patients had marked relief of pain and mammary tension after a few days of the treatment.

Two other groups have evaluated the usefulness of bromocriptine by double-blind crossover clinical trials. Anderson et al. (1) investigated 21 patients suffering from premenstrual syndrome during three successive menstrual cycles. After a control cycle, the patients were treated during the luteal phase either with 2.5 mg of bromocriptine twice daily or a placebo. They observed that the drug improved all the premenstrual symptoms but mastodynia was the only condition where the drug was significantly better than the placebo. Mansel et al. (8), using a similar approach, treated 29 women with cyclical mastalgia and 11 with noncyclical pain by a 5 mg/day dose of bromocriptine or placebo over six menstrual cycles. A significant improvement in breast symptoms, including pain, was observed in the group with cyclical pain. The treatment was unsuccessful in patients suffering from noncyclical pain.

Thus the usefulness of bromocriptine in the treatment of pronounced cyclic mastalgia is beyond question. However, the benefit is obtained at the expense of such side effects as nausea, dizziness, and a drop in blood pressure. These side effects are temporary and are observed mainly at the start of the treatment, so very few patients are unable to take the drug. There is some evidence that suggests the drug effects are temporary, in that in some patients, withdrawal of the drug results in a return of the symptoms. The mechanism by which pain relief is obtained also remains unclear. Most workers have measured plasma titers of prolactin both before and during the treatment and found that prolactin concentrations fall significantly on administration of bromocriptine in all cases. Since in patients suffering from noncyclical pain there was no pain relief, it is doubtful whether the lactogenic hormone was involved directly in the induction of pain due to cyclic mastalgia.

DANAZOL IN THE MANAGEMENT OF DISORDERS OF THE BREAST

Danazol is a synthetic derivative of 17α-ethinyl testosterone with, supposedly, antigonadotropin, weak androgenic and anabolic properties. It was developed mainly for use in patients suffering from gynecologic disorders. However, since the breast is a target organ for ovarian steroids, the usefulness of the drug has been investigated in patients suffering from disorders of the breast.

As early as 1971, Greenblatt et al. (6) treated 10 patients suffering from various complaints of the breast, such as gynecomastia, virginal breast hypertrophy, and chronic cystic mastitis, for varying lengths of time, and found the drug to be useful in most cases. These initial studies were then extended by Asch and Greenblatt (2) and Nezhat et al. (13), who treated a series of patients with a variety of benign breast disorders with varying daily doses of danazol (100–400 mg/day) for up to 10 months. Most patients had favorable responses and about 75 to 80% of them had complete relief of breast discomfort and pain, with the disappearance of clinical symptoms and a prolonged symptom-free period after discontinuation of the drug. Lauersen and Wilson (7) have also reported on a series of 40 patients with chronic cystic mastitis whom they treated with a 400 mg/day dose of danazol for up to 6 months. The data presented show that nearly all the patients had objective or subjective improvements or both in clinical symptoms. Similar findings have been reported by Baker and Snedecor (3) for patients suffering from severe fibrocystic disease.

As with bromocriptine, the administration of danazol also results in some transient side effects: muscle cramps, acne, oily hair, hot flushes, weight gain, hairiness, increased libido, and edema. However, most patients are able to tolerate the dosage and complete a 6-month course. About half the patients suffer from amenorrhea while on medication, but normal menses return with 2 to 3 months of withdrawal. Danazol is particularly effective in relieving symptoms of breast disorders in younger patients. In about one-third of the cases, there was some evidence of return of breast pain and tenderness on termination of the treatment. Some of the workers cited above have attempted to investigate the mechanism of drug action in terms of alterations to the endocrine environment.

There is general agreement among these workers that the drug fails to induce changes in plasma concentrations of estrogens or progesterone. Regarding gonadotropins, Greenblatt et al. (6) mention that the midcycle surge of follicle-stimulating hormone and luteinizing hormone was blunted by the administration of danazol, although the basal gonadotropin levels showed no significant changes. These findings were not confirmed by Lauersen and Wilson (7). This indicates that the drug action on the breast might not be mediated via alterations to endocrine function and that hormones probably play no direct major role(s) in pain relief. Whatever the mechanism of action of danazol and bromocriptine, it is clear that both bromocriptine and danazol are important drugs in the management of pain in patients with benign disorders of the breast.

CAUSES OF PAIN IN PATIENTS WITH CARCINOMA OF THE BREAST

Human breast cancer can be divided into four different phases: diagnosis of the primary and its removal, disease-free interval, detection of local or distant metastases, and relapse. Mastalgia, as a prominent complaint leading to the diagnosis of carcinoma, is noted in 10 to 15% of operable cases. In these patients, the presence of severe definite or diffused lumpiness is noted, and therefore pain must be classed as an infrequent symptom in primary carcinoma of the breast. On the other hand, it is a dominant feature of locally advanced inoperable disease in which the carcinoma has already invaded the brachial plexus and axilla. During the free period, a minority of patients occasionally complain of pain around the mastectomy scar. The exact reason for this complaint is not known, since in many of these cases there is no clinical evidence of local metastases. It may be that after mastectomy the skin flaps have been closed tightly and this has created excessive skin stress. At the metastatic stage, pain is caused mainly by an invasion of bone, with or without fracture, by the carcinoma, or by increased intracranial pressure due to metastasis in the brain. In many centers with limited follow-up facilities, pain at these and other sites is taken as the first indication of metastases. After relapse, patients suffer from chronic and intractable pain due to the unabated growth of metastases.

TREATMENT FOR PAIN IN CARCINOMA OF THE BREAST

Although it has been obvious to many clinicians that some patients suffer cancer pain from diagnosis to death, until recently no serious attempts were made to control their pain, as relief of pain was observed automatically in patients with hormone-responsive or hormone-dependent metastases treated by additive or ablative endocrine treatments. Yet with careful management of patients, pain control can be achieved in all four stages. Since after the diagnosis of carcinoma most patients undergo some form of breast surgery, and since pain in these cases is usually located at or near the site of carcinoma, removal of either tumor or breast will automatically result in complete pain relief. Patients with locally advanced disease, because of their unsuitability for breast surgery, are treated by a combination of endocrine therapies and local irradiation and, if these therapies induce reduction in tumor mass and increase mobility, are then selected for breast surgery. Through these approaches, pain relief can be obtained in most cases. In the absence of any clear evidence of local metastases, patients complaining of pain around the mastectomy scar are usually treated with local irradiation and/or analgesics.

Although most patients with metastatic cancer suffer from pain, its intensity varies both with the site of metastases and between patients with metastases at the same site, so decisions regarding the complaint tended to be taken arbitrarily by the attending physicians. Furthermore, since pain relief was observed in most patients who responded to various treatments for the regression of tumor metastases, there was, and still is, a heavy emphasis on producing treatments that will induce these regressions; very rarely were patients treated specifically for pain. Therefore, failure to obtain tumor regressions meant unresponsive patients were treated with progressively increasing doses of analgesics as a last resort, although endocrine and other treatments are available for pain relief and will induce at least a subjective response in the terminal stages. Some of the endocrine treatments used in the past for pain and the mechanism(s) by which they induce relief are discussed in this section.

The anti-inflammatory properties of glucocorticoids have been used routinely to treat pain due to cranial metastases successfully. In these patients, the main cause of pain seems to be an increase in intracranial pressure due to edema. Therefore, treatment with these steroids will reduce edema and thus relieve pain. Levodopa administered every 4 hr has been reported to be an effective pain reliever in metastatic cancer; this subjective response was found to be indicative of likely objective response of metastases to endocrine ablations (10).

Bilateral adrenalectomy, although never evaluated as a pain therapy, has been found to be an effective treatment for pain in patients with hormone-responsive or hormone-unresponsive metastases. Similarly, hypophysectomy appears to produce analgesic effects that seem to be unrelated to tumor regression (17). Finally, neuroadenolysis, which is probably one of the few treatments used specifically for pain relief, appears to produce subjective responses in most patients with metastatic cancer (11).

Because endocrine ablations induced pain relief, it was believed that the inavailability of hormones normally secreted by the excised glands was somehow implicated in the subjective response. The fact that these patients were given replacement hormone therapies that failed to reverse pain relief, and that many additive therapies also induce tumor regression and therefore pain relief were largely ignored. However, the possibility of a role for endogenous hormones in pain could not be investigated thoroughly until a treatment that did not require endocrine ablations or additive hormone therapies was available for pain relief. Neuroadenolysis, in which alcohol is injected into the sella turcica, seems to be one such treatment in which there appears to be no immediate destruction of the pituitary gland, although post-mortem examination of the gland shows severe necrosis. This treatment, therefore, afforded a unique opportunity to examine the possibility of hormonal involvement in pain.

Our own studies so far indicate that the ability to secrete prolactin, thyroid-stimulating hormone (TSH), corticotropin, α-lipotropin, and α-endorphin remains intact after neuroadenolysis (4). Furthermore, the pituitary appears to respond to the exogenous stimulus provided by TSH releasing hormone

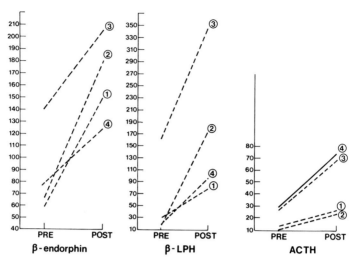

FIG. 1. Pre- and postneuroadenolysis changes in plasma titers of α-endorphins, α-lipotropin (α-LPH), and adrenocorticotropic hormone (ACTH) in four patients with metastatic cancer. The results are expressed as ng/liter.

by an increased release of prolactin and TSH. Plasma titers of corticotropin, α-lipotropin, and α-endorphin were found to be higher after neuroadenolysis than before the treatment (Fig. 1). Similar findings have been observed by others in cerebrospinal fluid (CSF) (F. Takeda, *personal communication*).

These findings indicate that instead of inhibiting the synthesis of any of the pituitary hormones, neuroadenolysis stimulated the secretion of adrenocorticotropic hormone (ACTH), α-lipotropin, and α-endorphin. Since α-endorphin is supposed to have analgesic properties, a rise in the plasma titer of the peptide would suggest the preneuroadenolysis levels were below the threshold required to maintain pain-free status and that neuroadenolysis raises the pain threshold through increased synthesis of the peptide. However, it is possible to argue against such a hypothesis on the grounds that, whereas pain relief observed after neuroadenolysis lasts for several weeks, administration of α-endorphin relieves pain for only a very short period. Further studies should reveal whether the raised plasma titers of these peptides are maintained for the duration of total pain relief.

In conclusion, there is as yet no published evidence that indicates direct involvement of hormones in pain relief, although this does not exclude the possibility of an indirect role in the induction of pain in both women with benign breast conditions and in breast cancer patients. Raised plasma and CSF concentrations of ACTH, α-lipotropin, and α-endorphin after neuroadenolysis suggest that the treatment might be acting on the mechanism in the hypothalamus that controls the secretion of corticotropin-releasing factor (CRF). Whether this rise in CRF interferes with neuronal pathways of pain by blocking pain signals remains to be explored.

ACKNOWLEDGMENTS

I am indebted to my colleagues: Prof. Guide Moricca, Prof. Franco Saullo, Prof. Luciano DiMartino, and Miss Irene Mitchell for their help in the preparation of this chapter.

REFERENCES

1. Andersen, A. N., Larsen, J. F., Steenstrup, O. R., and Nielsen, J. (1977): Effect of brom-ocriptine on the premenstrual syndrome. A double-blind clinical trial. *Br. J. Obstet. Gynaecol.*, 84:370–374.
2. Asch, R. H., and Greenblatt, R. G. (1977): The use of an impeded androgendanazol in the management of benign breast disorders. *Am. J. Obstet. Gynecol.*, 127:130–134.
3. Baker, H. W., and Snedecor, P. A. (1979): Clinical trial of danazol for benign breast disease. *Am. Surg.*, 45:727–729.
4. Cole, E. N., Selwood, R. A., England, P. C., and Griffiths, K. (1977): Serum prolactin concentrations in benign breast disease throughout the menstrual cycle. *Eur. J. Cancer*, 13:597–603.
5. Deshpande, N., Moricca, G., Saullo, F., DiMartino, L., and Kwa, G. (1981): Some aspects of pituitary function after neuroadenolysis in patients with metastatic cancer. *Tumori*, 67:355–359.
6. Greenblatt, R. B., Dmowski, W. P., Mahesh, V. B., and Scholer, H. F. L. (1971): Clinical studies with an antigonadotropin: Danazol. *Fertil. Steril.*, 22:102–112.
7. Lauersen, N. H., and Wilson, K. H. (1976): The effect of danazol in the treatment of chronic cystic mastitis. *Obstet. Gynecol.*, 48:93–98.
8. Mansel, R. E., Preece, P. E., and Hughes, L. E. (1978): A double blind trial of the prolactin inhibitor bromocriptine in painful benign breast disease. *Br. J. Surg.*, 65:724–727.
9. Martin-Comin, J., Pujol-Amat, P., Cararach, V., Davi, E., and Robyn, C. (1976): Treatment of fibrocystic disease of the breast with a prolactin inhibitor: 2Br-alpha-ergocryptine (CB-154). *Obstet. Gynecol.*, 48:703–706.
10. Minton, J. P. (1976): Precise selection of breast cancer patients with bone metastasis for endocrine ablation. *Surgery*, 80:513–517.
11. Moricca, G. (1977): Neuroadenolysis in the treatment of intractable pain from cancer. In: *Persistent Pain*, edited by S. Lipton, pp. 149–173. Grune & Stratton, New York.
12. Mussa, A., and Dogliotti, L. (1979): Treatment of benign breast disease with bromocriptine. *J. Endocrinol. Invest.*, 2:87–91.
13. Nezhat, C., Asch, R. H., and Greenblatt, R. B. (1980): Danazol for benign breast disease. *Am. J. Obstet. Gynecol.*, 137:604–607.
14. Preece, P. E., Mansel, R. E., Bolton, P. M., Hughes, L. E., Baum, M., and Gravelle, I. H. (1976): Clinical syndromes of mastalgia. *Lancet*, 2:670–673.
15. Schulz, K. D., Del Pozo, E., Lose, K. H., Kunzig, H. J., and Geiger, W. (1975): Successful treatment of mastodynia with prolactin inhibitor bromocriptine (CB-154). *Arch. Gynecol.*, 220:83–87.
16. Sitruk-Ware, R., Sterkers, N., and Mauvais-Jarvis, P. (1979): Benign breast disease. I: Hormonal investigation. *Obstet. Gynecol.*, 53:457–460.
17. Wilson, C. B., and Fewer, D. (1971): Role of neurosurgery in the management of patients with carcinoma of the breast. *Cancer*, 28:1681–1685.

*Advances in Pain Research
and Therapy, Vol. 7,*
edited by C. Benedetti et al.
Raven Press, New York © 1984.

Role of Neurosurgery in Cancer Pain: Reevaluation of Old Methods and New Trends

Carlo Alberto Pagni

*2nd Chair of Neurosurgery and Aldo Pasetti Center for Pain Research and
Therapy, University of Turin, 10126 Turin, Italy*

In the past, ablative neurosurgical procedures for pain relief have been based on the hypothesis that pain is due to activation of specific fibers, tracts, and centers whose destruction would block nociceptive impulses. However, if pain were simply a sensory modality conducted along such specific systems, we should be able to relieve patients permanently by appropriate destruction of these pathways somewhere in their course. As is now well known, this is not the case. What is worse, activity in sensory relays does not disappear after interruption of afferent systems. On the contrary, after such procedures, activity can be triggered by nonnoxious stimulation and exaggerated by deafferentation (58).

In the last decade or so, evidence has been adduced that pain is not due simply to activation of specific fibers in peripheral nerves or tracts in the central nervous system (these are long, ascending fibers with a common origin, function, and termination, which are collected in discrete regions of the neuraxis) or to activation of centers located in specific thalamic nuclei or cortical areas where sensory impulses are brought to consciousness to produce pain (25,58). Sensory mechanisms for localization of the source of painful excitations are only part of the many systems that subserve pain and its affective components. Nociceptive transmission involves not only the long afferents but also short neurons that extend from the spinal cord to the hypothalamus and terminate not only in pain "centers" but also activate a large number of subcortical and cortical structures (31). Moreover, neuronal systems subserving pain are open to many excitatory and inhibitory influences coming from many sources (nociceptive and other neural systems) that can enhance or block nociceptive impulses at every level of the central nervous system. Thus it seems that pain is due to the activation of many diffuse paths and of many gating mechanisms that allow patterns of activity to develop in widespread subcortical and cortical structures.

In less than 75 years, about 15 different neurosurgical operations have been devised to treat intractable pain. Certain procedures have been abandoned temporarily in favor of a new one and then resumed to avoid the drawbacks of the latest procedure. Moreover, the good results reported with a new operation often keep eluding surgeons who try to duplicate them. The obvious conclusion is that surgical procedures for pain do not produce as satisfactory relief as claimed by their proponents. In this chapter, I will attempt to give a brief overview and evaluation of the most widely used ablative procedures for cancer pain based both on personal experience and data found in the literature. These will include: (a) neurotomy and sympathectomy; (b) rhizotomy of the spinal and cranial nerves with neurolytic agents and by surgical section; (c) thermocoagulation of cranial nerves; (d) spinothalamic tractotomy, including open and percutaneous tractotomy of the spinal cord, and mesencephalic tractotomy; (e) commissural myelotomy; (f) stereotactic thalamotomy; and (g) psychosurgery. This chapter is an update of previous ones published in this series (58,59) and elsewhere (60).

NEUROTOMY AND SYMPATHECTOMY

Resection of peripheral spinal or cranial nerves, although simple, is rarely indicated for cancer pain because the procedure produces only very limited analgesia for a short period, followed by a regeneration with possible consequent pain (85). Moreover, it can be done only in purely sensory nerves, such as the branches of the trigeminal nerve, or in mixed nerves, such as the intercostal nerves, where interruption of motor pathways is insignificant. In such circumstances, neurolytic block is preferable because it is simpler and produces less morbidity. Similarly, section of afferent (pain) fibers in the splanchnic nerves (splanchnicectomy) supplying the upper abdominal viscera may be considered in managing severe pain from cancer of the pancreas or other visceral tumors, but neurolytic block of the celiac plexus is equally effective, is simpler, and produces less morbidity than the open operation (see Chapter by D. C. Moore, *this volume*).

CHEMICAL RHIZOTOMY

Spinal Dorsal Rhizotomy

Chemical destruction of the dorsal roots of spinal nerves as a substitute for surgical rhizotomy was first proposed in 1931 by Dogliotti (15), who reported the successful injection of alcohol into the subarachnoid space in treating intractable cancer pain. In 1955 Maher (46) reported the successful use of chemical rhizotomy achieved with injection of hyperbaric phenol solution. Of these two methods, I prefer to inject 5 to 10% phenol in glycerine. To achieve optimal results requires: (a) knowledge of the vertebral level at which nerve rootlets attach to the spinal cord; (b) having the patient in a special position in order to enhance the diffusion of hyperbaric phenol to reach the target rootlets; (c) the injection of the agent in small increments to avoid extensive diffusion of the agent to uninvolved neural structures; and (d) having the patient remain in the position for 30 to 45 min for the neurolytic agent to fix.

Properly administered, this is a simple and safe procedure, even in patients in very poor physical condition and with a very short life expectancy, and the procedure can be repeated in order to achieve longer and/or more extensive analgesia. Disadvantages are: (a) difficulty of blocking a large number of roots, (b) onset of motor and sphincter complications if high concentrations of phenol are used to obtain marked denervation, and (c) pain relief usually is not permanent but lasts some 2 to 4 months or perhaps longer. Recurrence of pain may be due to one or more of the following reasons: (a) the phenol producing an incomplete denervation of the painful area with insufficient reduction of nociceptive afferent input; (b) the abolition of pain in a given area of the body "unmasking" pain in another region, which before the block was not perceived by the patient who may have been preoccupied with the more severe pain; (c) the progressive spread of the tumor to produce pain in the undenervated area; and (d) the pain in the midline, such as it occurs with metastasis of the vertebra.

Despite these limitations, chemical rhizotomy has a definite place in cancer pain therapy. I have used subarachnoid block with 5 to 10% phenol in glycerine in 30 patients with severe cancer pain. All of these patients had been managed with multiphasic drug therapy (MDT), as suggested by Twycross (82) and Pagni and Franzini (61) in an attempt to control the various sources of the pain. Multiphasic drug therapy has included: (a) The use of nonsteroidal anti-inflammatory drugs (NSAID), which have a unique role in treating moderate to severe pain due to bone metastasis. Many of these drugs induce the production of prostaglandins that cause osteolysis and lower the threshold nociceptors. Since aspirin and NSAID are potent prostaglandin-synthetase inhibitors, they produce specific analgesic and anti-inflammatory effects and, in some instances, have antitumor effects in patients with bone metastasis. (b) Steroids to potentiate the actions of NSAID and to reduce soft-tissue swelling and inflammation in relatively circumscribed areas. They have also been used to enhance a sense of well-being. (c) Tricyclic antidepressants and phenothiazines, which have been found useful against denervation dysesthesia. (d) Carbamazepine and phenytoin, which have been found useful in relieving paroxysm of pain. (e) Psychotropic drugs to interrupt the vicious circle of pain, anxiety, and depression. (f) Adrenocorticotropic hormone (ACTH). When the MDT regimen did not produce complete pain relief, the patients were submitted to subarachnoid injection of phenol. Of these, 21 received a single injection and 9 received a second injection either because of appearance of pain in a previously apparently unaffected region or because of the recurrence of pain.

The results were as follows. Seven patients who achieved excellent relief from pain were lost at follow-up. Five patients, 2 of whom had a second injection, died pain-free 5 to 23 days after the injection. Six patients, 2 of whom had a second injection, achieved excellent and complete relief for the duration of the follow-up, which lasted up to 40 days. Twelve patients, including 5 who had a second injection, had recurrence of pain 3 to 30 days after the last block. In all of these patients, the MDT was resumed after the injection, and among those who had good results from a block, a satisfactory and practically complete control of pain was obtained for periods up to 5 months with a combination of block and MDT. On the basis of this experience, another 10 patients were managed by the combined use of MDT and neurolytic blocks, with excellent relief up to 5 months or until death.

In conclusion, subarachnoid block with phenol is very useful in managing patients with localized pain including low chest pain, abdominal and low back pain, pain in the inguinal and thigh region, and sacrococcigeal, rectal, and vaginal pain. The procedure is less effective in pain in the neck, upper limb, shoulder, and upper part of the chest. In managing patients with pain in the lower limb, there is significant risk of impairment of skeletal muscle function and sphincter control. It deserves reemphasis that pain relief usually lasts 30 to 40 days. Best results are achieved by combining subarachnoid phenol with MDT because the drugs control certain components of cancer pain not amenable to treatment with peripheral denervation.

Chemical Cranial Rhizotomy/Neurotomy

Five patients were submitted to cranial nerve blocks with 7.5 to 10% phenol alcohol according to the technique suggested by Bonica (6,7,45). Excellent results were obtained by combining this with MDT in 4 patients. One patient with carcinoma of the larynx and cervical metastatis who had received cobalt therapy with consequent submandibular and cervical scarring was given a phenol block of the third division of the trigeminal nerve without any relief, and subsequently was submitted to multiple surgical cranial rhizotomy.

PERCUTANEOUS THERMOCOAGULATION OF CRANIAL NERVES

Patients with malignancies of the face, head, and neck often suffer severe pain. Commonly at the beginning surgery, chemotherapy and radiotherapy can afford satisfactory relief of pain. Intense intractable pain, as a rule, arises only in advanced stages of the disease, especially if, after radiation therapy, fibrosis ensues with the formation of scleroatrophic or scleroneoplastic "plastrons" that damage major nerve trunks.

In the advanced stages, pain usually is referred to large areas in the peripheral fields of multiple cranial or cervical nerves bearing no relation to the original tumor site. Patients complain of persistent, progressively increasing pain. In cancer of the larynx, oropharynx, and posterior third of the tongue and mouth, pain is referred mainly to the area of the distribution of the glossopharyngeal and vagus nerves. In cancer of the mouth and anterior two-thirds of the tongue, gums, maxilla, orbit, nose, and sinuses, pain is referred mainly to the trigeminal nerve distribution. Very often patients complain of pain in the occiput and neck due both to lateral cervical metastasis and to fibrosis consequent to radiation.

The symptomatology is characterized by paroxysmal bouts of pain in the face, throat, tonsil, base of the tongue, and ear, provoked by talking, mouth movements, or swallowing (preventing food intake, which worsens the patient's condition). These agonizing bursts are similar to the paroxysmal pain of trigeminal and glossopharyngeal neuralgia. Burning sensations often are referred to the pharynx. Deep-seated pain in the ear is one of the most serious complaints. Other distressing symptoms include difficulty in swallowing, breathing, and talking; loss of taste; and dread of repeated bleedings, suffocation, and imminent death. These cause the patient to be depressed and anxious.

These patients are often referred to the neurosurgeon for treatment of pain. In the past, many surgical approaches have been proposed: (a) surgical rhizotomy of the trigeminal, glossopharyngeal, and cervical roots; (b) trigeminal tractotomy, including fibers of cranial nerves VII, IX, and X (35,87); (c) stereotactic thalamotomy (59) and mesencephalotomy (48,53); and (d) psychosurgical operations (87). Recently, percutaneous radiofrequency thermocoagulation of the roots of the trigeminal and glossopharyngeal nerves have been used for the treatment of severe cancer pain (10,36).

Percutaneous Thermocoagulation of the Trigeminal Nerve

Four patients were submitted to percutaneous thermocoagulation of the gasserian ganglion and rootlets. The operation was performed under local anesthesia with a Radionics FG5™ apparatus. Patients were premedicated with benzodiazepine and atropine. The electrode was introduced by the anterior approach of Hartel through the foramen ovale into the gasserian ganglion and rootlets. The position of the electrode was checked radiographically and by electrical stimulation (for review, see 77). Under ultra-short-acting barbiturate sedation, one or more thermocoagulations at high temperature (80–90°C) for 1 min were performed until complete analgesia and anesthesia were obtained in the target division(s). The results are summarized in Table 1A.

Percutaneous Thermocoagulation of Cranial Nerves IX and X

Four patients were submitted to thermocoagulation of cranial nerves IX and X using the technique described by Tew (80) and also by Broggi and Siegfried (10). The procedure, which was carried out with neuroleptoanal-

TABLE 1. *Percutaneous thermorhizotomy of cranial nerves*

Sex	Age	Diagnosis	Site of pain	Operation	Results
			A. Trigeminal ganglion and root		
Male	64	Carcinoma of the right lower gum	Lower half right face	Thermocoagulation of right trigeminal (+ MDT)	Excellent relief
Male	68	Carcinoma of the tongue	Right mouth, gum, tongue: continuous pain with paroxysmal bouts radiating to the ear	Thermocoagulation of right trigeminal	Excellent relief
Male	66	Pancoast syndrome with metastasis & Wegener granuloma	Right upper part of the face and head; slight pain left face	Thermocoagulation of right trigeminal (+ MDT)	Excellent relief; some discomfort from other pain controlled with MDT
Female	78	Squamous cell carcinoma of the right cheek	Right trigeminal area (especially 1st branch); slight in the right ear and throat	Thermocoagulation of right trigeminal	No relief; submitted to phenol gasserian ganglion block
			B. Thermorhizotomy of cranial nerves IX and X		
Male	53	Cancer of larynx; right cervical metastasis	Right pharynx, throat, root of the tongue, deep in ear; paroxysmal pain	Thermocoagulation of nerves IX and X	Total relief; only 15 days of follow-up

C. Glossopharyngeal and vagus nerves

Sex	Age	Diagnosis	Location	Procedure	Outcome
Female	80	Carcinoma right pharynx	Right ear, tonsil	Thermocoagulation of nerves IX and X (+ MDT)	Total relief; 2-mo follow-up
Male	57	Carcinoma left tonsil, pharynx	Left pharynx, tonsil; deep in left ear; pain paroxysms increased by swallowing	Thermocoagulation of nerves IX and X (+ MDT)	Total relief; 21-days follow-up; swallowing disturbances worsened
Male	65	Carcinoma of the posterior third of the tongue	Deep in the right ear and throat; swallowing makes pain worse	Thermocoagulation of nerves IX and X	Nearly total relief; swallowing disturbances worsened

D. Combined thermorhizotomy of cranial nerves and roots of cervix

Sex	Age	Diagnosis	Location	Procedure	Outcome
Male	68	Carcinoma left tonsil, pharynx, cervical metastasis	Left pharynx & tonsil; deep in left ear; left occiput & cervical region	1. Thermorhizotomy of the left nerves IX & X 2. Thermorhizotomy of the left cervical roots 3. Phenolic block of the left cervical roots (+ MDT)	Satisfactory relief of pain in the ear & throat; incomplete relief of neck & occipital pain; swallowing disturbances; 3-mo follow-up
Male	68	Metastasis of pulmonary cancer to the base of skull	Right face; proxysmal pain deep in right ear	1. Thermocoagulation of nerve V 2. Thermocoagulation of complex of nerves IX & X (+ MDT)	Complete relief from pain; paralysis of right nerve VI

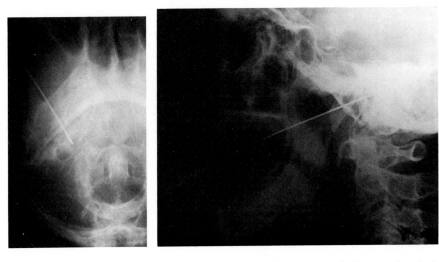

FIG. 1. The thermocoagulation probe is in the pars nervosa of the right foramen jugularis in this 65-year-old man.

gesia, entailed the insertion of an insulated needle with a bare tip of 5 mm through the skin overlapping the second upper molar tooth about 2.5 cm from the corner of the mouth and directed posteriorly, medially, and superiorly. Under fluoroscopic control, the needle is advanced so that in the frontal plane its point is directed to the center of the pupil of the ipsilateral eye similar to the needle insertion for gasserian ganglion block; in the lateral view, the needle is directed to the external acoustic meatus. The needle is advanced until its tip reaches the neural part of the posterior foramen lacerum. The position must be checked with repeated radiographs in frontal and lateral projections (Fig. 1). When the needle tip reaches cranial nerves IX and X, there is a sudden slowing of pulse (up to 20 per sec), with occasional bouts of irregular pulse or short periods of asystole that are followed in a few seconds by restoration of the normal frequency. As the point of the needle approaches the nerve, the patient may experience pain deep in the ear, throat, and tonsils of the same side. Then an electrophysiologic control is carried out to confirm the correct position of the needle by means of electrical stimulations, which produce paresthesia referred deep in the ear and less often in the upper pharynx.

Once the probe is in the correct position, a thermocoagulation is performed after producing sedation with an intravenous thiobarbiturate. Sudden rise of the temperature up to 50 to 55°C usually gives rise to slowing of the heart rate. Therefore it is important to increase the temperature very slowly in order to reach the therapeutic level. Two successive coagulations with the temperature of the probe at 80 to 90°C during 60 sec are performed. The results are summarized in Table 1B.

Combined Thermorhizotomy of Cranial Nerves V, IX, and X

This procedure was carried out in 2 patients: one had excellent relief, and the other had good but incomplete relief (Table 1C). In patients in whom the pain spreads to the neck, it will be necessary also to carry out thermorhizotomy of the upper cervical nerves or neurolytic blocks of these structures.

SURGICAL RHIZOTOMY

Surgical Cranial Nerve Rhizotomy

Patients in good physical condition and with a long life expectancy can be managed by surgical section of the roots of cranial nerves V, IX, and/or X alone or in combination with section of the roots of the upper cervical nerves. These procedures ensure complete and long-lasting relief, which in my experience persists for many months. I have used these procedures in 14 patients who had operation under general anesthesia with controlled respiration. A suboccipital craniectomy and unilateral or bilateral cervical laminectomy are performed via a midline cervical incision, which is curved laterally along the occipital region to the base of the mastoid process. The use of magnifying eyeglasses or the operating microscope greatly facilitates identification of the structures. The results obtained are shown in Table 2. It deserves reemphasis that these operations are stressful and carry certain operative risks. In this series, 12 patients had marked deterioration of their general physical condition in the postoperative period and 4 patients died 5 to 21 days after the operation.

Spinal Dorsal Rhizotomy

Dorsal rhizotomy of spinal nerves was the first operation successfully used in the surgery of pain. However, accurate analyses of long-term results were not attempted until recently. These have shown that the results are not as good as might be expected after complete denervation of a painful area produced by cutting an adequate number of nerve roots. Usually the operation has been an immediate, complete success, but in a few months patients start to complain of pain again (43).

In an analysis of the results in a group of patients, Loeser (43) found no technical factors accounting for the lack of long-term success of rhizotomy; therefore he suggested that abnormal physiologic phenomena are at work. Coggeshall et al. (12) suggested that some unmyelinated nociceptive fibers arising from cells of the dorsal ganglion but running in the anterior roots might be responsible for the recurrence of pain. Consequently, Osgood et al. (55) introduced the technique of posterior root "ganglionectomy," which

TABLE 2. *Surgical rhizotomy of cranial and cervical sensory roots*

Sex	Age	Diagnosis	Site of pain	Operation	Results
Male	69	Carcinoma larynx; cervical metastasis; swallowing increases pain; roentgen therapy	Left mandibula, occiput, neck; drug dependence	Left trigeminal, glossopharyngeal, C2–C3	Complete relief from pain until death 15 days later due to hemorrhage from tumor
Male	41	Carcinoma lip; cervical metastasis; roentgen therapy	Left mandibula, face, neck; drug dependence	Left trigeminal, glosso-pharyngeal, upper vagal rootlets. C2–C5	Complete relief; died 15 days later from hemorrhage from tumor & bronchopneumonia
Male	52	Carcinoma pharynx; cervical metastasis; cobalt therapy	Left occiput, throat	Left glossopharyngeal, C2–C4	Complete relief when discharged; no follow-up
Male	56	Carcinoma larynx; tracheostomy; submandibular scarring; cobalt therapy	Right neck under mandible, base of tongue, throat; swallowing brings on paroxysms of pain	Right glossopharyngeal, right and left C2–C3	Complete relief persisting at follow-up 16 mo later
Male	56	Carcinoma larynx; cervical metastasis; tracheostomy; cobalt therapy	Right mandibula, throat, ear occiput; swallowing increases pain	1. Left trigeminal 2. Left glossopharyngeal, C1–C3 & right C2–C3	Satisfactory results; pain in occiput, mandible, & throat abolished; pain in ear recurred but reduced; 3-mo follow-up until death
Male	59	Carcinoma pharynx; tracheostomy	Right head, mouth, throat, ear, & occiput; swallowing increases pain; drug dependence	Right trigeminal, glossopharyngeal, upper vagal rootlets, intermedius, & C2–C4	Relief of pain; postoperative death on 5th day from pneumonia & hemorrhage
Male	40	Carcinoma larynx; cervical metastasis; tracheostomy; cobalt therapy	Bilateral occiput & throat; swallowing brings on neuralgic pain paroxysms; drug dependence	Bilateral glossopharyngeal & C2–C4	Drug dependence made evaluation difficult; neuralgic pain fully abolished; some discomfort persisted; died 32 days after surgery

Sex	Age	Diagnosis	Pain distribution	Nerves sectioned	Outcome
Male	67	Carcinoma larynx; cervical metastasis; roentgen therapy	Right neck & ear; drug dependence	Right trigeminal glossopharyngeal, intermedius, C2–C4	Complete relief; postoperative pneumonia; death on 21st day from sudden cardiac failure
Female	37	Angiosarcoma of face; cobalt therapy	Left face & ear, with scalp diffusion	Left glossopharyngeal, trigeminal, intermedius, C2–C3	Complete freedom from pain until death 8 mo later; since 4th mo scanty, unpleasant, not painful sensation on the mandibular border
Male	47	Cancer of larynx, right laterocervical metastasis	Right face, ear, meatus acusticus and neck; paroxysmal bouts in right mandible; NSAID + morphine ineffective	Right trigeminal, glossopharyngeal upper vagal rootlets, C2–C5; left C2–C4	Total relief; died 2 mo later
Male	55	Carcinoma larynx; cervical metastasis; cobalt therapy; left laterocervical & submandibular scarring	Left face, ear, tongue, throat; NSAID + morphine ineffective	Left trigeminal, glossopharyngeal, intermedius C2–C4	Excellent relief when discharged; no follow-up
Male	59	Carcinoma larynx	Right face, ear, neck	Right trigeminal, glossopharyngeal, upper vagal, intermedius, C2–C5	Excellent relief; some "stabbing" persisted at vertex of head; died 45 days after operation
Male	52	Carcinoma larynx; cervical metastasis; tracheostomy	Left face, throat, neck, deep in ear; swallowing increases pain	Left trigeminal, glossopharyngeal, upper vagal rootlets, intermedius, C2–C4; right C2–C3	Total relief when discharged; no follow-up
Female	62	Sarcoma of left orbit	Left face	Left trigeminal	Excellent relief, mild dysesthesia & paroxysmal pain persisting in left face & ear some months after surgery; MDT provided nearly total relief

should interrupt even the sensory fibers that pass through the anterior root. However, evidence to support this hypothesis is still lacking. Failures from dorsal rhizotomy also are accounted for by the fact that cancer is a progressive disease that spreads and involves adjacent nerves that have not been interrupted surgically. Although this is undoubtedly true in certain cases, failures have been observed even if the denervation was adequate. Pain "recurs" even in permanently denervated and analgesic areas.

In such cases, there is not recurrence of the original pain; an entirely new, strange, annoying, burning, or aching, unbearable sensation develops, which the patient never had before. The abnormal sensation is referred to the anesthetic area or deep under the anesthetic skin. Sometimes denervated limbs feel like a painful phantom (58). In other words, recurrence of "pain" really represents the development of "anesthesia dolorosa": the source of pain does not lie in the peripheral nerves or roots, but in the central nervous system. Initially deafferentation is followed by decrease of activity in the deafferented central sensory pathways; later spontaneous, persistent, abnormal firing patterns develop, which give rise to the sensations patients call pain (for literature, see 58). Furthermore, cancer may damage nerve trunks with consequent loss of large, myelinated axons followed by disinhibition of small fibers, resulting in excessive neuronal firing in central pain pathways, which contributes to the pain. Further deafferentation by rhizotomy could exaggerate the abnormal firing.

In contrast, nearly four decades ago, Ray (65), and recently Barrash and Leavens (1), reported good results following extensive dorsal rhizotomy. However, Ray did not mention long-term results. The opinions of Barrash and Leavens are based on 72 cases of cancer pain: 40 patients were completely relieved and 10 were satisfactorily relieved. They believe that rhizotomy is a safe and effective procedure for severe intractable pain, including that caused by cancer.

I noted favorable results with extensive rhizotomy used to relieve cancer pain in the trunk, upper limb, and shoulder, but only in patients who survived less than 4 months. If survival was longer, there was pain recurrence or painful anesthesia. In patients with cancer pain in the face, head, and neck, rhizotomy of cranial nerves and cervical spinal roots sometimes gives longer relief. Moreover, denervation of the neck is well tolerated, and suppression of shooting pains is sufficient to make patients more comfortable (59,62). Rhizotomy can be used successfully even in pain limited to the perineum and sacrococcygeal region due to rectal and anal carcinoma in patients submitted to colostomy (19,34). Bilateral rhizotomy from S5 to S2 (some of which are to be spared on one side if there are no bladder disturbances) can afford complete relief. The area of perineal and perianal anesthesia is small and well tolerated without anesthesia dolorosa (19,34). Unfortunately, if carcinoma spreads to invade lumbar spinal nerves or roots, the operation proves inadequate.

A significant disadvantage of dorsal rhizotomy is massive denervation of an arm or leg, which makes the limb virtually useless. To avoid this, Sindou et al. (73) introduced the "selective spinal posterior rhizotomy" or "radicletomy" or "rhizidiotomy." With the aid of the operative microscope, only small-caliber fibers, which as the rootlets enter the cord are collected in a small lateral bundle, are cut; the large, myelinated fibers bound for the posterior funiculi, collected medially, are spared. Only pain sensation should be abolished, leaving intact other sensory modalities. The purposes of the operation are to spare inhibitory input on nociceptive afferents, thus preventing failures due to deafferentation, and to avoid functional impairment of limbs due to massive denervation. Sindou et al. (73,74) reported that, among the 20 patients subjected to this procedure, 13 obtained complete relief and 3 partial relief of pain. They concluded that the best indication for this procedure is pain in the upper limb due to cervical root involvement (e.g., Pancoast-Tobias syndrome) in which high cervical cordotomy is often ineffective and extensive posterior rhizotomy too drastic (74). Vlahovitch and Fuentes (83) share this opinion, although in their patients they combined "radicletomy" and total rhizotomy. Experience with the procedure is, however, limited.

SPINOTHALAMIC TRACTOTOMY

Spinothalamic tractotomy, sometimes referred to as anterolateral cordotomy, sections the spinothalamic tract in the anterolateral quadrant of the cord, wherein are located the ascending pathways that primarily transmit nociceptive information coming from the opposite side of the body. In patients with pain in the upper extremity and neck, the spinothalamic tract may be interrupted in the medulla or mesencephalon. The indications, technique, and complications of this procedure will not be discussed. Comments will be limited to the efficacy of open cordotomy and percutaneous cordotomy, with some comment on the problem of recurrence on long-term follow-up. Moreover, medullary and mesencephalic tractotomy will be mentioned briefly.

Open Cordotomy

Complete unilateral transection of the anterolateral quadrant at upper thoracic or cervical levels produces, in nearly every patient, analgesia in the contralateral half of the body, and bilateral section produces bilateral analgesia. Immediate relief of pain is achieved in nearly 60 to 80% of patients (64,87). However, the number of failures rises at long-term follow-up. Generally speaking, the incidence of recurrence of pain is about 30 to 50%. Unfortunately, details are often lacking in the published reports. Criteria for evaluation of the results and the length of survival are quite different in the various published series, thus precluding comparison of them. My personal experience is based on 28 patients I have been able to follow up personally. Among this group, more than 75% of the patients had recurrence of pain 3 months after the procedure was done. This statistic is higher than currently estimated in the literature. However, it compares quite well with Bohm's report (5), which, oddly enough, is never quoted even in the most complete reviews on the subject. He reported that out of 29 patients who had bilateral thoracic cordotomy, 20 had recurrence of pain at $3\frac{1}{2}$-months follow-up; 9 patients who survived only 2 months died free from pain. In other words, there was a recurrence of pain in all surviving patients at $3\frac{1}{2}$ months. No better were the results noted by Siegfried and Krayenbühl (72), who reported that 50% of the patients had recurrence of pain after a few weeks.

The obvious question is "Why the disappearance of analgesia?" Incomplete section of the spinothalamic tract with only temporary damage to ascending fibers has been blamed for the recurrence. Although this may be true in some cases, neuroanatomic studies have shown that fading of analgesia occurs even with complete bilateral sections of the anterolateral quadrant (11,26,58,87). Moreover, usually there is not simple recurrence of the pain for which the patient was operated on; patients complain of a new kind of pain, of disagreeable, unbearable sensations (dysesthesia). Peripheral stimuli can give rise to hyperpathia. These symptoms are identical to those of "central pain" and often are more annoying and sometimes more excruciating to the patients than the original cancer pain (11,56,58). Recovery of sensibility and the related symptomatology are not due simply to recovery of function of injured long ascending fibers, but in part to transmission of impulses by other multisynaptic or alternative spinal pathways, which can and often do display abnormal spontaneous activity (11,31,58). These pathways are diffuse and intermingled with other cord tracts. Total interruption of them will never be possible without severe impairment of other functions.

Reliable information is scanty about the effectiveness of cordotomy at C1–C2 for the relief of pain in the shoulder and upper arm. The number of patients reported is usually small (5,8,23,54), or the problem is not thoroughly discussed (48,50). White and Sweet (87) concluded that cervical cordotomy does not produce lasting analgesia of the arm. Schürmann (69) reported that with cervical cordotomy at level of C1–C2 permanent analgesia very rarely extends higher than C8–D1 and therefore is ineffective in providing pain relief in the shoulder and upper limb. None of the 6 patients I was able to follow up personally for more than 3 months obtained permanent analgesia of pain and good relief of pain in the shoulder and arm. In the opinion of White and Sweet (87), shoulder and upper limb pain is treated better by some form of leucotomy or thalamotomy; others prefer selective posterior rhizotomy (41,74,83) or mesencephalic tractotomy (48). The mechanisms of fading of analgesia, recurrence of pain, and occurrence of central pain are probably the same as in thoracic cordotomy.

Percutaneous Cordotomy

In 1963, Mullan et al. (52) introduced the technique of percutaneous cordotomy. The procedure, refined by others (24,39,42), entails the interruption of the anterolateral quadrant of the cord by percutaneous insertion of a coagulating probe in the spinal cord at upper or lower cervical level. It is a relatively minor surgical procedure; operative mortality seems very low (1 to 3%) even after bilateral procedures, and complications are fewer than those occurring with open cordotomy (66). Percutaneous cordotomy seems to offer the patients the same pain relief as open cordotomy (24,66), with a rate of immediate success up to 96% (79). However, long-term follow-up studies do not always detail precise results.

Impressive large series of cases are only of moderate interest because pain relief seems to have been assessed only at discharge (24,79), and correlations between survival and pain relief are sometimes lacking (24,39). Only Rosomoff (66) made an accurate study of 100 cases of bilateral cordotomy at long-term follow-up. Cancer pain and noncancer pain were grouped together, with results not given separately for pain in the upper or lower half of the body. Rosomoff (66) obtained "complete relief" postoperatively in 80 (80%) of 100 cases; at 6-weeks follow-up, 42 (67%) of 63; at 6 months, 18 (50%) of 36 of the patients remained pain-free; at 1 year, 30% were still relieved. It seems, therefore, that results of percutaneous cordotomy are neither better nor worse than those of open cordotomy. There is no report in the literature containing a detailed analysis of long-term results and failures in patients with pain of the upper limb and shoulder. Lorenz and associates (44) reported that failures and bad results were mainly due to difficulties in achieving permanent elimination of pain arising from the brachial plexus and from insufficient levels of analgesia.

Rosomoff (66) reported the use of percutaneous cordotomy in 34 patients who died within 6 weeks and in another 13 who died between 6 weeks and 3 months (i.e., high-risk patients in poor condition). He reported that the majority of patients had died pain-free. The best definition of the role of percutaneous cordotomy in surgery for pain was given by Mullan (51) who believes that this procedure extends the indication for cordotomy to those patients who are too ill for the open surgical procedure. Mullan emphasized that the procedure is not useful for the relief of pain which does not respond to the classical "open" method. Another important advantage is that the procedure may be repeated if necessary. This led to the extension of indications to many patients with advanced cancer who had only a few days or weeks of life expectancy. That could explain why percutaneous cordotomy "seems" to afford higher success rate than open cordotomy even in upper-half body pain. Clearly an operation that abolishes pain for 2 to 3 weeks in a patient who will survive for such a short time may not be as successful in relieving pain and suffering if the patient had lived 4 to 6 weeks or longer.

In summary, success of cordotomy—by open or percutaneous method— is tied strictly to the duration of survival of the patient. As to when either open or percutaneous cordotomy is indicated, if the patient is in fair condition with several months of life expectancy, the open technique done with the aid of the operative microscope, which allows better visualization of anatomic landmarks and more complete transection of anterolateral quadrant, is preferred. In patients with very short life expectancy, when limited damage to the anterolateral quadrant is sufficient to relieve pain during the last few days or weeks of life, percutaneous cordotomy is preferred.

Mesencephalic Tractotomy

Spinothalamic tractotomy at the mesencephalic level was introduced by Dogliotti (16) and Walker (84). The operation entails high operative mortality, complications, and frequent occurrence of central pain and dysesthesia (58,62). Thus it was abandoned even though it seemed indicated for face, neck, and upper limb pain.

The introduction of stereotactic technique by Spiegel et al. (76) renewed interest in mesencephalotomy. In fact, stereotactic midbrain tractotomy is an operation with low mortality and rare complications (58,62). Furthermore, the stereotactic lesion can be extended beyond the spinothalamic tract to impinge on the reticular formation where polysynaptic pain pathways are supposed to exist (88). The hope was it would be possible to obtain longer relief of pain and to avoid risk of central pain. The method was used only in small series of patients with cancer pain (25,28,53,88). Opinions about the efficacy of the operation differ. Some writers reported only poor results (88); others believe mesencephalotomy is the technique of choice for the treatment of pain in the head, neck, and arm (53). Still others believe that for relief of pain due to cancer, it is necessary to combine mesencephalotomy with bilateral cingulotomy (81).

In 1976, Mazars et al. (48) reported they had performed 224 stereotactic mesencephalotomies of which eight were done bilaterally. Of this group, 152 patients had cancer pain and in most of these patients the pain relief was prompt and excellent, especially in patients with cervical and cephalic pain which had not been relieved by other procedures. Relief was permanent and complete even in the upper thoracic region and the incidence of complications was very low; statistical analysis of the results, however, was not reported. Mazars et al. believe that cordotomy is still more effective than mesencephalotomy for pain in the lower half of the body (48). The results reported by Mazars and his colleagues are impressive and suggest further trial of the method.

Commissural Myelotomy

Commissural myelotomy consists of section of the pain fibers at the midline of the cord where they cross to ascend in the contralateral anterior quadrant. This procedure was expected to produce large bands of bilateral analgesia in the torso and/or limbs, depending on the cord-splitting level. It then would seem possible to obtain bilateral pain relief with a single operation, without damage to other spinal tracts and major complications. Unfortunately, success of the procedure has been rather elusive. Only Wertheimer and Lecuire (86) reported satisfactory results in a large series of cases submitted to lumbar myelotomy for bilateral pain of the legs, pelvis, and perineum. The incidence of complications, consisting of operative death, radicular pain, leg dysesthesia, paresis, and bladder or bowel dysfunction, was high. Of 80 patients followed up, 27 (34%) were completely relieved and 25 (31%) were improved; the procedure failed in 28 (35%). In 1963, Dargent et al. (15) reviewed the same series and concluded that commissural myelotomy is effective only for vaginal and visceral pain, and that cordotomy is preferred for rectal and leg pain.

This operation seemed a matter of only historic interest rather than of practical value when, in 1964, Lembcke (38) reported impressive results in 12 patients submitted to cervical myelotomy. All the patients were relieved and analgesia persisted up to 10 years in 6 long-term survivors; no serious complication occurred. This prompted new interest in the procedure, which was used both for pain in the lower half of the body (9,13,33,41,48,75) and for cervical, upper limb, and thoracic pain (29,63,70). Wertheimer and Lecuire's (86) standard incision was 2 to 3 cm long and a few millimeters deep. Currently most surgeons try to produce a deeper incision with complete splitting of the cord in two halves for several centimeters (9,13,33,63,75).

As is always the case in surgery for pain, some investigators are happy with the results and others are not. The former group includes Lembcke (38) and Broager (9), who state they gave up bilateral cordotomy in favor of commissural myelotomy. In contrast, Papo and Luongo (63) reported that although pain was completely relieved in all patients, it remained absent for only several weeks; severe pain recurred within 2 months.

It is generally agreed by those who have performed commissural myelotomy that (a) despite extensive splitting of the cord, defects in pain and temperature appreciation are relatively mild; (b) no permanent extensive analgesia ensues; and (c) hypalgesia, when present, fades away in a few weeks. On the contrary, disturbances due to dorsal column injury (loss of positional sense, tactile hypoesthesia, dysesthesia, tingling, ataxia) are frequent and may be marked (41,63). The mechanism by which myelotomy abolishes pain, even if temporarily, is far from clear. Schvarcz (70) suggested pain relief was due to interruption of extralemniscal polysynaptic pathways close to the central gray matter of the spinal cord; myelotomy acts like an intralaminar thalamotomy. Sourek (75) and Papo and Luongo (63) report that a close correlation exists between signs of posterior column damage and pain relief. When these fade away, pain usually recurs, suggesting a role of injury or irritation of dorsal column system responsible for the relief of pain. It seems to me that myelotomy is a rather mysterious operation whose mechanisms, indications, and results are far from clear.

TABLE 3. *Stereotactic thalamotomies*

Sex	Age	Diagnosis	Site of pain	Operation: target	Nuclei totally or partially destroyed	Results and postoperative findings[a]
Male	41	Carcinoma of tongue	Right root of tongue & throat; trisma	1st op: Left VPM		Relief of pain for 4 mo: recurrence C: none; SF: none
				2nd op: Left VPM		Immediate relief; roentgen therapy: satisfactory relief for 40 mo
Male	61	Cancer of right maxillary sinus	Right face	Left CM		Immediate relief C: none; SF: none
Male	58	Cancer of the nasopharynx	Right face	Left VPM-CM		Immediate relief
Male	61	Carcinoma of pharynx	Left face & ear; swallowing brings on pain	Right VPM	VPM + VPL	Immediate relief; roentgen therapy: free from pain at 20 mo follow-up C: transitory paresthesia left hand; SF: left hypalgesia & tactile & thermal hypesthesia; position sense reduced & astereognosia on left
Female	56	Breast carcinoma; metastasis to Gasserian ganglion	Right face & tongue	Left CM, Pf, VPM, VPL	CM, Pf (+ limitans), VPM + part of VPL, DM, VL, LP, Pulvin	Total pain relief; died 18 days later following hypophysectomy C: right arm ataxia; SF: total sensory loss in right face, marked sensory changes in right arm & leg

[a] C = complications; SF = sensory findings.

Sex	Age	Diagnosis	Symptoms	Operation	Structures	Results
Male	60	Carcinoma of larynx	Right throat & tongue; swallowing increases pain; drug dependence	Left CM, VPM	CM, VPM	Total relief; submitted 15 days later to gastrostomy because feeding by natural way or by means of nasogastric tube was impossible, died without pain C: slight right arm ataxia
Male	66	Carcinoma of pharynx	Left face & head; trismus; swallowing increases pain; drug dependence	Right CM, VPM & mesencephalotomy	CM, Pf (+ limitans), VPM, VPL; spinothalamic tract, medial lemniscus reticular substance at mesencephalon	Total relief; died 21 days after operation: hemorrhage from tumor C: slight left arm ataxia; SF: left total anesthesia
Male	58	Sarcoma of parotid gland	Left face, head, neck; swallowing is difficult; drug dependence	Right CM, VPM, VPL	CM, Pf (+ limitans) intral, VPM, VPL + part of LP, DM, Pulvin	Total relief of pain; died 56 days after operation as a result of broncopneumonia ab ingestis C: moderate thalamic syndrome; the patient does not complain of pain; SF: left hypesthesia to light touch, pain, head; astereognosis & abolition of proprioception
Male	50	Carcinoma of pharynx; right pleuritis	Right face, ear, head; swallowing exacerbates pain; right chest; drug dependence	Left CM	CM	Total relief of facial pain for 8 mo: thereafter total recurrence; chest pain unchanged: phenolization C: none; SF: none
Male	62	Carcinoma of gum, jaw, cheek	Left face & mouth; drug dependence	Right CM	CM	Relief of pain for 3½ mo: thereafter recurrence

Continued

TABLE 3. (*Continued*)

Sex	Age	Diagnosis	Site of pain	Operation: target	Nuclei totally or partially destroyed	Results and postoperative findings[a]
Male	70	Carcinoma of pharynx	Left tongue, gums, mouth, face, concha; drug dependence	Right CM	CM, Pf, + very small part of VPL	C: slight ataxia left hand for 4 days postop; SF: none Partial recurrence of pain in 5 days; died 18 days postop: cachexia C: none; SF: none
Male	53	Carcinoma	Left face, head, ear; trismus	1st op: Right CM	CM	Total relief; recurrence between 12th & 22nd day after operation C: none; SF: none
				2nd op: Right VPM	VPM, VPL	Total relief of pain during 30-day follow-up C: moderate painful thalamic syndrome on left body; SF: left hypalgesia & tactile & thermal hypesthesia; position sense reduced on left
Male	40	Ethmoidal carcinoma	Left jaw, eye, head, occiput, radiation to shoulder; drug dependence	Right CM	CM, VPM, VPL	Relief of pain, recurrence on 14th day, radiotherapy with good result during next 2 mo C: left transitory paresis; hyperpathic response to cold stimuli in left face, neck, arm, which disappeared in a few

Sex	Age	Diagnosis	Symptoms	Target	Nuclei	Results
						days; SF: transitory hypalgesia & tactile hypesthesia on left face & arm, persistent reduction of proprioceptive sensations & graphesthesia
Male	62	Carcinoma of gum	Right tongue, mouth, head; trismus; swallowing exacerbates pain	Left CM	CM, Pf intral. DM	Relief of pain for 2 days; total recurrence; died of disease in 42 days C: none; SF: none
Male	42	Carcinoma of tonsil	Right face & throat; swallowing worsens pain; drug dependence	Left CM, VPM	CM, Pf (+ limitans), VPM, VPL	Total relief until death 49 days after operation (hemorrhage from tumor) C: none; SF: transitory hypalgesia & tactile thermal hypesthesia on right face, arm
Female	79	Carinoma of parotid	Left face; trismus; swallowing increases pain	Right CM, VPM	CM, VPM, VPL	Drug dependence made difficult evaluation C: none; SF: hypalgesia & tactile hypesthesia on left face, shoulder, arm
Male	63	Cancer of maxillary sinus involving palate & nose	Deep in the face bilaterally	Bilateral pulvinectomy		Excellent relief for 2 mo; then lost at follow-up; no sensory defects; mild psychic disturbances: temporal disorientation

Stereotactic Thalamotomy/Hypothalamatomy

In patients in poor physical condition with a short life expectancy who have diffuse pain in the face, head, neck, and upper limb, stereotactic surgery to produce thalamic lesions should be considered. This includes lesions of the following nuclei: ventralis posteromedialis/ventralis posterolateralis (VPM/VPL); centromedian (CM); parafascicularis (Pf)/intralamina and limitans contralateral to the painful side (3,21,32,60). In my experience these procedures produce excellent short-term relief, but at long-term there is recurrence of pain (cases 54 and 55) or the occurrence of thalamic hyperpathia (Table 3) (47,57,60,78). Hypothalamotomy, which entails a lesion of the posteromedial hypothalamus, has been reported by Fairman (17) to provide long-term relief of cancer pain in a group of 125 patients and by Sano (67) in a small group of patients. Thalamolaminotomy, which entails a lesion in the internal medullary lamina of the thalamus, has been reported by Sano (67) to be effective in relieving severe cancer pain in the majority of a small group of patients. These results suggest that these techniques deserve a further trial.

Psychosurgery

Since the original report of Freeman and Watts (22) of excellent results with lobotomy for the relief of intractable pain, this procedure has been limited to patients with severe cancer pain, not relieved by other methods. Lobotomy seems to work in that it...changes the attitude of the patient toward pain (22), removes the anticipation and memory of the pain (71), and alters affective and emotional response to it, but it does not alter the perception of pain.

Unfortunately, bilateral lobotomy invariably produces apathy and severe psychologic deterioration. Because of this serious complication, less destructive procedures were introduced: unilateral lobotomy (68), undercutting of the frontal cortex (49), progressive radiofrequency frontal lobotomy (27), bilateral frontal topectomy (37), and dorsomedial stereotactic thalamotomy (76). However, even with those procedures, pain relief invariably seems to be associated with, and depends on, severe emotional and mental defects. Pain is relieved only so long as changes of personality persist; should they subside, there is recurrence of complaints.

To avoid psychic disturbances, White and Sweet (87) introduced graduated bilateral coagulation of medial frontal white matter. In this procedure, small areas of frontothalamic projection fibers are destroyed in successive steps at intervals of several days. In this way it seems possible to afford pain relief without severe mental deterioration. Bertrand et al. (2) attempted to obtain the same result by means of stereotactic section of the frontothalamic pathways. Lindstrom (40) performed frontal lobotomy by means of ultrasonic beam; "considerable relief from pain" was obtained in 45 of 48 patients thus treated without the mental defects of frontal lobe surgery.

In 1962, Foltz and White (20) introduced "cingulotomy." In the cingulum run pathways mediating activities of the limbic system to the entire forebrain; these pathways play a major role in emotional behavior. The hope was to modify emotional reaction to pain, relieving suffering with minimal psychic impairment. Foltz and White (20) reported excellent relief at 6-months to 1-year follow-up in a group of patients who showed marked emotional reaction to pain. Hurt and Ballantine (30) used bilateral cingulotomy in 32 patients with cancer pain and noted they were not able to document undesirable changes in intellect, memory, personality or other psychologic functions of these patients. Marked to complete relief was experienced by 37% of the patients, slight to moderate by 28%; but they noted a trend to progressive decrease in the initial degree of pain relief (30). It seems, therefore, that cingulotomy has, at least partially, fulfilled expectations. Duration of relief, however, is briefer than following more mutilating frontal operations with the attendant persistent mental impairment.

My experience is limited to four cases of frontothalamic section (2), four cases of cingulotomy (20), four of graduated frontal coagulation, and two of dorsomedial thalamotomy (76). As far as I can judge by this limited experience, relief of suffering was achieved only with concomitant personality changes and mental deterioration. Thus, I am rather inclined to agree with Falconer (18), who considers frontal surgery a procedure of therapeutic desperation. The less-mutilating procedures in more experienced hands might afford satisfactory relief with only minor personality changes.

REFERENCES

1. Barrash, J. M., and Leavens, M. E. (1973): Dorsal rhizotomy for the relief of intractable pain of malignant tumor origin. *J. Neurosurg.*, 38:755–757.
2. Bertrand, C., Martinez, N., and Hardy, J. (1966): Frontothalamic section for intractable pain. In: *Pain*, edited by R. S. Knighton and P. R. Dumke, pp. 531–535. Little, Brown, Boston.
3. Bettag, W. (1966): Results of treatment of pain by interruption of the medial pain tract of the brain stem. *Excerpta Medica Int. Cong. Series*, 110:771–775.
4. Birkenfeld, R., and Fisher, R. G. (1963): Successful treatment of causalgia of upper extremity with spinothalamic tractotomy. *J. Neurosurg.*, 20:303–311.
5. Bohm, E. (1960): Chordotomy for intractable pain due to malignant disease. *Acta Psychiatr. Scand.*, 35:145–155.
6. Bonica, J. J. (1953): *The Management of Pain*. Lea & Febiger, Philadelphia.
7. Bonica, J. J. (1979): Introduction to management of pain of advanced cancer. In: *Advances in Pain Research and Therapy, Vol. 2*, edited by J. J. Bonica and V. Ventafridda, pp. 115–130. Raven Press, New York.
8. Brihaye, J., and Rétif, J. (1961): Comparison des résultats obtenuse par la cordotomie anterolaterale au niveau dorsal et au niveau cervical. (À propos de 109 observations personnelles). *Neurochirurgie*, 7:258–277.
9. Broager, B. (1974): Commissural myelotomy. *Surg. Neurol.*, 2:71–74.
10. Broggi, G., and Siegfried, J. (1979): Percutaneous differential radiofrequency rhizotomy of glossopharyngeal nerve in facial pain due to cancer. In: *Advances in Pain Research and*

Therapy, Vol. 2, edited by J. J. Bonica and V. Ventafridda, pp. 469–473. Raven Press, New York.

11. Cassinari, V., and Pagni, C. A. (1969): *Central Pain. A Neurosurgical Survey.* Harvard University Press, Cambridge.
12. Coggeshall, R. E., Appelbaum, M. L., Facem, M., Stubbs, T. B., III, and Sykes, M. T. (1975): Unmyelinated axons in human ventral roots, a possible explanation for the failure of dorsal rhizotomy to relieve pain. *Brain*, 98:157–166.
13. Cook, A. W., and Kawakamy, Y. (1977): Commissural myelotomy. *J. Neurosurg.*, 47:1–6.
14. Dargent, M., Mansuy, L., Colon, J., and De Rougemont, J. (1963): Les problémes posè par la douleur dans l'evolution des cancer gynècologiques. *Lyon Chir.*, 59:62–83.
15. Dogliotti, A. M. (1931): Traitement des syndromes douloureux de la peripherie par l'alcoolisation subarachnoidienne des racines posterieures a leur emergence de la moelle epiniere, *Presse Med.*, 39:1249–1252.
16. Dogliotti, A. M. (1938): First surgical section in man, of the lemmiseus lateralis (pain-temperature path) in brainstem, for the treatment of diffuse, rebellious pain. *Anesth. Analg. (Cleve.)* 17:143–145.
17. Fairman, D. (1976): Neurophysiological basis for the hypothalamic lesion and stimulation by chronic implanted electrodes for the relief of intractable pain in cancer. In: *Advances in Pain Research and Therapy, Vol. 1*, edited by J. J. Bonica and D. Albe-Fessard, pp. 843–847. Raven Press, New York.
18. Falconer, M. A. (1948): Relief of intractable pain of organic origin by frontal lobotomy. *Res. Publ. Assoc. Res. Nerv. Ment. Dis.*, 27:707–714.
19. Felsööry, A., and Crue, B. L. (1976): Results of 19 years experience with sacral rhizotomy for perineal and perianal cancer pain. *Pain*, 2:431–433.
20. Foltz, E. L., and White, L. E. (1966): Rostral cingulotomy and pain "relief." In: *Pain*, edited by R. S. Knighton and P. R. Dumke, pp. 469–491. Little, Brown, Boston.
21. Fraioli, B., and Guidetti, B. (1975): Effects of stereotactic lesions of the pulvinar and lateralis posterior nucleus on intractable pain and dyskinetic syndromes in man. *Appl. Neurophysiol.*, 38:23–70.
22. Freeman, W., and Watts, J. W. (1950): *Psychosurgery in the Treatment of Mental Disorders and Intractable Pain.* Charles C Thomas, Springfield, Ill.
23. French, L. A. (1974): High cervical tractotomy: Technique and results. *Clin. Neurosurg.*, 21:239–245.
24. Gildenberg, P. L. (1974): Percutaneous cervical cordotomy. *Clin. Neurosurg.*, 21:246–256.
25. Glees, P. (1953): The central pain tract. *Acta Neuroveg.*, 7:160–174.
26. Graf, C. I. (1960): Consideration in loss of sensory level after bilateral cervical cordotomy. *Arch. Neurol.*, 3:410–415.
27. Grantham, E. G. (1951): Prefrontal lobotomy for relief of pain, with a report of a new operative technique. *J. Neurosurg.*, 8:405–410.
28. Helfant, M. H., Leksell, L., and Strang, R. R. (1965): Experiences with intractable pain treated by stereotaxic mesencephalotomy. *Acta Chir. Scand.*, 129:573–580.
29. Hitchcock, E. (1974): Stereotactic myelotomy. *Proc. R. Soc. Med.*, 67:771–772.
30. Hurt, R. W., and Ballantine, H. T. (1974): Stereotactic anterior cingulate lesions for persistent pain: A report on 68 cases. *Clin. Neurosurg.*, 21:334–351.
31. Kerr, F. W. L. (1975): Neuroanatomical substrates of nociception in the spinal cord. *Pain*, 1:325–356.
32. Kim, Y. K., and Umbach, W. (1972): Comparative evaluation of different psychosurgical methods. In: *Present Limits of Neurosurgery*, edited by I. Fusek and Z. Kunc, pp. 465–469. Avicenum, Praha.
33. King, R. B. (1977): Anterior commissurotomy for intractable pain. *J. Neurosurg.*, 47:7–11.
34. Kühner, A. (1976): La valeur des interventions sur les racines sacreés dans le traitement des syndromes douloureux du bassin. *Neurochirurgia (Stuttg.)*, 22:429–436.
35. Kunc, Z. (1964): *Tractus spinalis nervi trigemini. Fresh anatomic data and their significance for surgery.* Nakladatelstvi Ceskoslovenske Akadamie, Ved, Praha.
36. Lazorthes, Y., Verdie, J. C., and Lagarrigue, J. (1976): Thermocoagulation percutanée des nerfs rachidiens à visée analgésique. *Neurochirurgie*, 22:445–453.
37. Le Beau, J., Bouvet, M., and Rosier, M. (1950): Traitment des douleurs iréducibles par la topectomie. *Sem. Hop. Paris*, 24:1946–1952.

38. Lembcke, W. (1964): Über die mediolognitudinale Chordotomie im Halsmarkbereich. *Zentralbl. Chir.*, 89:439–443.
39. Lin, P. M., Gildenberg, P. L., and Polakoff, P. P. (1966): An anterior approach to percutaneous lower cervical cordotomy. *J. Neurosurg.*, 25:553–560.
40. Lindstrom, P. A. (1972): Prefrontal sonic treatment: Sixteen years' experience. In: *Psychosurgery: Proceedings of the Second International Congress on Psychosurgery*, edited by E. Hitchcock, L. Laitinen, and K. Vaernet, pp. 357–376. Charles C Thomas, Springfield, Ill.
41. Lippert, R. G., Hosobuchi, Y., and Nielsen, S. L. (1974): Spinal commissurotomy. *Surg. Neurol.*, 2:373–377.
42. Lipton, S., Dervin, E., and Heywood, O. B. (1974): A stereotactic approach to the anterior percutaneous electrical cordotomy. In: *Advances in Neurology, Vol. 4*, edited by J. J. Bonica, pp. 689–694. Raven Press, New York.
43. Loeser, J. D. (1972): Dorsal rhizotomy for the relief of chronic pain. *J. Neurosurg.*, 36:745–750.
44. Lorenz, R., Grumme, T., Herrmann, D., Palleske, H., Kühner, A., Stende, U., and Zierski, J. (1975): Percutaneous cordotomy. In: *Advances in Neurosurgery, Vol. 3*, edited by H. Penzholz, M. Brock, J. Hamer, M. Klinger, and O. Spoerri, pp. 178–185. Springer, Berlin.
45. Madrid, J. L., and Bonica, J. J. (1979): Cranial nerve blocks. In: *Advances in Pain Research and Therapy, Vol. 2*, edited by J. J. Bonica and V. Ventafridda, pp. 347–355. Raven Press, New York.
46. Maher, R. M. (1955): Relief of pain in incurable cancer. *Lancet*, 1:895–898.
47. Maspes, P. E., and Pagni, C. A. (1974): A critical appraisal of pain surgery and suggestions for improving treatment. In: *Recent Advances on Pain: Pathophysiology and Clinical Aspects*, edited by J. J. Bonica, P. Procacci, and C. A. Pagni, pp. 201–255. Charles C Thomas, Springfield, Ill.
48. Mazars, G., Merienne, L., and Cioloca, C. (1976): État actuel de la chirurgie de la douleur. *Neurochirurgie [Suppl.]*, 1:1–164.
49. McKissock, W. (1951): Rostral leucotomy. *Lancet*, 2:91–94.
50. Mullan, S. (1971): The surgical relief of pain. *Clin. Neurosurg.*, 18:208–224.
51. Mullan, S. (1974): Percutaneous cordotomy. In: *Advances in Neurology, Vol. 4*, edited by J. J. Bonica, pp. 677–682. Raven Press, New York.
52. Mullan, S., Harper, P., Hekmatpanah, J., Torres, H., and Dobbin, G. (1963): Percutaneous interruption of spinal pain tracts by means of a strontium 90 needle. *J. Neurosurg.*, 20:931–939.
53. Nashold, B. S. (1972) Extensive cephalic and oral pain relieved by midbrain tractotomy. *Confin. Neurol.*, 34:382.
54. Ogle, W. S., French, L. A., and Peyton, W. T. (1956): Experiences with high cervical cordotomy. *J. Neurosurg.*, 13:81–87.
55. Osgood, C. P., Dujovni, M., and Faille, R. (1976): Microsurgical lumbosacral ganglionectomy: technique, anatomic rationale, and surgical results. In: *Advances in Pain Research and Therapy, Vol. 1*, edited by J. J. Bonica and D. Albe-Fessard, pp. 855–862. Raven Press, New York.
56. Pagni, C. A. (1974): Place of stereotactic technique in surgery for pain. In: *Advances in Neurology, Vol. 4*, edited by J. J. Bonica, pp. 699–706. Raven Press, New York.
57. Pagni, C. A. (1977): Central pain and painful anesthesia. In: *Pain: Its Neurosurgical Management. Part II. Central Procedures*, edited by H. Krayenbühl, P. E. Maspes, and W. H. Sweet, pp. 132–257. Karger, Basel.
58. Pagni, C. A. (1979): General considerations on ablative neurosurgical procedures. In: *Advances in Pain Research and Therapy, Vol. 2*, edited by J. J. Bonica and V. Ventafridda, pp. 405–423. Raven Press, New York.
59. Pagni, C. A. (1979): Therapy of cancer pain in the head and neck. Role of Neurosurgery. In: *Advances in Pain Research and Therapy, Vol. 2*, edited by J. J. Bonica and V. Ventafridda, pp. 543–552. Raven Press, New York.
60. Pagni, C. A. (1981): Il ruolo della neurochirurgia nella cura del dolore incoercibile. In: *Progressi nella Fisiopatologia e Terapia del Dolore*, edited by E. Ciocatto, pp. 337–450. Ciocatto, Edizioni Medico Scientifiche, Torino.
61. Pagni, C. A., and Franzini, A. (1981): Strategia terapeutica nel dolore da cancro. *Minerva Med.*, 72:1–16.

62. Pagni, C. A., and Maspes, P. E. (1970): Problems in the surgical treatment of pain in malignancies of the head and neck. In: *Current Research in Neurosciences, Vol. 10*, edited by H. T. Wycis, pp. 138–153. Karger, Basel.

63. Papo, I., and Luongo, A. (1976): High cervical commissural myelotomy in the treatment of pain. *J. Neurol. Neurosurg. Psychiatry*, 39:705–710.

64. Piscol, K. (1975): Open spinal surgery for intractable pain. In: *Advances in Neurosurgery, Vol. 3*, edited by H. Penzholz, M. Brock, J. Hamer, M. Klinger, and O. Spoerri, pp. 157–169. Springer, Berlin.

65. Ray, B. S. (1943): The management of intractable pain by posterior rhizotomy. *Res. Publ. Assoc. Res. Nerv. Ment. Dis.*, 23:391–407.

66. Rosomoff, H. L. (1969): Bilateral percutaneous cervical radiofrequency cordotomy. *J. Neurosurg.*, 31:41–46.

67. Sano, K. (1979): Stereotaxic thalamolaminotomy and posteromedial hypothalamotomy for the relief of intractable pain. In: *Advances in Pain Research and Therapy, Vol. 2*, edited by J. J. Bonica and V. Ventafridda, pp. 475–485. Raven Press, New York.

68. Scarff, J. E. (1950): Unilateral prefrontal lobotomy for the relief of intractable pain. Report of 58 cases with special consideration of failures. *J. Neurosurg.*, 7:330–336.

69. Schürmann, K. (1972): Fundamental principles of the surgical treatment of pain. In: *Pain— Basic Principles—Pharmacology—Therapy*, edited by R. Janzen, W. D. Keidel, A. Herz, and C. Steichele, pp. 181–193. Thieme, Stuttgart.

70. Schvarcz, J. R. (1976): Stereotactic extralemniscal myelotomy. *J. Neurol. Neurosurg. Psychiatry*, 39:53–57.

71. Scoville, W. B. (1972): Psychosurgery and other lesions of the brain affecting human behavior. In: *Psychosurgery: Proceedings of the Second International Congress on Psychosurgery*, edited by E. Hitchcock, L. Laitinen, and K. Vaernet, pp. 5–21. Charles C Thomas, Springfield, Ill.

72. Siegfried, J., and Krayenbühl, H. (1972): Clinical experience in the treatment of intractable pain. In: *Pain—Basic Principles—Pharmacology—Therapy*, edited by R. Janzen, W. D. Keidel, A. Herz, and C. Steichele, pp. 202–204. Thieme, Stuttgart.

73. Sindou, M., Fischer, G., Goutelle, A., and Mansuy, L. (1974): La radicellotomie postérieure sélective. Premiers résultats dans la chirurgie de la douleur. *Neurochirurgie*, 20:391–408.

74. Sindou, M., Fisher, G., and Mansuy, L. (1976): Posterior spinal rhizotomy and selective posterior rhizidiotomy. In: *Pain: Its Neurosurgical Management, Part I: Procedures on Primary Afferent Neurons*, edited by H. Krayenbühl, P. E. Maspes, and W. H. Sweet, pp. 201–250. Karger, Basel.

75. Sourek, K. (1977): Mediolongitudinal myelotomy. In: *Pain: Its Neurological Management. Part II: Central Procedures*, edited by H. Krayenbühl, P. E. Maspes, and W. H. Sweet, pp. 15–34. Karger, Basel.

76. Spiegel, E. A., Wycis, H. T., Szekely, E. G., and Gildenberg, P. L. (1966): Medial and basal thalamotomy in so-called intractable pain. In: *Pain*, edited by R. S. Knighton, and P. R. Dumke, pp. 503–517. Little, Brown, Boston.

77. Sweet, W. H., and Wepsic, J. G. (1974): Controlled thermocoagulation of trigeminal ganglion and rootlets for differential destruction of pain fibers. Part 1: Trigeminal neuralgia. *J. Neurosurg.*, 39:143–156.

78. Talairach, J., Hecaen, H., David, M., Monnier, M., and de Ajuraguerra, J. (1949): Recherches sur la coagulation therapeutique des structures souscorticales chez l'homme. *Rev. Neurol. (Paris)*, 81:4–24.

79. Tasker, R. R. (1977): Open cordotomy. In: *Pain: Its Neurosurgical Management. Part II: Central Procedures*, edited by H. Krayenbuhl, P. E. Maspes, and W. H. Sweet, pp. 1–14. Karger, Basel.

80. Tew, J. J. (1976): Percutaneous rhizotomy in the treatment of intractable facial pain (trigeminal, glossopharyngeal and vagal nerves). In: *Current Techniques in Operative Neurosurgery*, edited by H. H. Schmidek and W. H. Sweet, pp. 409–426. Grune & Stratton, New York.

81. Turnbull, I. M. (1972): Bilateral cingulotomy combined with thalamotomy or mesencephalic tractotomy for pain. *Surg. Gynecol. Obstet.*, 134:958–962.

82. Twycross, R. G. (1979): Overview of analgesia. In: *Advances in Pain Research and Therapy, Vol. 2*, edited by J. J. Bonica and V. Ventafridda, pp. 617–633. Raven Press, New York.

83. Vlahovitch, B., and Fuentes, J. M. (1975): Résultats de la radicellotomie sélective postérieure à l'étage lombaire et cervical. *Neurochirurgie*, 21:29–42.
84. Walker, E. A. (1942): Mesencephalic tractotomy. A method for the relief of unilateral
intractable pain. *Arch. Surg.*, 44:953–962.
85. Wall, P. D. (1979): Changes in damaged nerve and their sensory consequences. In: *Advances
in Pain Research and Therapy, Vol. 3*, edited by J. J. Bonica, J. C. Liebeskind, and D.
Albe-Fessard, pp. 39–51. Raven Press, New York.
86. Wertheimer, P., and Lecuire, J. (1953): La myélotomie commissurale postérieure. À propos
de 107 observations. *Acta Chir. Belg.*, 52:568–574.
87. White, J. C., and Sweet, W. H. (1969): *Pain and the Neurosurgeon. A Forty Years Experience*. Charles C Thomas, Springfield, Ill.
88. Wycis, H. T., and Spiegel, E. A. (1962): Long-range results in the treatment of intractable
pain by stereotaxic midbrain surgery. *J. Neurosurg.*, 19:101–107.

Advances in Pain Research
and Therapy, Vol. 7,
edited by C. Benedetti et al.
Raven Press, New York © 1984.

Treatment of Cancer Pain with Hypophysectomy: Surgical and Chemical

Allan B. Levin and Lincoln L. Ramirez

Department of Neurosurgery, University of Wisconsin Clinical Science Center, Madison, Wisconsin 53792

The role of hypophysectomy in the treatment of cancer pain has been debated for several years. Although transcranial hypophysectomy for the treatment of malignant tumors was first described in 1952 (31,36), it was originally conceived as a means of achieving objective regression of metastatic prostate and breast carcinoma. The procedure was a logical extension of the hormonal manipulation by gonadectomy and/or adrenalectomy pioneered by Huggins (12). It was soon found that hypophysectomy, like its antecedent operations, relieved pain of metastatic breast and prostate carcinoma more consistently than it produced objective tumor regression. With the advent of stereotactic and open transsphenoidal hypophysectomy, pituitary ablation could be accomplished with greater safety. Similarly, the introduction of chemical hypophysectomy by Moricca in 1963 (29) offered another nonoperative route for pituitary destruction. These types of surgery and their variations became a practical option for relieving pain, not only for patients too debilitated by advanced cancer to undergo craniotomy, but also for those who previously were considered candidates for craniotomy.

In this chapter we will summarize: (a) the published results of surgical and chemical hypophysectomy; (b) the technique of stereotactic chemical hypophysectomy; and (c) the various suggested mechanisms of cancer pain relief with these procedures.

PAIN RELIEF FOLLOWING SURGICAL HYPOPHYSECTOMY

Over the past 14 years, six studies have been published describing the results of stereotaxic cryohypophysectomy (46), transcranial hypophysectomy (40), or open microsurgical hypophysectomy (7,38,41,42) specifically performed for the pain relief in patients with metastatic breast or prostate carcinoma. In four additional studies (14,24,37,48), pain relief was not the primary goal of hypophysectomy, but this therapeutic effect was discussed in some detail. In these combined studies, there was a total of 334 patients. Of these, 43% had metastatic breast carcinoma; the other patients had metastatic prostate carcinoma. In these studies, significant pain relief ranged from 60 to 90%; across the studies, 70% of the patients experienced significant pain relief. In 50% of the patients reporting pain relief, objective tumor regression also occurred.

In prostate cancer there was no definite correlation between the clinical results of castration or exogenous endocrine manipulation and pain relief after hypophysectomy (24,37,38,42). An exception to this view has been presented by Thompson et al. (40). Opinion varied as to whether tumor regression after hypophysectomy favored longer pain relief and survival than that found in patients demonstrating pain relief alone. Postoperative pain relief in prostate cancer averaged 7 months, whereas survival in these same patients averaged 11 months. Failure of the tumor to regress, unrelieved pain, or both reduced survival to less than 4 months.

Comparable information on breast cancer is not well documented. Reports on the use of transsphenoidal hypophysectomy for relief of pain in breast cancer have included few (7,41) or no details (14,48) on duration of relief or postoperative survival. This information may not be accurately derived from other reports in which hypophysectomy has been used for palliative treatment of metastatic breast cancer. In these latter reports, although pain relief was a frequent and welcome benefit, patients were not selected primarily due to intractable pain. In patients undergoing transsphenoidal hypophysectomy specifically for intractable pain, disease is far advanced and postoperative survival short. In published data on survival in the patient population obtaining pain relief, postoperative survival was only about 6 months (7,41). No data are available on duration of pain relief. Failure to develop tumor regression and/or pain relief diminished survival to less than 4 months.

In breast cancer, opinion varied as to whether a previous clinical response to castration or exogenous endocrine manipulation favored objective tumor remission after hypophysectomy (2,3,14,18,33). No direct information is available as to whether a response to endocrine manipulation in the patient with intractable pain favors the development of pain relief. However, since pain relief usually accompanies objective remission, a good response to endocrine manipulation in breast cancer would favor the development of pain relief following hypophysectomy. Pain relief can still result in cases without a positive clinical response to endocrine manipulation.

The effect of hypophysectomy on cancer pain seems mysterious for two reasons: pain relief usually occurs within hours of the operation, preceding objective remission, and, in previous studies, half of the patients who obtain pain relief ultimately show no obvious tumor regression. The absence of objective tumor regression does not exclude the possibility that pain may be relieved by very slight degrees of regression, undetectable by radiographs. The apparent dissociation between pain relief and objective tumor regression suggests hormonal sensitivity of the tumor may not be an adequate predictor of the pain relieving potential. This is supported by the finding that pain relief may develop in cases of hormone-independent breast and prostate cancer. Although tumor regression may prolong pain relief, the two processes of regression and pain relief may be independent. This raises the issue of whether hypophysectomy may relieve pain caused by other cancers. There are a few reports in the literature of the occasional use of surgical hypophysectomy in cases of malignant melanoma, hypernephroma, reticulum cell sarcoma, and cancer of the pancreas (19), but these have examined tumor regression rather than pain relief.

PAIN RELIEF FOLLOWING CHEMICAL TRANSSPHENOIDAL HYPOPHYSECTOMY

Chemical hypophysectomy has been used for pain relief in metastatic tumors of many types, including hormone-independent tumors (21,23,25, 26,29,47). In this technique, a hypophyseal lesion is produced by injecting alcohol into the sella turcica by a transsphenoid route. The volume injected varies among clinicians, ranging from 1 to 5 ml. Up to a point, the volume of injected alcohol must correlate with the degree of hypophyseal damage. There is, however, inadequate endocrinologic and anatomic (postmortem) data correlated with pain relief to serve as a guide in determining how much to inject. Clinicians who have used volumes of 1 to 2 ml (23,25,26,29) have sometimes found it necessary to repeat alcohol injections because inadequate relief has been achieved by the first procedure.

By 1978, Miles (26) and his colleagues had performed chemical hypophysectomy on 122 patients with all forms of cancer, of which 56% were of either the breast or the prostate. Of these, 42% obtained excellent pain relief and an additional 33% (a total of 75%) acquired sufficient relief to discontinue narcotic analgesics. To achieve these results, 30% of patients required a second injection, and 9% a third injection. The mean duration of pain relief was between 2 and 3 months. Duration of pain relief did not significantly correlate with the type of cancer. The period of survival was not reported.

Madrid (25) had treated 329 patients with this technique by January 1978. Patients with metastatic breast and prostate carcinoma constituted 80% of his cases. Of the total number of patients, 67% had complete relief and an additional 27% had partial relief. To achieve these results, 25% of patients required a second injection and 3% required a third injection. No data were given correlating relief to tumor type and no information was available on either duration of relief or postoperative survival. Moricca's (29) rate of success appears to be good, but details correlating tumor-type to pain relief, the role of multiple injections, and duration of relief are not available.

Stereotactic Chemical Hypophysectomy

Levin et al. (15,21) introduced the stereotactic approach to chemical hypophysectomy because of a desire to improve the technique in two specific

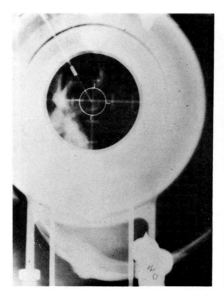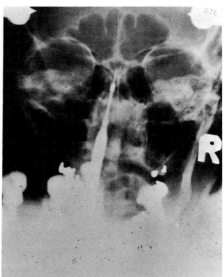

FIG. 3. Right: anterior-posterior view of needle at target. **Left:** lateral view of needle at target.

The AP radiographs and lateral fluoroscopy of the route of the 18-gauge needle should show that it has reached the floor of the sella turcica without deviation from its intended path. Upon entry of the 20-gauge needle into the sella turcica, AP radiographs should confirm the needle has not deviated from its path toward the midline target. Once this is confirmed, further advancement of the needle under lateral fluoroscopy will verify its approach to the target. When the needle has reached the target, confirming AP and lateral radiographs are made (Fig. 3). In only rare cases has it been difficult for the 18- and 20-gauge needles to penetrate the appropriate bony pathway. In such cases, a small hole was drilled using a Kirschner wire. The diameter of the Kirschner wire is just slightly larger than that of the spinal needle.

Once the position of the needle at the target is confirmed, the stylet is withdrawn and up to 2 ml of absolute alcohol is deposited. Injection under fluoroscopic monitoring allows one to see the small air bubbles that were trapped in the needle enter the sella turcica. The patient's pupils are checked after injection. Although it is believed that the alcohol stays within the sella turcica, rapid enlargement of the pituitary gland from the quantity of fluid injected can cause the pituitary to swell laterally and compress the nerves to the extraocular muscles lying within the cavernous sinus. It is also possible to get upward extension of the swelling and compress the optic chiasm. If there have been no pupillary changes or deviation of the eyes from the midline, the needle is withdrawn to a point approximately halfway between the initial target and the floor of the sella turcica and a second injection of 1 to 2 ml of absolute alcohol is injected. Again, the pupils are checked.

Providing there are no changes, the needle is again withdrawn to a point halfway between the second injection and the floor of the sella turcica, and a third dose of 1 to 2 ml of absolute alcohol is injected. The needle is then withdrawn to just above the floor of the sella turcica and approximately $\frac{1}{2}$ ml of alpha-ethyl cyanoacrylate (slow polymerizing) is injected as the needle is being withdrawn through the floor of the sella turcica. This seals the single hole in the floor of the sella turcica. After the needle is withdrawn, the needle guide is then removed from the nostril. If there is evidence of bleeding from the nasal passage, it is packed with gauze impregnated with petroleum jelly. If there is no significant bleeding, no packing is used. The patient is awakened, extubated, and watched carefully for the next 24 to 48 hr for the onset of diabetes insipidus. Patients are routinely placed on hydrocortisone supplement. With diabetes insipidus that cannot be controlled by oral intake, DDAVP (1-desaminocysteine-8-D-arginine vasopressin) is used. Thyroid supplement is also started several days into the postoperative period.

Results

Only one CSF leak in 85 patients undergoing this procedure has been found. In this patient, who was early in the series, the tumor had metastasized and invaded the floor of the sella. The CSF leak was sealed by injection of alpha-ethyl cyanoacrylate into the sella turcica. Since then, with routine use of alpha-ethyl cyanoacrylate, there have been no CSF leaks. Other complications include five ocular nerve palsies, of which three cleared completely. Four patients had bilateral or unilateral temporal field loss with associated ocular nerve palsies. One of these cleared completely, and two cleared partially. It is interesting to note that all of the complications occurred in the first 40 patients. There have been no complications since, and no procedure-related deaths have occurred in the entire series.

To date, stereotactic chemical hypophysectomy has been performed on 82 cancer patients. Breast and prostate cancer comprise 63% of the cases, whereas lung, kidney, and other tumors comprise the remainder. Preoperatively all patients were unable to achieve acceptable pain control despite large doses of parenteral narcotics. The results of chemical hypophysectomy are presented in Table 1. Good results were obtained in 84% of cases. This category represents patients reporting either satisfactory pain control with no analgesics or ability to achieve control with nonnarcotic analgesics or codeine. Six patients (four prostatic and two mixed) transiently obtained good pain relief (lasting at least one month) but later required cordotomy (five patients) or reinjection of alcohol (one patient) to achieve longer-lasting pain relief. These six patients are not included in the good result category. There was no significant difference ($p > 0.1$) in the response rate between the prostatic, breast, or mixed series.

For most patients who could be followed carefully, duration of relief was limited by death due to underlying neoplastic disease rather than recurrence

TABLE 1. *Pain relief following chemical hypophysectomy in 82 patients*

	Total no. of patients	Pain relief	Percent
Prostatic series			
Good	42	35	83
Transient exacerbation	35	10	29
Breast series			
Good	21	20	95
Transient exacerbation	20	3	15
Lung, kidney, and others			
Good	19	14	74
Transient exacerbation	14	3	21
Overall			
Good	82	69	84
Transient exacerbation	69	16	23

of pain. The mean postoperative survival was 5 months. The postoperative level of pain relief varied from day to day. Often there were minor variations in the level of relief necessitating nonnarcotic analgesics or codeine some days, and no drugs on other days. In 23% of the patients, occasional transient exacerbations of a more substantial nature typically lasted 1 to 5 days before spontaneously remitting. In one-third of the patients, the exacerbations were multiple, occurring about once a month. The cause of these transient exacerbations is unknown, but may be due to development of new metastasis or enlargement of already present metastasis.

Summary

In summary, chemical hypophysectomy has produced relief from pain caused by both hormone-dependent and hormone-independent tumor. The number of useful published studies is too limited to permit rigid conclusions. Few reports have provided a definition of pain relief. There has been rare use of independent observers (21). Although no systematic attempt has been made to provide detailed information on the type of pain that may be relieved by hypophysectomy, it is the impression of some investigators (21) that the pain most susceptible to relief comes from bone metastases. In chemical hypophysectomy, the initial success rate appears slightly better than that of surgical hypophysectomy for breast and prostate cancer. However, both duration of relief and survival appear to be shorter following chemical hypophysectomy. This may be a reflection of inadequate numbers of patients observed in clinical reports, or a reflection of far advanced disease present at the time of neurosurgical referral.

MECHANISM OF ACTION

The mechanism of relief in chemical hypophysectomy seems as mysterious as that following transsphenoidal hypophysectomy. Advocates of chemical hypophysectomy have proposed that the effect is due to concomitant hypothalamic injury (21,26,29) and suggested this operation may be qualitatively different from transsphenoidal hypophysectomy.

Pituitary Ablation

The mechanism by which pain is relieved in either chemical or surgical hypophysectomy is unknown. Unlike either cingulotomy or subcaudate frontal leucotomy, hypophysectomy does not produce relief by primarily allaying psychological suffering, nor does it alter normal sensitivity to pinprick or the appreciation of pain from acute injury (29,39). This goes against the theory that pain relief may be related to changes in peripheral pain receptor sensitivity (26). Additional evidence against this theory is found in a recent report on the successful use of chemical hypophysectomy in three patients with thalamic pain (22).

Humoral or neural modulation of central pain-inhibiting neurons would be a more plausible mechanism of action. According to that hypothesis, pain relief may result from excitation of central pain suppressor mechanisms either by means of a humoral agent distributed by the CSF (26,42) or by a direct neural stimulus. Hypophysectomy, it is reasoned, either eliminates a hormone responsible for pain augmentation produced by the pituitary, or induces (possibly by elimination of feedback suppression) a neural or humoral response originating from the hypothalamus that is responsible for pain suppression.

Oophorectomy (17), adrenalectomy (13), and orchiectomy (43) have long been known to produce relief of pain (usually within hours) in some patients suffering from metastatic breast or prostate carcinoma. The onset of this relief precedes objective remission by a considerable length of time: It may occur despite failure of objective remission, and appears similar in its time of onset to that following hypophysectomy. These observations imply there is a mechanism of pain relief common to all four operations distinct from pain relief attendant to tumor regression. Such a mechanism might be a hypothalamic pain-suppressing response activated by the elimination of hormonal feedback.

The foregoing raises the possibility that pain relief after hypophysectomy may be the result of stimulation of hypothalamic function rather than the elimination of pituitary function. There is additional support for this view. Several lines of evidence cast doubt on the notion that pain relief from hypophysectomy is directly related to the expected fall in levels of *known* pituitary hormones. First, pain relief occurs in cases of malignancies not known to be hormone dependent (21,25,38,41) and also in patients with breast and prostate carcinoma unresponsive to hormone manipulation (14,24,38,41). Second, although there exists a minimal level of hypophyseal damage sufficient to produce pain relief (46), beyond this point pain relief does not appear to be correlated with the completeness of ablation of known pituitary endocrine function (20,21,23,24,46,47). Third, patients may obtain relief despite failure to obtain an objective remission (7,14,24,38,41). Fourth, pain relief may occur promptly following oophorectomy (17), orchiectomy (43), or adrenalectomy (13) by increasing the level of the appropriate pituitary trophic hormones. Fifth, pain relief occurs after stalk section (20), a procedure that normally elevates prolactin blood levels (44). Sixth, pain relief occurs with administration of L-DOPA (27), a procedure that normally stimulates human growth hormone secretion (5).

Effects on Hypothalmus

The idea that pain relief after hypophysectomy may be unrelated to the hypophysectomy led some investigators to look for concomitant damage in other neural structures. Lipton et al. (23) provided evidence that alcohol injected into the sella extends up the pituitary stalk into the hypothalamus and third ventricle where damage has been found on postmortem examination. Levin (21) performed postmortem examinations in four cases of alcohol hypophysectomy for cancer pain. These revealed subependymal gliosis along the floor of the third ventricle, considerable cell loss in the supraoptic and paraventricular nuclei, and damage to the median eminence. The importance of the posteromedial hypothalamus in pain control was emphasized by Sano (35) and Fairman (6), who demonstrated that lesions in the posterior inferior peri-third ventricular area produced good relief in over 70% of patients whose pain was due to malignant tumor.

Despite the apparent success of posteromedial hypothalamic lesions in producing relief from pain of malignancy, open transsphenoidal microsurgical hypophysectomy for metastatic prostate and breast cancer to provide good pain relief has also been reported in 70 to 90% of patients (7,14,38,41,42). In this procedure, the likelihood of direct hypothalamic injury would be small. Daniel and Prichard (4) examined the hypothalamus and pituitary stalk of 59 patients who had undergone one of three pituitary ablative procedures—transfrontal pituitary stalk section, transfrontal hypophysectomy, or transsphenoidal hypophysectomy—and reported significant cell loss in both the supraoptic (SON) and paraventricular (PVN) nuclei due to retrograde degeneration. Other nuclei of the hypothalamus, however, did not show any obvious postoperative abnormalities. Regardless of which operative procedure was used, the only hypothalamic abnormalities observed lay anteriorly.

The relationship of anterior hypothalamic dysfunction to pain relief has not received extensive comment in the literature but may be inferred in part from studies examining the relationship between diabetes insipidus and pain relief. Lipton et al. (23) found no correlation between diabetes insipidus and pain relief. Levin et al. (22) performed chemical hypophysectomy in three patients with thalamic pain, achieving good relief in all three. The patients in this study recovered from diabetes insipidus within 1 year (two patients recovered within 6 months). Despite this, pain relief persisted. The failure of pain relief to correlate with this aspect of anterior hypothalamic dysfunction is in contrast to earlier speculation (21) of such correlation in a study of 29 patients with cancer pain. The life expectancy of the patient population in the earlier study was apparently too short to permit observations on pain relief persisting after recovery from diabetes insipidus.

It appears that overt hypothalamic damage, apart from retrograde cell loss in PVN and SON, may not be required in order to obtain prompt pain relief. Hypophysectomy, even when anatomically (30) and endocrinologically (20,21,23,24,46,47) incomplete, appears sufficient. This raises the question of whether chemical hypophysectomy is a unique neuroablative technique, or if it is simply another form of hypophysectomy, as they all act by a similar mechanism. The success of stereotactic chemical hypophysectomy on hormone-independent tumors may encourage the use of stereotactic thermal and cryohypophysectomy, as well as open transsphenoidal hypophysectomy on similar tumors. The results of such trials could settle the question.

Endogenous Opiate Involvement

Naloxone, a specific antagonist for morphine and its analogues, was administered to patients whose pain was relieved by hypophysectomy in an attempt to restore the pain. The object was to determine if hypophysectomy, like stimulation-induced analgesia (1,10), produces pain relief by augmenting endogenous opiate release. Thus far, the evidence does not favor an opioid-mediated mechanism, but this evidence is preliminary. Naloxone failed to reverse the pain relief achieved by chemical hypophysectomy in 29 cancer patients and 3 patients with thalamic pain in studies by Levin et al. (21,22). Miles (26) reported that of 12 patients who underwent chemical hypophysectomy for cancer, 8 failed to experience pain restoration following naloxone, whereas 4 did. Misfeldt and Goldstein (28) administered naloxone to a patient following transsphenoidal hypophysectomy for metastatic prostate and renal carcinoma. Naloxone did not cause the pain to return. An extensive trial of naloxone testing after surgical hypophysectomy has not been published. One difficulty with interpreting naloxone studies is that there are several different classes of opiate receptors, each with a varying affinity for naloxone (9). Naloxone insensitivity could be a reflection of limited affinity rather than an argument for a non-opioid mechanism. Failure to demonstrate pain restoration with naloxone may not exclude an opiate-mediated effect.

There is, however, additional evidence that opioid mechanisms may not serve an important role in this form of pain inhibition. This comes from studies in humans and rats. Miles (26) assayed metenkephalin and beta-endorphin in human lumbar CSF before, immediately after, and 5 hr after chemical hypophysectomy and failed to show elevation of either endogenous opiate. Hypophysectomy in rats diminishes plasma levels of beta-endorphin (8,11), and may either have no demonstrable effect on brain tissue beta-endorphin levels (11,34) or may actually decrease the beta-endorphin content of mediobasal hypothalamus (45) and periventricular tissue (32).

Stress-Induced Analgesia and Hypophysectomy Analgesia

The arguments presented here are consistent with a mechanism of pain relief in which hypophysectomy induces a pain-suppressing response mediated by the hypothalamus. This response may bear a relationship to stress-induced analgesia. In this phenomenon, an animal exposed to a novel stressor may demonstrate what appears to be an insensitivity to noxious stimuli that outlasts exposure to the stress (16). Not all stressors induce analgesia and not all noxious stimuli are equally affected by stress-induced analgesia. An animal may display pain sensitivity under certain circumstances and pain insensitivity under others. Being capable of two fundamentally different pain responses could be of profound evolutionary adaptive value. Normal pain sensitivity, for example, would be valuable in avoiding minor environmental dangers. In contrast, pain insensitivity activated by the stress of life-threatening predation would allow the animal to channel all energy into fight or flight. The existence of stress-induced pain insensitivity in humans has been inferred from observations on soldiers and athletes who sometimes report no pain despite having sustained demonstrably painful injuries. Stress evokes a characteristic integrated defense response of autonomic and neuroendocrine function orchestrated by the hypothalamus. It should not be surprising that analgesia may be a part of this repertoire of defense mechanisms. Stress-induced analgesia and posthypophysectomy analgesia may both arise from similar pain-suppressing hypothalamic mechanisms.

CONCLUSION

Surgical and chemical hypophysectomy are fundamentally similar procedures that relieve pain equally often. When allowance is made for the stage of disease at the time of neurosurgical referral, the duration of pain relief and survival are probably comparable. Although the mechanism by which pain relief is achieved is unknown, it is probably not directly related to the expected fall in levels of known pituitary hormones. Instead, pain relief may be the direct result of a hypothalamic pain-suppressing capability triggered by hypophysectomy. It is unclear if this capability is related to augmentation of endogenous opiates.

REFERENCES

1. Akil, H., Richardson, D. E., Hughes, J., and Barchas, J. D. (1978): Enkephalin-like material elevated in ventricular cerebrospinal fluid of pain patients after analgesic focal stimulation. *Science*, 201:463–465.
2. Atkins, H. J. B. (1963): Hypophysectomy for advanced cancer of the breast. *Proc. R. Soc. Med.*, 56:389–390.
3. Conway, L. W., and Collins, W. F. (1969): Results of transphenoidal cryohypophysectomy for carcinoma of the breast. *N. Engl. J. Med.*, 281:1–7.
4. Daniel, P. M., and Prichard, M. M. L. (1972): The human hypothalamus and pituitary stalk after hypophysectomy or pituitary stalk section. *Brain*, 95:813–814.
5. Eddy, R. L., Gilliland, P. F., and Ibana, J. D., Jr. (1974): Human growth hormone release. Comparison of provocative test procedures. *Am. J. Med.*, 56:179–185.
6. Fairman, D. (1972): Hypothalamotomy as a new perspective for alleviation of intractable pain and regression of metastatic tumors. In: *Present Limits of Neurosurgery*, edited by I. Fusek and Z. Kunc, pp. 525–528. Avicenum, Prague.
7. Gross, C., Frerbeau, P., Privat, J. M., and Benezeca, J. (1975): Place of hypophysectomy in the neurosurgical treatment of pain. In: *Advances in Neurosurgery, Vol. 3*, edited by H. Penzholz, M. Brock, J. Hamer, M. Klinger, and D. Spoerri, pp. 264–272. Springer-Verlag, Heidelberg.
8. Guillemin, R., Vargo, T., Rossier, J., Minick, S., Ling, N., Rivier, C., Vale, W., and Bloom, R. (1977): Beta-endorphin and adrenocorticotropin are secreted concomitantly by the pituitary gland. *Science*, 197:1367–1369.
9. Hill, R. G. (1981): The status of naloxone in the identification of pain control mechanisms operated by endogenous opioids. *Neurosci. Lett.*, 21:217–222.
10. Hosobuchi, Y., Adams, J. E., and Linchitz, R. (1977): Pain relief by stimulation of the central grey matter in humans and its reversal by naloxone. *Science*, 197:183–186.
11. Houghten, R. A., Swann, R. W., and Li, C. H. (1980): Beta-endorphin: Stability, clearance behavior, and entry into the central nervous system after intravenous injection of the tritiated peptide in rats and rabbits. *Proc. Natl. Acad. Sci. USA*, 77:4588–4591.
12. Huggins, C. (1966): Endocrine induced regression of cancers: Nobel prize lecture 1966. *Cancer Res.*, 27:1925–1930.
13. Huggins, C., and Bergenstal, D. M. (1952): Inhibition of human mammary and prostatic cancers by adrenalectomy. *Cancer Res.*, 12:134–141.
14. Kapur, T. R., and Dalton, G. A. (1969): Transphenoidal hypophysectomy for metastatic carcinoma of the breast. *Br. J. Surg.*, 56:332–337.
15. Katz, J., and Levin, A. B. (1977): Treatment of diffuse metastatic cancer pain by instillation of alcohol into the sella turcica. *Anesthesiology*, 46:115–121.
16. Kelly, D. D. (1982): The role of endorphins in stress-induced analgesia. *Ann. NY Acad. Sci.*, 398:260–271.
17. Kennedy, B. J. (1960): Hormonal therapy of mammary carcinoma. In: *The Treatment of Cancer and Allied Diseases, Vol. 4, The Breast, Chest and Esophagus*, edited by G. T. Pack and I. M. Ariel. Harper, New York.
18. Kennedy, B. J., and French, L. (1965): Hypophysectomy in advanced breast cancer. *Am. J. Surg.*, 110:411–415.
19. Kennedy, B. J., French, L. A., and Peyton, W. T. (1956): Hypophysectomy in advanced breast cancer. *N. Engl. J. Med.*, 255:1165–1172.
20. LaRossa, J. T., Strong, M. S., and Melby, J. C. (1978): Endocrinologically incomplete transethmoidal, transphenoidal hypophysectomy with relief of bone pain in breast cancer. *N. Engl. J. Med.*, 298:1332–1335.
21. Levin, A. B., Katz, J., Benson, R. C., and Jones, A. G. (1980): Treatment of pain of diffuse metastatic cancer by stereotactic chemical hypophysectomy: Long term results and observations on mechanism of action. *Neurosurgery*, 6:258–262.
22. Levin, A. B., Ramirez, L. F., and Katz, J. (1983): The use of stereotaxic chemical hypophysectomy in the treatment of thalamic pain syndrome. *J. Neurosurg.*, 59:1003–1006.

23. Lipton, S., Miles, J., Williams, N., and Bark-Jones, N. (1978): Pituitary injection of alcohol for widespread cancer pain. *Pain*, 5:73–82.
24. Maddy, J. A., Winternitz, W. W., and Norrell, H. (1971): Cryohypophysectomy in the management of advanced prostatic cancer. *Cancer*, 28:322–328.
25. Madrid, J. L. (1979): Chemical hypophysectomy. In: *Advances in Pain Research and Therapy, Vol. 2*, edited by J. J. Bonica and V. Ventafridda, pp. 373–380. Raven Press, New York.
26. Miles, J. (1979): In: *Advances in Pain Research and Therapy, Vol. 2*, edited by J. J. Bonica and V. Ventafridda, pp. 373–380. Raven Press, New York.
27. Minton, J. P., Bronn, D. G., and Kibbey, W. E. (1976): L-dopa effect in painful bony metastases. *N. Engl. J. Med.*, 294:340.
28. Misfeldt, D. S., and Goldstein, A. (1977): Hypophysectomy relieves pain not via endorphins. *N. Engl. J. Med.*, 297:1236–1237.
29. Moricca, G. (1976): Neuroadenolysis for diffuse unbearable cancer pain. In: *Advances in Pain Research and Therapy, Vol. 1*, edited by J. J. Bonica and D. Albe-Fessard, pp. 863–866. Raven Press, New York.
30. Norrell, H., Albes, A. M., and Winternitz, W. W. (1970): A clinicopathologic analysis of cryohypophysectomy in patients with advanced cancer. *Cancer*, 25:1050–1060.
31. Perrault, M., LeBeau, J., and Klotz, B. (1952): L'hypophysectomie totale dan le traitment du cancer sein: Premier cas francais: avenir de la method. *Therapie*, 7:290–300.
32. Przewlocki, R., Millan, M. J., Gramsch, C. H., Millan, M. H., and Herz, A. (1982): The influence of selective adeno- and neurointermedio hypophysectomy upon plasma and brain levels of beta-endorphin and the response to stress in rats. *Brain Res.*, 242:107–117.
33. Ray, B. S., and Pearson, O. H. (1962): Hypophysectomy in the treatment of disseminated breast cancer. *Surg. Clin. North Am.*, 42:419–433.
34. Rossier, J., Vargo, T. M., Minnick, S., Ling, N., Bloom, F. E., and Guillemin, R. (1977): Regional dissociation of beta-endorphin and enkephalin content in rat brain and pituitary. *Proc. Natl. Acad. Sci. USA*, 74:5162–5165.
35. Sano, K. (1977): Intralaminar thalamotomy and posteromedial hypothalamotomy in the treatment of intractable pain. *Prog. Neurol. Surg.*, 8:50–103.
36. Scott, W. W. (1952): Endocrine management of disseminated prostate cancer, including bilateral adrenalectomy and hypophysectomy. *Trans. Am. Assoc. Genitourin. Surg.*, 44:101–104.
37. Scott, W. W., and Schirmer, H. K. A. (1962): Hypophysectomy for disseminated prostatic cancer. In: *On Cancer and Hormones*, pp. 175–204. University of Chicago Press, Chicago.
38. Silverberg, G. D. (1977): Hypophysectomy in the treatment of disseminated prostate carcinoma. *Cancer*, 39:1727–1731.
39. Sweet, W. H. (1980): Central mechanisms of chronic pain. In: *Pain*, edited by J. J. Bonica, pp. 287–303. Raven Press, New York.
40. Thompson, J. B., Greenberg, E., Pazianos, A., and Pearson, O. H. (1974): Hypophysectomy in metastatic prostate cancer. *NY State J. Med.*, 74:1006–1008.
41. Tindall, G. T., Ambrose, S. S., Christy, J. H., and Patton, J. M. (1976): Hypophysectomy in the treatment of disseminated carcinoma of the breast and prostate gland. *South. Med. J.*, 69:579–583.
42. Tindall, G. T., Payne, N. S., and Nixon, D. W. (1979): Transsphenoidal hypophysectomy for disseminated carcinoma of the prostate gland. *J. Neurosurg.*, 50:275–282.
43. Trunnell, J. B. (1962): The role of hormonal therapy in neoplasms of the prostate. In: *Treatment of Cancer and Allied Diseases, Vol. 7: The Male Genitalia and the Urinary System*, edited by G. T. Pack and I. M. Ariel, pp. 104–137. Harper, New York.
44. Turkington, R. W., Underwood, L. E., and Van Wyk, J. J. (1971): Elevated serum prolactin levels after pituitary stalk section in man. *N. Engl. J. Med.*, 285:707–710.
45. Vermes, I., Mulder, G. H., Berkenbosch, F. J. H., and Tilders, F. J. H. (1981): Release of beta-lipotropin and beta-endorphin from rat hypothalami in vitro. *Brain Res.*, 211:248–254.
46. West, C. R., Avellanosa, A. M., Bremer, A. M., and Yomada, K. (1979): Hypophysectomy for relief of pain of disseminated carcinoma of the prostate. In: *Advances in Pain Research and Therapy, Vol. 2*, edited by J. J. Bonica and V. Ventafridda, pp. 393–400. Raven Press, New York.

47. Williams, N. E., Miles, J. B., Lipton, S., Hipkin, L. J., and Davis, J. C. (1980): Pain relief and pituitary function following injection of alcohol into the pituitary fossa. *Ann. R. Coll. Surg. Engl.*, 62:203–207.
48. Zervas, N. T. (1969): Stereotaxic radiofrequency surgery of the normal and the abnormal pituitary gland. *N. Engl. J. Med.*, 280:429–437.

Advances in Pain Research
and Therapy, Vol. 7,
edited by C. Benedetti et al.
Raven Press, New York © 1984.

Neuroadenolysis of the Pituitary of Moricca: An Overview of Development, Mechanisms, Technique, and Results

Giancarlo Gianasi

Service of Anesthesia and Intensive Therapy, Section of Analgesia, Bellaria Hospital, Bologna, Italy

For three decades, Bonica (3–6,9) has repeatedly called attention to the treatment of cancer pain as being one of the most important, albeit one of the most difficult, problems encountered in clinical practice. This is especially true in patients with advanced cancer who have widespread metastasis causing pain in multiple sites that is diffuse, not clearly localized, and that eventually progresses to become the main symptom of the disease. The difficulty in managing such widespread diffuse pain is not only due to the variety of the quality and sites of the pain but also to the progressive nature of the disease.

C. Benedetti and J. J. Bonica (*this volume*) state one of the important and basic principles in the management of patients with cancer-related pain: the therapist must have thorough knowledge of all therapeutic modalities. It is essential to know not only the analgesic efficacy and advantages but also the limitations, disadvantages, side effects, and complications of each procedure. Only with such knowledge integrated with information obtained from the history and physical examinations is it possible to determine the best method(s) to relieve cancer pain. In these patients, perhaps more than others, it is essential to assure a quality of life that, in turn, is determined by the degree of pain relief and, at the same time, conserves the patient's individuality and mental capabilities—conditions that may not be possible with the use of sedatives and narcotics given in sufficient quantity to provide effective relief.

Among the various therapeutic modalities that should be available, neuroadenolysis of the pituitary (NALP) has an important place in the armamentarium of the oncologic algologist. Unfortunately, in the past there have been misconceptions about the technical aspect of the procedure and, particularly, the results pertaining to its analgesic efficacy, side effects, and complications. Indeed, some authorities who did not have ample experience with the technique wrote erroneous and misleading assessments of the procedure. Consequently, NALP has been the subject of national and international debates, and has not received the widespread use it deserves. In view of these and other factors, it seems useful in this chapter to (a) briefly describe the chronology of the development of the technique, focusing on the work of Prof. G. Moricca; (b) describe Moricca's technique in detail, including selection of patients, preparation for the procedure, equipment to be used, and other specific technical details; (c) summarize the results obtained by Moricca and others with regard to its analgesic efficacy, side effects, and complications; and (d) briefly discuss the hypothesis for the rapid, intense, and widespread pain relief achieved with the procedure.

HISTORICAL PERSPECTIVE

The history of the destruction of the pituitary for pain relief began with the early work of Huggins (32) who showed that hormonal manipulation through gonadectomy and/or adrenalectomy to produce regression of cancer of the breast and prostate was often followed by relief of pain. In 1952, several groups including Le Beau et al. (36,83), Luft et al. (45,46), Shimkin et al. (90), and Scott (89) published reports on the use of transcranial hypophysectomy for the treatment of breast and/or prostate cancer. This procedure represents the practical application of the then well-known fact that the hypothalamic-pituitary axis constitutes the integrating and coordinating center for the entire endocrine system. Although these early workers carried out surgical hypophysectomy primarily to produce objective regression of metastatic breast/prostatic carcinoma, they noted that reduction or elimination of pain was a more consistent effect than tumor regression.

These early reports apparently did not arouse as much interest as might be expected, in part, because such major surgical operations in patients with advanced metastatic cancer had certain limitations. Among the most important of these is that such major surgical procedures cannot be performed on very poor risk patients for whom any major operation may be contraindicated. Cancer patients with visceral metastases, especially to the brain, were generally regarded by neurosurgeons as unsuitable candidates for the operation. Consequently, less stressful methods of pituitary inactivation were devised. In 1955, Forrest and Brown (24) published a report on their experience with insertion of radon into the pituitary via a rhinotransphenoidal approach. Later, Lewis and Baxton (40) studied the results of treating hormone-dependent tumors by insertion of radioisotopes or ligature of the peduncle of the pituitary or injection of alcohol into the gland.

During this time Moricca, working at the National Cancer Institute Regina Elena in Rome, was evaluating surgical adrenalectomy, oophorectomy, and hypophysectomy for the therapy of advanced breast cancer with diffuse metastasis. He soon realized that the surgical procedures, especially hypophysectomy, presented serious problems in patients in poor physical condition. Because of his extensive experience with neurolytic blocks (52), achieved by "blindly" injecting alcohol through a percutaneously placed needle, he began to consider the injection of alcohol into the pituitary through a needle passed into the gland via the rhinoethmoidosphenoid route. Before using the technique in patients, he carried out studies on cadavers to determine the best approach for insertion of the needle via this route. He inserted 2 needles, 1 in each nostril, and with the aid of successive radiographs as guides in directing the needles into the sella turcica, he was able to devise a technique to accurately place the needle into the pituitary gland.

In 1958, as part of his anatomic studies, he injected from 2 to 3 ml of alcohol tinted with methylene blue and noted the solution diffused not only along the peduncle of the gland but also to suprasellar spaces. Subsequent examination of the anatomic specimens confirmed the needles had penetrated the sella turcica through the transethmoidosphenoidal route. That same year he performed the procedure in 7 patients with encouraging results. At the same time Greco et al. (29), independent of Moricca but following the suggestions of Lewis and Baxton, injected alcohol into the pituitary gland of 5 patients with cancer. From the report of Greco et al. (29), one is unable to ascertain follow-up results, but the technique was very different from the one described by Moricca (55–57,87,88). In the last paper published in 1965 (28), Greco reported on 150 patients and then apparently discontinued use of the procedure, presumably as it appeared to be ineffective.

Moricca continued to use and improve the technique; in 1963, he first reported on its application in 37 patients (13). Five years later he described the technique in more detail (53) and emphasized that the procedure was highly effective in promptly eliminating the pain of hormone-dependent tumors, such as those of breast, prostate, thyroid, and uterus, that had progressed to an advanced phase of visceral and bony metastases. In many of these patients, the severe intractable pain could only be partially and/or transiently relieved by more aggressive, neurosurgical ablative procedures and could not be controlled by large doses of morphine or other potent narcotics.

During the early years, the technique consisted of injecting from 1.6 to 2 ml of alcohol at the initial treatment, followed a week later by a second injection of 0.8 to 1 ml of the neurolytic agent. A third injection was carried out 2 months later. At the time, he used the technique only for hormone-dependent tumor and noted the procedure had therapeutic benefits other than pain relief. It was not until 1974 that Moricca (58) published his experiences with the procedure in the treatment of cancer pain caused by advanced nonhormonal-dependent tumors.

The use of the procedure initiated an intense controversy and long debate, especially in Italy. Oncologists and neurosurgeons preferred to use other methods to remove or inactivate the pituitary gland. The advent of stereotactic surgery and microsurgery caused some clinicians to replace the classical hypophysectomy via craniotomy with the use of the rhinotransphenoidal route. Others technicians have included stereotactic cryohypophysectomy, open microsurgical hypophysectomy, thermal coagulation of the pituitary via the transphenoidal route—techniques which made pituitary ablation presumably safer than the classic surgical procedure (cf. A. Levin, *this volume*, for review). Others advocated pituitary inactivation through conventional roentgenotherapy, external irradiation with heavy particles (especially alpha rays and protons), and ultrasonic destruction of the pituitary. Still others used direct implantation of radioactive substances, such as seeds or pellets of ^{90}Y, ^{198}Au, and ^{32}P, into the sella turcica (25).

Moricca has always maintained (55,56) that these interventions compare unfavorably with neuroadenolysis since they have the same limitations as surgical hypophysectomy or require very sophisticated or very expensive material. Others entail long surgical procedures requiring deep and prolonged anesthesia that is dangerous to poor risk patients. In particular, Moricca has commented (53,60) on the limitation and disadvantages of radioisotopes (^{90}Y, ^{32}P, and ^{198}Au) inserted into the pituitary via a transphenoidal route because they involve several problems; the main difficulty lies in determining the proper dosimetry required to produce necrosis of the gland without damaging the surrounding tissue. This problem is closely linked with the question of positioning. Frequently, it is difficult to position such radioactive pellets in the desired site in the sella turcica; even if this succeeds, the pellets tend to shift after they have necrotized the immediately adjoining tissues. Implantation of additional pellets, besides being technically difficult because the sella is already occupied by the first pellets, might increase the incidence of complications. As a result, adequate inactivation of the pituitary is frequently not achieved. Histologic examination of the pituitary gland of patients treated with ^{90}Y implantation has clearly shown that the fibrotic area is limited to the tissues closely adjoining the ^{90}Y pellets.

A number of these problems are not inherent in Moricca's technique, and in the hands of a specialist who follows Moricca's technique correctly, the procedure provides a rapid, simple, and relatively inexpensive method of pain relief. The procedure does not require expensive equipment and can be practiced in any hospital where physicians with skill and expertise in the technique can carry it out, even in patients in serious physical condition. Above all, the procedure has the advantage that it can be repeated freely as the need arises, either for recurrence of the pain or manifestation of new signs of tumor growth (58,59,61,63), without impairing the patient's mental faculties as may occur with large doses of opioids and/or neuroleptic agents (65,67,74–78).

Some comments about terminology are in order. In 1981 Moricca (69,70) stated that diffusion of alcohol, which he first studied and noted in 1958, "left people rather perplexed on the true extension of the damage: therefore the first term 'chemical hypophysectomy' was adopted more for convenience, rather than to indicate the mechanism of action." The terms Moricca used subsequently, such as *pituitary alcoholinization* and *pituitary chemolysis*, before settling on the definitive term *neuroadenolysis of the pituitary* reflected the uncertainty of the mechanism of action, which even today is not completely understood. However, his immense experience and subsequent studies caused him to consider that the primary action of the alcohol is on the structures above the pituitary (55,57). Moreover, he insisted that no other technique of hypophysectomy, whether it be medical, surgical, or other, has the pain-relieving effect of NALP, even if surgical procedures may be slightly more effective in reducing the tumor progression (93,95). Following the earlier publication, Moricca continued to carry out the procedure in an increasing number of patients. In 1978, he reported on 2,202 patients who had received a total of 8,155 NALPs (64,67,68,70). The most recent papers (66,74,76,78) contain definitive refinements of the technique that make it safe when performed by a clinician who not only has acquired experience with the procedure but is able to prevent ocular complications, and if they do occur, the clinician is able to promptly and effectively treat them.

Finally, some comments about Moricca's attempts to try to understand the mechanism of action of NALP. It is obvious that in the 1960s, it was difficult to carry out studies entailing measurements of levels of hormones and biochemical agents. Consequently, it was necessary to rely on interpretation of results derived from anatomic and pathologic observations that involved, among other things, the injection of alcohol tinted with methylene blue. With foresight, he proceeded to introduce alcohol in quantities greater than the volume of the sella turcica, intuitively understanding that it is the diffusion of the alcohol into structures above the pituitary that is responsible for more complete pain relief and, therefore, control of the hormone-sensitive tumors (55). Earlier, he reasoned that injecting an incompressible liquid, such as alcohol, into an inextensible structure (the dura mater and bone of the sella turcica) in quantities larger than the capacity of the sella will result in escape of fluid from the sella through the only orifice available, the peduncle of the pituitary.

In considering the mechanism of action of neuroadenolysis in 1972 (55), Moricca stated the effects from this procedure were obtained from

> different mechanisms: compression produced by the injection, since the pituitary gland is contained in an almost enclosed space; subcapsular necrosis is thereby induced; direct chemical action represented by ethanol dehydration followed by tissue necrosis; action on blood vessel with thrombosis and subsequent cellular necrosis.

Moricca (55) also suggested that since the pituitary stalk represents an important pathway connecting the pituitary with the hypothalamus, the alcohol has "action on the hypothalamus." Alcohol marked with ^{14}C, injected into the sella of guinea pigs which had "dirtied" (diffused to) the entire area, was not a technical error but a typical effect of the NALP technique (76). Moricca's precocious conceptualization that the hypothalamus might be involved in the mechanism of action of the procedure has recently received support from studies by Deshpande et al. (18) who found that pituitary function in experimental animals, as judged by the plasma concentration of prolactin and thyroid-stimulating, follicle-stimulating, and luteinizing hormones, remains intact and the ability of the pituitary to respond to hypothalamic-releasing factors remains unimpaired. On the other hand, ACTH, beta-lipoprotein, and beta-endorphin concentrations are raised from the treatment. This led them to conclude that the procedure mainly effects the hypothalamus rather than the pituitary.

Finally, it must be emphasized that despite the disbelief and skepticism of some recognized authorities, Moricca has had the conviction, motivation, and interest to continue his steadfast, persistent, and intense efforts to spread the technique worldwide. The results have been a large number of international contributions (25,26,82,86,98) and the excellent results achieved in many centers of pain and cancer therapy (14–16,20,22,30,33,34,37,38,43,47–49,80,84,93).

CLINICAL APPLICATION

A comparison of this procedure to any other technique intended to "inactivate" the pituitary gland should no longer be considered, because, as mentioned above, inactivation of the pituitary is not the mechanism by which NALP produces pain relief. More appropriate and profitable would be a discussion of the role of NALP among the therapeutic modalities used in patients with advanced hormone-dependent cancers and among these, the suitable modalities to relieve patients with diffuse neoplastic pain, no longer controlled with other neurolytic or pharmacologic methods. The primary consideration is the indication for the procedure, i.e., the type of pain, type of cancer, and the optimal time for its application. A more diffuse and early application of the procedure consistently produces good pain relief, provided one avoids application of the procedure outside its field of action and protocol, and avoids techniques different from those advocated by Moricca, whose techniques remain the simplest and most effective, producing the best results.

Obviously, precise and rigid criteria for the selection of the best method(s) of pain control in cancer pain that apply to the entire general cancer population do not exist. For this reason, it is essential that the physician avoid generalization and select the method(s) that will assure the patient maximum, persistent pain relief, the method(s) that will exact the least physiologic and economic cost and minimal risk of severe morbidity or mortality. Equally important, it is essential that physicians accurately and honestly evaluate their own abilities with the various technical procedures.

In the selection of the method, the most important considerations are the following (67,70):

1. The intensity, quality, distribution, and duration of the pain assessed by objective as well as subjective means

2. The location or sites of the pain and the presumable cause(s)

3. The daily consumption of systemic analgesics and other pharmacologic agents for pain relief and treatment of the cancer

4. Physical, mental, and emotional condition of the patient and predicted life expectancy

5. Long-term pain-relieving effect as well as residual side effects and/or complications which provide the best benefit–cost ratio

6. Capability of the algologist to carry out the various therapeutic modalities for cancer pain.

Assuming the algologist is experienced and skilled with NALP, the procedure is an important and indispensable instrument to deal with bilateral diffuse pain, especially resulting from hormone-dependent tumors. Moricca's technique should be used when all antiblastic methods have been exhausted and diffuse pain persists or has recurred after other pain-relieving methods have been used. The general condition of the patient is not an absolute contraindication to NALP. Furthermore, it can always be repeated when the pain recurs or if there is no arrest in the progression of the tumor. Of course, ethical and humane limits to any technique are present in cancer patients in the terminal phase of the disease when there is loss of consciousness and death is likely in a few days (54,65,72,85). Yet, NALP can and should be used in monolateral pain, presumably hormone-dependent cancer, not only to provide pain relief but due to its possible neoplastic-arresting action. Finally, it can be used on cancer pain caused by visceral and/or peripheral neurogenic factors to reduce local compression/irritation of the neuroanatomic structures caused by the proximity of the tumor.

When, on consideration of the above factors, the algologist concludes that the patient may benefit from the procedure, then explicit informed consent must be obtained from the patient and/or family. Informed consent implies the patient and/or family has been thoroughly informed about the procedure and possible benefits, as well as side effects, possible complications of the technique, and, if necessary, of other applicable modalities. Once informed consent has been obtained, it is essential the algologist carry out a thorough preoperative evaluation and preparation of the patient, followed by consideration of the anesthetic techniques that will be used, the technical aspects of the procedure, the intraoperative side effects and complications, postoperative sequelae and postoperative evaluation of the patient, and the results obtained from the procedure.

Preoperative Evaluation and Preparation

The physiologic and psychologic evaluation of the patient with cancer-related pain, as well as assessment of the pain as summarized by C. Benedetti and J. J. Bonica (*this volume*), should be carried out prior to selection of the method of pain relief. In patients selected for NALP, it is especially

TABLE 1. *Equipment for neuroadenolysis (NALP)*

For needle placement	Auxiliary equipment
2 Moricca's needles	Disinfection equipment for nasal cavity
2 Bayonet forceps	Disposable suction catheter for the nasal
1 Small metal hammer	cavity
1 2-ml Tuberculin syringe	Bayonet forceps
1 Long Killian forceps	Antiseptic solution
1 Long Klemmer forceps	Gauze: squares, strips
1 Spinal needle	Drugs
	Steroids: hydrocortisone/methylprednisolone
	Absolute alcohol
	Coagulants

important to evaluate the physical, neurologic, and psychologic condition; the results of laboratory studies; and the analgesic modalities the patient has been subjected to in the past, especially the current form of pain therapy with particular emphasis on problems with narcotic dependence. Also essential is an assessment of the function of the ocular nerves.

Radiographs of the cranium in the anterior, posterior, and lateral projections are useful but not indispensable since they do not always show an "empty sella" which is the only contraindication to the procedure. Moreover, a visual assessment of the anatomic radiologic condition is obtainable before the beginning of the procedure while the image intensifier is being positioned. Bony abnormalities of the cranium do not contraindicate the technique but may create difficulties in positioning the needle in the sella turcica. Finally, it deserves emphasis that the equipment used for preoperative X-rays may produce images slightly different from those produced with a portable apparatus.

Anesthesia

The anesthesiologist must administer an anesthetic that is simple and produces the fewest side effects (Table 1). Moreover, it should permit prompt emergence from anesthesia and consciousness so the patient can be properly assessed. Avoid any drug that impairs the pupillary reflex especially at time of assessment after emergence from the anesthesia. These include atropine-like drugs and neuroleptic analgesics with central action. As part of the preanesthetic preparation, it is essential to withhold food for 3 hr; dairy products for at least 8 hr. I employ the following technique of anesthesia. The patient is given a small (3 mg) dose of *d*-tubocurarine to prevent fasciculation from succinylcholine chloride and is given with 100% oxygen for 3 min. This is followed by a modest sleep dose of thiopental sodium, administered as a 2.5% solution, followed by administration of 50% nitrous oxide and 50% oxygen with succinylcholine chloride, and orotracheal intubation with a cuffed tube. Maintenance of anesthesia is achieved with nitrous oxide/oxygen and succinylcholine by continuous drip or in doses of 20 to 25 mg, and ventilation is assisted or controlled to assure adequate oxygenation and CO_2 elimination. The very light, balanced anesthesia is continued during introduction of the Moricca needle until its point is in the desired position in the sella turcica. Once X-ray controls show the bevel of the needle in the proper place, the patient is ready to be extubated and awakened. Prior to extubation, thorough cleaning of the tracheobronchial tree and the pharynx is carried out. Extubation is performed only when the pharyngeal and laryngeal reflexes are active, because a laryngoscope cannot be used as it carries the risk of displacing the needle. Soon after extubation, the patient awakens and is able to cooperate with the algologist.

Equipment

The equipment in the operating room is very simple and modest; indeed, the procedure can be done outside an operating room. The only indispensable items are (a) an operating table with a headrest that is radiotransparent; (b) free access to radiologic equipment for the head of the patient on a transverse plane to the patient; and (c) a sharp focusing flashlight and a room in which it is possible to beam the lights. Of course, apparatus and instruments to administer anesthesia, instrument tables, and suction apparatus should be available. Members of the team should wear lead aprons or other means of radiation protection.

The instruments needed for the procedure are placed on 2 separate tables, on opposite sides of the operating table as listed in Table 1 above. The Moricca needle is made of stainless steel and has a stylet to prevent any obstruction by blood clots. The visible surface is smooth with the exception of 5 or 6 notches at the proximal quarter that serve as a reference point in the event it is necessary to make minor adjustments following introduction into the sella turcica. Obviously, before the procedure is started, all the instruments must be tested to assure their proper function and the X-ray apparatus placed in position.

Position of the Patient and Other Preparations

Accurate positioning of the patient is essential to the correct and rapid execution of the procedure. The patient is placed supine on the operating table with head semiflexed on a radiotransparent headrest that allows the patient to be comfortable and, at the same time, holds the head steady in the needed position. The operator should have unobstructed, direct visualization of the forehead (glabella) of the patient and good visibility of the region of the sella during the use of the image intensifier. Once the patient is in the proper position, a catheter is introduced into the nasal cavity op-

TABLE 2. *Steps for introduction of Moricca's needles*

---

1. The needle is introduced through the disinfected nasal cavity and directed posteriorly, superiorly, and slightly medially toward the glabella when viewed from the frontal plane and toward the midpoint of the zygomatic arch when viewed from the side.
2. The needle is inserted through the mucous membrane of the posterior nasal cavity toward the sphenoid process and advanced through the base of the cranium with very light strokes of the hammer. Passage through the various structures can be ascertained by noting variation in resistance and in the tone of the percussion.
3. Once the base of the sella is perforated, the stylet is retracted slightly and the needle is advanced by slight percussion of the hammer. Once the resistance of the dorsum sella is reached, the stylet is advanced but it should not be made to enter the entire length of the needle.
4. X-Ray of the position of the needle is taken in the anterior, posterior, and lateral view.
5. The Queckenstedt maneuver is performed.

---

posite the one through which the needle will be introduced. The nasal cavity and pharynx are aspirated and the catheter is left in place. (Earlier, Moricca had used both nasal cavities to insert needles, but soon noted the same effect could be achieved by introducing 2 or more needles through the same nostril so one nostril is plugged in the postoperative period, causing less discomfort to the patient.) An antiseptic solution consisting of 20% chlorexidine gluconate in 0.5% aqueous solution and 10% polyvinylpyrrolidone is applied widely to the skin around the nares and into the nasal cavity into which the needle will be introduced. Prior to application of the antiseptic solution, the patient's eyes are closed and a wet gauze placed over them, to avoid irritation. Just before the introduction of the needle, the excess antiseptic in the nasal cavity is removed with gauze.

Introduction of Moricca's Needle

The introduction and positioning of the Moricca needle, if done properly, require only relative and brief use of the image intensifier because there are numerous clinical signs that are of objective value. The steps used in introducing the Moricca needle and placing it in the exact position are listed in Table 2. Progression of the needle is checked by means of the image intensifier until its point reaches the proper position. The point of the needle in relation to the anterior and posterior clinoid processes should be assessed through the lateral view. It is especially important to know if the point of the needle lies in the center of the sella in the anterior or posterior view plane (78). The point of the needle should be in close proximity to the posterior wall of the sella to favor the diffusion of alcohol along the pituitary stalk and involve the pituitary hypothalamic structures (Figs. 1 and 2). Once the needle has been properly positioned, a Queckenstedt maneuver is performed to ascertain if cerebrospinal fluid or blood flows from the hub of the needle. A negative Queckenstedt assures that there is no damage to the dural sleeve of the sella, that the point of the needle is not in a vessel, and that the sella is not "empty." If the maneuver produces blood, the needle is moved slightly; however, in the event that cerebrospinal fluid is obtained, the procedure must be abandoned and is considered a "traumatic" NALP. On the other hand, fluid flowing from the needle may be other than cerebrospinal fluid and, therefore, should be examined for density and consistence. For example, in cases of a cystic adenoma or arachnoid pseudocyst of the sella, fluid may be obtained that is not cerebrospinal fluid. In any event, the procedure must be abandoned, even if radiologically the needle is fixed in the center of the sella.

Injection of Alcohol

Once proper positioning of the needle is ascertained, the patient is awakened sufficiently to be able to cooperate and collaborate adequately with the operator. At this point, injection of the alcohol is initiated. It deserves emphasis that the absolute alcohol must be of the highest purity and in containers that prevent evaporation and dehydration, such as Moricca's container. If ampules are used, each one is opened just prior to use. Prior to aspirating alcohol into the syringe, the plunger should be rinsed in alcohol to wash off any talcum powder from the operator's glove or residue from heat sterilization. Two milliliters of the alcohol are aspirated into the syringe, the syringe is then adapted carefully to the needle so as not to displace it and the injection initiated. The alcohol should be injected in fractional doses of approximately 0.25 ml at intervals of 15 to 20 sec. During the entire period, the diameter of the pupil and the pupillary reflex response to light are continuously monitored, best done in a darkened room. To avoid clots in the needle, reinsert the stylet of the needle between injections. The injection should be done gently and slowly to avoid a transient headache referred to the glabella. After 2 ml of alcohol have been injected, the needle is withdrawn slightly and another series of injections may be carried out if deemed necessary. Indeed, a third series of injections to a total of 6 ml of alcohol may be used during the first treatment. After the injection of alcohol is completed, the stylet is reintroduced into the needle and the needle withdrawn gently by rotating maneuvers. After the needle has been withdrawn, nasal tamponade is achieved with sterile gauze soaked in antiseptic.

At this point, some questions remain unanswered regarding the quantity of alcohol to introduce during a single sitting, the number of procedures to carry out, and the total amount of alcohol used to achieve the desired results. The following points are relevant to these questions: there are no criteria, including the size of the sella, to indicate the optimal quantity of alcohol to use during a single NALP. On the other hand, there is an absolute contraindication to continue injecting alcohol whenever anisocoria is observed and/or when there is impairment of the pupillary reflex response to light. The exception to this rule is when these complications are transient. Caution should also be used in continuing the injection in the presence of diffuse persistent headache that develops after one or more fractions of the alcohol injections. Such headaches sometimes precede the appearance of impairment of ocular reflexes, although there is no evidence this is due to an increase in intracranial pressure.

Generally, a single NALP procedure is terminated once 6 ml of alcohol have been injected. If we are dealing with a form of cancer that is not hormone-dependent, such as cancer of the lung, it is rare to inject amounts larger than 6 ml during the entire NALP.

The degree and duration of prompt pain relief after a single procedure do not closely correlate with the quantity of alcohol introduced. Indeed, transient analgesia can occur after a traumatic NALP where no alcohol has been injected.

Postoperative Care

During the immediate postoperative period, it is essential to carefully monitor fluid intake and output, vital signs at least twice a day or more if necessary, and carry out certain laboratory studies including blood glucose, blood and urinary electrolyte contents, and creatinine. It is also important to watch for metabolic alterations frequent in patients with disorders of certain organs, either due to the cancer or as a result of chemotherapy or other anticancer therapeutic procedures. Three to six hours after the procedure, the patient is allowed oral intake, first pure liquids and later food. The following day the patient may ambulate, if able to do so before the procedure was carried out.

Subsequent Therapy

Several conditions or criteria may indicate a second, a third, and even a fourth procedure. First, if the total quantity of alcohol, considered as minimal dose (6 ml) was impossible to inject during the initial procedure, a second NALP is performed in 48 to 72 hr. The number of NALP procedures that will be performed in a cycle depends on (a) the total dose of alcohol one wants to inject; (b) if during the initial procedure, the occurrence of ocular side effects intraoperatively caused suspension of the procedure before the total amount was injected; (c) the degree and duration of the pain relief achieved with the preceding injections; and (d) the general status of the patient. It deserves reemphasis that repetition of the procedure is always possible from a technical standpoint, since past experience and studies suggest the introduction of the needle causes no structural changes in the cranium that would create technical difficulties for subsequent injections. Certainly, additional procedures should be carried out whenever there is recurrence of the pain from cancer and whenever there are signs of an active, neoplastic invasion, provided the condition of the patient has *not* become terminal. In general, a dose of 3 ml of alcohol is sufficient to reestablish analgesia obtained from preceding cycles of the NALP procedures.

Complications

Like many other procedures or pharmacologic agents used to produce pain relief, the NALP procedure is not without risk. Some of the causes of intraoperative complications are due to gross technical error or unforeseen anatomic anomalies which result in malposition of the needle. These include insertion of the needle point beyond the roof of the sella suggested by the presence of cerebrospinal fluid during the Queckenstedt maneuver; the needle point in the internal carotid artery suggested by spurts of arterial blood when the stylet is removed; the presence of the needle point in the cavernous sinus suggested by a steady flow of blood; and the same sign of blood if the needle point is in a branch of the pituitary portal venous system. In the latter case, visualization of the needle position with radiographs shows that in the lateral position, the point is quite far from the dorsum sella, but in the anteroposterior projection it is very close to or completely in the midline. This rare, undesirable occurrence is corrected with a simple move- ment of the needle; however, in all other cases, the NALP must be aban- doned and the patient should be carefully observed neurologically. Thus, the needle must be positioned on the saggital midline plane to keep the procedure's risk at a minimum.

The most frequent and important complication of NALP is due to the introduction of alcohol when the point of the needle is *not* in the center of the sella (78). This is often due to rapid and superficial evaluation of the position of the needle or repeated difficulty in obtaining proper positioning. Under such circumstances, the procedure should be abandoned because the patient should never pay the price of ocular dysfunction. The serious intra- operative complications of NALP are usually due to the diffusion of alcohol to the parasellar region with consequent involvement of the extrinsic ocular nerves. These include impairment or damage to the optic, trochlear, or ab- duceus nerve, but these are rare. I have seen two patients with transient damage to the fourth and sixth cranial nerves unilaterally.

An intraoperative complication that is not unusual is irritation to the optic nerve and, more often, to the oculomotor nerve. This may occur even when the needle is correctly positioned, especially when there is increased intra- cranial pressure that may be caused by venous hypertension, hypercapnia, or inadequate anesthetic technique. Involvement of the oculomotor nerve is manifested by a slight anisocoria, which may progress to a reduced pup- illary reaction to light on the affected (midriatic) side and subsequent loss of reflex of the pupil to light. Sometimes some of these phases are skipped, but this is not necessarily related to the total dose of alcohol injected or with

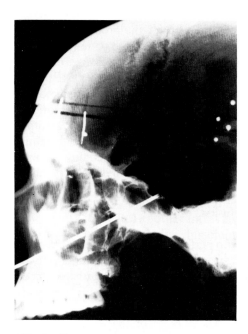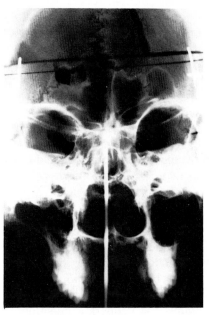

FIG. 1.   Roentgenograms depicting the correct position of the Moricca needle in the sella turcica prior to the injection of alcohol.   **Left:** Lateral view showing the tip of the needle close to the posterior wall of the sella to favor the diffusion of alcohol along the pituitary stalk and involve the pituitary-hypothalamic structures.   **Right:** Anteroposterior view of the same.

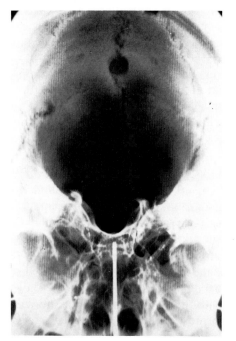

FIG. 2.   Roentgenograms showing correct position of the needle in the sella turcica prior to the injection of alcohol, prior to achieving neuroadenolysis.

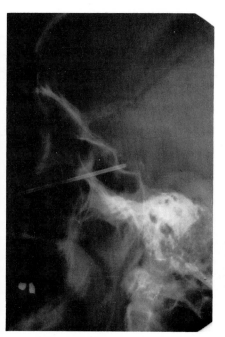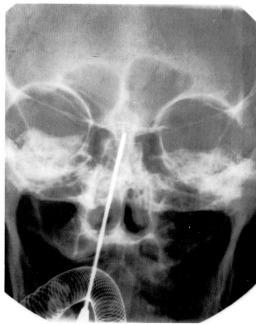

FIG. 3. Left: Lateral projection. The point of the needle is clearly at the level of the adenohypophysis. This is not the most advisable position. **Right:** Anteroposterior projection (same patient as on left). The point of the needle appears well positioned in the center of the sella, but the needle will have to be inserted further in order to obtain a better position of the point in relation to the posterior wall of the sella. It will therefore be necessary and in anteroposterior control, since the point of the needle could have moved from the center of the sella.

posterior projection, and other points. A certain symmetry of the sella is not infrequent. Therefore, positioning the point of the needle in the midline does not mean the point itself is exactly at the center of the sella turcica. Also, the structures around the sella could be symmetrical in respect to the cranium or to other endocranial structures, rather than the sella itself. Thus, in order to determine the most useful projection and judge if the point of the needle is at the center of the sella in a specimen with the cranium devoid of the upper portion, a stylet is inserted from above, at the center of the sella; subsequently, over it a needle is fixed using the transsphenoidal route until the point of the needle is positioned in the most posterior part of the sella at the limit between the superior half and inferior half of the lamina quadrilatera. Subsequently, an X-ray is taken in the lateral projection; in the anteroposterior projection, in which the sella is seen as a curved line with convexity toward the upper part with the point of the needle transfixed at the center; and finally, in the anteroposterior position with a 35-deg inclination (projection of Towne), which allows good identification of the sella.

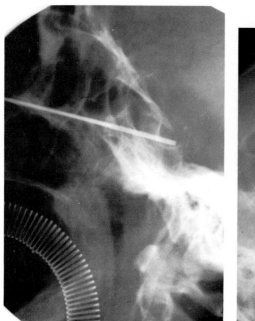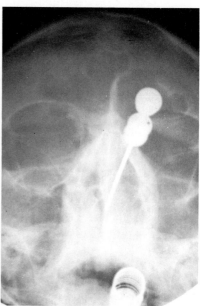

FIG. 4. Left: Lateral projection. The needle does not appear in the optimal position (it appears too low on the floor of the sella). **Right**: Fronto-occipital projection. The needle appears to be in the midline. This projection, however, does not verify if the point of the needle is exactly at the center of the sella.

RESULTS

As Bonica (7–9) warned, to evaluate the efficacy of a pain-relieving modality in cancer patients, it is necessary to assess the quality, intensity, duration, and distribution of the pain; the pathophysiology caused by the cancer; and the physical, emotional, mental, and moral condition of the patient. In patients in whom the pain is associated with anxiety, depression, and other psychologic effects, modalities that interfere with the mental and emotional condition of the patient (e.g., opiates) provide better pain relief than techniques that do not. However, pharmacologic agents rarely *completely* relieve severe or very severe cancer pain.

In this regard, the NALP procedure has a particularly important role because when properly carried out, it provides effective relief of severe, widespread diffuse pain, which only morphine can relieve to a satisfactory degree when it is still efficacious (23,56,57,64). It produces these beneficial effects without altering the function of the peripheral or central nervous system. Unfortunately, the beneficial results obtainable with NALP are not confirmed at the same level of efficacy by every author; nevertheless, they all recognize that in at least one-third of patients in whom every other pain-

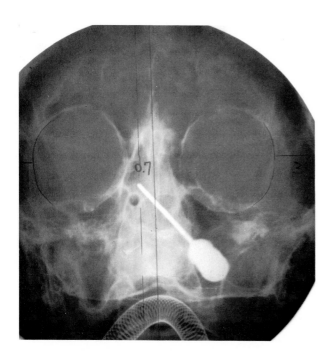

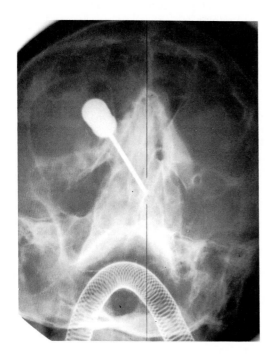

FIG. 5. Top: Anteroposterior projection. The point of the needle appears to be 0.7 cm from the midline. This results from the head of the patient not properly positioned. In fact, the distance from the lateral board of the temporal plate is 2 cm on the right side and 3 cm on the left side. **Bottom:** Anteroposterior projection (same patient as at top). The head is now properly positioned: the point of the needle now appears to be on the midline.

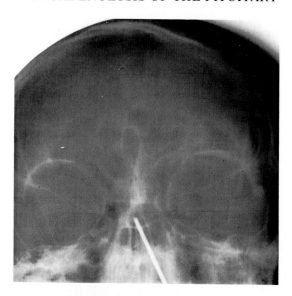

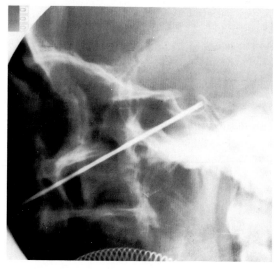

FIG. 6. **Top:** Anteroposterior projection. The point of the needle is at the center of the sella: proper positioning. **Bottom**: Lateral projection. The point of the needle is in the proximity of the posterior wall of the sella: proper positioning.

relieving modality has failed, the NALP procedure was able to produce effective pain relief (12,14,15,20–22,26,30,33,34,37,38,41–44,47–49,68–70,74,76,82,84,86,93,95,96,98,102).

An attempt to provide a complete overview of every publication is difficult because (a) not all published material is at our disposal; (b) some case reports have been compiled with objectives other than pain relief; and (c) not all

TABLE 3. *Moricca's results with NALP (1963–1978)*

Total number of patients treated	2,202
Hormone-dependent cancer	91.6%
Nonhormone-dependent cancer	8.4%
Complete pain relief	
After first NALP	59.2%
After second NALP	9.5%
After third NALP	27.7%
Total	96.4%
Incomplete pain relief after third NALP	3.6%
Ethanol injected (during each session)	2–5 ml

data acquired with NALP have been published. Moreover, much of the published data are difficult to analyze because they suffer from one or more of the following defects in reporting:

1. The NALP technique is not described in detail and/or is different from the one described by Moricca, particularly in relation to the position of the needle and the quantity of alcohol.

2. The number of patients who had undergone other ablative procedures without positive results but still responded to NALP are rarely documented.

3. A follow-up of acceptable duration was not done, in part, due to the death of the patient soon after the procedure was carried out.

4. Many reports do not describe the protocol followed to verify the results; or the protocols are different from one another, and therefore the data cannot be compared.

5. A significant number of reports do not provide information on whether the pain was due to the cancer or to other causes.

6. In publications reporting incomplete pain relief with NALP, many do not describe what pain characteristics were not relieved.

7. Finally, most reports do not indicate if the NALP affected the evolution of the tumor.

Considering the published results and the descrepancies noted above, it is understandable why different published sets of data give different results regarding analgesic efficacy and incidences of complications. To obtain comparative evaluation, it is necessary to compare only those results having a uniform choice of patient, identical positioning of Moricca's needle, and the injection of similar quantities of alcohol. To provide comparative data, four tables are reproduced: Table 3 contains data obtained from a paper of Moricca et al.; Table 4 contains results I obtained with NALP performed using the Moricca technique described above; Table 5 is a combination of these two tables with data obtained from a number of published papers; and Table 6 contains a list of side effects and complications that I have encountered when performing the NALP or consequent thereto.

The data contained in these tables on the results of the NALP merit some brief comments. First, it is important to clarify the issue of the total number

TABLE 4. *Statistics with NALP (1979–1982)*

Patients treated	109	
With hormone-dependent tumors	73	(67%)
Very poor risk patients	83	(76.2%)
Age (years)	66	(52–78)[a]
Procedures performed		
Total	248[b]	
Average per patient	2.27	
Ethanol injected (ml)		
Per procedure		3.18 (0.5–7.2)[a]
Total per patient		5.09 (0.5–11.4)[a]
Procedures not completed[c]	16	
Follow-up to 3 months or death	93	
Total pain relief	82	(88.2%)
Partial pain relief	11	(11.8%)
Total pain relief in hormone-dependent cancer	60/64	(93.8%)
Total pain relief in hormone-autonomous cancer	22/29	(75.9%)

[a] Average values with range in parentheses.

[b] This total includes 17 NALPs that were repeated to control the pain which had returned after the first set of NALPs had controlled it for a significant period of time.

[c] These are cases where it was not possible to perform a sufficient number of NALPs to introduce 6 ml of ethanol.

of patients and the total number of NALPs performed by Moricca, and the percentage of patients who obtained pain relief after each injection of alcohol in the pituitary gland (Table 3). The table shows that good pain relief was obtained by 59.2% of patients after the first procedure, by 9.49% of the patients after the second, and by 27.71% of the patients after the third procedure. Regardless of the effect on the pain, Moricca repeated the NALP until a total of at least 6 ml of alcohol was injected. This constitutes a cycle of therapy, and 96.4% of patients obtained good pain relief from the first cycle of NALP. However, in a certain percentage of these patients, pain recurred several months to years later at which point another cycle of NALP can be repeated.

As regards the incidence of complications, the following can be stated:

1. The most recently published statistics and the most numerous number of patients are those with the least number of complications.

2. The more Moricca's technique is not followed, the greater the incidence of complications.

3. The incidence of serious metabolic alterations seems related to the state of the hypothalamic-pituitary axis, to the evolution of the cancer, and to the previous form of therapy, but is not predicted with the usual laboratory examinations.

4. All of the sequelae and/or the described complications, except for traumatic NALP and the hemorrhage from Moricca's needle, are independent from the pain-relieving effect of alcohol.

In comparing the table that includes the statistics of Moricca and the one summarizing the data of others, some specific points may be noted that will

TABLE 5. *Pain relief with NALP*

Author (Country)	Number of patients	Number of NALPs	Percent of pain relief		
			Complete	Partial	None
Corssen (United States)	32	34	69	28	3
Grünwald (Uruguay)	60	110	65	25	10
Levin (United States)	82	82	34	56	10
Lipton (United Kingdom)	187	292	40	30	30
Lloyd (United Kingdom)	25	34	74	0	26
Miles (United Kingdom)	104	161	47	37	16
Takeda (Japan)	102	136	80	10	10
Gianasi (Italy)	109	248	88	12	0
Romoli (Italy)	40	51	65	20	15
Ischia (Italy)	75	87	57	32	11
Total Average	816	1,235	62	25	13
Moricca	2,202	8,155	96	4	0

help understand the differences in results reported by different authors. Careful consideration of various factors reveals that the results are not as different from each another as the numbers shown suggest. For example, the choice of the patient and the quantity and quality of pain relief and other criteria permit one to move cases from one column to another, rendering the data on the pain-relieving efficacy of the procedure more uniform, decreasing the differences between the reports of others and those of Moricca. Indeed, it is important to remember that although the earlier experience entailed the use of a single NALP and the injection of from 1 to 2 ml alcohol, Moricca has used (and has never stopped stressing the need to use) a larger amount of alcohol, even if this required performing additional NALPs.

Moricca has not published in detail the amount of alcohol he has been able to inject with the first, second, third, or subsequent NALPs in the several thousand patients he has treated. The thing he has stressed is that pain relief improves as more alcohol is introduced into the sella, even though the desired results may be achieved with only one NALP. If we examine the incidence of pain relief reported by Moricca after each NALP, we see that his results are not much better than those of other authors. In fact, immediate and complete pain relief was achieved in only 59.2% of the pa-

TABLE 6. *Side effects and sequelae observed in 248 NALPs performed on 109 patients*

Traumatic NALP (empty sella)	4	(1.6%)
Headache (usually frontal and short-lasting)	101	(40.7%)
Ocular disturbance	68	(27.4%)
Short-lived anisocoria	49	(19.6%)
Anisocoria which disappears within 1 week	13	(5.2%)
Irritation of perisellar nerves	6	(2.4%)
Hemianopsia	0	
Palpebral ptosis	0	
Cerebrospinal fluid leakage	1	(0.4%)
Hemorrhage from Moricca's needle	1	(0.4%)
Meningitis	0	
Diabetes insipidus	107	(43.2%)
Resolved in 1 month	23	(9.3%)
Late appearance (over 1 week)	8	(3.2%)
Hyperthermia (37.7°–40.2°C)	67	(27.0%)
Lasting over 3 days	3	(1.2%)
Endocrine-metabolic imbalance	32	(12.9%)
Coma and death	19	(7.7%)
Hemiparesis	0	
Decreased awareness	13	(5.2%)
Convulsions	0	
Nursing error	12	(4.8%)
Hyperphagia	0	
Hypothyroidism	1	
Hypoadrenalism	0	
Hypogonadism	?	

tients after the first procedure; the percentage increased to 68.7% with the second procedure, and an additional 27.7% required a third or more procedures, in order to achieve a success rate of 96.4%. To achieve such a high percentage, he injected not less, and often more, than 6 ml of alcohol.

Other reasons for discrepancies between Moricca's results and others is that reports by those with limited experience could reflect results of pain relief in the initial phase of the application of the technique before it was perfected. Another point to be made is that only a few authors in a small number of cases reported pain relief achieved in patients with cancers that were hormone-dependent separately from those of nonhormone-dependent tumors; however, the authors did recognize that differences exist between these two cancers. Still another reason for differences is that the follow-up reported in the table averages several months, but only 4 authors repeated the NALP procedure when it became necessary because the pain recurred. That Moricca carried out nearly 4 NALP procedures for each patient reflects the fact that he recalled the patient for follow-up repetition of the procedure in a large percentage of patients. Therefore, lower success results will show up if the procedure was not repeated when necessary and the patient survives for a long period of time. Not only did the majority of authors use only a single procedure, but the interval between increments of injections is so long as to preclude sufficient diffusion of the alcohol to achieve the desired results. Thus, the reported statistics on any pain-relieving results would show a lower success rate also when smaller quantities of alcohol were used. The above considerations suggest that the incidence of partial and complete pain relief together produces results similar among the different authors.

Another important point is that any liquid introduced into the sella before the injection of alcohol will dilute the neurolytic agent. Madrid (47) first injected a contrast medium in a quantity equal to one-tenth of the alcohol with consequent dilution of the neurolytic agent from 98 to 88%. Miles and Lipton (50) introduced a radiopaque solution equal to two-fifths of the amount of alcohol injected that became diluted to 62%.

Another issue that may help explain the difference in results is that only a few authors indicate the best position to have the point of the needle prior to injecting the alcohol into the sella turcica. This omission may be due to the fact that they presumed the published X-rays in their reports would be sufficient to show the position of the needle or perhaps, they did not give enough importance to this issue, although they do emphasize that proper position of the needle is necessary to avoid damage to the ocular nerves. In contrast, I maintain, in agreement with Moricca, that the position of the needle at the posterior limit of the sella between one-third and two-thirds distance from the quadrilatera lamina may have a significant influence in diffusion of the alcohol to the suprasella area where it has its primary pain-relieving action. I have noted that the more anterior position into the adenohypophysis, in the course of performing the procedure, has resulted in unsatisfactory pain relief. In addition, a very wide sella with, possibly, an incomplete dural cuff would be conducive to more frequent instances of complications and severe headache when the alcohol is injected rapidly.

With regard to the effect of the NALP on the evolution of the tumor, the data in the literature are not conflicting but simply insufficient, presumably due to the difficulty of collecting a proper data base or some of the authors being interested only in the effect of NALP on pain.

The data reported in this paper are only from papers that fulfilled some of the aforementioned criteria and that were available. I wish to give special mention to the data of Fujita et al. (25) who repeated the procedure and were able to obtain 82% complete pain relief. Other publications that confirm the high efficacy of NALP in relieving cancer pain are so numerous it is not possible to cite them all (9–11,17,23,82,92; and C. Benedetti and J. J. Bonica, *this volume*). Indeed, the procedure was the subject of a signed letter in the *Journal of the American Medical Association* (12). Many have considered the advent of NALP as a milestone of modern pain therapy, and on the occasion of the Congress in Rotterdam (102), it was reported that over 14,000 patients "suffering from unbearable and intractable pain" have been treated with NALP, reaffirming that this method "is established as a safe and effective method to provide immediate, complete and often prolonged pain relief when all other modalities to obtain relief have failed."

The efficacy of the procedure on relieving diffuse cancer pain has been admitted by some persons who, early in the development of the procedure, expressed skepticism. Pagni (81), who has spent much of his professional career managing patients with pain and whose neurosurgical bias is differently oriented from that of an anesthesiologist-algologist, states:

> the neuroadenolysis . . . is able to produce analgesia in the diffuse pain especially those caused by tumor which are hormone dependent [with] . . . minimal surgical trauma . . . [is] . . . applicable also in very poor risk patients; . . . if the tumor is also hormone-dependent, besides a regression of the pain, there is also a beneficial effect on the evolution of the tumor.

Ventafridda and De Conno (99) have not obtained the best results with NALP, favoring cancer pain control with drugs instead of different neurolytic techniques; nevertheless, they recognized that "for diffuse pain caused by hormone-dependent tumors, in particular cancer of the prostate and of the breast, when MAP at high dosages has not been effective, one should consider the Moricca procedure for neuroadenolysis."

If others who for different reasons practice different types of antalgic therapy come to this conclusion, it means that much of the opposition to NALP is without scientific basis. The algologist must always make available to the patient with cancer pain any modality that may be found efficacious in relieving the patient's pain.

MECHANISMS OF PAIN RELIEF BY NALP

Despite the great advances in research on acute pain during the past decade and the vast amount of new information acquired, and the attempts of several workers to elucidate on it, the mechanism by which NALP produces pain relief remains unknown (17,18,35,39,41). This is due, in part, to the great voids in our knowledge of the neuropathophysiology and biochemistry of cancer pain. As emphasized by Bonica, these voids in our knowledge are due to lack of research on the basic mechanisms of cancer pain. To date, no publication is available that reports on scientific research specifically directed to the basic mechanism of cancer pain. In view of this, and since A. B. Levin and L. L. Ramirez (*this volume*) summarize the hypotheses that have been proposed on the mechanisms of action of NALP, I will limit my comments to a few relevant points.

First, much skepticism about the efficacy of NALP stems from there being no changes in the function of the peripheral nociceptive system following the procedure, yet the patient experiences pain relief. This skepticism early in the development of the procedure prompted Moricca to carry out the aforementioned anatomic (60), pathologic (71), and histochemical (71) studies and, later, studies entailing the use of the somatosensory evoked potentials (100).

Second, most investigators are tempted to explain the pain relief achieved with NALP by hypothesizing a single mechanism. Some have suggested that the procedure eliminates hormones produced by the pituitary that are re-sponsible for enhancement of nociceptive transmission (91,101). Other in-vestigators have suggested that NALP disturbs the hormonal balance through effects on certain parts of the central nervous system (27,79), or that it directly or indirectly influences the ubiquitous dopaminergic endor-phinergic receptors in the structures affected by the alcohol (19,51). Still others implicate certain structures in the hypothalamus and third ventricle (10,11,17,18,31,50,55,62,69,70,73,94,97).

Since 1970, Moricca has maintained the hypothesis that NALP acts on the hypothalamic and other suprasellar structures rather than on the pitui-tary, and his recent studies carried out in collaboration with Deshpande, already cited (17,18), support this idea. As previously mentioned, they found that following NALP, pituitary function as measured by the plasma con-centration of prolactin and thyroid-stimulating, follicle-stimulating, and lu-teinizing hormones remain intact and the ability of the pituitary to respond to hypothalamic releasing factors remained unimpaired. On the other hand, ACTH, beta-lipoprotein, and beta-endorphin concentrations were raised after the treatment. This led them to conclude that the procedure effects the hypothalamus rather than the pituitary. What is left is to elucidate on the relationship between the increased levels of these peptides and possible changes in nociceptive transmission at the level of the spinal cord, brainstem, and brain. This and many other questions need to be answered to clarify this issue.

Although none of the studies to date have defined the precise mechanisms of NALP, clinicians should not be deterred from using the procedure. After all, general anesthesia has been used for nearly a century and a half, and we still do not know the precise mechanism of its action. Moreover, the lack of information of the action of the procedure should spur researchers to exert even greater efforts in studying this issue. In addition, since NALP produces such impressive, dramatic pain relief, this procedure might be useful as a research tool in studying the mechanisms of nonmalignant chronic pain and cancer pain, and perhaps the mechanisms of action of other an-algesic therapies.

SUMMARY

Neuroadenolysis was first introduced and repeatedly advocated by Mor-icca as an effective modality in relieving the pain of cancer. Although it appears to be more effective in hormone-dependent cancer, it has also been found to provide effective relief of pain caused by nonhormonal tumors. To obtain optimal results with the ablative procedure, it is essential to closely follow Moricca's technique which, among other things, includes the precise placement of the needle point in the sella turcica and the injection of incre-ments of 0.25 ml of alcohol at intervals of 15 to 20 sec, until at least 4 ml (preferably 6 ml) of solution is injected. Moreover, in a significant percentage of patients, it is necessary to carry out a second, third, or additional injections. Equally important is the careful monitoring of the patient both during the injection to prevent the development of serious ocular complications and after the injection to treat the side effects and sequelae of the procedure. The published data suggest that if these guidelines are followed, over 90% of patients with diffuse cancer pain will obtain effective relief.

REFERENCES

1. Bernard, L., Donzelle, G., and Deumier, R. (1980): L'hypophysiolyse dans le traitement des douleurs cancéreuses. *Anesth. Analg. (Paris)*, 37:345–352.
2. Bonica, J. J. (1953): *Management of Pain*. Lea & Febiger, Philadelphia.
3. Bonica, J. J. (1954): The management of cancer pain. *GP*, 10:34–43.
4. Bonica, J. J. (1978): Cancer pain. A major national health problem. *Cancer Nursing J.*, 4:313–316.
5. Bonica, J. J. (1979): Importance of the problem. In: *Advances in Pain Research and Therapy*, Vol. 2, edited by J. J. Bonica and V. Ventafridda, pp. 1–12. Raven Press, New York.
6. Bonica, J. J. (1979): Cancer pain. In: *Pain*, edited by J. J. Bonica, pp. 337–362. Raven Press, New York.
7. Bonica, J. J. (1980): Pain research and therapy: Past and current status and future needs. In: *Pain, Discomfort and Humanitarian Care*, edited by J. J. Bonica and L. K. Y. Ng. Elsevier/North-Holland, Amsterdam.
8. Bonica, J. J. (1982): Introduction: Management of cancer pain. *Acta Anaesth. Scand. [Suppl.]*, 74:5–10,75–82.
9. Bowsher, D. (1978): Effects of naloxone on patients who have had malignant pain achieved by pituitary alcohol injection (abstract). Second World Congress on Pain, Montreal.
10. Casini, O., Massidda, B., Moricca, G., Muggiano, A., and Pellegrino, A. (1978): (a) Tassi plasmatici di prolattina e somatotropina in pazienti trattati con neuroadenolisi per incoercibili algie neoplastiche. *Acta Anaesthesiol. Ital.*, 29:833–844.
11. Casini, O., Massidda, B., Moricca, G., Muggiano, A., and Pellegrino, A. (1978): Modificazioni del tasso serico delle gonadotropine LH e FSH in pazienti neoplastici sottoposti a neuroadenolisi a scopo antalgico. *Acta Anaesthesiol. Ital.* 29:813–824.
12. Check, W. A. (1979): Alcohol injection relieving intractable pain. *J.A.M.A.*, 2164–2165.
13. Ciocatto, E., Moricca, G., and Cavaliere, R. (1963): Terapia del dolor en el enfermo canceroso. Relazione IX Conr. Argentino Anest., Buenos Aires.
14. Corssen, G., Adward, T. W., and Ford, A. (1984): Control of intractable cancer pain in man: further experimental and clinical experiences with pituitary neuroadenolysis (NALP). In: *Pituitary Neuroadenolysis in Cancer Pain in Hormone-Dependent Tumors*, edited by S. Ischia, S. Lipton, and G. F. Mattezzoli. Edizione Librera, Verona. (*in press*)
15. Corssen, G., Holcomb, M. C., Moustapha, I., Langford, K., Vitek, J. J., and Ceballo, R. (1977): Alcohol-induced adenolysis of the pituitary gland: A new approach to control of intractable pain. *Anaesth. Analg. (Cleve.)*, 56:414–421.
16. Corssen, G., and Yanagida, H. (1979): How does clinical adenolysis of the pituitary gland control intractable cancer pain? Abstr. Corso Aggiornamento Terapia Antalgica, Tropea.
17. Deshpande, N., Moricca, G., Saullo, F., Di Martino, L., and Kwa, G. (1981): Some aspects of pituitary function after neuroadenolysis in patients with metastatic cancer. *Tumori*, 67:355–359.
18. Deshpande, N., Moricca, G., and Di Martino, L. (1982): Pituitary function after neuroadenolysis in patients with metastatic cancer suffering from intractable pain. Proceedings of the XIII International Cancer Congress, Cat. Card N. 82, 082833.
19. De Wied, D. (1976): Hormonal influence on motivation learning and memory processes. *Hosp. Pract.*, 11:123–131.
20. Editorial (1981): Pituitary ablation for pain relief. *Lancet*, 1:1348–1349.

21. Evans, P. J. D., Lloyd, J. W., Moore, R. A., and Smith, R. F. (1982): Pituitary function following hypophysectomy for pain relief. *Br. J. Anaesth.*, 54:921–925.
22. Farcot, J. M., Habener, J. P., Laugner, B., Schoeffler, P., Farny, J., and Lafaye, P. (1979): Les douleurs des cancers metastases hormono-dépendants. Leur traitement par l'hypophysiolyse a l'alcool. *Anaesth. Analg. (Paris)*, 36:323–329.
23. Farcot, J. M., Habener, J. P., Laugner, B., and Muller, A. (1981): L'hypophysiolyse a l'alcool. Indications, techniques et résultats. Observations sur le mécanisme d'action (27 cas). *Anaesth. Analg. (Paris)*, 38:361–364.
24. Forrest, A. P. M., and Brown, D. A. (1955): Pituitary radon implant for breast cancer. *Lancet*, 1:1054–1059.
25. Fujita, T., Kitani, Y., Tozawa, R., and Takeda, F. (1980): Mode of pain relief on recrudescence after alcohol hypophysectomy. Proceedings of the VII World Congress on Anaesthesiology, Hamburg.
26. Gianasi, G. C. (1984): Neuroadenolisi pituitaria. A nalisi dei risultati clinici in un gruppo di pazienti ad alto rischio. In: *Pituitary Neuroadenolysis in Cancer Pain in Hormone-Dependent Tumors,* edited by S. Ischia, S. Lipton, and G. F. Mattezzoli. Edizione Librera, Verona. (*in press*)
27. Gilad, I., Locatelli, V., Cocchi, D., Carminati, R., Arezzini, C., and Muller, E. E. (1978): Effect of hyperprolactinemia and 2-Br-alpha-ergocryptine on neuroendocrine mechanism(s) for gonadotrophin control. *Life Sci.*, 23:2245.
28. Greco, T. (1965): L'alcoolizzazione dell'ipofisi. Vantaggi di questo metodo nel trattamento dei tumori maligni avanzati e delle loro riproduzioni. *Urol. Int.*, 19:54–57.
29. Greco, T., Sbaragli, F., and Cammilli, L. (1957): L'alcolizzazione della ipofisi per via transfenoidale nella terapia di particolari tumori maligni. *Settim. Med.*, 45:355–356.
30. Grunwald, J. (1984): Pituitary neuroadenolysis. Two years experience treating cancer pain and hormone-dependent tumors. In: *Pituitary Neuroadenolysis in Cancer Pain in Hormone-Dependent Tumors,* edited by S. Ischia, S. Lipton, and G. F. Mattezzoli. Edizione Librera, Verona. (*in press*)
31. Gybels, J., Drianenses, J., and Cosyns, P. (1976): Perspective in cancer research. Treatment of pain in patients with advanced cancer. *Eur. J. Cancer*, 12:341.
32. Huggins, C. (1966): Endocrine-induced regression of cancer: Nobel prize lecture 1966. *Cancer Res.*, 27:1925–1930.
33. Ischia, S., Maffezzoli, G. F., and Pacini, L. (1984): NALP: Personal experience and results. In: *Pituitary Neuroadenolysis in Cancer Pain in Hormone-Dependent Tumors,* edited by S. Ischia, S. Lipton, and G. F. Mattezzoli. Edizione Librera, Verona. (*in press*)
34. Katz, J., and Levin, A. B. (1977): Treatment of diffuse metastatic cancer pain by instillation of alcohol into the sella turcica. *Anesthesiology*, 46:115–121.
35. Kosayaschi, R. M., Palkovits, M., Miller, R. J., Chang, H. J., and Quatrecasas, P. (1978): Brain enkephalin distribution is unaltered by hypophysectomy. *Life Sci.*, 22:597.
36. Le Beau, J., and Perrault, M. (1953): A propos de l'hypophysectomie totale dans le traitement du cancer. *Sem. Hop. Paris*, 29:1096.
37. Levin, A. B., and Katz, J. (1979): Stereotaxic chemical hypophysectomy in the treatment of diffuse metastatic cancer pain (abstract). International Symposium on Pain, Sorrento.
38. Levin, A. B., Katz, J., Benson, R. C., and Jones, A. G. (1980): Treatment of pain of diffuse metastatic cancer by stereotactic chemical hypophysectomy: Long term results and observations on mechanisms of action. *Neurosurgery*, 6:258–262.
39. Lewis, J. M. (1981): Hypophysectomy differentially affects morphine and stress analgesia. *Proc. West. Pharmacol. Soc.*, 24:333.
40. Lewis, J. L., and Baxton, L. (quoted from Greco, T.) (1958): Discussione dell'Adunanza Scientifica del 21 dicembre 1957. *Boll. Mem. Soc. Tosco-Umbra Chir.*, 19:78.
41. Lipton, S. (1976): Transnasal pituitary injection. In: *Recent Advances in Anaesthesia and Analgesia,* edited by H. C. Langton and R. S. Atkinson, pp. 249–250. Churchill Livingstone, Edinburgh.
42. Lipton, S. (1979): The injection of alcohol into the pituitary fossa (Moricca operation). In: *Relief of Pain in Clinical Practice,* pp. 178–220. Blackwell, Oxford.
43. Lipton, S., Miles, J. B., Williams, N., and Bark-Jones, N. (1978): Pituitary injection of alcohol for widespread cancer pain. *Pain*, 5:78–82.
44. Lloyd, J. W., Rawlinson, W. A. L., and Evans, P. J. D. (1981): Selective hypophysectomy for metastatic pain. A review of ethyl alcohol ablation of the anterior pituitary in a Regional Pain Relief Unit. *Br. J. Anaesth.*, 53:1129–1133.

45. Luft, R., and Olivecrona, H. (1955): Hypophysectomy in man. Experiences in metastatic cancer of the breast. *Cancer*, 8:261–270.
46. Luft, R., Olivecrona, H., and Sjogren, B. (1952): Hypophysectomy in man. *Nord Med.*, 47:351.
47. Madrid, A. J. L. (1979): Chemical hypophysectomy. In: *Advances in Pain Research and Therapy*, Vol. 2, edited by J. J. Bonica and V. Ventafridda, pp. 381–391. Raven Press, New York.
48. Madrid, A. J. L. (1984): Pituitary neuroadenolysis (NALP). Immediate and long term results. In: *Pituitary Neuroadenolysis in Cancer Pain in Hormone-Dependent Tumors,* edited by S. Ischia, S. Lipton, and G. F. Mattezzoli. Edizione Librera, Verona. (*in press*)
49. Miles, J. (1979): Chemical hypophysectomy. In: *Advances in Pain Research and Therapy*, Vol. 2, edited by J. J. Bonica and V. Ventafridda, pp. 373–380. Raven Press, New York.
50. Miles, J., and Lipton, S. (1976): Mode of action by which pituitary alcohol injection relieves pain. In: *Advances in Pain Research and Therapy*, Vol. 1, edited by J. J. Bonica and D. Albe-Fessard, pp. 867–869. Raven Press, New York.
51. Misfeldt, D. S. (1977): Hypophysectomy relieves pain not via endorphins. *N. Engl. J. Med.*, 297:1236.
52. Moricca, G. (1961): Ulteriori acquisizioni sulle terapie di blocco nelle algie neoplastiche. Atti Corso Aggiorn. Tumori, Roma, Nicolai, Roma, pp. 129–154.
53. Moricca, G. (1968): The management of cancer pain. *Proceedings of the IV World Congress on Anaesthesiology, London*, pp. 266–270. Excerpta Medica, Amsterdam.
54. Moricca, G. (1971): Conclusioni. In: *La Valutazione del Rischio Operatorio*, pp. 545–551. Ambrosiana, Milano.
55. Moricca, G. (1972): Chemolysis of the pituitary in the management of cancer pain. *Proceedings of the V World Congress on Anaesthesiology, Kyoto*, pp. 271–281. Excerpta Medica, Amsterdam.
56. Moricca, G. (1973): La neuroadenolyse de l'hypophyse dans les algies rebelles. *III Symp. Intern. Soc. Anesth.*, Charleroi, Wepion, Namur, pp. 305–308.
57. Moricca, G. (1974): Neuroadenolysis for the antalgic treatment of advanced cancer patients. In: *Recent Advances on Pain*, edited by J. J. Bonica, P. Procacci, and C. Pagni, pp. 313–328. Charles C Thomas, Springfield, Ill.
58. Moricca, G. (1974): Neuroadenolysis of the pituitary in diffuse and so-called intractable cancer pain. *IV European Congress on Anaesthesiology*, pp. 7–10. Excerpta Medica, Amsterdam.
59. Moricca, G. (1975): La neurolyse hypophysaire dans les algies diffuses des cancéreux. *Cah. Anesthesiol.*, 23:815–818.
60. Moricca, G. (1976): Neuroadenolysis for diffuse unbearable cancer pain. In: *Advances in Pain Research and Therapy*, Vol. 1, edited by J. J. Bonica and D. Albe-Fessard, pp. 863–866. Raven Press, New York.
61. Moricca, G. (1976): Neuroadenolysis (Alcoholinisation of the Pituitary) for intractable cancer pain. *Proceedings of the IV World Congress on Anaesthesiology*, pp. 319–328. Excerpta Medica, Amsterdam.
62. Moricca, G. (1977): Pituitary neuroadenolysis in the treatment of intractable pain from cancer. In: *Persistent Pain*, edited by S. Lipton, pp. 149–173. Academic Press, London.
63. Moricca, G. (1977): La neuroadenolisi nel dolore intrattabile da cancro. In: *Convegno Nazionale sul Dolore nelle Neoplasie,* edited by G. Martinelli, L. Vecchiet, and L. Basilico, pp. 127–130. Tipo Erre, Grugliasco.
64. Moricca, G. (1979): Il ruolo della neuroadenolisi e die blocchi antalgici nelle algie neoplastiche. In: *La Terapia del Dolore in Oncologia*, edited by D. Amadori and A. Ravaioli, pp. 53–58. Tipografia Moderna, Forli.
65. Moricca, G. (1980): Discussion about terminal patient. In: *Atti 1st Corso Pratico Intern. Aggiornamento sulla Terapia del Dolore*, edited by R. Rizzi and M. Visentin, pp. 69–75. Vincenza.
66. Moricca, G. (1980): Blocchi nervosi e neuroadenolisi pituitaria del dolore oncologico. La misura del Colore. In: *Elementi di Fisiopatologia Clinica e Terapia del Dolore*, edited by E. Arcuri, F. Calabresi, and G. Moricca, pp. 53–61, 207–226. Aipe's, Roma.
67. Moricca, G., Arcuri, E., and Moricca, P. (1979): Attuale ruolo dei blocchi antalgici nella strategia terapeutica in oncologia. In: *La Terapia di Supporto al Paziente Oncologico*, pp. 347–369. AIOM, Roma.

68. Moricca, G., Arcuri, E., and Moricca, P. (1979): Neuroadenolysis. In: *The Continuing Care of Terminal Cancer Patients*, edited by R. G. Twycross and V. Ventafridda, pp. 155–163. Pergamon, Oxford.
69. Moricca, G., Arcuri, E., and Moricca, P. (1981): Neuroadenolysis of the pituitary. *Acta Anaesthesiol. Belg.*, 1:87–99.
70. Moricca, G., Arcuri, E., and Moricca, P. (1981): Neuroadenolisi pituitaria. In: *Progressi nella Fisiopatologia e Terapia del Dolore*, edited by E. Ciocatto, pp. 235–246, Edizioni Medico Scientifiche, Torino.
71. Moricca, G., Bigotti, A., and Cavaliere, R. (1970): The alcoholization of the hypophysis in the management of cancer pain. In: *Xth International Cancer Congress*, edited by R. W. Curnley and J. E. McGay, pp. 540–548. Medical Arts, Houston.
72. Moricca, G., and Clausi Schettini, C. (1976): Neurochirurgia. In: *Terapia del Dolore Cronico Tumorale e Terapia di Supporto*, edited by P. Periti and S. Monfardini, pp. 653–661. Roma.
73. Moricca, G., and Colistro, F. (1974): Hormonal control of malignant tumors. In: *Characterization of Human Tumours*, edited by W. Davis and C. Maltoni, pp. 218–232. Excerpta Medica, Amsterdam.
74. Moricca, G., and Gianasi, G. C. (1981): Neuroadenolysis of the pituitary. In: *Endocrinology and the Anesthetist*, edited by T. Oyama. Elsevier, Amsterdam.
75. Moricca, G., and Gianasi, G. C. (1984): La neuroadenolisi pituitaria nel trattamento del dolore de cancro e del tumore ormono-condizionato. In: *Pituitary Neuroadenolysis in Cancer Pain in Hormone-Dependent Tumors,* edited by S. Ischia, S. Lipton, and G. F. Mattezzoli. Edizione Librera, Verona. (*in press*)
76. Moricca, G., and Gianasi, G. C. (1981): Terapie antalgiche particolari: la neuroadenolisi pituitaria. In: *Trattato Enciclopedico Italiano di Anestesia.*, pp. 331–340. Piccin, Padova.
77. Moricca, G., and Gianasi, G. C. (1984): Neuroadenolysis of the pituitary (NALP) in treatment of cancer pain. Acta 1st Intern. Symp., History Modern Anaesthesia, Rotterdam (*in press*).
78. Moricca, G., and Gianasi, G. C. (1984): Neuroadenolysis of the pituitary (NALP) for the treatment of cancer pain and metastatic hormone-dependent tumors. In: *Trattato di Oncologia*, Buraresti, (*in press*).
79. Neri Serneri, G. G., Masotti, G., Gensini, G. F., Poggesi, L., Abbate, R., and Mannelli, M. (1981): Prostacyclin and thromboxane A_2 formation in response to adrenergic stimulation in humans: a mechanism for local control of vascular response to sympathetic activation? *Cardiovasc. Res.*, 15:287–294.
80. Newfield, P., Maroon, J. C., and Albin, M. S. (1977): Pituitary adenolysis. *Anaesth. Analg.* (*Cleve.*), 56:879.
81. Pagni, C. (1980): Alcuni aspetti della neurochirurgia del dolore In: *Elementi di Fisiopatologia Clinica e Terapia del Dolore*, edited by E. Arcuri, F. Calabresi, and G. Moricca, pp. 163–183. Aipe's, Roma.
82. Pasqualucci, V., Paoletti, F., and Bifarini, G. (1978): Risultato della neuroadenolisi ipofisaria in un primo gruppo di pazienti enoplastici. *Minerva Anestesiol.*, 44:263–272.
83. Perrault, M., Le Beau, J., and Klotz, B. (1952): L'hypophysectomie totale dan le traitment due cancer sein: Premier cas francais: avenir de la method. *Therapie*, 7:290–300.
84. Roberts, M. T. (1981): Pituitary fossa injection with alcohol for widespread cancer pain. *N.Z. Med. J.*, 93:1–8.
85. Romano, C., Guardabasso, B., and Campana, A. (1982): Nuove ipotesi di colpa professionale in oncologia. *Boll. Ist. Tumor Napoli*, 39:227–239.
86. Romoli, M. (1984): La nostra esperienza nella neuroadenolisi pituitaria nel trattamento di alcune forme neoplastiche. In: *Pituitary Neuroadenolysis in Cancer Pain in Hormone-Dependent Tumors,* edited by S. Ischia, S. Lipton, and G. F. Mattezzoli. Edizione Librera, Verona. (*in press*)
87. Sbaragli, F., and Mininni, D. (1961): L'alcoolizzazione della ipofisi nel trattamento dei tumori maligni in fase avanzata o delle loro riproduzioni. *Osp. Ital. Chir.*, 4:470–479.
88. Sbaragli, F., and Mininni, D. (1961): La tecnica della alcoolizzazione ipofisaria per via naso-transfenoidale. *Osp. Ital. Chir.*, 4:551–559.
89. Scott, W. W. (1952): Endocrine management of disseminated prostate cancer including bilateral adrenalectomy and hypophysectomy. *Trans. Am. Assoc. Genito-Urinary Surg.*, 44:101–104.

90. Shimkin, M. B., Boldrey, E. B., Kelly, H., Bierman, H. R., Ortega, P., and Naffziger, H. C. (1952): Effects of surgical hypophysectomy in man with malignant melanoma. *J. Clin. Endocrinol.*, 12:439.

91. Sicuteri, F. (1982): Novita sull'emicranai: nocipatia o "malattia del dolore", una nuova concezione nosologica. *Federazione Med.*, 35:212–218.

92. Sypert, G. W. (1980): Comment on "Treatment of pain of diffuse metastatic cancer by stereotactic chemical hypophysectomy . . .". *Neurosurgery*, 6:262.

93. Takeda, F. (1984): Results of cancer pain relief and tumour regression by pituitary neuroadenolysis and surgical hypophysectomy. In: *Pituitary Neuroadenolysis in Cancer Pain in Hormone-Dependent Tumors,* edited by S. Ischia, S. Lipton, and G. F. Mattezzoli. Edizione Librera, Verona. (*in press*)

94. Takeda, F. (1984): Some considerations on the mechanism of pain relief by means of pituitary neuroadenolysis. A clinical investigation. In: *Pituitary Neuroadenolysis in Cancer Pain in Hormone-Dependent Tumors,* edited by S. Ischia, S. Lipton, and G. F. Mattezzoli. Edizione Librera, Verona. (*in press*)

95. Takeda, F., Fujii, T., Uki, J., Tozawa, T., and Fuse, Y. (1983): Cancer pain relief by means of pituitary neuroadenolysis and surgical hypophysectomy. *Neurol. Med. Chir.*, 23:41–49.

96. Takeda, F., Uki, J., Fuse, Y., Kitani, Y., and Fujita, T. (1982): The pituitary as a target of antalgic treatment for intractable cancer pain. Proceedings of the XIII International Cancer Congress, Seattle, Cat. Card N. 82-08283.

97. Takeda, F., Uki, J., Fujii, T., Kitani, Y., and Fujita, T. (1983): Pituitary neuroadenolysis to relieve cancer pain. Observations of spread of ethanol instilled into the sella turcica and subsequent changes of the hypothalamopituitary axis at autopsy. *Neurol. Med. Chir.*, 23:50–54.

98. Valle Gil, C., Herrera Vargas, R., and Flores, F. (1980): La neuroadenolisis y c.a. avanzado. *Anestesiologia*, Vol. 7, edited by G. Vasconcellos, pp. 169–173. Editores Medicos, Mexico City, Mexico.

99. Ventafridda, V., and De Conno, F. (1981): Strategia terapeutica nel dolore da cancro avanzato. *VIII Corso Agiornamento Oncologia Medica,* Vol. 1, pp. 315–328. Pitostampa, Perugia.

100. Yanagida, H. (1979): Alcohol-induced pituitary adenolysis: How does it control intractable cancer pain? An experimental study using tooth pulp-evoked potentials in rhesus monkeys. *Anesth. Analg. (Cleve.)*, 58:279–285.

101. Yanagida, H., and Corssen, G. (1980): How does clinical adenolysis of the pituitary gland control intractable pain? (abstract). VII World Congress on Anaesthesiology, Hamburg.

102. Yanagida, H., and Corssen, G. (1982): The history of alcohol-induced pituitary neuroadenolysis (abstract). First International Symposium on History Modern Anaesthesia, Rotterdam (*in press*).

Subject Index